Handbook of
Drug and Chemical Stimulation of the Brain
Behavioral, Pharmacological and Physiological Aspects

Handbook of
Drug and Chemical Stimulation of the Brain

Behavioral, Pharmacological and Physiological Aspects

R. D. Myers

VAN NOSTRAND REINHOLD COMPANY

NEW YORK   CINCINNATI   TORONTO   LONDON   MELBOURNE

MEDICAL ECONOMICS BOOK DIVISION, INC.

ORADELL, NEW JERSEY

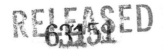

Van Nostrand Reinhold Company Regional Offices:
New York Cincinnati Chicago Millbrae Dallas

Van Nostrand Reinhold Company International Offices:
London Toronto Melbourne

Manufactured in the United States of America

Published by Van Nostrand Reinhold Company
450 West 33rd Street, New York, N.Y. 10001

Published simultaneously in Canada by Van Nostrand Reinhold Ltd.

15 14 13 12 11 10 9 8 7 6 5 4 3 2 1

Library of Congress Cataloging in Publication Data

Myers, Robert D   1931–
   Handbook of drug and chemical stimulation of the
brain.

   1. Psychopharmacology.   I. Title. [DNLM: 1. Brain
—Drug effects.   2. Stimulation, Chemical. WL300 M996h]
RM315.M93   615'.78   74-10564
ISBN 0-442-25622-1

DEDICATED WITH DEEP AFFECTION

to

MARGIE

and to

BOB, JIM, DEDE, ANNE

Preface

Ever since its inception in 1969, my intent in writing this book has been to present a comprehensive and up-to-date survey of the world's literature that pertains to the direct action of a drug or other chemical on the brain. Since experiments using the method of chemical stimulation have blossomed forth so readily in the past few years, this is indeed an appropriate time to take stock and review the exciting endeavors in this field and their present status.

Many of the research papers which are based on the application of a chemical to cerebral tissue have made substantial advances to our overall understanding of brain function. As such, they should be brought to light in the perspective of their own specific discipline. In view of this, it is my frank hope that this survey will be of value to every student interested in any of the intriguing issues of brain function, whether he be an inquisitive beginner or an established neuroscientist.

Each chapter is organized on a functional basis according to major physiological and behavioral systems. In this way, the facts which can be gleaned from the text should bring to the academician and clinician alike a keen awareness of the unique way in which a given chemical or drug can affect a distinct cerebral structure. A worker in one field of physiology, psychology, pharmacology or medicine hopefully will become cognizant of the enterprising activity of a worker in an entirely different area even though both may utilize the same experimental means to an end.

This book also seeks to point out some of the directions that a researcher may take in the future. In every chapter, the care and controls that are necessary in this proliferating field are emphasized so as to help the reader make a sensible interpretation of the series of isolated observations about a specific topic. Inasmuch as instances of controversy are not uncommon, I have attempted to evaluate critically the source of discrepancy which often rests simply in a difference in laboratory procedure.

In addition to the recent studies describing the action that a drug exerts on a specific cerebral structure, the early research reports of the German, Swiss and Japanese workers at the turn of the century are included. Since an attempt has been made to include every pertinent paper written on this topic, any omission from the reference citations is certainly unintentional. Should the reader be aware of any paper which ought to be incorporated in the future version of this survey, I would be most grateful if the information is forwarded to me.

In general, a rule of thumb was followed to exclude from either the text or the master summary tables an abstract or summary written for the proceedings of a meeting, a conference, symposium or colloquium. Ordinarily, such an abstracted account is characterized by insufficient experimental detail, an inadequate analysis of the results or another shortcoming. Obviously, arbitrary exceptions to this rule had to be made. Although the basic reference list was completed in 1971, I have nevertheless included as many reports published in 1972 as possible.

I am deeply indebted to a great number of individuals who contributed in so many diverse ways to every aspect of this book. It is truly a pleasure to thank my professional colleagues and friends, both in England and America, who shared their valuable ideas on this subject, gave of their own personal insights and who offered the most salutary criticisms. My technicians and several other members of my laboratory staff kindly participated in the tracking down of articles, the redrawing of figures, and the reading and proofreading of the manuscript. Many authors not only gave generous permission to use their figures but often forwarded their own photographs or line drawings. The cooperation of the librarians and their various staff members of Purdue University, Indiana University Medical Center, National Institute for Medical Research (London), U.C.L.A. Brain Information Service, and University College (London) is deeply appreciated.

My secretary, Miss Jorga Fielder, typed the final draft of the book in its entirety with never-ending patience and a willingness for which I am sincerely grateful. Each of my four children always extended an amicable and helping hand whenever and in whatever direction it was needed. Finally, the cheerful and untiring efforts of my wife in typing the initial drafts, collating the references, in attending to hundreds of inconspicuous details and in offering inestimable encouragement have made this book possible.

R. D. MYERS

Lafayette, Indiana

Contents

Handbook of
Drug and Chemical Stimulation of the Brain

Behavioral, Pharmacological
and Physiological Aspects

1 Principles of Chemical Stimulation of the Brain

"To deride the hope of progress is the ultimate fatuity, the last word in poverty of spirit and meanness of mind. There is no need to be dismayed by the fact that we cannot yet envisage a definitive solution of our problem, a resting-place beyond which we need not try to go . . ."   P. B. MEDAWAR (1972)

I. INTRODUCTION

The incomparable challenge inherent in the manifold mysteries of brain function has led to one of the most fascinating experimental endeavors in all of the neurosciences. Essentially this widespread quest has centered on a prodigious attempt to "decode" the chemical fabric of a discrete collection of neurons. The logistics of such a decoding enterprise rests on the fundamental principle that an artificial alteration of the biochemical environment of a distinct region of the brain will produce a specific functional change in an animal. If such a change is evoked and is clearly repeatable, the response must make immutable sense in terms of the anatomy of the nervous system. In fact, the reaction to an alteration in the local chemical milieu of the brain may correspond directly with the acknowledged function of that morphological area. Or it may not correspond with the general knowledge about the structure which has been derived from the more traditional neurological approaches based on ablation or electrical stimulation.

Admittedly, any new method whereby a compound is applied directly to brain tissue, particularly of a wide-awake and behaving animal, is open to criticism. As we shall see in Chapter 2, the vast number of bench-top problems attendant to the technique itself is impressive. However, Sir Peter Medawar's statement at the heading of this chapter reflects with great insight the spirit in which the experimental evidence of an encoded functional system should be examined. The progress has been painfully slow and often obfuscated by an experimental or technical limitation rather than by an impoverished theoretical viewpoint. But the hope of understanding the neurochemical attribute of each of the complex

1

networks of neurons is notably profound, particularly if the concepts based on chemical stimulation are linked together with those derived from other experimental sources including those of histochemistry, transmitter dynamics and drug action.

In a word then, the overall purpose of this decoding endeavor is to contribute to the neuroscientist's goal of unraveling the mechanisms and even perhaps the circuitry that underlie the intricate processing of information of which the vertebrate brain is so capable. The chemical signal which triggers a response, the chemical reaction which inhibits that response, the balance and the interplay between the two, and the action which an individual substrate may have on another chemical system—all of these constitute a part of the questions raised when one stimulates the brain with a chemical substance.

II. WHY CHEMICAL STIMULATION?

The rationale upon which the laboratory usage of chemical stimulation of the brain is based can be subdivided into two major parts. The first is concerned with the anatomical locus and cellular mechanism of any of the endogenous humoral factors. These substances that occur naturally in brain tissue include the biogenic amines, peptides, and steroids. A second and entirely different purpose centers on the localization of a possible central site of action of a chemical or drug that is administered systemically. From behavioral observations, many of these artificially synthesized compounds appear superficially to exert a direct effect on some part of the central nervous system. On the basis of these two fundamental points and because of the attractive analogies that can often be drawn with the responses evoked by electrical stimulation of brain tissue (Myers, 1971a), the theoretical principles and procedures of chemical stimulation have evolved.

A. Definition

In the broad context of general physiology, we shall use the term chemical stimulation to apply to any class of neuronal events that is brought about when an endogenous or synthetic substance is applied locally within a given structure of the brain. Although a multitude of compounds may affect nervous tissue in a way that is not necessarily excitatory in the sense of membrane physiology, the reaction observed by the scientist is indicative of a local perturbation of that tissue reached or touched upon by the chemical.

For example, some of the endogenous hormones, when deposited in the brain, appear to inhibit rather than stimulate neural elements in a manner similar to that of electrical current. Moreover, certain drugs act to hyperpolarize or depolarize a neuron by altering the flux of cations across the axonal membrane. Still other compounds may either block or enhance the action of a transmitter substance or another humoral factor that is released into the synaptic cleft between two or more nerve cells. Rather than compartmentalizing the effect of a locally applied substance into functional categories, which in themselves would often be *ad hoc* and arbitrary, the term chemical "stimulation" is retained in this book for descriptive purposes.

B. Comparison with Ablation and Electrical Stimulation

Defying all reason is a question that is argued rather vehemently in some circles by a few investigators. Is chemical stimulation "more physiological" or "less physiological" than some other laboratory procedure used in the exploration of brain function? Plainly, at the very moment when an experimental neurosurgeon enters the cranium, a nonphysiological state is created. Beyond this, the logic of the debate degenerates into a matter of relativity. The implantation or insertion of any device into any part of the brain results in a pathological circumstance. Taking the question of relative "physiological-ness" a step further, almost any neurobiological technique, except perhaps a skull X-ray, can interfere to some degree with normal function. Even the ingestion of an ordinary pill by mouth is viewed as unphysiological by certain naturopathic practitioners, who happily are in the minority.

Scientists who utilize the method of chemical stimulation ordinarily follow certain principles of neuroanatomy and exercise basic neuropharmacological controls. By staying within these principles, this approach to studying the brain can be as valid as any other that seeks a specific functional answer in the realm of an unknown cerebral process. If performed properly, the analytical exploration of a reaction of a given structure to a chemical can supplement in a very vital way the information that is already known from other studies of that region. In the broad purview of stimulating tissue that is intrinsically excitable, the topical application of a chemical does permit a fine grain resolution of the characteristics of a collection of neurons that are seemingly delegated to a specific function. Why is this so?

First, on the basis of the biochemistry of cortical and subcortical structures, we know that endogenous substances such as amines, amino acids and hormones are present in varying concentrations in separate parts of the brain (e.g., Hebb, 1970; McEwen *et al.*, 1972). Second, cytochemical studies of individual fiber systems show that individual amine pathways are laid down anatomically in unique patterns (e.g., Fuxe *et al.*, 1966; Shute and Lewis, 1967). Third, the membrane of an individual neuron that lies contiguous to another possesses a special sensitivity to different molecules, as demonstrated by the technique of iontophoresis. Logically, one can deduce that within a single collection of neurons each cell possesses: (a) distinct chemoreceptors; (b) the capacity to convey an impulse to another cell by virtue of the release of an endogenous substance; or (c) a mechanism in the form of the release of a humoral factor for altering the depolarization threshold of an adjacent cell.

What happens when we either ablate this collection of neurons or pass electrical current through it? These events can be conceptualized by considering a schematic representation portrayed in Fig. 1-1 of a hypothetical collection of nerve cells in an unspecified area of the mammalian brain. Let us assume that three separate pathways traverse this structure. Pathway A is excitatory and mediated by an excitatory substance at synapses A_1 and A_2 to stimulate functional system

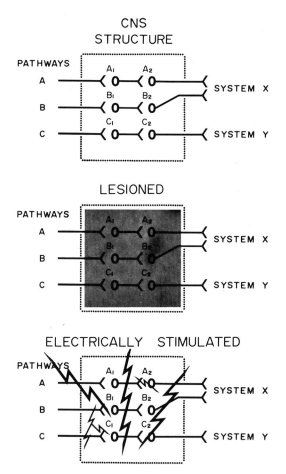

Fig. 1-1 A hypothetical structure in a mammalian central nervous system (CNS). Three separate pathways mediated by three individual sets of synapses traverse this structure. When the structure is lesioned (*middle*), all of the pathways are transected and the synapses are destroyed. When electric current is passed through the structure (*bottom*), all of the pathways are excited homogeneously in an undifferentiated manner.

X. Pathway B is mediated by an inhibitory substance at synapses B_1 and B_2 to block functional system X. Pathway C is mediated by an excitatory substance at synapses C_1 and C_2 to stimulate functional system Y.

If this hypothetical structure contained within the dotted block is lesioned, as denoted by the shading, obviously all three pathways which carry separate messages are destroyed. Therefore, it would be impossible to ascertain which pathway is responsible for a designated part of the system. Further, total obliteration of the pool of neurons, as in the case of certain structures in the limbic system, may result in a functional self-cancellation of both excitatory and inhibitory elements contained within the structure.

If the same set of neurons illustrated in Fig. 1-1 is stimulated with an electric current, the net result may be a most complicated and variable depolarization of all of the pathways in that region. Simultaneous changes in the ion flux of each nerve membrane would occur altogether in this segment of the three pathways. The point is simply that such a sequence of events makes it impossible to make any sort of functional differentiation between the distinctive nature of each pathway.

Based on studies using electrical stimulation, Valenstein and his colleagues have presented strong evidence that several neuronal systems in the brain-stem of the rat are closely overlapping if not entirely intermingled. The upshot of this experimentally troublesome situation is the fact that eating, drinking, preening and gnawing behavior may be elicited by electrical stimulation of the same diencephalic site but with no consistency (Valenstein et al., 1970). What is worse, the animal's behavior can switch without an alteration in the parameters of the electrical stimulus. To overcome part of the obstacle of evoking a more discriminable effect, Miller (1965) has described how he resorted to the use of smaller and smaller electrodes until he eventually saw no effect at all. Even in an animal much larger than a rat and with considerably greater mass of brain tissue, the problem of obtaining a consistent response to electrical stimulation, time after time, is just as great. As a result, Robinson and Mishkin devised a probabilistic model to account for the irksome variability in a monkey's response to electrical stimulation (Robinson, 1964; Robinson and Mishkin, 1968). However, this innovative approach fails to provide a sufficient resolution to the intertwined characteristics of the anatomical pathways in the brain.

Largely because of this irreconcilable experimental situation, the recourse of injecting a chemical into brain tissue has evolved. To sort out and distinguish between various interlaced networks of neurons, the method of chemical stimulation makes four basic assumptions: (1) that the neuronal membrane at the dendritic junction will be sensitive to a chemical; (2) that the cells in another functional category in the surrounding tissue will remain "quiet" while the excitation of an individual set of neurons takes place; (3) that a specialized receptor to a specific substance or class of compounds recognizes the presence of the molecule; (4) that among a group of cells, a collective excitation or inhibition will occur in synchrony. As will be evident in the text to follow, these assumptions are often but not always borne out.

III. LEVELS OF CHEMICAL ANALYSIS

A multi-disciplinary approach has characterized the investigation of the brain from the standpoint of its structural features. The diversity of the anatomical components of the brain is as remarkable as the distinctive chemical properties of individual structures. At the cellular level, the ultrastructural components of a nervous pathway are unusually diverse; as such they perform unique functions. Figure 1-2 presents a schematic diagram of the connections of a neuron with two other neurons. The sub-cellular configuration is, of course, not the same for any two neurons. In fact, as is well-known from the research in the field of neurogenesis of Weiss, Pomerat and others who have studied the living neuron in

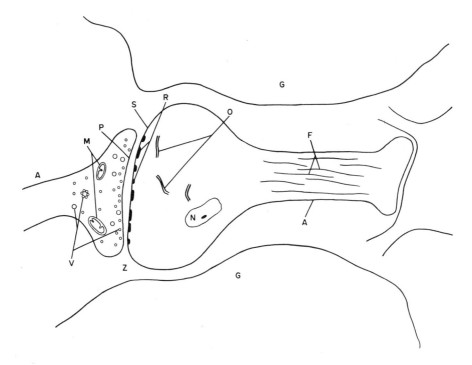

Fig. 1-2 A schematic representation of a neuron positioned between the axonal ending of a second neuron and the dendritic process of a third. The fine detail of the synaptic coupling and other ultrastructural elements are illustrated which could be affected by the chemical applied to this tissue. Abbreviations are as follows: A. axon membrane; F. neurofibril; G. glial cell; M. mitochondrion; N. nucleus; O. organelle; P. presynaptic membrane; R. receptor site; S. post-synaptic membrane; V. vesicle; Z. synaptic zone or cleft.

tissue culture (Weiss, 1970; Pomerat *et al.*, 1967), the internal elements of the cytoplasm are in a constant state of flux. The metabolic attribute of each neuron is also characterized by kinetics that are ever changing. Nevertheless, Fig. 1-2 serves to illustrate how many different sub-cellular elements a chemical can affect when applied directly to neuronal tissue.

Some years ago, Roth and Barlow (1961) described the then startling fact that both enzymes and substrates in the brain differ greatly from region to region; based on content analysis alone, the endogenous concentration of metabolically active substances in cerebral tissue such as ACh, cholinesterase, dopamine, norepinephrine, serotonin, neutral and acid amino acids is not at all uniform from one structure to the next (e.g., Richter, 1964; Lajtha, 1969). It is a well accepted dogma today that each amine, for example, possesses a unique patterning of concentration in the brain. Furthermore, many necrotizing compounds including arsenic salts, carbon disulfide and gold thioglucose have a special affinity for restricted parts of the brain. This again attests to the distinctiveness of the chemical organization with respect to cerebral structures.

If such a regional biochemistry of brain tissue is taken as the starting point, how can we attack the problem of determining why there is a finite distribution of neurohumoral substances? Of what significance is this distribution of each chemical substance to the life and well-being of an animal? Logically, there is a continuum of points of entry into the so-called "black box" which ranges from the most molar or systemic approach to the extremely reductionistic or molecular. Above all are two vital questions: (1) Where can the scientist obtain the most information along the continuum? (2) At that level, does the experimental yield of information contribute measurably to an overall comprehension of brain function? The following sections describe and evaluate five of the possible levels of scientific approach to the analysis of neurochemical mechanisms.

A. Systemic Administration of a Chemical

There are several advantages of using one of the systemic routes to administer a drug which has a potent action on the nervous system. Each one is simple, fast and convenient. By taking behavioral and neurological measures, a first estimate can be obtained of the effect that any chemical compound exerts on the nervous system. To illustrate an extreme view, a well-known pharmacologist once remarked to the author that "giving a CNS stimulant orally or by other systemic means is the only way to study the drug, because that is the only way a drug acts!" To those concerned with the CNS mechanism of drug action, the illogical facets inherent in such a statement are at once apparent.

Because the blood-brain barrier retards or prevents the entry into the CNS of a great many molecules even of low weight, it is often impossible to establish whether a compound has a direct action on the CNS. One is always reminded of the somewhat embarrassing situation in the 1950s concerning the notion that the epinephrine secreted from the adrenal glands into the bloodstream during stress has an immediate and direct energizing effect on the neurons of the reticular formation. Later it was shown that at plasma levels adrenaline, like so many biogenic amines, does not penetrate the blood-brain barrier. Even those compounds such as alcohol or barbiturates which do enter readily into the brain parenchyma from the vasculature may have a selective affinity for a certain structure, although as anesthetics their neurochemical similarities are striking.

Many neuropharmacologically active substances can exert simultaneous peripheral effects on the autonomic ganglia and at the neural effector junction. Even by using a pharmacological gimmick such as the comparison of the effects of two salts of a drug (e.g., atropine) which pass the blood-brain barrier differentially, the complex actions of both agents on all organ systems outside the nervous system are inordinately difficult to interpret.

One type of systemic route that can help to eliminate some of the inconclusiveness about the peripheral versus central action of an agent is that of close intra-arterial injection. For example, if a drug is injected unilaterally into one of the vertebral arteries, the directness of action on an area of the brain can be ascertained particularly if the latency of response corresponds to the lag in the circulation time. Ordinarily, the close intra-arterial approach requires death-defying surgical procedures used on an anesthetized preparation, which in itself can limit an extrapolation to the conscious animal.

In addition to the methodological weaknesses, it must be recognized that the lack of anatomical specificity represents the most serious deficiency in any of the systemic approaches. Because the blood supply disperses so efficiently any test substance that is able to penetrate the barriers of the brain, it is conceivable that all neuronal systems are affected indiscriminately. The hope of localizing an effect of a drug or of characterizing a discrete set of receptors within a part of the brain is utterly lost.

Equally as important is the finding that the same endogenous substrate can be utilized for more than one function. To illustrate an instance of biological parsimony, the peripheral and central effects of epinephrine may be entirely dissimilar. Given intraperitoneally in the rat, epinephrine is a puissant anorexogenic agent (Russek and Piña, 1962; Russek et al., 1967). Injected at circumscribed sites in the brain-stem, however, this same catecholamine evokes intense feeding behavior in the same species (Chapter 7). Administered peripherally, epinephrine is also one of the most potent thermogenic agents known, but injected at an anatomically restricted site in the brain, epinephrine produces a fall in body temperature (Chapter 6). These striking differences in mode of action reveal at once the overwhelming necessity for the anatomical localization of the effect of a chemical. Autoradiographic studies in which radioactive drugs are able to pass through the cerebral barriers indicate that one substance may penetrate the brain tissue quite differently from another and even accumulate unevenly at different anatomical loci (Roth and Barlow, 1961).

B. Cerebral Ventricular Route

The traditional approach to studying the direct effect of a chemical substance on the brain has been to inject the substance into the cerebrospinal fluid (Chapter 2). By 1960, over 200 research papers had been written that dealt primarily with the physiological changes produced by all kinds of compounds after they were injected into the cerebral ventricle in all manner of animals (e.g., Schain, 1960; Winterstein, 1961). The importance of this approach cannot be underestimated. Because the route of entry, by its very nature, circumvents opportunely the blood-brain barrier, the immediate effect of a substance may yield some initial estimate of its central function or its regional mechanism of action. Feldberg (1963) has elaborated upon the points of contrast arising when a single chemical is given by way of the cerebral ventricles as opposed to a peripheral route. As one would imagine, the effects are often opposite.

Some qualitative differences in the effect of a drug can be observed when it is given in various parts of the fluid cavities, i.e., the lateral as opposed to the fourth ventricle (Feldberg, 1963). The reason for a different response is the higher regional concentration of the drug in the structure contiguous to the site of injection. Methods for the perfusion of separate parts of the ventricular cavity enable the investigator to isolate often quite clearly the general anatomical locus upon which a drug acts (Carmichael *et al.*, 1964; Feldberg and Myers, 1966; Myers, 1972). To prevent the admixture of CSF in one ventricle with the CSF in another ventricle into which a chemical is injected, Herz *et al.* (1970) have utilized a eucerine plug inserted into the lumen so as to occlude the passage of fluid from one region to another. This clever intra-lumenal stopper is suitable only for an acute preparation because of the regional hydrocephalus which would develop in the wake of such an occlusion.

Whenever an injection is made into the ventricle, there is always the question of the patency of the indwelling cannula. In fact, it is known that what are assumed to be ventricular injections are at least partially tissue injections. Further, after a variable interval of time, which is certainly capricious, the tip of a ventricular cannula usually becomes blocked. Thereafter, a volume of a drug that is injected seeks the path of least resistance, which is usually around the external shaft of the cannula and dorsalward into the subarachnoid space.

Overall, the ventricular approach is best considered as a highly useful but provisional one at least anatomically. Time and again, the experimental results generated by the use of ventricular injections of a drug are only a temporary scaffolding that admittedly cannot be removed until the construction of a morphological map of the chemical's action is completed. Such a mapping is accomplished by local chemical stimulation. Based on the results of a ventricular injection, it is perfectly reasonable to set forth general hypotheses and theories. Thus, one can extrapolate provisionally from a "general pot of stew to a specific vegetable." When definitive information is finally obtained on the anatomical nature of a specific "vegetable," then more information about the stew is only redundant and of secondary importance. This critique has serious implications for a model builder whose theoretical position stems solely from experiments utilizing the ventricular approach. For as soon as the results from a micro-injection or other regional anatomical analysis become available, then this less specific model is superceded or replaced in its entirety. How can this be justified?

There are several important papers documented in the chapters ahead in which a single substance has been shown to exert one effect when acting from the ventricle but an opposite action when injected or deposited in different anatomical areas of the brain. Moreover, the classical categorization of a neural receptor for an adrenergic substance, originally differentiated on the basis of peripheral experiments, may not even apply to neurons in the brain which line the walls of the ventricle (Grunden, 1969). Finally, if the stereotaxic technology is available in a laboratory and preliminary information is known about the central action of a compound, then the intraventricular approach should be replaced by direct stimulation. This permits precise anatomical localization and a more accurate estimate of the actual physiological concentration of a given substance that evokes an effect.

C. Direct Stimulation of Tissue

With the advent of sophisticated stereotaxic techniques for the accurate cannulation of a specific structure in the brain of at least a dozen species, many facets of regional neurochemistry can be explored without difficulty. As described in Chapter 2, by injecting a solution or depositing crystals of substance in a region, it is possible to mimic the function of an endogenous substrate, stimulate local metabolic activity, characterize the intracerebral receptor sites, and above all, localize anatomically each of these effects. The fact that the local effect of a chemical on a tiny portion of brain tissue can be witnessed in terms of its action on the entire organism is the very essence of this book.

D. Iontophoretic Application

A fourth and still more molecular approach is provided by a technique in which a chemical is applied by iontophoresis to a single cell in the brain through a micropipette. At first glance, this would seem to be a most attractive way of manipulating the chemical environment of only one neuron or at least a very small group of neurons. At different intervals, selected by the experimenter, one, two or more substances in solution can be ejected into the extra-neuronal space from the tips of a fused array of multi-barrelled pipettes. A simultaneous recording of the change in the extracellular potential of a single neuron and a change in its discharge characteristics can indicate whether the ejected substance affects the membrane as an excitant or depressant. Information about the post-synaptic excitability of the membrane, its impedance and other characteristics can be ascertained if proper controls are exercised.

Perhaps the very appeal of the technique does not sufficiently herald its drawbacks which stem principally from the standpoint of scientific control. For example, the concentration of the substance ejected cannot be specified. The local pH, the trauma to tissue pCO_2 level, and an anesthetic or paralyzing action of the solution cannot be determined. Apart from these limitations, membrane effects other than those of dendritic origin can disturb the potential (Curtis and Crawford, 1969).

However, the major weakness of the technique of iontophoresis is a very simple one. Molecularly, it is an isolated preparation. An iontophoretically-induced change in the firing pattern of a single neuron may tell much about that cell but reveal very little about the relationship of that neuron to others in the same substructure. More remote is the role of the stimulated cell in a chain of interconnecting neurons. As such, information on the relationship between that cell and its role in a systemic function or behavior is hard to derive. Although this inherent biological difficulty may be overcome in the future, it is essentially common to most all of the current microanalytical methods used to study brain function. Nevertheless, the value offered by the technique in uncovering a fundamental property of a neuron, including the elucidation of its chemical sensitivity or the demonstration of a transmitter-like sequence, is self-evident.

E. Tissue Analysis

The tools of analytical chemistry have provided a wealth of important facts in many species about the biochemical make-up of every segment of brain tissue. The *in vitro* analysis of neural tissue embraces many subdisciplines including: the histochemical tracing of fiber systems from one region to another; the estimate of the content of an endogenous substrate; the assay of its metabolites; and the approximation of the turnover of a neurohumoral factor. Biological or radio-assay of the effluent collected from either the ventricle or tissue is another way of determining the regional activity of a given substance, but a live animal is used in this case.

There are several clever ways of combining one or more of these techniques with the more traditional ones already mentioned. For instance, the usage of a small and discretely placed lesion in one part of the CNS has been found to be valuable for tracing a pathway in the brain-stem that contains an amine (Harvey *et al.*, 1963). The push-pull perfusion of an isolated part of the brain of an animal to which a stimulus is applied has also been useful in the *in vivo* analysis of the moment-to-moment changes in neurochemical activity (see Chapter 2).

The most widely practiced procedure still used today by neurochemists is the *in vitro* analysis of the content of a specific compound in the brain. Although a plethora of humorous anatomical malapropisms exists in the neurochemical literature,[1] the analysis of whole-brain homogenates may nevertheless constitute an important first step. An equally important second step may be the chromatographic or other assay of different parts of the brain that are dissected on a gross scale with frequent imprecision. As long as a functional extrapolation is not taken with dogmatic finality, the direction can be pointed to the next step—a physiological analysis.

Unfortunately, the assay of a fraction of the whole brain of either an individual animal or of a pooled sample of brains can utterly obscure the discrete variation in the chemical topography of the brain. As is clear now, each of these variations may have great functional significance. For this reason, the uniform analysis of the chemical content of a single structure such as the hypothalamus has been deprecated (Myers, 1969a). Simply put, this structure alone serves a multiplicity of functions simultaneously. It contains at least five amines and nine polypeptides that are located in different nuclei, each implicated in a divergent process. From this, it is easy to understand how misleading a single chemical measure of whole-brain or whole-region may be.

IV. CHEMICAL SENSITIVITY OF BRAIN TISSUE

Any compound, whether in a high or low concentration, can excite or depress a neuron or collection of neurons in the brain. It may also alter the temporal firing characteristics of the neurons. These changes may either relate to the passage of a depolarizing current from one cell to the next or are totally unrelated to the process of synaptic transmission.

The phenomenon of chemical sensitivity of brain tissue is divided here into two categories: (1) *endogenous* sensitivity in which the activity of a group of neurons is altered by natural substances synthesized within the body; and (2) *exogenous* sensitivity in which the neuronal activity is affected by synthetic compounds that are able to pass the blood-brain barrier.

A. Sensitivity to Endogenous Factors

Compounds that are synthesized within the brain parenchyma of the mammal can be differentiated according to their functional role from those manufactured outside of the central nervous system. Of course, a compound belonging to either category may act upon elements in the nervous system.

Many of the neurohumoral factors within the brain are viewed popularly as

---

[1]What is designated as "cortex" is really the cerebrum. Or "cortex," "midbrain" and "the rest" may mean (1) cerebrum, (2) diencephalon and mesencephalon, and (3) cerebellum, pons and medulla.

possessing the attributes of the synaptic transmitter. A telling point to be emphasized here is that simply because a substance affects the properties of a neuron in one direction or another does not in any sense imply that it is a transmitter substance. As discussed in the Epilogue, it may well be that only one chemical compound found naturally in mammalian brain tissue, acetylcholine (ACh), can indeed be regarded as a chemical transmitter. Although not widely adopted, there is even a reasonable argument documented lucidly by Nachmansohn (1971) against the notion, usually accepted on faith, that ACh does play a transmitter role in the CNS.

1. *Substances Within the Brain*

Whether or not a chemical has an action within the synaptic junction is contingent ordinarily upon three main criteria set forth here as questions: (1) Does the substance occur naturally at the nerve ending by being synthesized endogenously? (2) When applied postsynaptically, does the compound depolarize the membrane of the neuron and evoke a supra-threshold change in a potential that is propagated? (3) Is the substance released presynaptically from intracellular vesicles onto postsynaptic sites located on a contiguous cell that are uniquely sensitive to that substance?

Dating back to Florey (1960), numerous essays and accounts have been published about the criteria necessary for a substance to be considered as a synaptic transmitter in the invertebrate or vertebrate nervous system. The subject has probably been treated most comprehensively by Werman (1966) who has contended that many of the standard criteria are of interest only insofar as the biological function of the synapse. These include the presence of a synthesizing enzyme, an inactivating enzyme, and pharmacological identification through the usage of receptor blocking agents. In fact, Werman (1972) now believes that only two of the major criteria need to be satisfied beyond doubt: (a) "identical action" and (b) "collectability of the transmitter." At once, it is easy to see how this view could be conceptually restrictive if one attempts to formulate a set of principles that applies to the mammalian synapse. For example, there are many substances such as polypeptide hormones that exert a marked local action on a specific group of neurons. The effect is often identical to that evoked by a natural peptide [Criterion (a)]. At the same time, the peptide can be collected and isolated from the self-same tissue. Yet, it would be difficult to envisage such a substance as a synaptic transmitter.

Nevertheless, Werman's conceptualization of "identical actions" must be regarded as a powerful criterion with which to examine the local synaptic action of a compound. The potential of this criterion is enhanced further not only if the substance is present naturally but if the enzyme systems for its manufacture and degradation are firmly established.

The criterion of identical actions is the basic one upon which many of the studies employing chemical stimulation are based. The stimulation or mimicry of synaptic activity in a large group of neurons is certainly one of the main objectives of applying a given chemical to a specific structure in the brain. One supposition inherent in the theory that embodies this approach is that a certain group of cells displays a special sensitivity to the compound while others are either insensitive or react to the artificial application of the endogenous chemical in some way other than depolarization.

Without prior biochemical information about the content, synthesis, metabolic turnover, and mechanism of degradation of an endogenous compound, the criterion of "identity of action" can also be deceptive. If the criterion is considered *in vacuo*, one could easily promulgate, by demonstration alone, the ludicrous concept that formaldehyde is a transmitter substance at the neuromuscular junction. The rhythmic fasciculations of the target muscle, twitching and even gross limb movement that follow an arterial perfusion of a formalin solution can be used beguilingly as convincing evidence to a casual and uninformed onlooker of its "transmitter" property.

Similarly, many chemicals applied to nerve tissue in a relatively high dose can inhibit the discharge of a neuron in several ways including the hyperpolarization of the membrane or the total swamping of receptor sites on the postsynaptic membrane. Unfortunately, individual cholinomimetic compounds which do fall categorically into a criterion of identical action may possess this inhibitory action. An excellent illustration of this is found in the drug, carbachol, used widely as a cholinomimetic for activating cholinergic receptors in brain tissue. Its pharmacological and toxicological properties include effects on pH, the binding of cations, permeability of the axonal membrane, synaptic blockade and an exceptional resistance to hydrolysis. For this reason, anatomical and pharmacological controls are necessary requisites for establishing veraciously the identical action criterion for acetylcholine.

2. *Substances Outside the CNS*

Substances that are not present in the synaptic vesicles or storage granules within the terminal bouton of a nerve nonetheless may exert a potent pharmacological effect on the dendritic process or on the cell body of the neuron. As cited frequently in the following chapters, different classes of neurons have been rather well documented on the basis of their response to these compounds. Through microelectrode analysis, these units are observed to alter their firing pattern in response to a local change in the blood concentration of sodium, glucose, steroid hormones, CO_2, amino acids, foreign protein such as a pyrogen, peptides and other factors. Circumscribed regions or nuclei in the brain contain a disproportionately high density of individual cells that have been characterized variously as detectors, sensors or receptors for a given chemical. Ordinarily, the location of these neurons corresponds with the recognized function of that region of the brain.

Somewhat related to these chemo-detectors are other kinds of neurons that have been identified and differentiated, again by microelectrode studies. On the basis of their reactivity to a specific physical stimulus of a given magnitude or threshold value, these neurons are implicated in the sensing of changes in temperature of the blood, osmotic tension and possibly hydrostatic pressure. Having either sort of specialized sensitivity to a systemic factor, each of these individual neurons is believed to be able to contribute to the overall monitoring of a specific aspect of the physico-chemical state of the blood that surges through the micro-circulation contiguous to the cell.

B. Sensitivity to a Synthetic Compound

Should they be capable of penetrating the blood-brain barrier, certain drugs or chemicals may exert a nonspecific effect on the central neuron. Other compounds have a special affinity for cells distributed in various regions of the brain. For example, salts such as monosodium glutamate that are (or were believed to be) innocuous because of their widespread usage (Olney and Sharpe, 1969) and highly toxic compounds such as gold thioglucose may attack only restricted parts of the nervous system under certain conditions (Chapter 7).

Alterations in the function of a given group of neurons can be caused by the direct action of a compound on one of a number of cellular elements or processes (Fig. 1-2). Certain toxins affect the axonal membrane or the binding of molecules to the surface of the membrane. Or they may interfere with the cell's natural permeability to ions or molecules. Some drugs affect the ability of a neuron to release a humoral factor from its terminal ending, while other chemicals prevent the re-uptake into the neuron of the factor after it is released presynaptically. Blocking agents may compete with a natural substance for receptor sites on a neuron as indicated in Fig. 1-2.

Still other compounds interfere with the metabolism of the constituents of the cytoplasm by inhibiting enzyme synthesis or the intracellular catalyzing mechanism involving substrate oxidation. Stimulants, convulsants, depressants, anesthetics or other anatomically nonspecific drugs can exert a multifaceted action on several aspects of neuronal function. However, in each case, the pharmacological action of a chemical depends on its structural characteristics. A subtle modification in the molecular configuration will alter a compound's specificity, efficacy and overall potency.

C. Scope of Chemical Sensitivity

A remarkable illustration of the variety of individual chemosensitivity which brain tissue possesses is contained in Table 1-1. It was constructed from the studies included in Chapters 3 through 12. As a requisite for inclusion in the Table, each chemical substance had to have produced some effect when injected,

TABLE 1-1 Summary of Commonly Used Substances That Exert Specific Effects After Injection or Application to Brain Tissue. The General Classification is Based on the Primary Effect of the Substance

I. Cholinergic Homologues

Agonists	Blockers	Anticholinesterases
Acetylcholine (ACh)	Hemicholinium	Physostigmine (Eserine)
		Neostigmine (Prostigmin)
Carbamylcholine (Carbachol)		Diisopropylfluorophos-phate (DFP)
Nicotine	Hexamethonium	
	Mecamylamine	
	Tetraethylammonium	
Muscarine	Atropine	
Methacholine (Mecholyl)	Scopolamine	
Bethanechol	Methyl atropine	
Pilocarpine	Methyl scopolamine	
Arecoline		
Oxotremorine		

II. Catecholamines and Sympathomimetic Homologues

Agonists	Blockers	Monoamine Oxidase (MAO) Inhibitors
Norepinephrine (α)	Dibenamine	Iproniazid
L-Dopa	Phenoxybenzamine (Dibenzyline)	Amitriptyline
Dopamine	Phentolamine (α)	Imipramine
	Tolazoline	Desipramine (DMI)
	Yohimbine	
		Nialamid
Epinephrine (α and β)	Dichloroisoproternol (DCI)	Tranylcypromine
Isoproterenol (β)	Propranolol (β)	
Phenylephrine		
Naphazoline		
Tetrahydrozoline		
Ephedrine		
Amphetamine		

III. Indole and Other Amines

	Blockers
Serotonin (5-HT)	Methysergide
	BOL (LSD)
5-Hydroxytryptophan (5-HTP)	
Melatonin	
5-Hydroxytryptophol (5-HTOL)	

TABLE 1-1   *(Continued)*

III. Indole and Other Amines
5-Methoxytryptophol
   (5-MTOL)
Histamine

IV. Endocrine and Other Hormonal Factors
L-Thyroxine
Triiodothyronine
Growth Hormone (GH)
Adrenocorticotrophic
   Hormone (ACTH)
Cortisol (Hydrocortisone)
Cortisone
Corticosterone
Dexamethasone
Antidiuretic Hormone
   (ADH, vasopressin)
Angiotensin I and II
Renin

V. Hormones of Reproduction
Follicle Stimulating
   Hormone (FSH)
Luteinizing Hormone
   (LH)
Estrogen
Estradiol
Estrone
Estriol
Hexestrol
Stilbestrol
Progesterone
Norethindrone
Chlormadinone
Testosterone
Cyproterone
Androstenedione

VI. Amino Acids
Glutamine
Gamma-Amino Butyric Acid
   (GABA)
Aspartic acid

VII. CNS Stimulants or Convulsants	CNS Relaxants (Anti-Parkinson)	Local Anesthetics
Metrazol	Trihexyphenidyl	Cocaine
Leptazol	Benztropine	Procaine (Novocaine)

(Continued)

TABLE 1-1 *(Continued)*

VII. CNS Stimulants or Convulsants	CNS Relaxants (Anti-Parkinson)	Local Anesthetics
Strychnine	Biperiden	Lidocaine (Xylocaine)
Picrotoxin		Tetracaine
Tubocurarine		Dibucaine
Oxotremorine		
Nikethamide (Coramine)		

Narcotic and Other Analgesics	Hypnotics and Sedatives
Morphine	Pentobarbital sodium
Nalorphine	(Nembutal)
Apomorphine	Chloralose
Salicylate	Ethyl alcohol

Psychotropic Drugs	Neurotoxins, Pathogens, Glycosides, etc.
Chlorpromazine	S. typhosa
Perphenazine	E. coli
Promazine	Sh. dysenteriae
Reserpine	Capsaicin

Diuretics	Gold thioglucose
Ouabain	2-Deoxy-D-glucose
Digitoxin	Penicillin
Chlorothiazide	Na fluorocitrate
Hydrochlorthiazide	Na fluoracetate
Diamox (Acetazolamide)	Cobalt
Mercuric Acetate	Alumina cream
Chlormerodrin	6-Hydroxydopamine
Ethacrynic Acid	(6-OHDA)

Hypoglycemics

Insulin
Tolbutamide
Chlorpropamide

applied, deposited or implanted in a particular structure or region of the brain of an experimental animal.

At once it is clear that nearly every major class of neurogenic or neuroactive compound has been tested regionally. To other substances not necessarily associated with a central function or control system, the brain also shows a special sensitivity. Although some substances in several of the classifications cited might act on neurons in a nonspecific manner, many compounds such as the toxins and pathogens evoke a pattern of response that differs in degree as well as in the kind of symptoms observed.

V. CHEMICAL RECEPTORS IN THE BRAIN

The capacious theorizing about receptors in the central nervous system that are sensitive to certain chemical complexes is intellectually intricate. The main reason for this is twofold. First, the principles underlying pharmacological receptor theory have evolved from diverse experiments on autonomic ganglia and cardiac, smooth and skeletal muscle. They are often accepted tacitly as being equally applicable to nerve cells in the mammalian brain. Second, although great progress has been made to date in isolating and characterizing macromolecules with a special affinity for a candidate transmitter (see Duncan, 1967), an actual receptor has never been physically visualized or otherwise identified.

A. Receptor Criteria

When evaluating the studies on chemical stimulation in the following chapters, it is conceptually helpful to have a basic grasp of the properties of a biological receptor that is chemosensitive in contrast to one specially sensitive to light, sound or other physical stimuli. Ehrenpreis *et al.* (1969) have outlined perspicuously the criteria of a receptor complex on a cell. These criteria take into account the phenomenon of the combining of biogenic amines, vasoactive polypeptides and hormone-binding proteins with chemically specific receptor sites.

First, the receptor complex must have the property of chemo-recognition either for a specific class of endogenous molecules or the exogenous molecules of a synthetic drug. Second, the chemo-recognition of a receptor macromolecule is a genetically determined property in that the species-specific response is more common than atypical. Third, when an agonist binds to the receptor molecule in sufficient quantity, a perturbation in the state of the molecule arises which initiates a change in the function of that cell. Fourth, the binding of an agonist to a receptor does not require an alteration in the structural conformation of the substance.

One outstanding feature of a receptor is its capacity to bind a specific antagonist as well as the corresponding agonist. What determines the selective affinity of a given compound for a specific binding site is the chemical structure of the compound. Today, much research is devoted to disentangling the structure-activity interaction. Frequently, an antagonist which competes with an agonist for the same receptor site is structurally similar to that agonist, which itself has the capacity to elicit a cellular change. Although several kinds of receptors are proposed from studies of ganglionic transmission and the actions of drugs on the three types of muscle tissue, as yet there is only the most circumstantial evidence that a similar class of receptor exists in the CNS. Whether they function in a distinctive way can be judged by the reader in the chapters to follow.

For purposes of illustration, two major categories of receptors will be described briefly because of the amount of research that has been completed on their local action on cerebral structures.

B. Characterization of Neural Receptors

The catecholamine receptors in the periphery have been divided into alpha and beta, corresponding in most cases to their respective excitatory and inhibitory actions. For example, when a catecholamine agonist binds to an alpha adrenergic receptor, vasoconstriction, contraction of the membrane and dilation of the pupil occur. If these effects on muscle tissue are blocked by pretreatment with a specific antagonist that combines with these receptors, the antagonist is classified as an alpha adrenergic blocking agent.

Beta receptors within the same tissue seem to mediate the dilatation of vessels in skeletal muscle, bronchial relaxation, and an increase in the animal's heart rate. A drug which prevents these effects is termed a beta adrenergic blocking agent. Although norepinephrine acts predominately on alpha receptors and is classified as an alpha agonist, whereas epinephrine acts on both types of receptors, this convenient dichotomy may be somewhat of an oversimplification even in peripheral tissue. In contemplating the existence of a system of adrenergic receptors in the central nervous system, the dual category of action may apply only partially to some structures and not at all to others (e.g., McLennan, 1963, 1970; Grunden, 1969). Research in this area is still in its infancy.

The distinction of two kinds of cholinergic receptors is based on the interesting predilection of two substances that occur in nature to mimic certain of the effects of acetylcholine on peripheral organs. Depending on the dose used, nicotine stimulates or blocks synaptic transmission in autonomic ganglia and at the motor end-plate. Muscarine stimulates smooth and cardiac muscle as well as the exocrine glands. Each of the *nicotinic* effects can be blocked by hexamethonium at the sympathetic ganglia or by tubocurarine applied to skeletal muscle. The *muscarinic* effect can be blocked by atropine. Therefore, there appear to be three types of receptors: two are nicotinic, one is muscarinic. Each is respectively sensitive to, and in turn blocked by, one of the three classes of cholinergic antagonists. Caution must be exercised in interpreting stimulation experiments, since this rudimentary view of the cholinergic receptor system is really an historical one (Koelle, 1965). In all likelihood, there are counterparts in the central nervous system, but other aspects of this categorization of receptors may not be comparable to the periphery.

As long as sight is not lost of the fact that the classification or designation of a receptor site on the basis of an antagonist is really the contrivance of human ingenuity, it is legitimate to play the pharmacological game inside the central nervous system with agonists and antagonists. Clear insight about an action of a chemical may be gained if pharmacological relationships can be established in terms of potency of action. However, to construct a model of synaptic function in a region of the brain or to base a theory of a functional mechanism solely on the findings of an agonist is in either case a provisional endeavor. For instance, if isoproterenol, a beta adrenergic agonist, produces a specific dose-dependent effect after it is micro-injected into brain tissue, and this response is abolished by propranolol, a beta receptor antagonist, then the possibility exists that a beta receptor is involved in the effect. If so, then epinephrine or possibly norepinephrine injected in the same way should exert an identical effect as isoproterenol. Moreover, the response to epinephrine should again be antagonized equally as well by propranolol. If such a test is not conducted at a local site in the brain, the validity of any conclusion is seriously jeopardized. Why?

In reality, the main issue is always whether or not the *endogenous* substrate itself evokes a specific and repeatable response that is concentration dependent. Since isoproterenol and propranolol are not present naturally in the brain, a physiological model based strictly on the response to the synthetic compound is as artificial as the substance injected.

VI. ANATOMICAL BASIS OF CHEMICAL STIMULATION

In this book, the results obtained on all mammalian and nonmammalian species have been included. However, because of the wide variations in the dimensions and morphological relationships between each of the brains in which chemicals have been applied, it is impossible to describe a generalized neuroanatomical schema. Fortunately, under each major topic of enquiry, a reasonable number of anatomical reconstructions have been completed so that most regions having a noteworthy affinity or sensitivity to a compound are presented.

Table 1-2 designates each of the structures into which a chemical has been given according to the major anatomical designation: telencephalon (cerebrum), diencephalon, mesencephalon (midbrain), or rhombencephalon. In a significant proportion of all research papers utilizing the chemical stimulation method, the site of stimulation was in the hypothalamus, a major diencephalic structure. For this reason, the hypothalamic nuclei and the general regions that cannot be designated as nuclei are further subdivided. Several other major structures have been similarly divided.

A. Relative Position of Major Structures

The gross morphological features of the mammalian brain are presented in Fig. 1-3A. This schematic diagram represents a prototype integrated by Nauta and Karten (1970) for all mammals, in that the structures are placed in zones of suggestive rather than literal size and position. Figure 1-3B portrays the major

TABLE 1-2 Structures in Which Chemical Substances Have Been Injected,
Applied or Deposited

Major Cranial Subdivisions	Structure	Sub Part
Telencephalon	Pyriform lobe (Splenium)	
	Cingulate gyrus	
	Corpus callosum	
	Corpus striatum	
	Caudate nucleus	
	Dorsal, ventral	
	Putamen	
	Globus pallidus	
	Hippocampus	
	Dentate fasciculus	
	Septum	
	Lateral, medial	
	Amygdala	
	Dorsal, ventral	
	Olfactory bulb	
	Medial Forebrain Bundle (MFB)	
	Fornix	
Diencephalon	Thalamus	N. reuniens, Ventral N., Anterior N., Centromedian N., Reticular N., Dorsomedial N.
	Hypothalamus	Preoptic area, Lateral, Dorsomedial, Ventromedial, Posterior, Anterior, Mammillary bodies, Median eminence, Arcuate N., Paraventricular, N., Periventricular N., Supraoptic N., Tuber cinereum, Anterior Commissure.
	Medial Forebrain Bundle (MFB)	
	Fornix	
Mesencephalon	Substantia nigra	
	Zona incerta	
	Red nucleus	
	Interpeduncular nucleus	
	Superior colliculus	
	Periaqueductal gray	
	Reticular formation	
	Habenula	
	Dorsal tegmentum	
	Ventral tegmentum	
Rhombencephalon	Medulla	
	Pons	
	Reticular formation	

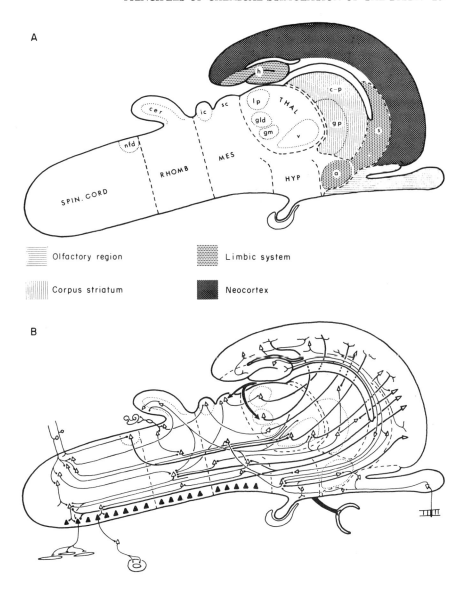

Fig. 1-3 Schematic drawings representing the mammalian brain. In comparison with the nonmammalian brain, the most pronounced differences appear in the composition of the pallial mantle in which the general cortex has become replaced by neocortex; the apparent absence of the nonmammalian external striatum; and the appearance of a circumscribed somatic sensory nucleus (v) in the thalamus receiving, among other somatic sensory lemnisci, part of the spinothalamic tract and most of the medial lemniscus originating in the nuclei of the dorsal funiculus (nfd). Major conduction pathways afferent and efferent

(*Caption continued*)

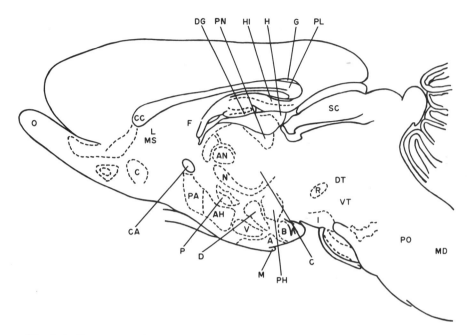

Fig. 1-4 Structures of the rat's brain viewed in a sagittal plane about 0.5 mm from the midline. Abbreviations are as follows: A. arcuate nucleus, AH. anterior hypothalamus, AM. amygdala, AN. anterior thalamic nuclei, B. mammillary bodies, C. centromedian nucleus, CA. anterior commissure, CC. corpus callosum, CN. caudate nucleus, D. dorsomedial hypothalamus, DG. dentate gyrus, DM. dorsomedial thalamus, DT. dorsal tegmentum, F. fornix, G. cingulate gyrus, GP. globus pallidus, H. habenula, HI. hippocampus, I. interpeduncular nucleus, L. lateral septum, M. median eminence, MD. medulla, MS. medial septum, N. nucleus reuniens, O. olfactory bulb, P. paraventricular nucleus, PA. preoptic area, PH. posterior hypothalamus, PL. pyriform lobe (splenium), PN. periventricular nucleus, PO. pons, PU. putamen, R. red nucleus, RF. reticular formation, RN. reticular nucleus, SC. superior colliculus, SN. substantia nigra, V. ventromedial hypothalamus, VN. ventral nucleus, VT. ventral tegmentum, Z. zona incerta.

(*Fig. 1-3 caption continued*)

to the neocortex have been indicated in a slightly bolder line. Abbreviations: a, amygdala; cer, cerebellum; c-p, caudoputamen; gld, lateral geniculate body; gm, medial geniculate body; gp, globus pallidus; h, hippocampus; HYP, hypothalamus; ic, inferior colliculus; lp, nucleus lateralis posterior of thalamus; MES, mesencephalon; nfd, nuclei of the dorsal funiculus; RHOMB, rhombencephalon; s, septum; sc, superior colliculus; SPIN. CORD, spinal cord; THAL, thalamus. (From Nauta and Karten, 1970)

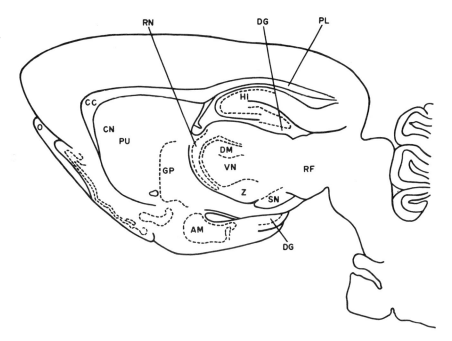

Fig. 1-5 Structures of the rat's brain viewed in a sagittal plane about 2 mm from the midline. Abbreviations as in Fig. 1-4.

conduction pathways for afferent and efferent systems. This schematized representation depicts the trajectories associated with the neocortex as well as those within and between structures inferior to the cortex.

Since 56% of all studies involving chemical stimulation of the brain have been carried out with the laboratory rat, two sagittal views of the brain of this mammal are shown in Figs. 1-4 and 1-5. The structures indicated in Fig. 1-4 represent their size and relative relationship just off the midline. By comparison, Fig. 1-5 reveals many of the same structures as well as others present in a sagittal plane viewed approximately 2.0 mm from the midline.

1. *Structures of the Forebrain*

A side view of the general schema of rhinencephalic structures which encompass much of the limbic system is presented in Fig. 1-6. The more detailed relationships between the large internal fiber systems that link key structures to each other are illustrated schematically in Fig. 1-7. Arising from the hippocampus is a conglomerate of fibers that pass through a large and discernible myelinated structure—the fornix. Collaterals from the fornix pass into the septal nuclei and arise from this structure. From the main body of the fornix, fiber systems diverge rostral and caudal to the anterior commissure. Part of this fornical sys-

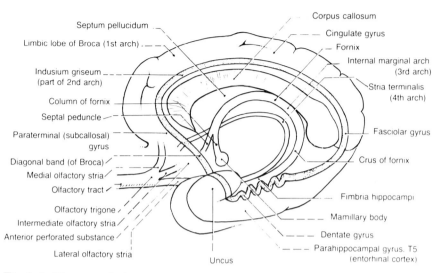

Fig. 1-6 Diagram of the concentric rhinencephalic formations. (From Bossy, 1970)

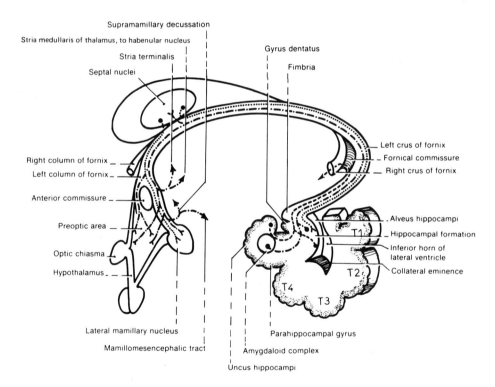

Fig. 1-7 Fornix. (From Bossy, 1970)

tem extends into the mammillary bodies which form the caudal portion of the inferior hypothalamus.

2. Structures of the Diencephalon

A modified, in depth view in the frontal plane of major thalamic nuclei and their tracts of connection is given in Fig. 1-8. Lying directly beneath the thalamus is the hypothalamus, which is comprised of nuclei which are designated strictly on

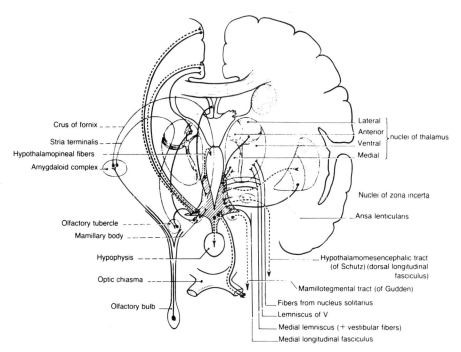

Fig. 1-8 Main cerebral pathways of the autonomic nervous system. (From Bossy, 1970)

the basis of their anatomical position or relationship to other structures. These include the optic tract, optic chiasm, third cerebral ventricle, and the fornix.

Figure 1-9 portrays the approximate position of each nucleus in a schematic representation of the hypothalamus. The prominent nature of the median eminence-tuberal region at the base of the hypothalamus reveals the intimate morphological relationship of the hypothalamus with the pituitary gland. In every chapter of this book, studies are described in which one or more of the individual structures of the hypothalamus have been stimulated with a chemical substance.

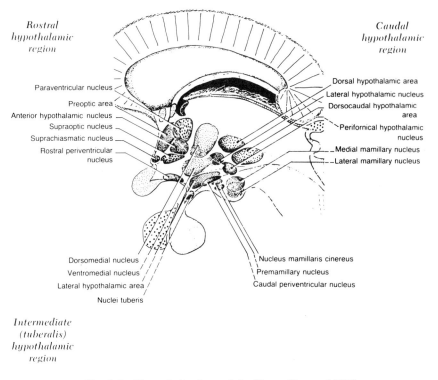

Rostral hypothalamic region

Caudal hypothalamic region

Paraventricular nucleus
Preoptic area
Anterior hypothalamic nucleus
Supraoptic nucleus
Suprachiasmatic nucleus
Rostral periventricular nucleus

Dorsal hypothalamic area
Lateral hypothalamic nucleus
Dorsocaudal hypothalamic area
Perifornical hypothalamic nucleus
Medial mamillary nucleus
Lateral mamillary nucleus

Dorsomedial nucleus
Ventromedial nucleus
Lateral hypothalamic area
Nuclei tuberis

Nucleus mamillaris cinereus
Premamillary nucleus
Caudal periventricular nucleus

Intermediate (tuberalis) hypothalamic region

Fig. 1-9   Hypothalamic nuclei. (From Bossy, 1970)

3. *Interconnecting Pathways*

Whereas the pyramidal system links the primary motor cortex directly to motor nuclei in the spinal cord and hence to their respective muscle groups, the extra-pyramidal system consists of a far more diffuse set of efferent pathways. Figure 1-10 illustrates diagrammatically both of these complex major motor systems and many of the structures upon which they impinge and synapse. The pyramidal pathways connect the large motor neurons of the precentral gyrus to the thalamus and thence to the bulbar pyramids. These corticofugal fiber networks supply several sets of cranial motor nuclei. However, the principal level at which the system has been defined remains the bulbar pyramids, chiefly because rostral or caudal to the pyramids, the interconnections even in the decussation of fibers are hopelessly interwoven with other fiber bundles (Patton and Amassian, 1960).

The intricate afferent and efferent connections of the extrapyramidal pathways are also depicted in Fig. 1-10. The rich anatomical relationship between the caudate nucleus, putamen, nuclei of the thalamus, red nucleus and the mesencephalic reticular formation with the motor regions of the cortex are of

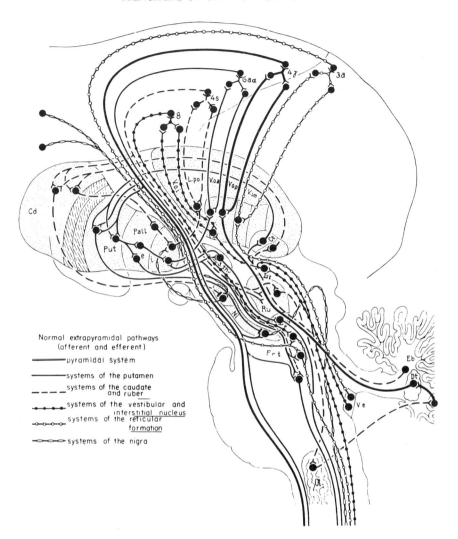

Fig. 1-10 Fiber connections of the extrapyramidal motor system with the afferent and efferent pathways. Abbreviations are as follows: Cd, caudatum; Ce, centrum medianum; Dt, dentate nucleus; Eb, emboliform nucleus; F.rt, reticular formation; Ist, interstitial nucleus; L.po, lateropolaris; Ni, nucleus niger; Ol, inferior olive; Pall.e, pallidum externum; Pall.i, pallidum internum; Put, putamen; Ru, red nucleus; S.th, subthalamic nucleus; Ve, vestibular nuclei; V.im, ventrointermediate nucleus of the thalamus; V.o.a, ventro-oral thalamic nucleus (anterior); V.o.i, ventro-oral nucleus of thalamus; V.o.p, ventro-oral thalamic nucleus (posterior) (Jung and Hassler, 1960).

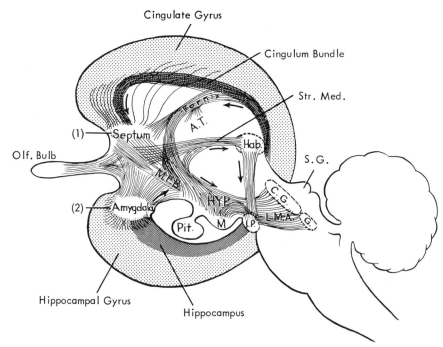

Fig. 1-11 MacLean's schemata for limbic system organization. The upper figure identifies projections by a variety of divergent pathways from olfactory bulb and brain-stem into the limbic system. The lower figure identifies limbic outflow by way of fornix, medial forebrain bundle, and habenulo-peduncular tract to brain-stem. The anteriomedial region of this circuit, in the vicinity of the septum (1), is identified by MacLean as relating predominately to survival of the species. The anterolateral region of this circuit, in the vicinity of the amygdala (2), is identified by MacLean as relating predominately to survival of the individual. (Livingston, 1967; from MacLean, 1958)

Fig. 1-12 Diagrammatic representation of the connections between some limbic forebrain structures and the midbrain. Broken lines indicate projections to central and lateral regions of the brain-stem tegmentum. Pathways distributing to medial tegmental regions are indicated by solid lines. A: descending pathways from limbic system to midbrain-fornix, medial forebrain bundle, and mammillo-tegmental tract. B: pathways to stria medullaris and fasciculus retroflexus. C: ascending projections from midbrain to limbic system: dorsal longitudinal fasciculus, medial forebrain bundle and mammillary peduncle. Anatomical abbreviations are as follows: A. anterior thalamic nuclei, AM. amygdala, AVT. ventral tegmental area of Tsai, CA. anterior commissure, CI. inferior colliculus, CO. optic chiasma, CS. superior colliculus, GC. central gray substance, Hb. habenula, Hip. hippocampus, HL. lateral hypothalamic area, HPV. paraventricular hypothalamus, IL. intralaminar thalamus, IP. interpeduncular nucleus; Mm. mammillary bodies, NCS. nucleus centralis superior, NGD. dorsal tegmental nucleus of Gudden, NGP. ventral tegmental nucleus of Gudden, RPO. preoptic region, S. septum. (Modified after Nauta, 1958; from Zanchetti, A., 1967. *In* Quarton *et al.* (eds.) *The Neurosciences.* New York, Rockefeller University Press, p. 607)

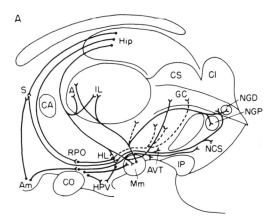

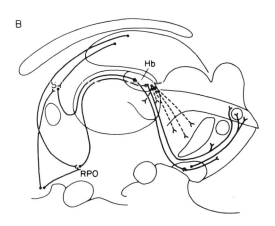

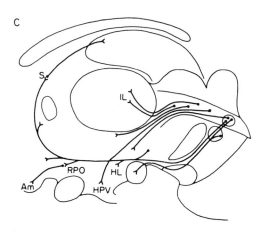

special importance (Jung and Hassler, 1960). When the functional aspects of sensory-motor integration are considered from a chemical viewpoint, the underlying morphology depicted in Fig. 1-10 is particularly significant for such physiological responses described in Chapter 10 as tremor, stereotyped behavior and epileptiform seizures. Interestingly, the cerebellum sends ascending fibers to the thalamus where a subsequent distribution and relay connection to other areas are made. Statokinetic systems are thereby served in large measure by the extrapyramidal network of fibers.

Just as closely organized are the structures which comprise the limbic system. As shown in Fig. 1-11, the major projections of the fornix, stria medullaris, medial forebrain bundle and habenular pyramidal tract integrate the outflow of the rhinic or limbic lobe. Working in harmony, these structures were identified by Papez (1937) as having as much or more to do with an emotional experience and its expression as with olfaction, thought originally to be the primary function of this lobe. MacLean (1970) has suggested that in the limbic system, the circuit linking the septum, amygdala and hypothalamus with other structures is associated with different aspects of emotional behavior. But by virtue of the richness of the interconnections, the limbic lobe is anatomically integrated.

A closer and more detailed analysis of the ascending and descending pathways of the limbic system has been completed by Nauta (1958). What has been designated conventionally as the Nauta circuit is illustrated in Figs. 1-12A, B and C, which are based on the histological tracing with silver stain of degenerating fibers. Diagrammatically, these sagittal sections recapitulate the anatomical articulation of both the amygdala and hippocampus via the fornix, in the lateral plane of the septum and preoptic area (Fig. 1-12A). The medial forebrain bundle and the mammillo-tegmental pathway form two other strong associations between the more caudal limbic structures. The dorsal aspect of the stria medullaris (Fig. 1-12B) synapses in the habenula and continues via other pathways to the midbrain. The afferent network of fiber bundles that feeds the limbic system originates in the mesencephalon in the central gray matter and in the nuclei found in the dorsal and ventral tegmentum.

B. Pathways of the Biogenic Amines

Extensive studies of amine-containing neurons using the techniques of chemical staining and histochemical fluorescence have uncovered two major neuronal systems in the mammalian brain: (1) cholinergic and (2) monaminergic.

1. *Cholinergic Systems*

Shute and Lewis have identified histochemically an ascending cholinergic reticular system and a separate collection of pathways in the limbic system that is also cholinergic (Shute and Lewis, 1967; Lewis and Shute, 1967). Using acetylcholine esterase (AChE) staining procedures following selectively placed lesions,

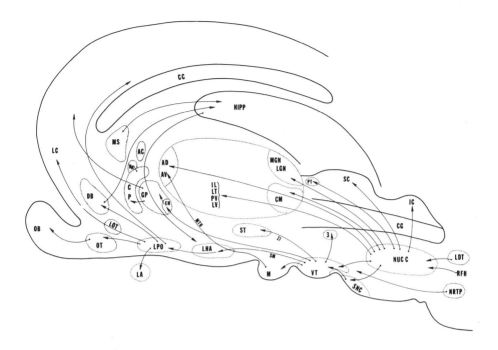

Fig. 1-13 Diagrammatic representation of the ascending cholinergic reticular system of Shute and Lewis showing the two components of this system, i.e., the dorsal tegmental pathway and the ventral tegmental pathway. The dorsal pathway emanates predominantly from the nucleus cuneiformis (Nuc C) of the mesencephalon and projects diffusely to the anterior (SC) and posterior (IC) colliculi, pretectal area (PT), medial (MGN) and lateral geniculate (LGN) nuclei (especially the ventral nucleus of the LGN), centre median (CM) and intra-laminar thalamic nuclei (IL), several specific thalamic nuclei including the lateral ventral (LV) and posterior ventral (PV) nuclei, and the anterior thalamic nuclei, especially the antero-dorsal (AD) and antero-ventral (AV) groups. The nucleus cuneiformis receives fibers from the latero-dorsal tegmental (LDT) area (including the locus coeruleus) and the reticular formation of the lower brain-stem (RFH). The ventral tegmental pathway emanates mainly from the ventral tegmental area of Tsai (VT) and the substantia nigra (SNC) and projects primarily to the subthalamus (ST), zona incerta (ZI), hypothalamus and basal forebrain areas. These projections, in part, pass via the supra-mammillary bodies (SM), mammillary body (M), lateral hypothalamic area (LHA), lateral preoptic area (LPO) to the olfactory tubercle (OT), nucleus of the lateral olfactory tract (LOT) and to limbic (LC) and other cortices. Direct fibers from this system supply the oculomotor nucleus (3). The entopeduncular nucleus (EN) and globus pallidus (GP) also receive direct fibers from this system, the latter, in turn, projecting to the caudate (C) and putaminal (P) formations, and nucleus accumbens (NA). Some connections via the lateral preoptic area, are made with the diagonal band of Broca (DB) and medial septum (MS), the latter being the origin of cholinergic hippocampal (Hipp) afferents. (From personal communication, with permission of Dr. Peter J. Morgane)

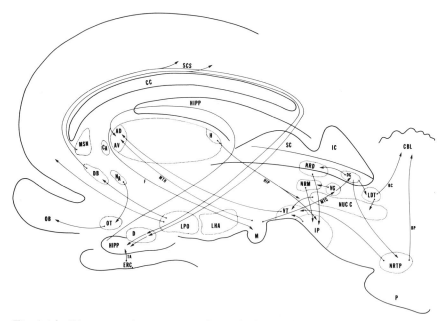

Fig. 1-14 Diagrammatic representation of the cholinergic limbic system of Lewis and Shute. Fibers of one group in this system are afferent to the hippocampal formation passing from the medial septal nucleus (MSN) and nucleus of the diagonal band of Broca (DB) to the dentate gyrus (D), hippocampus (Hipp) proper (dorsal and ventral hippocampus), and subiculum. A second group of fibers passes from the antero-dorsal (AD) and antero-ventral (AV) thalamic nuclei to the retrosplenial and cingular areas, respectively (not shown). From the nucleus accumbens (NA) fibers of this system project to the olfactory tubercle (OT) and bulb (OB). Another group of neurons are afferent to the cerebellum, with fibers originating in the dorsal tegmental nucleus of Gudden (DG) and thence projecting to the latero-dorsal tegmental nucleus (mainly locus coeruleus, LTD) and to cerebellum (CBL) via the brachium conjunctivum (BC). Another group of fibers from the dorsal nucleus of Gudden projects directly to the nucleus reticularis tegmenti pontis of Bechterew (NRTP) and, via the brachium pontis (BP), to the cerebellum. One group of neurons of this cholinergic limbic system is afferent to the dorsal tegmental pathway component of the ascending cholinergic reticular system. These run from the dorsal tegmental nucleus of Gudden to the latero-dorsal tegmental nucleus and thence to the nucleus cuneiformis (Nuc C). A second group is afferent to the ventral tegmental pathway as follows: they run from the dorsal (DG) and ventral (VG) nuclei of Gudden, via the nucleus raphé dorsalis (NRD) and nucleus raphé medianus (NRM), to the interpeduncular nucleus (IP). Included in this group are projections from the habenular nuclear area connecting with the dorsal nucleus of Gudden, and through this, with the latero-dorsal tegmental nucleus, nucleus cuneiformis and substantia nigra. Also in this group are projections to the dorsal tegmental nucleus of Gudden, thence to the nucleus reticularis tegmenti pontis of Bechterew and, through this latter, to the ventral tegmental area of Tsai (VT). Other abbreviations: SCS. supracallosal stria; CC. corpus callosum; ERC. entorhinal cortex; TA. temporo-ammoniac fibers; P. pons; HIP. habenulo-interpe-

they have delineated dorsal and ventral tegmental pathways. As presented in Fig. 1-13, the dorsal cholinergic system emanates from the cuneiform nucleus of the midbrain, and projects rostrally in a diffuse manner to a large number of thalamic nuclei and other structures. Figure 1-13 also shows that the ventral tegmental pathway extends anteriorly to the substantia nigra, subthalamus and hypothalamus passing dorsal to the mammillary complex. This AChE containing fiber system then projects via distinct pathways to the globus pallidus, caudate nucleus, putamen, and also to the limbic cortex as well as to the medial septum, which is the origin of a cholinergic afferent trajectory to the hippocampus.

A second major cholinergic system designated as such by Shute and Lewis links together the structures of the limbic system in terms of both afferent and efferent components. A close examination of Fig. 1-14 reveals the bi-directional pathways to and from the hippocampus that connect the septum, thalamus, preoptic area and mammillary bodies. Of significance are the connections to structures in the midbrain including tegmental nuclei and the raphé nuclei. Thus, the hippocampal formation is morphologically related to many structures in the forebrain and midbrain through a series of cholinergic projections.

2. Monoamine Systems

Based on the studies of Andén, Fuxe and many others who have employed histochemical fluorescence to trace the pattern of discrete amine-containing neurons, it appears that separate serotonergic, noradrenergic and dopaminergic pathways traverse the brain-stem (Fuxe et al., 1968). As conceptualized by Morgane and Stern (1972) in Fig. 1-15, as many as six chemical subsystems, characterized by the presence of the monoamines, innervate in a complex fashion a number of structures lying along the longitudinal axis. A large portion of the reticular formation of the mesencephalon is a norepinephrine-staining system of fiber bundles. The ventral noradrenergic pathway (A coding) passes all the way to the cortex, whereas the dorsal noradrenergic pathways are associated with the locus coeruleus (AG). This nucleus possesses distinct connections with the nuclei of the raphé complex (B coding) which in turn projects dorsalward to limbic-forebrain structures including the septum. This is shown also in Fig. 1-15.

Although undoubtedly having efferent connections, the ascending dopaminergic system arising in the mesencephalon traverses the internal capsule on its course through the globus pallidus to its termination in the corpus striatum, which consists of the putamen and caudate nucleus. The lesion studies of Morgane and Stern (1972) tend to bear out the anatomical principles of the mono-

---

duncular tract; MTG. mammillo-tegmental tract; SC. superior colliculus; IC. inferior colliculus; H. habenula; MTH. mammillo-thalamic tract; M. mammillary body; LHA. lateral hypothalamic area; LPO. lateral preoptic area; CA. anterior commissure; F. fornix. (From personal communication, with permission of Dr. Peter J. Morgane)

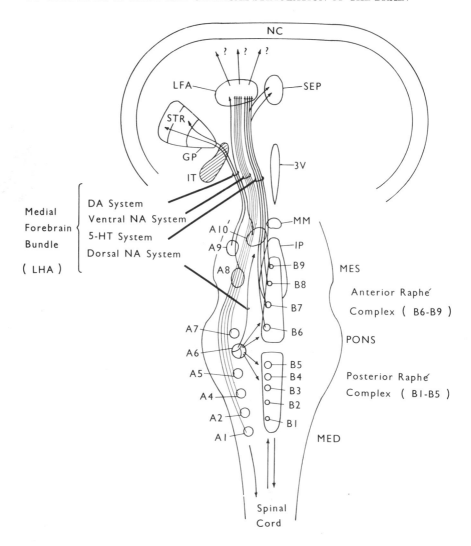

Fig. 1-15 Fiber pathways and nuclear assemblies comprising the serotonergic, noradrenergic, and dopaminergic systems in the brain. Note especially the latero-lateral stratification of the heterogeneous chemospecific circuits comprising the medial forebrain bundle. The locus coeruleus (Nucleus A6) has especially powerful relations with the raphé complex, and its rostrally projecting pathway comprises primarily the dorsal noradrenergic pathway of Fuxe. The ventral noradrenergic pathway originates in noradrenergic cell groups in the lateral reticular formation of the medulla, pons, and mesencephalon. Cholinergic systems also in this bundle are not shown. Abbreviations: NC. neocortex. SEP. septal area, LFA. limbic forebrain area, 3V. 3rd ventricle, STR. neostriatum (putamen and caudate nuclei), GP. globus pallidus, IT. internal capsule, DA. dopamine, NA. noradrenaline, 5-HT. serotonin, LHA. lateral hypo-

amine system although thorough-going studies utilizing anterograde and retrograde degeneration have yet to be completed.

VII. GENERAL CONSIDERATIONS

The method of chemical stimulation has been applied to a vast number of problems in the study of brain function. As long as one maintains a pharmacological propensity as each study is considered, the reaction that an individual drug produces can be more readily interpreted. For example, many of the compounds that have been injected into brain tissue, as described in the chapters ahead, exert a selective action only on an organ system outside of the brain. If such a compound appears to exert a central effect, two explanations usually can account for this action: (1) a metabolic by-product is the source of the effect after the compound undergoes partial degradation, usually in the liver, or (2) the drug acts primarily on the sympathetic or parasympathetic nervous system. In this latter case, autonomic feedback to the brain can delude the reader into a false interpretation of a direct action on CNS tissue.

A. Development of the Field

Many phenomena other than those included under the chapter topics have been investigated using the approach of chemical stimulation. For instance, the rate of axoplasmic flow of an amino acid following its injection into the reticular formation has been monitored in the rat (Foulkes and Robinson, 1968) as well as the spread of crystalline serotonin from the caudate nucleus (Cohen and Sladek, 1972). Important experiments have also been undertaken to determine the deleterious ultrastructural changes that accompany the local injection of compounds such as ouabain into the parietal lobe of the rat's cortex (Cornog et al., 1967), serotonin into the ectosylvian gyrus of the cat (Osterholm et al., 1969), or 6-hydroxytryptamine into the midbrain of the cat or rat (Poirier et al., 1972). Recently, the effects of crystals of biogenic amines have been analyzed in terms of their effect on the firing pattern of single neurons in the immediate vicinity of the implant (Kent, 1972).

---

thalamic area, MM. mammillary body, IP. interpeduncular nucleus, MES. mesencephalon, MED. medulla, B1–B9. coding of raphé nuclei (serotonergic neurons) according to histofluorescence mapping of Fuxe et al. (1968), A1–A10. coding of noradrenergic neuron groups of lateral reticular formation according to histofluorescence mapping of Fuxe et al. Question marks are placed on arrows between limbic forebrain area and neocortical formations because, although these pathways have been traced diffusely to the neocortex by histofluorescent mapping, they have not been identified by anterograde degeneration or other anatomical studies. (From Morgane and Stern, 1972)

Scientists have published their results on chemical stimulation of brain tissue in over 110 different journals. Quite remarkably, only 10 of these journals account for approximately 50% of all of the contributions made to this field. Table 1-3 presents the compilation of these journals together with the frequency of citation according to the percentage of the total articles. Interestingly, the journal that is the leading source of papers, *Physiology and Behavior,* is among the newest ones, having been founded in 1966. Another fact revealed by this analysis is that these 10 journals are international in scope as reflected by the respective scientific editorial boards. This underscores the fact that this field is not only interdisciplinary but has drawn great interest throughout the world.

TABLE 1-3 Ten Journals Most Commonly Used for Publication of Experiments on Chemical Stimulation Cited in Order of Frequency of Usage

Title of Journal	Number of Articles	Percent of Total Articles
Physiology and Behavior	59	8.4
Endocrinology	47	6.7
Journal of Comparative and Physiological Psychology	44	6.3
Neuroendocrinology	37	5.3
Neuropharmacology	31	4.4
Science	31	4.4
Journal of Physiology	27	3.8
American Journal of Physiology	26	3.7
Brain Research	24	3.4
Experimental Neurology	20	2.8

The wide spectrum of species used for the studies is illustrated in Table 1-4. As expected, the laboratory rat is the animal that dominates the experimental endeavors in this field. Surprisingly, the human ranks sixth among all species tested. The monkey ranks just behind the rabbit in frequency of use and well ahead of other less costly organisms including the guinea pig and two varieties of bird.

Finally, the explosive growth of this field which parallels in some respects the developments that have occurred in cognate disciplines has been astounding. Table 1-5 presents an historical tabulation of the frequency of citation of journal articles devoted to chemical stimulation. The interval is in five-year blocks except for the years of 1971 and 1972. In these two years alone, as many research papers have appeared as in all of the years prior to 1965.

It should be noted that most all of the related papers and reports have been excluded from the book that do not correlate the intracranial injection to an anatomical structure and for which no attempt at localization was made. The

TABLE 1-4   Ten Most Commonly Used Organisms in Chemical Stimulation Experiments.
(A citation is based on the number of individual journal articles in which the species was
the test subject)

Animal	Reference Citations
Rat	394
Cat	169
Rabbit	54
Monkey	42
Dog	12
Human	11
Chicken	8
Guinea pig	6
Pigeon	5
Goat	3

vast amount of experiments dealing with the intracerebral injection of viruses
and other material, usually into the rodent (e.g., Haley, 1957), is omitted. As
Mims (1960) demonstrated with the volumes typically infused by the virologist
into the mouse's brain, the solution always reaches the cerebral ventricles, subarachnoid space and usually the bloodstream. Except in instances in which a
research report may make a vital point, experiments also have not been included
in which a solution is injected into one of the ventricles, subarachnoid space,
cisterna magna or a region of the neuraxis caudal to the medulla.

TABLE 1-5   Frequency of Published Research in the Field of Chemical Stimulation of
the Brain According to 5-Year Blocks of Time

5-Year Interval	Number of Published Papers
1915	1
1916–1920	0
1921–1925	1
1926–1930	5
1931–1935	1
1936–1940	6
1941–1945	2
1946–1950	3
1951–1955	14
1956–1960	35
1961–1965	106
1966–1970	358
1971–1972	170

B. Usage of Master Summary Tables

At the end of each of Chapters 3 through 12, a Master Summary Table has been included. The general purpose of each of these tables is to give the reader an overall grasp of the extensive contributions made in each discipline. More specifically, the large variety of drugs and chemicals injected into all sorts of sites in different species can be recognized. As such, the tables can be used as a guide to what has been accomplished and to the scope of the experiments undertaken. In this connection, a word of caution is necessary in regard to their usage.

Although the text raises many critical points about the research *per se*, many of the variables that are crucial to interpretation are not included in the table. These are: (a) the number of animals used, which means that an entry in the table can be based on a single injection into one animal or on a summary of hundreds of observations on many animals; (b) the reliability of the procedure in terms of the number of times that a response was evoked after a specified chemical was applied to a single site; (c) the large number of drugs and chemicals that had no observable effect when injected or deposited similarly; (d) the precise magnitude of a given response; (e) the duration of the experiment in terms of whether the reaction was followed for 30 seconds, 30 minutes or 30 hours; (f) whether or not a statistical analysis, if appropriate, was carried out; (g) information about or examples of histological verification of the site of implantation, the zone of necrosis and the area of destruction; (h) the evidence of the spread or diffusion of the chemical or drug; (i) the usage of an anatomical control for morphological specificity; and (j) the usage of a drug control for pharmacological comparison.

As a result, the single most important misapplication of a given table would be to equate two entries by comparing one experimental observation with another, particularly if the directions of the responses are opposite. For example, contrasting the action of a single dose of carbachol given at one site in the rat's brain with a mapping analysis based on three doses injected at 100 sites scattered throughout the brain-stem of the dog is utterly insipid. As unimaginable as it may seem, there are cases in which the observed effect of an agonist at one site is published in one journal and the opposite effect of an antagonist in another journal, both observations having been made on the same animal.

Therefore, after an overview of general effects of a compound is obtained from a given table, the original reference is the best source for a full evaluation of the breadth, scope and quality of a specific report.

The state of the animal is given in each table as follows: U = unanesthetized and unrestrained; C = constrained, confined, curarized or not able to move about in its immediate environment; and A = anesthetized. The designation usually refers to the interval of observation. Thus, the effect of a hormone implanted under anesthesia but recorded post-operatively is categorized as U or unanesthetized.

The physical form in which a substance was delivered at a given site in the brain is denoted as being either in solution (liquid) or as a crystal (solid). Thus, a hormone or other substance that is prepared in a carrier medium of agar, gelatine, cocoa butter, sucrose, or other material is considered to be in crystalline form at the time of its insertion into brain tissue. A compound that may precipitate readily but yet is given in solution is likewise considered as a liquid injection. A question mark (?) indicates that the information was not given in the original article, whereas a dash (−) signifies that the dose (e.g., water or antibodies) is not calculable.

Experimental Methods for Stimulating the Brain with Chemicals

2

I. INTRODUCTION

The fundamental premise underlying the method of chemical stimulation is two-fold: (1) either to change the existing quanta of an endogenous substrate or other material, or (2) to introduce a synthetic compound within the brain parenchyma. Therefore, the chief emphasis of any experimental procedure is to deliver the substance to a discrete cerebral site in the hope of localizing its action.

The delivery system for the intracerebral administration of a chemical has become a rather sophisticated business in many laboratories. This is due mainly to some of the difficult questions raised in Chapter 1, as well as to the possible significance of the lesion produced by the injection tube, the diffusion of the material itself, and the effect that an exogenous chemical actually has on an individual nerve cell or a collection of neurons. Thus, the technical advances have been guided by the necessity of utilizing increasingly smaller-sized tubing and more diminutive amounts of the stimulating agent—solution or solid. As one would expect, these developments have accrued in large measure because of the improved technology in several fields of engineering, which have given us needle tubing of very fine gauge, miniature syringes of low volume and high delivery pressure, thread-like plastic tubing and highly reliable infusion pumps.

About 60 years ago, Hashimoto (1915), a Japanese scientist working in Vienna, described probably the first cannula system, which was devised for the injection of solutions into the diencephalon of the non-narcotized rabbit. The injector cannula was inserted through a guide as shown in Fig. 2-1. This historical achievement is particularly significant since the basic principles that were employed are the same as those that have "evolved" more recently. For example, the injector needle (B) contained a sleeve which fit snugly into the metal cylinder to provide a leak-proof seal. The metal cylinder served as a guide for the injector needle. Further, the cylinder was implanted always prior to an experiment and, by virtue of the threads cut at the base, was screwed tightly into the skull; it could not be cemented to the skull because dental acrylic had not yet been invented.

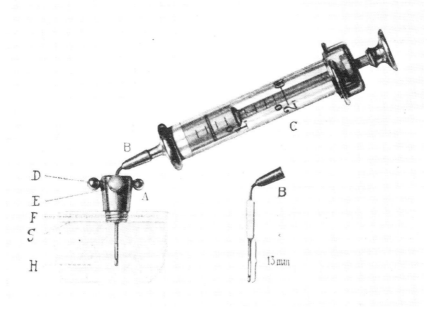

Fig. 2-1 A = Metal cylinder, B = Injection needle and connection to syringe, C = Pravatz syringe, D = Fastening head for the metal cylinder, E = Fastening screw for the metal cylinder, F = Skull, G = Dura mater, H = Brain matter. (From Hashimoto, 1915a)

Finally, the needle was removed from the cylinder after the injection had been made.

II. CANNULA DESIGNS

In the 1930s the technology of cannulation was advanced by Hasama (1930), Masserman (1937), and others whose pioneering work was unfortunately often marred by the ubiquitary nature of the large volumes injected. This in turn precluded any precise anatomical localization of drug action. However, Masserman (1937) developed what was later nicknamed a "chemitrode" for simultaneous bipolar electrical stimulation or injection of a chemical in solution, both of these through the same needle.

Two outstanding contributions were made in the 1940s. Comroe (1943) using a single needle implanted acutely into the brain-stem of the dog, examined the effect on respiration of a solution injected in a volume as small as 1 μl and no greater than 5 μl. He also called attention to the conceptual differences in the effects between an injection into tissue and the ventricle. In Scotland, Pickford (1947), again using a single needle in an acute preparation, was the first to make the salient point about dose-response and then illustrate a dose-dependent relationship of a chemical (ACh) given in a small and localizable volume in the brain-stem.

In 1953, a second "chemitrode" device was improvised by Liljestrand (1953) who drew a silver wire into a fine glass capillary tube. This was then used for either monopolar electrical stimulation or for the injection of a small volume of a chemical solution.

In 1956 Fisher introduced the use of the crystalline technique for depositing steroids and other substances in solid form into the hypothalamus of the rat.

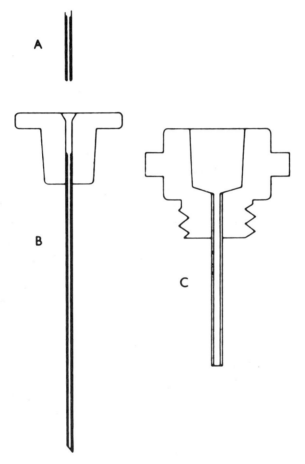

Fig. 2-2 Procedure for micro-injections in the conscious rabbit. The "guide" C, is screwed into the skull after stereotaxic positioning. The cannula B, is inserted by hand through the "guide." A, represents the specially ground end of the hypodermic needle attached to the micro-syringe. A fits tightly in the Perspex head of the cannula. (From von Euler and Holmgren, 1956)

In that same year, von Euler and Holmgren (1956) published what is considered to be a model cannula system. It has now become the standard configuration upon which all sorts of variations are based for either the injection of a solution or the application of crystals. The design of the cannula, illustrated in Fig. 2-2, is based on the principle of a permanently implanted guide tube (Fig. 2-2C) which is held in a base that is fastened by cement or screwed into the craniotomy hole. The needle (Fig. 2-2A) of the micro-syringe fits tightly into the head of the plastic insert to make a perfect coupling with the injector needle (Fig. 2-2B). After the injector needle is lowered through the guide, the injection is made. The depth of the locus of the injection is varied simply by altering the length of the injector needle (Fig. 2-2B). With the utilization of this almost universally adopted concept, a stereotaxic entry is provided by the stationary guide into a site that can be tested repeatedly in an unanesthetized animal. In fact, von Euler and Holmgren (1956) utilized rabbits in which this sort of cannula system had been implanted for up to 6 months.

A. Infusion of Solutions

Many minor or major modifications of this cannula design have been contrived. Specific details about the construction and experimental applications are reviewed comprehensively in *Methods in Psychobiology, Volume 1* (Myers, 1971a). For injecting a solution into the brain, a micro-syringe containing the solution is attached either directly to the external portion of the injector needle or connected to it via a length of polyethylene tubing. The great advantage of using flexible connecting tubing is that the plunger of the syringe can be impelled remotely by the experimenter, usually from outside the cage; thus, an injection can be made randomly at any time, without signaling the animal or disturbing it in any way.

1. *Single Cannula*

Some of the single cannula systems that are in widespread use today are presented in summary form in Fig. 2-3. The six different arrangements (Booth, 1968c) that are illustrated present some of the means for connecting a syringe to the needle. Several methods are also shown whereby the requisite fluid seal can be achieved in order to prevent unwanted backflow; this can also be accomplished by a diaphragm (Myers, 1971a) or a special silicone rubber sealant (Kottler and Bowman, 1968).

Another system employs a removable guide tube, the depth of which can be altered simply by loosening a set-screw inserted into the sleeve that fits over the guide (Cooper *et al.*, 1965). As shown in Fig. 2-4, the sleeve itself is screwed into a multi-holed skull plate which is fitted onto the surface of the bone. The depth of the injector needle can also be varied by an even smaller sleeve, the internal structure of which also serves to prevent backflow. The concept of

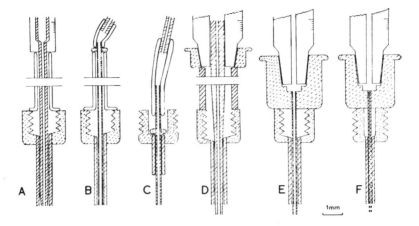

Fig. 2-3 Intracranial injection systems. Chronically implantable guide cannulae sketched with cap and attached insert removed and injection needle in operating position. A. Guide cannula made from 21-gauge needle; 10-μl syringe through polyethylene spacer cut for each guide. B. 23-gauge guide; 30-gauge injection pipette with soldered stop, through individual spacer. C. 30-gauge pipette soldered to 23-gauge support; PE 10 connector to 10-μl syringe. D. 21 guide, cut to standard length; μl syringe with tip ground to approximately 27 gauge, to 2 mm beyond guide tip, through 13 standard-length spacer needle. E. 23 standard-length guide; 33 standard-length needle to 2 mm beyond guide, Luer hub to 10-μl syringe. F. 27 standard-length guide; 34 needle to tip or 2 mm beyond, Luer hub to 10-μl syringe in repeating dispenser. The widths of the needles are drawn to the scale indicated but no other horizontal or vertical dimension is to scale. (From Booth, D. A. 1968c. *J. Pharmacol. Exptl. Ther.* **160**: 336–348. The Williams and Wilkins Co., Baltimore)

remote injection is also employed in that the polyethylene tubing connects the injector needle to the syringe. A special feature of a multi-holed skull plate, shown in Fig. 2-4, is that an entry into the brain can be made along different coronal and parasagittal planes, thus enabling the experimenter to explore different anatomical areas.

2. Multiple Cannulae

The necessity of performing anatomical controls in the same animal as well as the intriguing prospects involved in stimulating two sites simultaneously, has generated a number of multi-cannula systems in which up to eight guide cannulae are positioned in a predetermined array. One of the first multi-cannula units was devised by Hoebel (1964) for injecting solutions or applying crystals in the brain of a rat. In Fig. 2-5, the guide tubes are shown fastened to a phenolic plastic block according to stereotaxic coordinates calculated beforehand. The principal disadvantage of this system is that if there is an error in one coordinate, then all cannulae will be mis-positioned simultaneously.

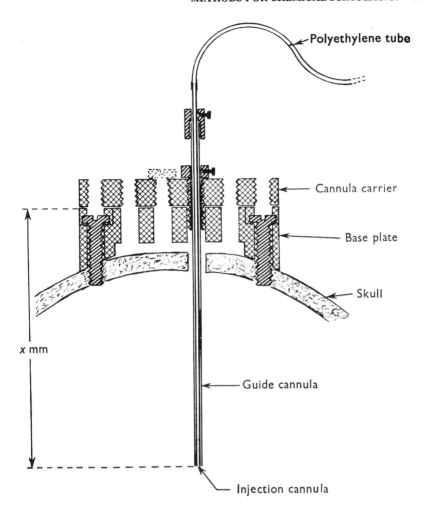

Assembly *in situ*

Fig. 2-4 Micro-injection assembly attached to skull, in cross-section. (From Cooper *et al.*, 1965)

An array that is made up of guide tubes implanted independently has been perfected for larger animals such as the cat and monkey (Myers, 1964a; Myers and Yaksh, 1969). Figure 2-6 illustrates how tubes are placed in the brain of a monkey. After each cannula has been lowered, the entire array is fixed permanently in place by cement. A polyethylene pedestal is screwed over the array, filled with cement and then capped to maintain a sterile preparation. The figure illustrates an injection being made into the left anterior cannula (lateral) with the two medial (posterior) guides not shown.

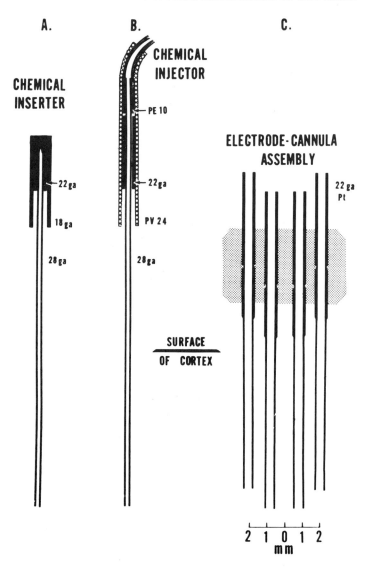

Fig. 2-5 A. Obturator for insertion of crystalline chemicals and for plugging an electrode-cannula when it is not in use. B. Chemical injector which fits inside an electrode-cannula for injection of fluid drugs from a remote micro-syringe. C. Assembly of four electrode-cannulae cast in a block of dental cement. (From Hoebel, B. G. 1964. *EEG Clin. Neurophysiol.* **16**: 399–402. Elsevier Publishing Co., Amsterdam, The Netherlands)

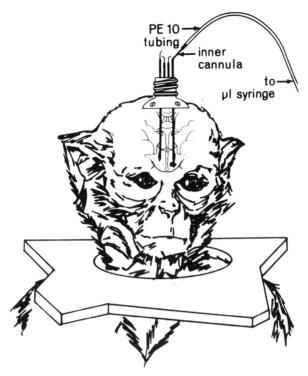

Fig. 2-6 Rhesus monkey acclimated to a primate chair. A bilateral array of 22 gauge outer micro-injection guides is implanted chronically with tips resting in different regions of the hypothalamus. The 28 gauge inner injector cannula, which is attached to a microliter syringe via PE 10 tubing, is lowered to a depth 1 mm below the outer cannula. Injections of chemicals in solutions in volumes of 0.5 to 1.0 μl enable precise localization of the chemical agent. (From Sharpe and Myers, 1969)

Variations on this basic idea have been published specifically for use in the chicken (Marley and Stephenson, 1968), rat or other animal, with light weight, ease of construction, simplicity of usage or even low-cost being among the principal justifications (e.g., Lilly, 1958; Epstein, 1960; Myers, 1963; Wagner and deGroot, 1963a; Decima and George, 1964; Valzelli, 1964; Nadler, 1965; Myers *et al.*, 1967; Khavari *et al.*, 1967; Grunden and Linburn, 1969; Ankier and Tyers, 1969; Meyer and Ruby, 1970; Altaffer *et al.*, 1970; Chisholm and Singer, 1970; Morris *et al.*, 1970; Russel *et al.*, 1972; DiStefano, 1972). A multipurpose concentric cannula has also been devised for the sterile micro-injection of a drug into the brain of a human (Heath and Founds, 1960).

A summary diagram showing one of the erudite approaches now being adopted to control for the problems of volume, diffusion and reliability is presented in

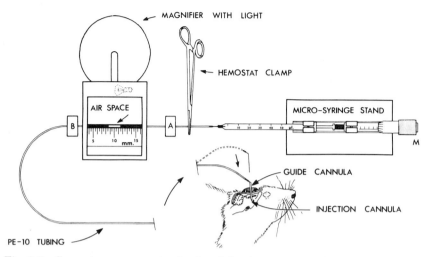

Fig. 2-7 General arrangement of micro-injection system. Fluid is injected by advancing a micrometer arm (M, as shown), by pushing the syringe piston manually, or by activating a calibrated infusion pump via an interval timer. Before and after each micro-injection, PE tubing is occluded by a hemostat clamp which has been modified to prevent damage to tubing by coating tips with epoxy and by bending the arms so that when shut the clamp closes just enough to prevent fluid from moving when syringe piston is advanced. Movement of a 2- to 3-mm air space in a calibrated segment of the tubing between pieces of tape A and B is used as a measure of the volume injected; reliance on syringe plunger advancement as read on the syringe volume scale may result in large errors. A piece of 30-gauge stainless steel tubing is epoxied into end of micro-syringe in place of a Luer-Lok hypodermic needle to reduce the possibility of air bubbles in the system. A 30-gauge stainless steel injection cannula inserted into a 23-gauge guide cannula permanently implanted stereotaxically with anchor screws and dental cement was used in these experiments although other sizes of tubing and cannula configurations may be used equally well in larger or freely moving animals. A micro-injection directly caudal to anterior commissure is shown in above drawing, which is not to scale. (From Swanson *et al.*, 1972)

Fig. 2-7, taken from Swanson *et al.* (1972). In this example, the micro-injection is made by rotating by hand the micrometer that drives the micro-syringe plunger. As the fluid advances, the air bubble inserted for monitoring purposes into the tubing line (Myers, 1971a) is tracked by a magnifying glass to reflect the movement of the solution out the injection cannula and into the brain.

A remote injection into the hypothalamus of the cat (Myers, 1971a) is illustrated in Fig. 2-8. The plunger of the micro-syringe is driven by the motor of a pump which is switched on by a timer placed several feet away from the animal. The duration of the injection, as well as the rate of inflow, is thereby precisely controlled. Furthermore, the animal is not disturbed by any movement of the experimenter, since the injector cannula is always inserted earlier. These two

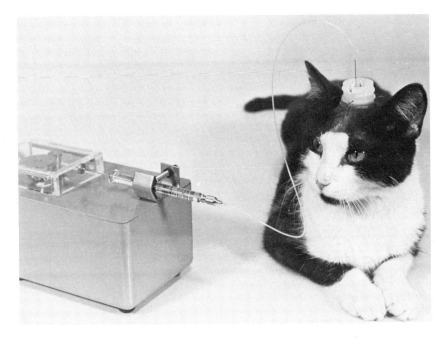

Fig. 2-8   Micro-injection of a putative transmitter into the hypothalamus of an unrestrained cat.   A four-cannula array, held in place by a plastic-bottle-top pedestal, had been implanted one week earlier.   The Sage pump is timed to deliver 0.8 μl over an interval of 36 seconds.   (From Myers, 1971)

latter approaches have made very accurate delivery of a chemical solution in a volume often a fraction of a microliter a commonplace in many laboratories throughout the world.

B. Application of Crystals

Although considered in some scientific quarters to be a less physiological approach to the stimulation of a structure, the use of chemicals in solid form rather than in solution is derived from three divergent premises, two practical, the other theoretical.

From a wholly practical standpoint, the usage of a substance in crystalline form is the only recourse when testing the efficacy of a compound that is virtually insoluble or dissolves at a low rate. Used in this form, its presence within tissue simulates, in broad terms, the relatively slow metabolic action of a substance such as a hormone. A second practical consideration is the experimental simplicity in terms of the ease of application. For testing a large number of animals, the use of a crystalline substance is surely a convenient procedure. However, whether the factor of convenience should determine an experimental approach to a scientific question is an equivocal point about which some wariness exists.

The third justification stems from the early work of MacLean and others on the problem of diffusion of liquids and the difficulty entailed in the localization of the liquid. It was, in fact, MacLean (1957a) and later Rech and Domino (1959) who condemned, nearly in their entirety, the procedures involving liquid injections into brain tissue. But as will be discussed in the following section, the reasoning that was at the root of the abjuration of the use of a solution was based on technical limitations of the period. Short of micro-iontophoresis, anatomical localization is readily possible if a small enough volume is employed. Thus, the criticism that was not trivial then is today merely of historical interest.

In the last decade, several different devices with the suffix "trode" have been described for depositing crystals of a given compound, e.g., "chemode," "oestrode," "chemitrode" and "omnitrode." These differ quite clearly in two main characteristics from the design of the needle utilized to inject a solution. First, the extracranial portion of the tube is closed-off or capped externally; second, the solid chemical is either fused to, drawn in or tamped into the tip of the injector needle. Once inside the lumen of the tube, the injector can be inserted into a guide and removed after a short interval, left in place for a long period or implanted into the tissue.

Following the design principle of the double-barrelled or concentric tubes of von Euler and Holmgren, a number of these cannulae have been developed. For example, MacLean (1957a) used a stylet wire inserted in the shaft of the injector needle to eject the crystals from the tip into which they had been tamped. Nashold and Gills (1960) later introduced the idea of sealing the tip of the injector with an inactive substance such as carbon which had the advantages of (a) preventing the escape of the drug as it was lowered into tissue, and (b) helping to mark the site of the implant. Grossman (1960) utilized the double-barrelled cannulae for repeated stimulation of the brain of the rat, and throughout the 1960s, the implantation of crystalline steroids and chemicals was done

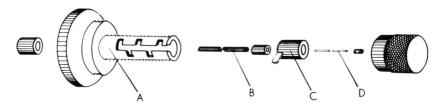

Fig. 2-9 A cannula system for the application of crystals at specific loci. The actual size of each part is indicated in brackets. A. The notched base for moving and locking in the cannula system at one mm depths (10 mm); B. The outer barrel of the guide cannula (22 to 25 mm); C. Exploring guide holder (about 5 mm); D. Tamping needle cannula which holds the crystals (22 to 25 mm). (From Hernández-Peón et al., 1963)

routinely in many laboratories, including those of Lisk, Harris, Hernández-Peón, Sawyer and Fisher.

A cannula used for placing crystals at different depths was devised by Hernández-Peón *et al.* (1963). As shown in Fig. 2-9, an exploring guide tube could be locked into place at any number of depths each separated by 1 mm. After a crystalline substance was tamped into an injector needle, the needle was lowered into the brain to a level limited by the lock guide tube. Using an injector needle of fixed depth, Ivaldi *et al.* (1964) added, in a clever fashion, the

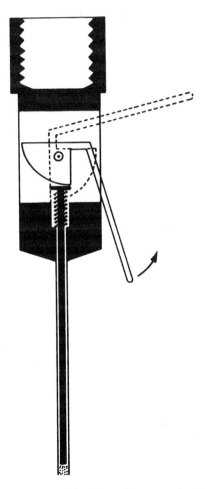

Fig. 2-10 Schematic drawing of implantation cannula. To eject a pellet, the stylet is pushed down. After deposition of the material the cannula is retracted. (From Smelik, P. G., 1967. *Neuroendocrinology* 5: 193–204. S. Karger, Basel, Switzerland)

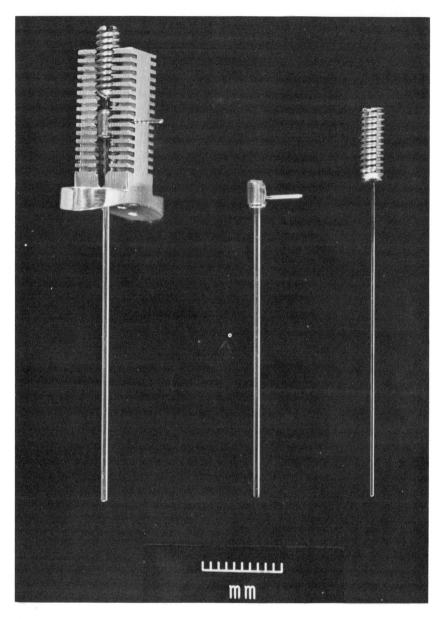

Fig. 2-11 The three major components of a double chemitrode, i.e., from left to right: chemitrode body, exploring guide and one cannula, and stilette with screw head. For illustrative purposes only one cannula is shown inserted through the skull plate. The screw head is not tightened down against the exploring guide in order to show them as separate components. (From Bronzino *et al.*, 1972a. *EEG Clin. Neurophysiol.* **32**: 195–198. Elsevier Publishing Co., Amsterdam, The Netherlands)

capacity for simultaneous bipolar recording or electrical stimulation by insulating the sides of both the injector and guide cannula.

To illustrate the extent of the remarkable developments that have occurred in cannula technology, Fig. 2-10 is a schematic diagram of a double-barrelled cannula made by Smelik (1967) in which the crystalline material is tamped into the outer guide tube before it is lowered into the brain. Then at any desired time in the course of an experiment or during surgery itself, the cylindrical pellet of crystals is ejected into the tissue simply by raising the lever on the side of the cannula base.

Evolving from the work in the laboratory of Hernández-Peón, other sophisticated chemitrodes have been introduced by Morgane and his colleagues (Bronzino et al., 1972a; Morgane et al., 1972). Figure 2-11 shows the three components of a chemical stimulation system in which the guide tube can be locked in at 15 different vertical planes within the brain. As a result, the injector needle containing the stimulating crystal at its tip is limited as to depth of penetration by the predetermined position of the guide cannula. With this device, the neural pathways or nuclei that fall into layers or strata in a given part of the CNS can be tested for their sensitivity to a chemical. Thus, the same principle is employed as that used for injecting a chemical prepared in solution at different depths, i.e., by a "spacer" placed between the injector and guide or by an injector needle of varying length.

Although it is nearly impossible to specify the absolute dose of a chemical applied in solid form, two methods have been utilized in such an attempt. Stein and Seifter (1962) showed that quantitatively different reactions in behavior can be demonstrated simply by the number of times the external tip of an injector needle is tapped by one's finger. The obvious questions concerning the reliability of such a tapping procedure have been raised (Myers, 1971a). Another method used frequently in neuroendocrinological studies is to vary the diameter of the injector needle. A cannula with a larger lumen tends to release the test hormone at a higher rate and dose (e.g., Lisk, 1969a). Again, quantitative differences in terms of the response of the organ system have been shown.

C. Regional Perfusion with Push-Pull Cannulae

There are two important physiological limitations of the aforementioned procedures for chemical stimulation. First, the duration of the stimulus is difficult to control since this parameter is dependent upon certain physical characteristics such as the rate of dissolution of the substance, its metabolic degradation and the extent of dispersion in the tissue (Folkman et al., 1968). Second, unlike electrical current applied to the tissue at the tip of the electrode, the chemical stimulus regrettably cannot be either turned on or switched off at will.

A technological advance, which may go far to exculpate the more traditional stimulation methods from this deficiency, is the technique of localized perfusion of a chemical in solution. Three distinct advantages of this technique exist in that: (a) the concentration of the stimulating agent can be precisely controlled; (b) the stimulation can be terminated quickly since the chemical is drawn off just as rapidly as it is infused; and (c) a lower concentration of a chemical can be used because the population of neurons is bathed by the perfusate continually during the interval of perfusion. An additional spin-off is that the collected

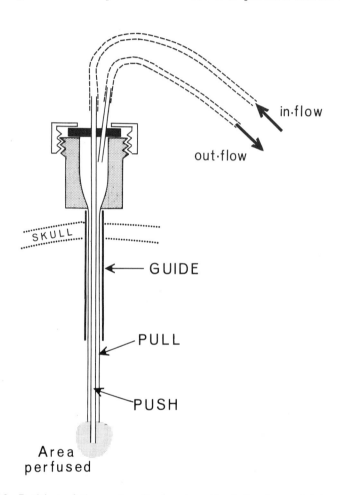

Fig. 2-12 Position of the push-pull cannulae after being lowered into a permanently implanted guide tube. Perfusate from the push syringe is pumped into the inflow tube, through the inner push cannula, and to the tip where a spherical area of tissue (1.5 mm dia) is perfused (shading). The perfusate is immediately withdrawn, at the same flow rate, into the space between the push and pull cannulae and into the body of the pull cannula. In the outflow tube, the perfusate flows back into the pull syringe. The diagram is not to scale because of the smallness of some of the parts. (From Myers, 1970)

effluent that has come in contact with the tissue can be saved and used in a number of ways: it can be re-perfused, assayed or transferred (transfused) to the same anatomical site in another animal (Myers, 1967a; Delgado *et al.*, 1972).

The history and the usage of the experimental procedure for a push-pull perfusion have been reviewed by Myers (1972). Essentially, two designs for push-pull cannulae have been developed for actual physiological studies: (1) the side-by-side design in which the push (inflow) tube is fastened directly to the pull (collecting) tube (Delgado, 1966); and (2) the concentric arrangement in which the push (inflow) tube is positioned inside the pull (outflow) tube (Myers, 1967a). Because the size of the lesion is much smaller, the localization is more circumscribed, and the chance of an occlusion is reduced, the concentric push-pull cannula system is more widely used today than the side-by-side configuration.

Recently, a removable push-pull assembly has been devised which has the benefits of the concentric design as well as other experimental advantages including that of varying the depth of perfusion (Myers, 1970a). As described in later chapters, it is used not only for chemical stimulation but also for studies on the release of endogenous factors from isolated portions of tissue in a given structure (Dudar and Szerb, 1970). Figure 2-12 shows the position of the push

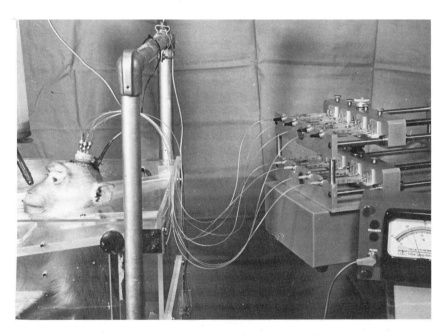

Fig. 2-13 Bilateral push-pull perfusion of the anterior hypothalamus and posterior thalamus of a rhesus monkey acclimated to a restraining chair. The inflow and outflow tubes from the cannulae are illustrated. (From Myers, 1972)

tube inside the pull cannula after both have been lowered through a guide tube that is implanted permanently. When the push-pull assembly is used with a precision infusion-withdrawal pump, this ensures that the perfusate is drawn off at the identical rate at which it is pumped in. The region of infiltration portrayed in Fig. 2-12 by the shading, i.e., the area of chemical stimulation, can be limited quite precisely by the distance between the tips of the push and pull tubes (Myers and Veale, 1970).

The application of the push-pull stimulation techniques for the monkey, cat or other large animal is straightforward as shown in Fig. 2-13. Recently, Myers (1972) and Veale (1972) have presented modifications suitable for the rat and rabbit, respectively. Figure 2-14 shows how a push-pull cannula assembly can be lowered through one of a series of guide tubes attached to a Monnier-Gangloff plate. By this procedure, numerous anatomical sites can be stimulated up to 10 times with a chemical, without any apparent loss in sensitivity of the site (Veale, 1972). Specific experimental findings utilizing these procedures are described in Chapters 6, 7, 9 and 11.

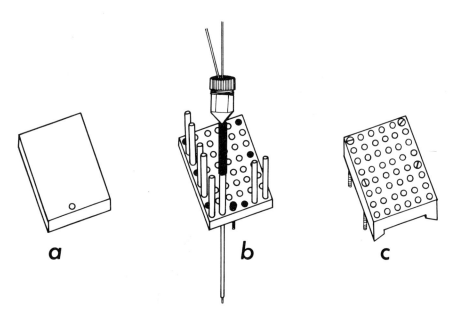

Fig. 2-14 Base-plate (c); guide plate with push-pull cannula assembly, anchor screw and spacer (b); Teflon cover (a). During perfusions, (b) is attached onto (c); between experiments, (a) is used to cover (c) which is attached to the skull. For illustration only 8 guide tubes are shown in the guide plate (b). One push-pull cannula is inserted through one of the guide tubes. (From Veale, W. L. 1972. "A stereotaxic method for the push-pull perfusion of discrete regions of brain tissue of the unanesthetized rabbit," *Brain Research*. 42: 479–481, fig. 1. Elsevier Publishing Co., Amsterdam, The Netherlands)

III. EXPERIMENTAL AND THEORETICAL ISSUES

A large number of technical factors serve to determine how an experiment is interpreted when a chemical is applied to brain substance. Many of these factors revolve about the kind of compound used for stimulation, the control substance, the volume and concentration of the drug, and the vehicle used as the carrier of the chemical. The following sections deal with both the theoretical and practical issues of the technique of chemical stimulation which will hopefully help the reader to evaluate the data in the chapters that follow.

A. Diffusion of a Chemical in Tissue

The validity of any conclusion about the morphological specificity of an effect produced by a chemical given locally is based solely upon the histological localization of the site of stimulation. Of major concern are the questions related to the degree to which a chemical spreads and whether the concentration of the compound at a secondary site remote from the actual stimulation locus will produce a detectable physiological response.

After MacLean (1957a) had shown the extent to which a solution in a volume as large as 20 μl would travel up and away from the tip of the injection, Rech and Domino (1959) made the additional observation that a volume "of as little as 10 microliters (sic!) produces a lesion." Harrison (1961) then demonstrated that 3.0 μl of radioactive thyroxine spread over a 5 mm area after injection into the brain of a rabbit. As shown by Fog and Pakkenberg (1971) 5 μl of tritiated dopamine injected into the corpus striatum spread sufficiently far in the brain of the rat, that the highest density of grains in the autoradiographs was in the superficial ipsilateral cortex. This is illustrated in Fig. 2-15. From all of these results, an infallible deduction is at once evident; the larger the volume injected, the greater the impossibility of localizing any action of the chemical.

An investigation of the physical spread of a chemical substance from the site of injection into the diencephalon of the rat has revealed the clear volume-spread relationship. When each of four different dyes was injected in five volumes ranging from 0.5 to 4.0 μl, the extent to which the dye spread within tissue correlated highly with the magnitude of the injected droplet (Myers, 1966). In fact, the distance that each marker-dye travelled through tissue exceeded the actual dimension of each of the different microliter droplets, as shown in Fig. 2-16. From these studies, the conclusion was reached that the volume injected into the brain of a small animal such as the rat should never exceed 0.5 μl and no more than 1.0 μl should be injected into the brain of a larger animal such as the cat.

Such a conclusion has generally been borne out in other studies of a similar sort. For example, when 1 μl of ^{14}C-morphine is injected into the hypothalamus of the rat, 90% of the radioactivity, i.e., that constituting the effective dose, is re-

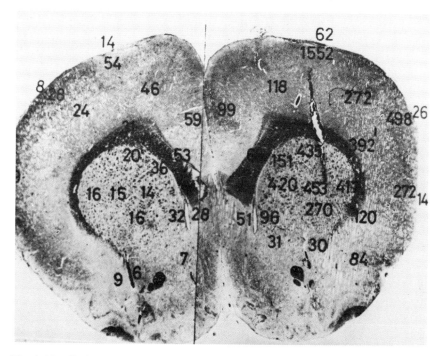

Fig. 2-15 Grain counting of an autoradiogram on a 10 μ transverse slice of rat brain. Intracerebral micro-injections were made into the center of the corpus striatum on both sides. On the right side, tritiated dopamine (200 μg = 5 μc in 5 μl) was injected; on the left side ordinary dopamine (200 μg in 5 μl) was injected. Fixation in formaldehyde; stained by Weil's method. The numbers are mean counts per area (3025 μ^2) in various parts of two brain slices cut around the injection site with an interval of 100 to 200 μ. The injection area is visible in the right hemisphere and is 1 mm anteriorly and 2.5 mm laterally to the bregma. (From Fog and Pakkenberg, 1971)

tained within 1 mm of the site of injection (Lomax, 1966a). Using autoradiography, Schubert et al. (1970) have shown that a much larger volume (2.5 μl) of ^{14}C-morphine solution infused into the diencephalon spread to a correspondingly greater degree. In other experiments in which scintillation spectrometry has been used, a 1 μl volume of ^{3}H-norepinephrine was found to remain within the region of the injection (Booth, 1968c; Javoy et al., 1970). Using ^{3}H-acetylcholine and ^{14}C-serotonin in addition to ^{3}H-norepinephrine, Myers et al. (1971d) have verified the view that most of the radioactivity of a biogenic amine contained in 1 μl remains within the general structure into which the injection is made, at least in a concentration which would have a physiological effect on the local pool of neurons.

Tracer studies involving the implantation of crystalline material show a pattern of spread in neural tissue that is nearly identical with that of solution. At a

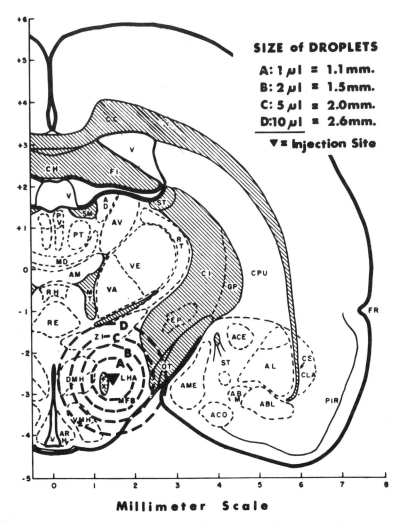

Millimeter   Scale

Fig. 2-16   Diagrammatic reconstruction from the de Groot atlas of the rat brain at the coronal level of AP 5.4. The volume of brain tissue which would be displaced by each microliter droplet is depicted by the dashed lines, if the microinjection were made in each case in the lateral hypothalamus. The actual size of each microliter droplet is given in millimeters in the legend. (From Myers, 1964a)

conference held in 1963, Michael reported that the radioactivity following the administration of ^{14}C-stilbestrol in the base of the brain fell off sharply about 0.6 to 0.8 mm from the site of the implant. Beyond this region, the grain counts reached background levels (Michael, 1966). A correspondingly sharp decline in the gradient of radioactivity also follows the implant of ^{3}H-estradiol, with only a minimal part of activity detected 2.0 mm away from the site of applica-

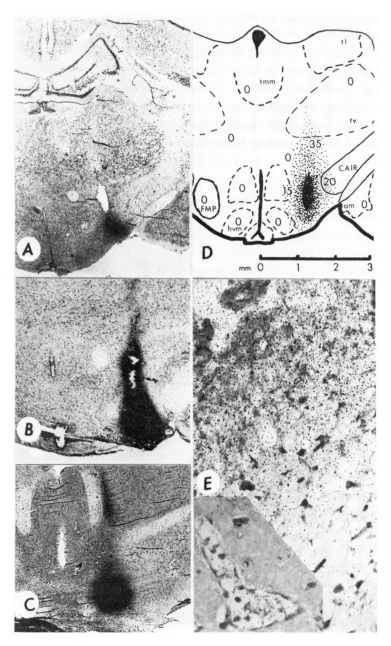

Fig. 2-17 Dry-mount autoradiograms of frontal sections from rat brain showing
the site of ^{3}H-atropine implantation in the centrolateral (A) or posterolateral
(B and C) hypothalamus. The black rounded areas indicate the spread of intense radioactivity. One hour (A) after the implantation, radioactivity is still

tion (Palka *et al.*, 1966). An autoradiographic analysis shown in Fig. 2-17 of the dispersion of tritiated atropine deposited in the hypothalamus revealed a lateral spread of activity of less than 1 mm, with but slightly greater dispersion along the needle track (Grossman and Stumpf, 1969).

The technique of histochemical fluorescence has also been employed to trace the movement of an implanted substance. Unfortunately, considerable controversy surrounds the report of the extensive transport of crystalline dopamine implanted in subcortical structures (e.g., Routtenberg *et al.*, 1968; Montgomery and Singer, 1969a). This is also true of the magnitude of the spread of biogenic amines given in solution (e.g., Ungerstedt *et al.*, 1969; Bondareff *et al.*, 1970). It is perhaps possible that some sort of technical problem is at the basis of this imbroglio, which additional research in different laboratories will undoubtedly resolve.

B. Delivery of the Chemical into the Brain

When a drug or chemical is injected into the brain, the vehicle ordinarily used for preparing the solution is physiological saline. For the control fluid, the saline alone is infused. Concern over the use of 0.9% saline as the carrier has continued to grow since sodium chloride itself can have a profound local effect on nerve tissue. The action of this salt is manifested in changes in an animal's body temperature, water intake and even in the animal's emotional state (Chapters 6, 8, 11). Even discrepancies reported in the literature following an intracerebral injection of the same substance have their origin simply in the carrier used: distilled water as opposed to artificial CSF (Kulkarni, 1967; Banerjee *et al.*, 1970). Moreover, the sodium cation may interact with a substance in such a way as to exaggerate its local effect or diminish it. For this reason, a

---

visible at the implantation site, although the diameter appears smaller than at 12 minutes (B) and at 5 minutes (C). Part D shows in a schematic drawing the results of silver grain counting (the numbers represent silver grain counts per 250 by 250 μm area) from autoradiograms obtained 2 minutes after implantation, when carbachol-induced drinking was first blocked. Two minutes after implantation, no radioactivity could be discovered in tissue structures more than 1 mm from the core of the implantation site, even after 2 months' exposure time of the autoradiograms. am, Nucleus amygdaloideus medialis; CAIR, capsula interna, pars retrolenticularis; FMP, fasciculus medialis prosencephali; hvm, nucleus ventromedialis hypothalami; tl, nucleus lateralis thalami; tmm, nucleus medialis thalami, pars medialis; tv, nucleus ventralis thalami. Part E is a dry-mount autoradiogram at a higher magnification ($\times$ 100) from a frontal section of the implantation area, obtained 2 minutes after ^{3}H-atropine implantation, exposure time 14 days. The inset at the bottom of part E demonstrates transport of radioactive material in a blood vessel, 24 days' exposure time, ($\times$ 200). All sections were 2 μm thick and were stained with methylgreen-pyronin. (From Grossman, S. P. and W. E. Stumpf. 1969. *Science.* **166**: 1410–1412. Copyright, 1969, by the American Association for the Advancement of Science)

suitable solvent contains isotonic concentrations of the essential cations including potassium, magnesium and calcium, in addition to sodium.

Another major point revolves about the tonicity and pH of the solution to be injected. If, let us say, an artificial CSF is used as the solvent, the addition in any large amount of a given solute can render the infusate sufficiently hypertonic that a solution of parallel hypertonicity is necessary as a control. Similarly, the pH of the injection fluid should be adjusted as closely as possible to that of cerebral tissue. When both factors of tonicity and pH are taken into account, two of the distinct advantages of using a solution for chemical stimulation are attained.

1. *Crystalline Technique*

On the crystalline side of the coin, some fascinating methods have been contrived for applying a solid chemical to brain tissue. For example, to prevent the rapid release or action of a steroid, Bohus and Endröczi (1964) dissolved the hormone in agar. Another vehicle that has been utilized for a similar purpose is cocoa butter (Fraschini *et al.*, 1968a and b) which has a convenient melting point of 35°C, just below that of body temperature. In both instances, the vehicle can be manipulated, weighed for the purpose of estimating the dose and placed in the injector needle. Paraffin wax, phenol, talc, gum arabic and other organic and inorganic compounds have also been employed as carriers for a crystalline deposit.

To prevent the crystal from being dislodged as it is implanted in the target site, a film of saturated sucrose solution is often applied at the tip. When dried, the thin layer of sucrose provides a durable coating which begins to dissolve on touching the brain parenchyma, thereby exposing the tissue to the chemical. Another procedure which has been followed widely for over a decade is to heat a weighed portion of the crystalline chemical just until it reaches the melting point. Then the syrupy chemical is drawn up into the hollow tube, allowed to dry by cooling and then implanted. Finally, different kinds of "cappings" have also been used for retarding the metabolic degradation of the chemical and for marking the site of application.

Curiously enough, there is still some disagreement about the best way to permit the substance to infiltrate into neuronal tissue. Most investigators either eject the crystal from the cannula or let it diffuse from the lumen of the injector needle after the tip has been extended through the mass of glial and fibrous tissue which surrounds the end of the guide tube. However, an alternative not commonly practiced is to keep the tip containing the crystalline material within the guide as much as 1.0 mm above the tip. The substance then diffuses only slowly through the glia after extracellular fluid has reached the implant.

2. *Technical Aspects*

Three major technical problems are associated with the use of solid chemicals. First, it is difficult to sterilize a crystal or pellet of material. When a non-

TABLE 2-1 Variables and Questions Comparing the Use of Solutions vs. Crystals for the Local Stimulation of Brain Tissue with a Chemical. (from Myers, 1971a)

Variable	Application of crystals	Micro-injection of solution*
1. Anatomical localization of action	Precise	Precise
2. Dose at site	Approximation only	Accurate estimation
3. pH	No control	Precise control
4. Temperature	Irrelevant (attains ambient level)	Irrelevant
5. Osmolarity (tonicity)	No control	Precise control possible
6. Lesion produced	Dependent on size of injection needle or amount of ejected crystals	Dependent on volume of injection
7. Sterility and pyrogen absence	Difficult	Easily accomplished
8. Necrotic tissue at site	Present	Present
9. Mechanical pressure or deformation	Minimal	Dependent on rate of injection
10. Diffusion	More gradual	More immediate but volume dependent
11. Convenience factor	More	Less
12. Use of compounds of low solubility	Possible	Difficult
13. Action of blocking agents at site	Effective	Effective
14. Control anatomical placements	Required	Required
15. Action via ventricular route	Ruled out or unlikely	Ruled out or unlikely
16. Dissolution of substance as injector is lowered through tissue	Possible	None

*Analysis based solely on use of ≤ 0.5 μl in an animal smaller than the rabbit and ≤ 1.0 μl in an animal the same size or larger than a rabbit. Use of larger volumes invalidates any such comparison.

sterilized substance is deposited in tissue, a local inflammation is often evoked and a proliferation of neuoglia and fibrous tissue occurs that is characteristic of a reaction to a foreign body. On successive applications of the same drug, the sensitivity of the locus of stimulation will decline or desist altogether.

Second, if the solid material to be placed in the brain is not pyrogen free, the long-term course of almost any experiment can alter dramatically, That is, if a fever develops within 10 to 100 minutes as a result of the implant, the animal usually shows signs of tremor or shivering, aphagia, either hyperdypsia or adypsia, and may even seek out a corner and huddle, lie down and fall asleep. Depending upon what the observer is looking for, an interpretation of one or more responses as being a primary effect of the drug would be incorrect because each reaction could simply be a secondary consequence of fever.

Third, many biologically active compounds are exceedingly thermolabile. As a chemical is melted for fusion into the tip of the cannula, its molecular configuration certainly may change depending on the intensity and duration of its exposure to the heat.

Other factors which will influence the outcome of an experiment in which the crystalline method is used are shown in Table 2-1. A comparison is presented here of the variables associated with the use of chemicals for stimulation in both solid and liquid forms. The reader should be cautioned that such a comparison is valid only if the volume of the solution injected is 0.5 μl or less in an animal smaller than a rabbit, or 1.0 μl or less in a larger animal.

C. The Problem of Dose or Concentration

A few pharmacologists, physiologists and other scientists see little utility in the method of chemical stimulation principally because a compound often must be injected or applied in an exceedingly high concentration to produce an effect. For example, the concentration of a substance such as norepinephrine that is used to obtain a quantifiable response in terms of micrograms of amine per gram of brain tissue frequently exceeds the entire quantity of norepinephrine found endogenously within the structure. In spite of this situation, to reject the whole method with a sweeping generality that "such a dose is unphysiological" would appear to be *de facto* premature. But if this is so, why then is such a high dose necessary?

Almost without exception, the concentration of an endogenous substance such as a biogenic amine forms the basis for the comparison between that and the dose level. This concentration is usually calculated from an assay performed on a block of tissue or from a gross measure of the concentration in whole brain. Without going into the infirmities pertaining to the assay of an entire brain, which has already been dealt with in terms of the disregard for anatomical specificity (Myers, 1969a), such a measure gives no consideration to certain important ultrastructural relationships.

Observations based on light and electron microscopy as well as histochemical fluorescence suggest that the concentration approaches saturation within the vesicles or granules containing an amine. If the quantitative estimates of a humoral factor in the nerve ending itself are contemplated, it is easy to understand how this tiny fraction of tissue contributes disproportionately to the value reported for the gross mass of tissue. Similarly, the subsynaptic membrane, adjacent to the nerve ending, upon whose receptors a substance acts when liberated presynaptically, occupies a correspondingly diminutive bit of tissue. When one considers the vast network of capillaries and blood vessels, neuroglia, extracellular fluid, dendrites, cell bodies and axon fibers, it is easy to imagine that far less than probably $\frac{1}{1000}$ of all tissue in the brain is comprised of the vesicle-membrane-receptor complex.

In the special case of steroid and perhaps polypeptide hormones, which may influence directly the inhibitory, releasing and other factors, there is evidence that postulated receptors on the proteinaceous membrane of a target cell may have only a secondary or indirect activity, or none at all. For example, radio assays of the hypothalamus show that estrogen is apparently taken up and bound by acceptors that are located not in the hypothalamic neuronal membrane but rather in the nucleus itself (Anderson, Peck and Clark, 1973, personal communication). The cellular remoteness of this sort of site could easily be related to the level of estrogen in brain tissue. This would seem to have some physiological significance.

Logically then, the significant issue at stake is the concentration of an amine, steroid or other humoral factor only at the receptor-end of the synapse. That is, the real question in this context centers directly on the actual amount of the substance within the axon bouton expressed in picograms of compound per nanogram of nerve terminal. Although such a stupendous question is now technically unanswerable, the ratio of the substance to tissue weight could well be close to unity. Therefore, one would logically deduce that the concentration of the factor reaching the receptors and subsequently attaching to the sites on the contiguous cell would approach a level close to saturation.

To simulate this synaptic condition with a chemical injection would in reality require an equally high concentration. The reasons are illustrated schematically in Fig. 2-18. One can see from this diagram that the hypothetical compound after injection travels widely around every structure and in every direction. However, only a very small fraction of the chemical in solution or in solid form would reach specific receptor sites. If a low dose of a substance is given, then the amount lost to the surrounding tissue would be so large that a concentration of sufficient potency to activate the postsynaptic receptors would not be achieved.

Related to this important theoretical issue is an equally noteworthy consideration on the other side of the conceptual fence. In actual experimental terms, the single factor of a high dose of a chemical used for stimulation can invalidate

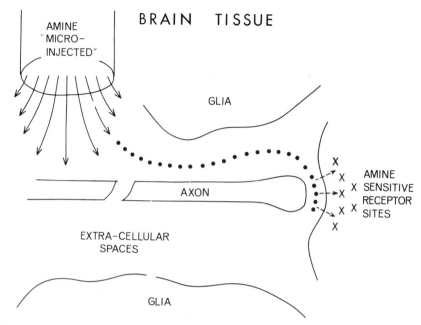

Fig. 2-18   A theoretical diagram to explain why a high pharmocological concentration of a neurotransmitter, such as an amine, is required to produce a physiological response. When an amine is micro-injected into brain tissue, it diffuses in every direction throughout the extracellular fluid spaces, onto glia and around axons and other nerve processes. Only the smallest fraction of the amine reaches (• • •) the amine sensitive receptor sites at a postsynaptic membrane to activate a neuron involved in a specific physiological system. (From Myers, 1970b)

an investigation. A legitimate interpretation is impossible under one or more of the following sets of circumstances when: (1) the same physiological or behavioral response is evoked by the chemical, no matter where in the central nervous system the chemical is applied or injected; (2) by halving or doubling the concentration or volume of the chemical applied to the tissue, there is, nevertheless, no evidence of a dose-response relationship; (3) a known neurotoxin, nerve blocker, anesthetic or similar substance has the same effect as the chemical used for stimulation; (4) a pharmacological antagonist or blocking agent, known to have a molecular specificity corresponding to the chemical, does not attenuate the effect, or exerts the same effect as the agonist; and (5) another chemical or chemicals that are structurally unrelated to the test substance produce the same response when deposited at the same site in the brain.

D. Cannula Lesions and Anatomy

The abhorrence espoused by some critics of this technique in which subcortical tissue is inescapably impaled by a cannula has no more relevance to the question of understanding brain function than the criticism of implanting a stimulating or lesioning electrode in the same manner. Surely, the reduction in the overall size of a lesion achieved through the cannulation of a ventricle rather than tissue is a weak trade-off against the very real potential for localizing and identifying the discrete anatomical site of action of a compound. Nevertheless, the reader's interpretation of each experimental result is always tinged by the underlying unknown of the degree of tissue destroyed in the region purportedly activated by the chemical that is injected.

For a start, a lesion produced merely by lowering a cannula through a mass of tissue transects materially many pathways and invades numerous nuclei. The smaller the size of the brain, the greater will be such a transection and invasion. In fact, as the ostensible neurochemical differences seem to be unfolded between two species—a small rodent and a larger feline—the possibility exists that the amount of viable tissue remaining in the smaller animal may in part be the basis for a dissimilarity.

If one considers, for example, the stimulation of the ventromedial hypothalamus (VMH) of a rat by means of an injector cannula that passes through a guide tube of larger gauge implanted just above the VMH (Epstein, 1960), it is apparent that such a cannula configuration, if positioned bilaterally, would do away entirely with the dorsomedial nucleus as well as parts of other midline structures of both the hypothalamus and thalamus. It is for this reason that the interpretation of a given research finding and any subsequent formulation of a model should depend upon the punctiliousness of the anatomical controls that are undertaken. The essential ones are as follows: (1) representative histological sections that display not only the entire cannula track but also the cytological condition of the stimulation locus (e.g., Hall and Myers, 1972); (2) control application of the chemical in an entirely different part of the brain to rule out a single nonspecific response due possibly to an irritative effect that occurs wherever the substance is applied (Rodgers and Law, 1968; Endröczi et al., 1963a); (3) morphological mapping of the sites of stimulation to show all sites which can be excluded, as well as implicated, in the mediation of the chemically-induced response (Booth, 1967); (4) validation of the specific effect produced by a chemical within a distinct anatomical structure in another species of animal, preferably one with a larger brain (Feldberg and Myers, 1965a; Myers and Yaksh, 1969); (5) an experimental verification of the diffusion or spreading of a substance with the scientist's own particular injection or implant procedure to provide an internal validation of the delivery system (Myers, 1966).

Other procedures now being established to augment the level of experimental validity include electron microscopy of the area of implant, analysis of the degeneration of fiber systems, and chemical assay to detect the changes in endogenous substances in the areas surrounding the implant. Finally, it should be mentioned that an anatomical survey of the results obtained with chemical stimulation often coalesces with the more traditional observations following ablation or electrical stimulation of the same structure (Gildenberg, 1957). In this respect, a careful examination of the pathways connecting the stimulated structure with other anatomical regions or trajectories is of the utmost importance. Thus, one is thereby able to perform a kind of functional "dissection" of a neural system based on a meticulous anatomical analysis of the sites sensitive to a specific chemical compound.

IV. CHEMICAL TRANSPORT HYPOTHESES

Does a chemical applied to a restricted portion of brain tissue actually exert its physiological effect there? Obviously, if a substance is given in a volume greater than a very small but critical amount, it will take the line of least resistance, as discussed previously, usually up the side of the guide cannula, and then spread out indiscriminately some distance over many structures. However, should the chemical be applied in crystalline form or in a minute volume, will the substance still act at a remote locus solely as the result of its transport or diffusion?

In the last decade, the validity of most experiments using chemical stimulation have been seriously challenged by two provocative hypotheses. Essentially, each proposes that a compound deposited within a given structure may not really exert its primary effect on neurons in that anatomical area but rather act at a second more sensitive region located at some distance from the point of application. How could this happen? According to one theory, the substance is believed to enter into the blood supply either by diffusion, active transport or other means, and is subsequently carried to the remote site by the circulation. In the second case, the carrier is instead the CSF contained within the cerebral ventricles.

Both of these notions are not without some reasonable foundation. Certainly no one would deny that a drug or chemical may exert a given effect on a neural system by acting either locally on the structures which form the walls of the ventricular cavities or from the capillary beds. Therefore, we shall examine in some detail the set of fundamental premises that would be required to fulfill logically the tenets of these two related hypotheses.

A. Chemical Transport via Blood

A certain degree of uptake of a chemical implanted in the brain parenchyma is bound to occur, since this is assuredly one route of elimination of a foreign substance (Averill, 1970). The question then centers on the amount of uptake. One unique possibility is as follows: even though a steroid hormone, for which this transport hypothesis was originally based, is implanted directly into the hypothalamus, it nevertheless could produce its effect by acting some distance away on the cells of the pituitary rather than on the adjacent nerve cells.

1. *The Implantation Paradox*

This "implantation paradox" was formulated by Bogdanove following two critical observations. First, a glandular (thyroid) transplant evokes a more intense localized cytological disturbance when grafted to the pituitary than when placed in the hypothalamus (Bogdanove and Crabill, 1961). Second, a glandular (ovary) graft or hormone (estradiol) implant in the pituitary again causes localized changes within the cellular elements of the pituitary that are directly proportional to the size of the deposit; however, the intrahypothalamic deposition of hormone or tissue affects the cytology of the pituitary only when placed in the median eminence in the region of the portal plexus. Figure 2-19 illustrates with remarkable clarity the reason why a hypothalamic implant could alter pituitary function. Succinctly stated, the intrapituitary pellet simply does not distribute the hormone moiety in as nearly an efficient way as the pellet placed intrahypothalamically. The latter chemical more readily enters the descending portal blood supply which flows directly to the pituitary. Then, the exogenous hormone is distributed by virtue of the capillary network throughout the pituitary—a primary and focal point of action (Löfgren, 1960).

Many scientists have shown a predilection to subjugate the importance of the blood transport hypothesis. Two major and almost steadfast positions have

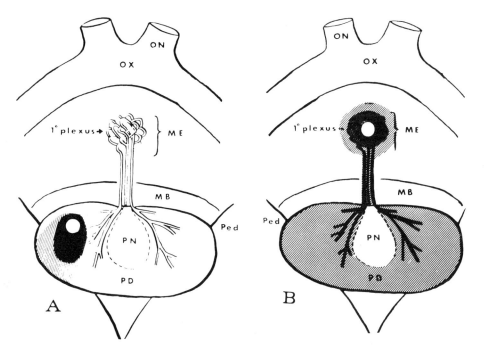

Fig. 2-19 Diagrams of the rat hypothalamus, hypophysis and pituitary portal vessels. ON, OX = optic nerve and chiasm. ME = median eminence. MB = mammillary body. Ped = cerebral peduncle. PN = pars nervosa. PD = pars distalis. Intrapituitary (A) and intrahypothalamic (B) hormone depot sites are shown in white. Postulated regions of high and low concentrations of hormone from the depots are shown by heavy and light shading, respectively. (From Bogdanove, 1963b)

been adopted. First, some sort of a local anatomical action of a hormone seemingly cannot be denied because a lesion placed in the implicated tissue severely impairs the function of the hormone system; what is more, the impairment is in the predicted direction. Other experiments based on electrical stimulation of the same site entrench this view even more deeply. Second, strong evidence has been obtained that there are specialized hormone receptors which must have some function. These receptors take up and bind steroids, again at sites that are homologous to those at which a hormone implant evokes a measurable response. However, an attitude of caution is mandatory because these observations constitute mainly circumstantial evidence upon which the acceptance or rejection of any hypothesis should not be based.

2. *Evaluation of the Transport Hypothesis*

A great deal of careful research has been initiated to ascertain the acceptability of the "implantation paradox." If the hypothesis is wholly or even partially valid, then all of the following propositions should be undeniably verified. As indicated, every proposition has been negated when put to the experimental test.

1. *If a hormone is deposited in the hypothalamus and causes a physiological effect via the pituitary, then it should be evenly distributed in the hypophysis.* This is untrue since Palka *et al.* (1966) found that radioactivity of a tritiated hormone that was implanted in the brain persisted in brain tissue. Moreover, the activity detected in the pituitary was distributed unevenly, being found only on the same side as the implant.

2. *If the plexus in the median eminence serves as the entry channel to the pituitary for hypothalamic implants, then the closer the implant site is to the plexus, the greater will be the (a) intensity and (b) proportion of endocrinological responses.* Lisk (1965b) and numerous others (see Chapters 4 and 5), using hormone implants, showed that the further away the steroid was from the median eminence and the closer it was to the mammillary complex, the greater the effectiveness in altering hormonal function.

3. *If a radio-labelled hormone that has a functional effect when applied intrahypothalamically acts only following its transport to the pituitary, then radioactivity should be higher in the hypophysis.* Chambers and Sobel (1971) failed to find any radioactivity whatsoever in the pituitary after an effective amount of the radio-labelled hormone had been deposited in the hypothalamus. Similarly, Lippert and Waton (1969) found no radioactivity in the hypophysis of the cat after ^{14}C-histamine had been micro-injected into either supraoptic or paraventricular nuclei.

4. *If the neural pathway to the median eminence from that part of the hypothalamus which has been stimulated with a hormone is cut by a miniature knife so as not to disturb the blood supply, the implant should still possess its effect if it acts at the pituitary rather than the neural level.* Knigge and Joseph (1971) demonstrated that the deafferentation of the projection of neurons to the basal

hypothalamus rendered a hormone pellet ineffective when it was deposited distal to the knife-cut and when the portal blood circulation was still intact.

5. *If the pituitary is removed from the sella turcica, thereby interrupting the portal blood supply, a hormone placed in the hypothalamus should have no effect.* Kajihara and Kendall (1969) found that a hormone placed in the hypothalamus nevertheless altered secondarily the secretions of a pituitary which had been transplanted under the kidney and obviously had no portal connection with the diencephalon.

6. *If a hormone is placed in a subcortical structure which has no direct blood supply to the pituitary but only a neural connection to the basal hypothalamus, the hormone should have no effect.* Slusher (1966) showed that a steroid placed in one subcortical region (hippocampus) could affect markedly the function of a gland (adrenal) peripherally.

Notwithstanding the foregoing evidence described here from lesion, stimulation and binding experiments, still other data at present weigh heavily against the concept of an "implantation paradox." How can we reconcile this conclusion with the data which led to a blood transport idea? On re-reading the papers of Bogdanove, one could imagine that the dependent variable—local cytological change—may be an appropriate end-point for the analysis of hypophyseal tissue but an inappropriate one for examining the response of hypothalamic cells. Why?

Although the presence of a fragment of gland may evoke reactive atrophy in the surrounding cells of a similar gland, the molecular "information" exuded by the tissue fragment may contain little or no pertinent "message" for a distinct group of nerve cells, at least when measured by histopathological techniques. Certainly, the glandular implant, because of its inherent biological complexity, does not mimic the local cellular condition which exists after a single steroid or chemical analogue is deposited in the brain or reaches the site of action via the normal channel of circulation.

Finally, the technique by which the question has been examined is just as important as the approach to the question itself. This is often the vital if not ultimate factor in the evolution of any tempting hypothesis which may explain to some satisfaction a result inconsistent with that of another scientist. Since some radioactivity may indeed be found in the hypophysis when labelled crystals of a hormone are tamped in the diencephalon, this story has not ended entirely. Even though an open mind must be maintained about this hypothesis, the belief that a hormone does indeed exert a direct and distinct effect on neural tissue has now become difficult to eschew.

B. Chemical Transport via CSF

Equally as provocative is the possibility that a chemical implanted or injected into brain tissue acts via the fluid contained in the ventricular cavities. This so-called "ventricular hypothesis" is contingent solely upon the process of passive diffusion or active transport away from the site at which the chemical is deposited.

Before the evidence for the hypothesis is examined, it should be emphasized that several confounding factors which have tended in retrospect to muddy the waters of logic should be considered first. Since the last century, it has been known that toxins and other substances given intrathecally possess a direct effect on nervous tissue (e.g., Roux and Borrel, 1898; Delezenne, 1900). By the same token, still other compounds such as adrenaline or Pituitrin given in the lateral ventricle can have an effect directly opposite to that seen when they are given by one of the systemic routes (e.g., Cushing, 1930; Light and Bysshe, 1933; Feldberg, 1963). In addition, if a large volume of a drug is injected into brain tissue, it is certain to spill out into the ventricle. When this happens, the same dose of a drug may appear to be equally potent if given by either the tissue or ventricular route (Morselli et al., 1968), because the injection volume or load in the tissue is equivalent to that of an intraventricular infusion. That is, if 500 μl are infused into tissue, probably $\simeq 495$ μl would empty into the ventricular cavity.

Finally, unless positioned with the utmost precision, the lumen of a cannula intended to be in the ventricle is likely to encroach upon neural tissue ventral or dorsal to the tip, particularly if an animal as small as the rat is the test subject. Hence, the droplet of drug solution or even a crystalline implant could, in fact, alter the neuronal activity locally before dispersing in the ventricular spaces.

1. *Evaluation of the Ventricular Hypothesis*

The requisite sequence of events underlying a ventricular hypothesis would be as follows: (a) a portion of the chemical reaches the ependymal wall; (b) this portion passes out into the cerebrospinal fluid; (c) it then undergoes dilution and (d) is carried "downstream" as CSF flow is only in the caudal direction; (e) the remainder of the substance attaches to or stimulates the receptors at the primary site of sensitivity; and (f) the biological response is evoked.

The feasibility of a substance acting in this anatomically circuitous fashion, in contrast to Bogdanove's hypothesis, has been discussed repeatedly by a number of authors to account for experimental results obtained mainly with a single drug, carbamyl choline (Komisaruk, 1966; Hull et al., 1967; Fisher and Levitt, 1967; Routtenberg, 1967; Baxter, 1967, 1968; Myers and Cicero, 1968; Khavari et al., 1968; Gloor, 1969). However, for the concept to be accepted as a working hypothesis possessing some element of generality, each of the following propositions should be verified experimentally. In each case, every one has been negated.

1. *If a drug deposited in brain tissue exerts its action via the CSF, then the intensity of the response will correlate positively and highly with the proximity of the site to the ventricular lumen.* Levitt et al. (1970) and others (see Chapters

7 and 8) have found no relationship between the distance of the injection site from the wall of the ventricle and the efficacy of the compound injected.

2. *If the CSF serves as a transport medium, then a radio-labelled chemical which has a physiological action when applied to tissue should be detected in the ventricle.* The radioactivity of three labelled putative transmitters (ACh, 5-HT and NE) injected in solution into a physiologically sensitive site (hypothalamus) was retained primarily in that tissue. Further, radioactive material sufficient to reflect a pharmacologically significant quantity of the compounds could not be detected in ventricular perfusates (Myers *et al.*, 1971). Similarly, crystals of a specific labelled chemical (atropine) do remain localized within a 1.5 mm sphere of tissue (Grossman and Stumpf, 1969).

3. *If a drug injected in cerebral tissue acts secondarily after diffusion into the ventricles and re-entry into other tissue, then the latency should be longer than when given directly in the ventricle.* In a large number of studies in which such comparisons have been made, an opposite temporal relationship has been uniformly demonstrated (see, for example, Chapters 6, 7 and 11). In every instance, the latency is as short or shorter when the test compound is applied to brain tissue.

4. *If a drug injected into tissue acts via the CSF, then a comparison of the two routes should show that the dose required to produce a given effect would always be less when the drug is given into the ventricle than that when injected via tissue, i.e., because the applied or injected chemical decreases in concentration as it disperses.* In all experiments in which such a comparison has been made, the concentration of a compound given by the ventricular route must always be as much as 100 times greater to produce the same functional response as that produced when the compound is injected directly into a sensitive site. To evoke a specific behavior such as drinking or a physiological response such as hyperthermia, a much higher dose of the effective compound must be given intraventricularly than in a structure sensitive to the drug (Feldberg and Myers, 1965a; Lovett and Singer, 1971; Routtenberg and Simpson, 1971).

5. *If a number of sites are found that are sensitive to a specific dose of a chemical in terms of a functional response, then a disparate proportion of these loci should be scattered around or near the ventricular lumen if the drug acts via that route.* A large number of histological studies in which sites of stimulation are localized by careful anatomical mapping (Chapters 4, 5, 6, 7 and 8) reveal that sites of maximum sensitivity to a chemical evoking a functional change are clustered in or around given nuclei, collections of terminal axons, or at the origin of a fiber system (e.g., Booth, 1967; Grant and Jarrard, 1968; Myers and Yaksh, 1969; Levitt, 1971; Yaksh and Myers, 1972).

6. *If a drug given in tissue acts via the ventricular route, it should have the same effect when given intraventricularly.* The same compound, e.g., nicotine, injected into a specific diencephalic structure may have an effect, when given in the cerebral ventricle, directly opposite to that evoked when the compound is

micro-injected into tissue (Hall and Myers, 1972). In both cases, the response is dose-dependent.

7. *If a drug or chemical acts at a distant site following diffusion or transport, a concentration of the compound above the pharmacologically effective threshold ought to be reached within that site.* With the exception of one laboratory group (Bondareff *et al.*, 1970), studies in which a radioactive substance is applied or injected into a structure in a small volume have shown consistently that the substance is compacted or retained principally within that structure (Michael, 1966; Palka *et al.*, 1966; Booth, 1968c; Grossman and Stumpf, 1969; Javoy *et al.*, 1970; Schubert *et al.*, 1970; Myers *et al.*, 1971). Although a dye injected in the same way as a radioactive tracer is useful primarily in estimating the physical characteristics of spread of a substance, the results obtained in experiments tracing the extent of the diffusion of a dye marker in brain tissue (Myers, 1966) and those employing labelled substances are strikingly concordant.

As in the case of the "implantation paradox," the great bulk of the experimental evidence does not favor the hypothesis of ventricular transport of a chemical injected into brain tissue. Of course, it is possible that such a phenomenon could occur in the special case of a single chemical, carbamyl choline, for which the hypothesis was in part originally evolved (Routtenberg, 1972). The wisdom of such a restricted generality would seem to be biologically unsound. Finally, one substance, dopamine, when applied to subcortical nuclei, has been reported to spread uncommonly, even transcallosally, by a process of "axonal streaming" (Routtenberg *et al.*, 1968; Bondareff *et al.*, 1970). Unfortunately, using the same technique of histochemical fluorescence, Ungerstedt *et al.* (1969) do not confirm this result but find, instead, that the uptake of dopamine is apparently concentrated in a well-defined network of nerve terminals.

V. CURRENT CONSIDERATIONS

If any central conclusion would issue forth from the points made in this chapter, it would be simply the necessity for punctilious control and a scrupulous design of every experiment involving an implantation or injection of a chemical into brain substance. To supplement existing knowledge about an anatomical structure and to implicate a given chemical mechanism in the function of that structure require much care and planning. Otherwise, one can never be even partially certain that an experimental observation does in fact reflect a localized phenomenon, intricate as it may be, or rather is the incommodious result of a chemically nonspecific, diffuse, and non-localizable effect.

That a technique or variation in some technical aspect of the chemical stimulation procedure may account for some of the curious if not baffling differences between species seen in this field is a very real possibility. Analytical comparisons between the methods employed and the circumstances under which an experiment is performed should always be made first and prior to a deduction that one species differs from another. As is discussed in the Epilogue, however, this is not to deny that the brain of each and every genus could be "coded" individually with a chemical architecture of unique design (Myers and Sharpe, 1968b).

In connection with this intriguing idea are two methodological observations of immense relevance. Miller *et al.* (1968) reported that within a single strain of rats, there were considerable differences in the endogenous content of two biogenic amines measured in discrete areas of the brain. However, the cause of the astounding irregularities in the content values was to be found in the source of the animals, i.e., the commercial breeder and supplier. In another study, a two- to fourfold difference occurred in the animals' cardiovascular responses to a cholinomimetic compound injected into brain tissue of rats of the same strain but which were, once again, obtained from different animal supply houses (Brezenoff, 1972).

These observations could almost serve to stagger the imagination in relation to the interpretation of an individual set of data. Clearly, each animal should be used, when possible, as its own control for each experimental aspect—anatomical specificity, chemical specificity, and pharmacological specificity. Quantitative relationships involving the dose, volume, toxicity, and pH of a chemical can then be ascertained between groups.

3 Cardiovascular, Respiratory and Other Vital Functions

I. INTRODUCTION

Intrinsic governing mechanisms operate autonomously 24 hours-a-day within the heart, vasculature, respiratory apparatus, gastrointestinal tract and other vital organs. Many physiologists have also demonstrated in the classical tradition the existence of extrinsic regulatory elements in the lower brain-stem, in certain subcortical structures and even in the cerebral cortex. Each of these regions may exert a direct influence over the control of the moment-by-moment function of an individual organ system. In fact, the extrinsic portion of the overall regulation may temporarily override the intrinsic automaticity extant at either the level of the organ itself or the autonomic ganglia, or both. Although the fluctuations brought about in the activity of a given organ system are largely reflexive in nature, the brain somewhat curiously occupies a pivotal role in the extrinsic regulation. There are several explanations for this.

First, there can be no doubt that a master monitor must serve each vital system independently and in some order of priority. For example, the survival of an organism, in a primitive or any other environment requires that consciousness be sustained throughout the waking period of life. Ordinarily, respiratory and cardiovascular systems provide a sufficient supply of O_2 to vital structures during exercise and at rest, during an interval of emotional stress, or under any one of a number of other imaginable circumstances. It would be difficult for these responses to originate from an intrinsic nerve network contained within an individual organ because the feedback response must be "on-line" and coordinated precisely in terms of reciprocal excitation and inhibition. As a result of a clear-cut reflexive system that is contained within the brain, the capacity for instantaneous mobilization of the appropriate sequence of responses is thus achieved.

Second the simultaneous integration of two or more of these vital organ systems is also a crucial factor to the survival of the animal. By having a multiple reflex representation in the central nervous system, the anatomical wherewithal

78

exists whereby: (a) the direction taken by a collection of reflexive responses is coordinated, since one group may oppose or complement another simultaneously: (b) the intensity of a battery of reflexes is coordinated; and (c) an individual reflex is coordinated with respect to one that is activated at the same time that another is inhibited.

Morphologically, the close proximity of each structure comprising the rhombencephalon as well as the pathways that link these lower brain-stem structures to other parts of the brain provide the basis for such a simultaneous integration. Thus, a parallel set of efferent motor responses is invariably characteristic of a unified autonomic discharge. The influence of this upon what is commonly referred to as the process of homeostasis is indeed profound.

Homeostasis, a generalization derived from the work of two "heroes" in the realm of physiology, Claude Bernard and Walter Cannon, remains a useful concept in the biological sciences. Homeostasis describes conceptually the equilibrium or balance between energy exchanges in the internal environment. The existence of receptors in each vital organ is the cardinal concept in the homeostatic process, since these detectors signal the onset of a state of imbalance. As to the integrative role played by the CNS, the neural receptors which are highly sensitive to a chemical or physical disturbance are located in circumscribed areas. They form the primary functional link in the chain of events leading to a restoration of the balance in energy exchange at each instance of almost perpetual disequilibrium. Undoubtedly, in the internal environment, a steady state of equilibrium or perfect stability is purely a hypothetical matter. However, it is one state in which unique cellular elements in specific parts of the brain act as constant comparators. As such, these cells are adjusting their output unendingly in typical feedback fashion to the immediate requirements of the organ system.

The investigation into the chemical mechanisms involved in the central component of homeostasis is the outgrowth of several lines of thought. From the observations based on lesions, we know that circumscribed regions within the lower brain-stem are essential for the regulation of the heart and respiratory systems. In the case of a cardioactive drug such as digitalis, a major question is whether a part of the agent's action is upon the region in the brain-stem implicated in the regulation of peripheral blood flow and cardiac function. Similarly, in connection with respiration are the levels of CO_2 in the systemic circulation monitored by the same region in the medulla oblongata that has been implicated in the ventilatory response? Do receptors in this region detect changes in CO_2 or plasma pH which in turn trigger a compensatory alteration in the respiratory sequence? Great experimental attention has also been given to the possibility that a neurotransmitter is released by neurons in the brain-stem in response to either afferent impulses or to an aberration in the constituents of circulating plasma. That is, one humoral factor may initiate the excitatory outflow and another substance, an inhibitory action. As such, this would represent a kind of central analogue to the peripheral sympathetic-parasympathetic duality of autonomic activity.

II. CARDIOVASCULAR CONTROL

The region containing the cerebral mechanism that affects circulation has been variously termed the "vasomotor center" or "bulbar cardiovascular center." It is located in the medulla oblongata. The evidence for its existence has a long history dating back to the 1870s with the work carried out in Ludwig's laboratory in Leipzig. There, Dittmar and Owsjannikow, using the method of successive transections of the neuroaxis, showed independently that a reflexive rise in blood pressure depended on the integrity of the bulbar (medullary) region. They found that progressive rostral to caudal transections of the brain-stem had no effect on vasoconstrictor reflexes or resting blood pressure until the level of the superior olive was reached (Bard, 1960). In 1916, Ranson demonstrated, again by lesions to the spinal cord, that afferent pressure impulses ascend via the spinal cord to the bulbar vasoconstrictor center where the primary pressor reflex arc is completed (Ranson, 1916). Clinical observations of the result of a pathological ablation to this region bear out these historical findings. For example, Baker *et al.* (1950) discovered that corresponding pathways in the medulla were involved in all of the deaths of poliomyelitis patients who experienced circulatory failure.

More recent knowledge about both the location of the vasomotor center in the bulb and the efferent impulses arising from the hypothalamus, which according to Manning (1965) and Peiss (1965) are equally as important as the medullary outflow, has been obtained primarily by the method of electrical stimulation. Ranson and Billingsly (1916) employed a fine needle electrode to differentiate discrete loci that, upon stimulation, gave either a rise or fall in blood pressure. Many classical papers have appeared by Bach, Monnier, Uvnäs, Wang, Hilton, Delgado and others using stimulating current, but Alexander (1946) mapped the entire bulbar-pontine region of the cat in order to localize and separate the pressor from depressor areas. A ventral view of these regions in the lower brain-stem is illustrated in Fig. 3-1. Of interest is the research of Pitts *et al.* (1939) who demonstrated the morphological independence of these spots from others in the medulla which alter respiration when stimulated similarly.

How the control exerted by the hypothalamus is functionally related to that executed by these two bulbar regions is still not certain. In their classical series of papers in the early part of this century, Karplus and Kreidl (1927) evoked strong pressor responses by stimulating electrically the basal portion of the hypothalamus. Later, Ranson and his colleagues (e.g., Ranson and Magoun, 1939), Hess (1954, 1957) and other investigators were able to identify a number

ANATOMICAL ORGANIZATION

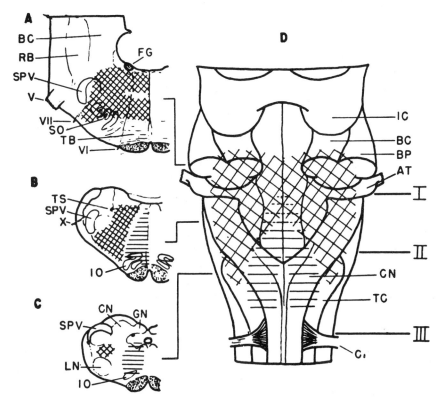

Fig. 3-1 Localization of pressor and depressor centers in the brain-stem of the cat. Pressor regions indicated by crosshatching; depressor regions by horizontal ruling. A–C: cross sections through medulla at levels indicated by guidelines to D; D: semidiagrammatic projection of pressor and depressor regions onto the dorsal surface of the brain-stem viewed with the cerebellar peduncles cut across and the cerebellum removed. AT: auditory tubercle; BC: brachium conjunctiva; BP: brachium pontis; C_1: first cervical nerve; CN: cuneate nucleus; FG: facial genu; GN: gracile nucleus; IC: inferior colliculus; IO: inferior olivary nucleus; LN: lateral reticular nucleus; RB: restiform body; SO: superior olivary nucleus; SPV: spinal trigeminal tract; TB: trapezoid body; TC: tuberculum cinereum; TS: tractus solitarius. V, VI, VII: corresponding cranial nerves; I, II, III: levels of transection. (From Alexander, 1946)

of regions in the diencephalon at which stimulation evoked a vasomotor change such as an elevation in blood pressure.

Disagreement about the specificity of these effects persists, however, since few if any loci in the hypothalamus mediate only an increment in the pressor response or heart rate without a simultaneous, more generalized discharge of the entire sympathetic nervous system (van Bogaert, 1936a and b). The characteristics of this reaction are often intense and include tachypnea, dilatation of the pupils, piloerection, salivation, rage and vocalization. Thus, the cardiovascular changes evoked by punctate stimulation may reflect the integrative capacity of the hypothalamus in regard to each of these functions. This is quite different from the role of the bulbar reflexive region. Electrical stimulation of the hypothalamus can also cause a drastic reduction of arterial blood flow, superficially seen during thermoregulation, which is not necessarily mirrored either in a record of cardiac rate or the pressure gradient in the same vessels.

Parts of the cerebral cortex and other structures are also thought to participate in the integration of circulatory control, particularly with respect to conditioned cardiovascular changes (Smith, 1965). For example, electrical stimulation of the sigmoid gyrus causes renal ischemia, whereas similar stimulation of the cingulate gyrus and amygdala may evoke pressor or depressor responses depending upon the locus of excitation. To evaluate these results with reference to an integrative versus direct reflex control over the circulatory system is difficult.

The investigations using chemical stimulation of the brain have been devoted largely to three main issues: (1) the anatomical aspects of cardiovascular control; (2) the site of action of vasoactive drugs; and (3) the possible endogenous neurohumoral substances in the brain that may mediate a change in blood pressure and heart rate.

A. Pressor and Depressor Responses

As early as 1936, a group of Chinese physiologists performed an elegant experiment to demonstrate that the iontophoretic application of acetylcholine on the surface of the medulla elevates the blood pressure of the dog (Suh *et al.*, 1936).

A set of investigations completed in Gellhorn's laboratory in the mid 1950s was among the first to deal with the possibility that a hypotensive drug exerts part of its effect by a direct action on the central nervous system. Although no localization was possible because of the inordinately large volume (40 μl) injected into the hypothalamus, Gellhorn and Redgate (1955) found that different groups of drugs can exert opposite actions on the blood pressure of the cat. In a dose smaller than that used to produce an equivalent effect via the cerebral ventricle, procaine or pentothal infused in a high concentration, purportedly into the posterior hypothalamus, augmented and prolonged the marked hypotensive response produced by ACh, mecholyl or histamine administered systemically. On the other hand, strychnine, Metrazol and Desoxyn, infused again in high concentration and in 40 μl volumes into the caudal hypothalamus, not only shortened the duration of the fall in the cat's blood pressure but, in fact, led to a hypertensive phase in the cat. In spite of the lack of localization, Gellhorn and Redgate interpreted these results as an indication of the importance of the posterior hypothalamus in mediating a sympathetic discharge which has a direct consequence on the animal's blood pressure.

Following up this proposition, Redgate and Gellhorn (1956a) then injected a nerve blocker or a barbiturate anesthetic, again into the posterior hypothalamus of the unanesthetized cat that had not been treated previously with a peripheral hypotensive agent. Using the same large 40 μl volume, they found that pentothal, Nembutal or procaine caused a sharp decline in both blood pressure and pulse rate. Thus, the view that phasic vascular reflexes come under the control of the posterior hypothalamus was given additional support. The local effect of each drug corresponded well with the result obtained from either lesioning or electrical stimulation of the caudal area, which depresses or elevates blood pressure, respectively.

An oversimplified but traditional belief held in the early 1950s was that the anatomical counterpart of the sympathetic controller in the posterior hypothalamus was a corresponding parasympathetic mechanism within the anterior hypothalamus. With this in mind, Redgate and Gellhorn (1956b) then repeated the same experiments as before but switched the locus of injection more rostrally. When Nembutal or pentothal was infused into the anterior hypothalamus in an unspecified dose and volume, the bradycardia induced by intravenous norepinephrine was attenuated. If either of these anesthetics was injected into the rostral hypothalamus, without prior treatment of the catecholamine, then the blood pressure and heart rate increased in 5 of 7 cats. The authors concluded that a tonic sympathetic mechanism in the posterior area is "released" or simply not inhibited when the anterior hypothalamus is suppressed. This then would account for the augmented cardiovascular activity.

Anatomical localization, a dose response function and pharmacological and other controls would be required to substantiate this conceptualization of the exceedingly complex cardiovascular control system. In this context, Bard (1960) has evaluated the rudimentary concept of sympathetic-parasympathetic excitation at the diencephalic level as follows:

> "As far as the circulatory system is concerned, the only established parasympathetic pathways of control are the vagal fibers to the heart, the sacral vasodilator outflow to the external genitalia and, in all probability, secretory fibers to salivary glands. In this connection, it is well to bear in mind that there is no valid experimental evidence that a reflex fall in arterial pressure can be due to any parasympathetic activity other than vagal cardiac inhibition."

According to Price et al. (1965), the anatomical distribution of independent sites in the bulbar region mediating either a rise in arterial blood pressure or a fall are not predictable stereotaxically. Using two vapor anesthetics commonly used in surgery and a local nerve blocker, they showed that in the anesthetized dog cardiovascular responses to electrical stimulation of pressor or depressor reflex areas in the medulla could be differentially modified. Cyclopropane equilibrated in saline and injected in a 5 μl volume had a much more potent effect on the vasodepressor than on the pressor neurons. However, halothane or procaine, also injected into the vasomotor area of the medulla, had an equally inhibitory effect on both pressor and depressor sites that had again been previously identified by electrical stimulation. Although numerous sensitive sites were found, the wide scattering of loci sensitive to each of the chemicals does not support the classical view of a "vasomotor-center." Such an interpretation would in itself be bolstered if Price *et al.* had used a somewhat smaller volume for their injections. Nevertheless, their results do explain the unusual potency of cyclopropane in causing the marked arterial hypertension seen in the dog.

1. *Hypertension and Angiotensin II*

Following the discovery of Goldblatt in the 1930s that a rise in blood pressure was produced by an interference with the circulation of the kidney (see Goldblatt, 1948), there is general agreement that hypertension caused by renal failure is due to a hormonal product of the kidney, renin. This substance is transformed in the blood to a polypeptide, angiotensin II (also called hypertensin), which is an exceedingly potent hypertensive agent. Presently, it is believed that angiotensin II vasoconstricts arterioles directly. In addition, this octapeptide may also act indirectly on the sympathetic nervous system.

Recently, Rosendorff *et al.* (1970) have shown that angiotensin II causes a sharp pressor effect after it is infused into the vertebral artery or injected into the cerebral ventricle of the rabbit. A comparison of the doses required to evoke the increment in blood pressure in the case of both routes of administration ruled out the possibility that the effect on brain tissue was due only to reabsorption into the cerebral blood supply. Yet because of the high dose necessary to induce transitory hypertension by either route, a whole host of questions is raised concerning angiotensin II's role in the central control of vasoconstriction.

In a similar study of the hypertensive action of angiotensin II in another species, Andersson *et al.* (1972) have infused the polypeptide into the third ventricle of the goat. Of critical importance was the finding that the pressor response to angiotensin II is pronounced and long-lasting when the peptide solution was made hypertonic with sodium chloride. The same dose of angiotensin II given in isotonic glucose surprisingly had no effect whatsoever on the goat's blood pressure. Therefore, it would appear that angiotensin II and sodium may act synergistically within the structures along the walls of the ventricular cavities to bring about the hemodynamic changes so crucial to the survival of the organism. The mechanism and reason why such a synergism exists are unknown at present.

A preliminary attempt to localize to the hypothalamus the sharp pressor response which occurs in the anesthetized cat following the injection of angiotensin II into the lateral cerebral ventricle was not successful (Severs *et al.*,

1966). The polypeptide was injected into the posterior hypothalamic area in a sufficiently large volume of 25 to 50 μl to diffuse into the ventricular system but was probably not in a high enough dose to act by this route.

In line with this is another failure to localize experimentally a central site sensitive to angiotensin II (Deuben and Buckley, 1970). When injected into the nucleus mesencephalicus profundus of the cat, angiotensin II did not elicit a pressor response which is obtained when the polypeptide is perfused through the aqueduct of Sylvius in the region of this nucleus. Therefore, the cells of the "pressor pathway," which ostensibly passes through this part of the mesencephalon, are not sensitive to angiotensin II, or at least not to its effect when acting directly on the brain parenchyma. Unfortunately, Deuben and Buckley

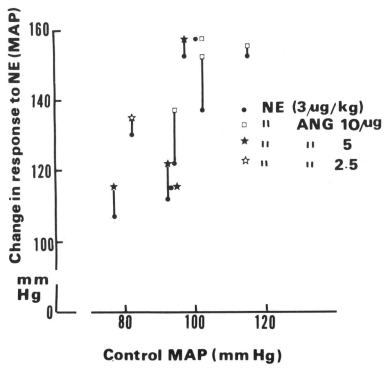

Fig. 3-2 Potentiation of the pressor response to norepinephrine (NE) by intrahypothalamic doses of angiotensin (ANG). Abscissa: control mean arterial pressure (MAP) ordinate: changes in MAP in response to NE. ●, the pressor response to NE (3 μg/kg) before administration of ANG. □, ★, ☆, pressor responses to the same dose of NE after administration of 10, 5 and 2.5 μg of ANG respectively. The vertical lines thus represent the magnitude of change in response to NE. (From Dutta, S. N. *et al.*, 1971. Responses to microinjections of angiotensin into the hypothalamus of cats. *Neuropharmacology*. **10**: 231–236. Pergamon Press, New York)

did not inject angiotensin II directly into the sub-nucleus medialis, the structure in the mesencephalon which they propose from lesion and perfusion experiments mediates the rise in blood pressure evoked by centrally applied angiotensin. However, pontine, medullary or other areas probably mediate the powerful central effect that angiotensin II exerts on blood pressure.

The search for the central site at which this potent vasoactive works was continued by Dutta *et al.* (1971) who also used the anesthetized cat. Following the injection of angiotensin II in a large (10 μl) volume into the ventromedial hypothalamus, a sharp rise in systolic and diastolic blood pressure occurred. A dose of 2.5 to 10 μg evoked the pressor response with a latency as short as 7 seconds. This was strangely *not* dose dependent except when angiotensin II was found to potentiate the rise in blood pressure evoked by systemic norepinephrine as shown in Fig. 3-2. Moreover, the hypertensive response was obtained in only 54% of the experiments, and a tachyphylaxis to repeated intrahypothalamic injections of the peptide also occurred. Although Dutta *et al.* believe that the ventromedial nucleus of the hypothalamus may be one site of action of angiotensin II, no anatomical controls or mapping of the injection sites were performed and the large volume injected would preclude precise localization. Curiously, they also found that 2 to 4 μg of angiotensin II injected into the cerebral ventricle caused a prolonged and intense pressor response. Since a higher dose was required in tissue than in ventricle to evoke the rise in blood pressure, the logic of localization of the effect is the wrong-way-around. Nevertheless, the latency of the response to an angiotensin II micro-injection would suggest that some of the polypeptide's effect is mediated by hypothalamic neurons located medially.

2. *Hypotensive Drugs*

Innumerable pharmacological agents used in the treatment of cardiovascular disease have an action on cardiac muscle, the vasculature or their sympathetic innervation. Recently, the possibility has also been raised that some of these compounds have a major effect on the central nervous system. Clonidine, an analogue of the sympathomimetic imidazoline derivatives, has a potent hypotensive action when used therapeutically in patients with high blood pressure. When injected into sites histologically identified as just dorsal to the mammillary bodies in the region of the mammillo-tegmental fasciculus, clonidine exerts a potent anti-hypertensive effect as shown in Fig. 3-3 (Struyker Boudier and van Rossum, 1972). In the anesthetized rat, 3 to 10 μg of clonidine lowers blood pressure and reduces significantly the animal's heart rate for up to 2 hours following the micro-injection. A dose as low as 1 μg reduced the rat's heart rate even though its blood pressure remained stable. Of interest is the fact that the sites of sensitivity to clonidine are homologous to a region of dense noradrenergic nerve terminals. Hence, clonidine may somehow act centrally to modify the aminergic activity of these neurons.

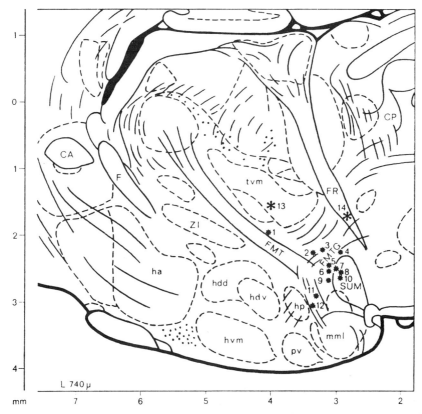

Fig. 3-3 Sagittal section through the hypothalamus of a rat with indications of the sites of injection. At the sites 2–13 clonidine causes both a reduction in heart rate and a fall in blood pressure. At 1 only a blood pressure fall was observed while at 13 and 14 no effect could be obtained or cardiovascular changes occurred after a latency of more than 30 minutes. (From Struyker Boudier and van Rossum, 1972)

Many of the toxic effects of digitalis and other glycosides are also presumed to be due to a direct action on the central nervous system. In the anesthetized cat, 5 to 20 μg ouabain were injected in a volume of 10 μl into the dorsal nucleus of the vagus or the nucleus of the tractus solitaris, both located within the medulla (Basu-Ray et $al.$, 1972a). In most of the cats, this glycoside evoked several distinct kinds of cardiac arrhythmias, illustrated in Fig. 3-4, when it was injected at either site. These included: bradycardia, atrio-ventricular blockade, paroxysmal ectopic beats and terminal ventricular fibrillation. A decline in respiratory rate usually accompanied the arrhythmias, probably because the large volume of ouabain injected impinged upon neurons also involved in respiratory function. Other concommitant symptoms observed were salivation,

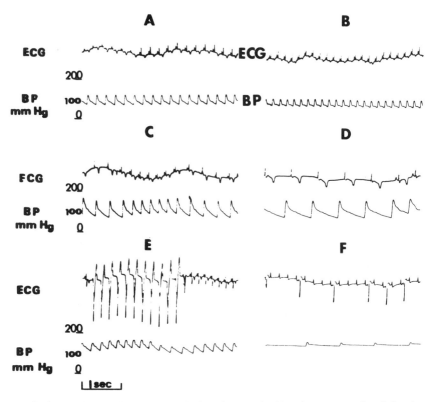

Fig. 3-4 Cardiac arrhythmias and the changes in blood pressure after injection of ouabain into the dorsal nucleus of the vagus of a cat. A, control, before normal saline; B, control, 10 minutes after normal saline; C, 10 minutes after 20 μg of ouabain; D, 10 minutes after cumulative dose of 40 μg of ouabain; E, 10 minutes after cumulative dose of 60 μg ouabain; F, before death. (From Basu-Ray, B. N. *et al.*, 1972a. *J. Pharmacol. Exptl. Ther.* **181**: 357–361. The Williams and Wilkins Co., Baltimore)

urination, spontaneous jerky movements of the forelimbs and the twitching of muscles of the ear and those surrounding the eye. Since a digitalis-like substance passes readily through the blood-brain barrier, it is conceivable that the cardio-toxic effect of these agents is mediated at least partially by sensitive cells in the medulla or in the diencephalon.

In an almost identical study, Basu-Ray *et al.* (1972b) repeated their experiments but this time injected ouabain in an even larger volume (20 μl) into the ventromedial hypothalamus. In 12 of 15 anesthetized cats, ouabain again produced a fall in blood pressure and in 10 of these animals heart rate also declined. Arrhythmias were observed that were characterized by impaired A-V conduction, cardiac block or extrasystole. The lethal effects of ouabain given by the hypothalamic, ventricular and intravenous routes are shown in Fig. 3-5. Unfor-

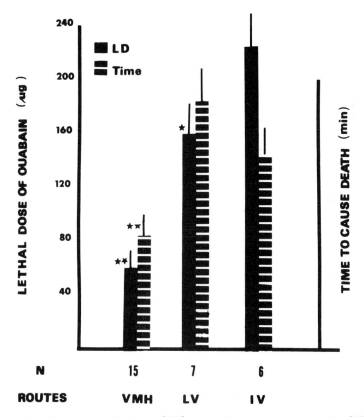

Fig. 3-5 Cumulative lethal doses (LD) and times to cause death (TD) in minutes after repeated injections of ouabain, at 20 minute intervals until death, into anesthetized cats. (VMH) injection into the VMH (20 µg each time); (LV) injection into the lateral ventricle (20 µg each time); (IV) intravenous injections (40 µg each time). N, number of cats. **P < 0.001 compared to LV and IV injections. *P < 0.05 compared to IV injections. ■ = LD. ▤ = TD. (From Basu-Ray et al., 1972)

tunately, anatomical controls were not undertaken. Because of the earlier findings that the infusion of ouabain, into the medulla, caused a similar cardiovascular dysfunction, the morphological specificity of the glycoside's action remains unclear particularly since an injection of ouabain in the same dose into the cerebral ventricle produced the identical effects.

B. Cholinergic and Adrenergic Action on Cardiovascular Mechanisms

A major puzzle yet to be solved centers on the specific transmitter or other humoral substances that are released presynaptically by the neurons in the medullary reflex arc in the hypothalamus and in somewhat higher "centers" which are involved in cardiovascular control.   An examination of the vast literature on the effects of different agents injected into the cerebral ventricles reveals essentially what one would expect: that a substance found endogenously within the brain will drastically alter an animal's heart rate and/or blood pressure.   The magnitude and direction of the change depend upon the substance given and the dose.   In the last ten years, a beginning has at least been made toward the understanding of a possible "coding" of both the pressor-depressor mechanism and accelerator-decelerator controller within the medulla, hypothalamus and other areas.

An initial comparison of the actions of biogenic amines infused in small volumes into the diencephalon of the unanesthetized cat showed that differential changes in cardiac activity were produced by cholinergic or adrenergic compounds (Myers, 1964a).   When micro-injected into the mesencephalon or anterior or lateral hypothalamus, ACh or carbachol accelerated the heart rate.   However, epinephrine injected into the medial hypothalamus lowered cardiac rate.   Since in both instances, the cholinergic or adrenergic substance also evoked other physiological or behavioral changes, often of a quite opposite nature, a shift in cardiac rate may have been of secondary consequence to an alteration in another autonomic system.

If the cholinergic activity of the anterior hypothalamic, preoptic area is altered similarly in the rat, cardiovascular changes are also seen (Macphail, 1968).   After carbachol was injected into the anterior preoptic area, the animal's heart rate declined.   The fall, in terms of beats per minute, was in some rats 25 to 62% of the normal rate and did not occur after the cholinomimetic was infused into the posterior hypothalamus.   This finding is in accord with the view that a part of the supraspinal control mechanism underlying parasympathetic activity is located in the rostral hypothalamus.

There is some uncertainty about the states of hyper- and hypotension that could be mediated by cholinergic receptors in the brain-stem, at least in terms of the local effect of nicotine when it enters the CNS via the cerebral circulation.   For example, Ingenito et al. (1972) found that nicotine perfused through the cerebral circulation of the anesthetized cat evoked mainly bradycardia and a hypotensive response.   Similarly, a fall in blood pressure without any remarkable shift in heart rate has been observed after nicotine was injected or perfused through different parts of the cat's cerebral ventricle (e.g., Armitage et al., 1967; McCarthy and Borison, 1972).

In an exploratory study based on a small number of experiments, Brezenoff and Jenden (1969) showed that the blood pressure of the anesthetized rat is influenced by a drug given locally in one region of the hypothalamus.   Usually carbachol, oxotremorine or acetylcholine mixed with eserine evoked a fall in arterial pressure, bradycardia and sometimes a decline in respiratory rate when they were infused in the posterior part of the hypothalamus.   Histamine injected in the same area, as shown in Fig. 3-6, evoked a hypertensive response,

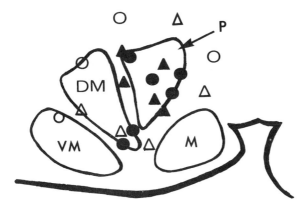

Fig. 3-6 Representative sites of drug injections. P = Posterior hypothalamic nucleus, DM = Dorsomedial nucleus, VM = Ventromedial nucleus, M = Mammillary nucleus. ▲ = Pressor effect of histamine, △ = No effect of histamine, ● = Hypotensive effect of carbachol except for the most dorsal site in P, which produced a delayed pressor response, O = No effect of carbachol. (From Brezenoff, H. E. and D. J. Jenden. 1969. Modification of arterial blood pressure in rats following microinjection of drugs into the posterior hypothalamus. *Int. J. Neuropharmacol.* **8**: 593–600. Pergamon Press, New York).

but norepinephrine had only a mild effect. When atropine was given intravenously, the cholinomimetic-induced hypotension was blocked or reversed. That the induced pressor phenomenon is more complicated than a simple activation of a muscarinic receptor system was evidenced by the delayed rise in blood pressure often seen following the injection of the drugs into the hypothalamus.

Following a series of additional experiments in which carbachol was injected into the fourth ventricle, Brezenoff and Jenden (1970) proposed that cholinergic vasodilator nerve fibers may exist centrally in the medulla. This was based on the localization of the sites of injection as indicated in Fig. 3-7, some of which apparently pierced the tissue beneath and above the ventricular space. The region of maximum sensitivity was the floor of the fourth ventricle, an area just rostral to the nucleus solitaris, which in itself is believed to play a role in the regulation of blood pressure, particularly with respect to the carotid sinus reflex. The long latency in the pressor response to carbachol may have been due to the diffusion time of the cholinomimetic to the nucleus solitaris. Since either mecamylamine or hexamethonium injected intraventricularly abolished the carbachol-induced hypertension, the central synapses which mediate the cardiac response could be classified as nicotinic. On the other hand, the central structures which activate the hypotensive response appear to be muscarinic. If oxotremorine, methacholine, or muscarine itself was injected into the posterior hypothalamus of the anesthetized rat, the typical drop in blood pressure occurred as shown in Fig. 3-8 (Brezenoff and Wirecki, 1970). Some weak pressor

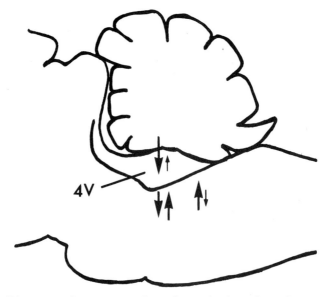

Fig. 3-7 Diagrammatic representation of a sagittal section of rat brain 1 mm lateral to the midline. Injection sites of carbachol are indicated by the arrows. The arrows also indicate the direction of the major (large arrows) and minor (small arrows) components of the biphasic changes in arterial blood pressure following micro-injections of carbachol. 4V = fourth ventricle. (From Brezenoff, H. E. and D. J. Jenden. 1970. Changes in arterial blood pressure after micro-injections of carbachol into the medulla and IVth ventricle of the rat brain. *Neuropharmacology*. **9**: 341–348. Pergamon Press, New York)

responses were observed in some of the rats following this muscarinic hypotensive effect, especially after oxotremorine was injected. Methacholine injected in very high doses had a much weaker hypotensive action than the other two compounds. Although atropine injected also into the hypothalamus produced no change in blood pressure *per se*, this muscarinic blocking agent did abolish the effect of all three agonists micro-injected 15 minutes later. Since these three pharmacological agents produce an atropine-sensitive hyperpolarization in sympathetic ganglia, the same sort of neuronal hyperpolarization may occur within the hypothalamic cells responsible for the evocation of hypotension.

In a further examination of the actions of cholinomimetic substances on the central control of blood pressure, Brezenoff (1972) found that either carbachol or neostigmine injected in a single high dose of 3 μg caused a hypertensive response when injected into the ventromedial or posterior part of the hypothalamus of the rat. On the other hand, when carbachol was infused into the dorsomedial or premammillary area, the rat's blood pressure fell, whereas neostigmine injected at the same site again caused a hypertensive response. As would be expected, the latency of the effect of the anticholinesterase was some-

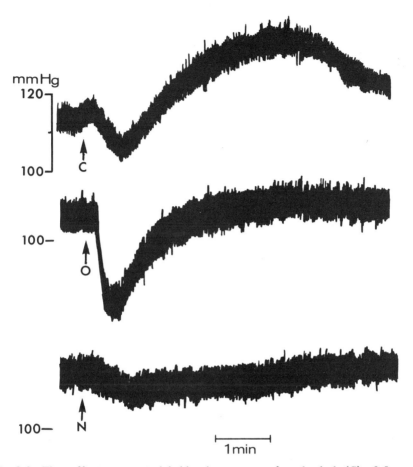

Fig. 3-8 The effects on arterial blood pressure of carbachol (C), 0.5 μg; oxotremorine (O), 1 μg; and nicotine (N), 3 μg; injected into the same site in the floor of the fourth ventricle. Injections were made at 90 minute intervals. (From Brezenoff, H. E. and D. J. Jenden. 1970. Changes in arterial blood pressure after microinjections of carbachol into the medulla and IVth ventricle of the rat brain. *Neuropharmacology.* **9:** 341–348. Pergamon Press, New York)

what longer. Large doses of two other cholinesterase inhibitors, physostigmine and edrophonium, produced the characteristic elevation in arterial pressure also when injected into the hypothalamus. Although the technical limitations imposed by giving a volume as large as 1 μl in the rat brain (Chapter 2) could explain the discrepancies in the locus of response to carbachol and neostigmine, the results do support the view that endogenous ACh may modulate the peripheral cardiovascular functions pertaining to arterial pressure and heart rate.

The role of a catecholaminergic mechanism in the brain-stem has also received some attention. When crystals of a beta receptor antagonist, propranolol, were placed either within the rostral hypothalamus or mesencephalon a gradual but pronounced bradycardia ensued that was not as intense as that observed when the same dose was given in the cerebral ventricles (Lavy and Stern, 1970). Deposits of carbachol in the cortex, hippocampus and cerebellum also caused, in most instances, an almost equal decline in heart rate. The authors conclude that the decrease in heart rate, caused when the beta blocker is given systemically, is due to this drug's action on the structures comprising the hypothalamus and mesencephalic reticular formation. However, because of the high dose of 1000 μg, the absence of anatomical specificity, and the lack of pharmacological controls other than saline, an alternative explanation is feasible. An intravenous injection of one-fourth of this dose, i.e., 250 μg, evokes an even greater bradycardia; therefore, the locally applied crystals most likely leaked into the bloodstream or were taken up by this route so that the drug would certainly have caused the bradycardia through its peripheral action.

In the baboon, heart rate and blood pressure are altered by norepinephrine infusion into the hypothalamus. Toivola and Gale (1970) found that the catecholamine suppressed cardiovascular function in this species of monkey in causing a bradycardia accompanied by hypotension. Although large volumes (15 to 30 μl) were infused into the rostral hypothalamus, this part of the diencephalon could be involved in the autonomic control of cardiac tone. A similar infusion of 5-HT or epinephrine in two of the monkeys also depressed the heart rate and blood pressure perhaps because of a nonspecific sedative effect caused by the experimental procedure itself.

1. *Regional Blood Flow*

An innovative approach to the study of local blood flow in a discrete part of the brain is the usage of infusion of labelled xenon into the hypothalamus of the rabbit (Cranston and Rosendorff, 1971). Changing the level of arterial pCO_2 caused a corresponding alteration in the rate of hypothalamic blood flow as measured indirectly by the local clearance of ^{133}Xe. Interestingly, an anesthetic altered the blood flow in the cerebral cortex while the hypothalamic flow rate was unchanged. This served to demonstrate autoregulation of vascular elements within brain tissue.

Using the ^{133}Xe clearance method again, Rosendorff and Cranston (1971) found that hypothalamic blood flow declined in a dose dependent fashion following the local injection in high doses of norepinephrine into the anterior hypothalamus of the rabbit. However, when only 1 μg of NE was injected in the same area, regional blood flow increased; 5-HT also had this opposite effect of augmenting blood flow. The constrictor action of the locally applied NE could be prevented by adding 50 μg of the alpha-adrenergic blocker, phenoxybenzamine, to 40 μg of NE and injecting both substances simultaneously into the anterior hypothalamus. Although a beta-antagonist control injection was not given, this result would imply that the receptors involved in the mechanism of vasoconstriction possess alpha receptor activity.

III. RESPIRATORY CONTROL

By circumscribed destruction or electrical stimulation of certain portions of the medulla, a so-called "respiratory center" has been localized in the lower brain-stem. Ever since the studies of Marckwald, Langendorff and others which date back to the 1880s, a functional separation into inspiratory and expiratory regions has been attempted in many kinds of investigation. On the basis of his lesion experiments done in the 1920s, Lumsden proposed the additional distinction of a gasping and an apneustic center (see Liljestrand, 1953). Using the procedures of electrical stimulation, Monnier (1938) differentiated a ventral medullary inspiratory region and a more dorsal expiratory area which were believed to control the efferent activity of the vagus nerve. Pitts *et al.* (1939), Liljestrand (1953) and many others have tried to elucidate rather precisely the points in the bulb at which electrical stimulation would induce or inhibit inspiration and expiration and would modify the rate of breathing.

Since the respiratory apparatus is sensitive to a large variety of stimuli, many parts of the CNS seem to be involved in the modification of ventilatory responses. For example, electrical stimulation of the sigmoid and other gyri of the cortex, as well as of the thalamus and hypothalamus, often produces changes in respiration. As in the functional control of circulation, these regions of the brain would seem, first, to be involved in the volitional aspect of respiratory control, and second, to participate in the integrated sequence of autonomic changes that occur during a more generalized sympathetic discharge of central origin.

A persistent issue in this field today is the identification of the anatomical area or areas which may be sensitive to a subtle alteration in pH or CO_2. The next sections describe the attempts to deal with this issue.

A. Sites Sensitive to Chemical Change

The important contributions of Winterstein, Leusen, Mitchell, Loeschcke, Severinghaus and others indicate that receptors on the surface of the medulla are sensitive to molecular CO_2 or to H^+ ions passing to this region via the arterial blood supply. The hypothesis that respiratory responses are controlled alone by the pH of the CSF bathing the bulbar region (see Leusen, 1972) has been questioned by Pappenheimer and his colleagues (Fencl *et al.*, 1966; Pappenheimer, 1967).

Although Pappenheimer *et al.* (1965) have been unable to determine the depth to which a substance must penetrate the medulla from the ventricular route to exert a ventilatory effect, Loeschcke *et al.* (1958), Mitchell *et al.* (1963) and others have found that chemoreceptive areas correspond with those delineated by electrical stimulation. These sensitive regions, located on the floor of the fourth ventricle, react to changes in pH, acid-base equilibrium, CO_2 pressure or all three. The regional perfusion or local application by cotton sponge of HCO_3^- or acid solutions to the ventrolateral area serves to depress or provoke respiratory responses (see Leusen, 1972). However, Borison *et al.* (1972) believe now that changes in chemical constituents of the CSF following intraventricular injections act as a result of their movement into the brain parenchyma rather than on specialized receptors located on the ependymal wall or the pial surface within the ventricular system.

Considered now to be classical experiments were those performed by Comroe in 1943 attacking the problem of the central monitor of CO_2 content in the blood. Using a micro-injection volume as low as 1 μl, he found that $NaHCO_3$ buffered to pH 7.4 by CO_2 was the most effective stimulus of respiratory activity when the bicarbonate solution was injected into the dorsal region of the medulla (obex) and into some sites within the pons, portrayed in Fig. 3-9. Many of the sites sensitive to an alteration in bicarbonate concentration were usually those at which electrical stimulation also produced hyperpnea. Solutions of lactic or hydrochloric acid (0.001 N to 0.1 N) failed to alter the respiratory function when injected at homologous loci. A number of other chemical substances were, on the whole, negative in their effect. Comroe's

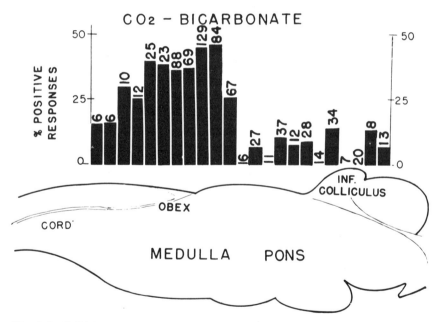

Fig. 3-9 Solid bars represent the percent positive responses to CO_2-bicarbonate solutions injected into the pons, medulla and upper portion of the spinal cord. Each bar represents injections made at 1 mm intervals into portions of the brain-stem represented immediately beneath the bar. The numbers above the bars indicate the total injections performed at that level, irrespective of distance from midline or below surface of the brain-stem. (From Comroe, 1943)

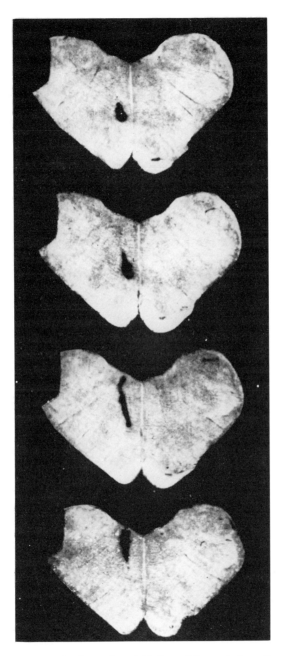

Fig. 3-10   Spread of 3 μl 1% osmic acid injected 3 mm below the surface of the ventricle. (From Liljestrand, 1953)

results provided the first direct evidence that, in addition to CO_2, the concentration of HCO_3^- ions in the bulbar region can play an important part in the control of respiratory activity. At the same time, Comroe rejected the acid-base theory of respiratory control proposed by Gesell (1940).

Although not named as such, one of the early so-called "chemitrodes," a glass capillary needle electrode through which an electrical pulse or a chemical could be delivered, was used to study respiratory function. Using osmic acid, Liljestrand (1953) was also the first investigator to show that 3 μl of this dye spread over a large area of tissue illustrated in Fig. 3-10, mainly by way of the cannula track. When bicarbonate was micro-injected in the medullary reticular formation overlying the inferior olive, the respiratory rate and sometimes the amplitude were stimulated after a short interval of apnea. Examples of this response which often persisted for several minutes after the intramedullary injection are shown in Fig. 3-11. At some points in the bulb, the chemically-elicited change in respiration did not coincide with any response to electrical stimulation. Careful controls with solutions of low or neutral pH also supported

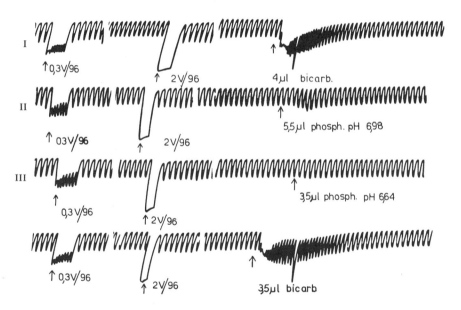

Fig. 3-11 Comparison of the specific respiratory action of $NaHCO_3$ and that produced by changes of pH. At I $NaHCO_3$ gives a strong respiratory response. Injections of phosphate buffer solutions of pH 6.98 and 6.64 at the same place (II and III) only induce insignificant or no responses. New bicarbonate injection again gives strong response. The unchanged electrical reactions serve as a control that the same place has been stimulated. Injected fluids: 1.3% $NaHCO_3$ of pH 8.3, 1/15 molar phosphate buffer solution. Numbers below the curves indicate the stimulus strength and pulses per second, or injected volume in μl. Each downstroke is an inspiration. (From Liljestrand, 1953)

Comroe's opinion that there are chemosensitive regions reactive to HCO_3^- ion concentration in the bulb that respond to the level of serum bicarbonate, which in turn stimulates ventilatory activity. In contrast to the morphological differences found by Comroe, Liljestrand localized the sites rather well probably because the injector needle used to deliver the test solution was so much smaller. However, the regions do not overlap anatomically with the previously described respiratory or pneumotaxic "center," thought to exist in the pons, the localization of which was derived largely by the lesion studies of Gesell (1940).

Another extensive study was carried out by Kim and Carpenter (1961) in an attempt to delineate specific sites that were chemosensitive to bicarbonate and other salts. HCO_3^-, HPO_4^{2-} and citrate salts of sodium were infused into the medulla of the anesthetized cat in a volume of 3 μl. So-called positive responses in terms of temporary respiratory arrest or apneusis occurred after 75% of the injections. As illustrated in Fig. 3-12, nearly all of the salt solutions were surprisingly effective in altering the cat's ventilatory responses. Further, Kim and Carpenter were unable to find a specific area that could be delineated anatomically which was particularly sensitive to any of the anions. However, they presented a thought-provoking explanation of the local effects of phosphate

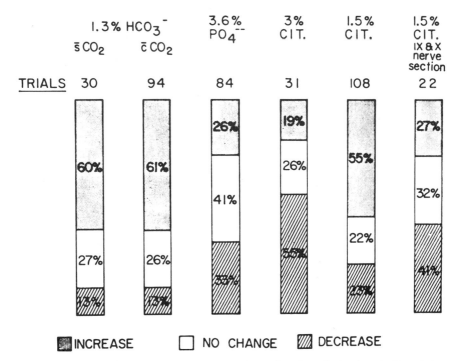

Fig. 3-12 Ventilatory responses to injections of various isotonic solutions into the medullary reticular formation. (From Kim and Carpenter, 1961)

or bicarbonate on the medullary neurons. Based on experiments using isolated nerve preparations, they hypothesized that each of the salts could exert a nonspecific action on the binding of calcium ions so that a non-ionized complex is formed. Thus, an elevated value of CO_2 in arterial blood could interfere with the normal stabilizing action of ionized calcium, which is removed by the local presence of citrate (DeHaven and Carpenter, 1964). Such a condition is apparently simulated by an intramedullary micro-injection of the salts.

As shown in an investigation of the central action of an anesthetic, the rostral hypothalamus may also have some direct or indirect relationship to the control of respiratory function. When 7 to 32 μg of chloralose were injected in the anterior part of the hypothalamus of the anesthetized cat, the rate of respiration declined sharply (Feldberg and Myers, 1965b). At the same time, however, body temperature also fell. Hypothermia in itself could account for a distinct change in the animal's breathing rate.

That respiratory control may be under the influence of a specific transmitter, ACh, has been hypothesized by Metz (1961) on the basis of the correlation between the level of ACh and acetylcholinesterase in cortical and subcortical areas and the condition of the respiratory reflex. In accord with this supposition, stimulation of a number of different diencephalic sites with cholinergic substances does alter the respiratory function of the conscious cat (Myers, 1964a). The micro-injection of ACh or carbachol into the anterior or lateral hypothalamus and the centro-lateral nucleus of the thalamus elevated the animal's respiratory rate. Conversely, an adrenergic substance, epinephrine, injected into the posterior or medial hypothalamus reduced the rate of breathing. In both instances, these changes were accompanied by alterations in behavior as well as generalized elevation in autonomic activity (see Chapter 10). Thus, it is difficult to know whether separate neuronal pathways for slowing or increasing ventilatory responses are triggered independently at this diencephalic level by different neurohumoral substances.

B. Pulmonary Edema

A large lesion of the anterior hypothalamic preoptic area produces a fatal pulmonary edema. Such a pathological condition has been duplicated by the technique of chemical stimulation of the same anatomical locus. An injection of aconitine in a large 20 μl volume into the rostral hypothalamus of the anesthetized rat produced edema of the lungs accompanied by froth and fluid in the trachea (Seager and Wood, 1962; Wood et al., 1964). The edematous reaction, which is almost always lethal, develops within a few hours after the injection, regardless of the type of anesthetic used. The response was not blocked by atropine given systemically to the rat. In an effort to find additional agents which evoke a similar edematous reaction, Seager and Wood injected some 30 other compounds in the same sites all without noticeable pathology.

The specificity of aconitine for producing edema is quite remarkable and is still, over ten years later, an unexplained phenomenon.

An independent confirmation of the findings of Seager and Wood has been reported by a group of Russian workers who extended the observation of aconitine's action to another species, the rabbit (Lazaris *et al.*, 1967). Although no volume was specified and hence no dose could be ascertained, aconitine again produced a lethal edema and widespread hemorrhage of the lungs in both the rat and rabbit when the chemical was injected into the hypothalamus. Prior to the death of each rabbit, which was attributed to convulsions, the animal's respiration deepened and its respiratory rate declined. Some rabbits held their breath and in others a blood-stained froth exuded from the nose. Evidence of the anatomical localization of this pathological effect was not presented although the points of injection were reported to fall along the medial portion of the hypothalamus. It is interesting that Rosenthal (1941) found that aconitine injected in nanogram doses into the infundibular region evokes bradycardia, extrasystoles, arrhythmias and a sino-auricular heart block.

Carbachol also produces the same sort of pathology as aconitine when this cholinomimetic is injected in very high doses and in large volumes into the preoptic area of either the rat or rabbit. Pulmonary edema, hemorrhage and a variety of autonomic effects occurred, which in some instances were lethal (Reynolds and Simpson, 1969a). If the injection sites were outside the lateral preoptic area, the effects were absent. As Seager and Wood showed earlier, norepinephrine and pentobarbital failed to produce the edema. Contrary to the findings of Seager and Wood, the peripheral administration of atropine blocked the edematous reaction. Similarly, a prior injection of 400 μg of atropine in the preoptic area prevented the pulmonary symptoms evoked by carbachol given later. Thus, the preoptic area apparently mediates the acute effects of carbachol on the respiratory system which may be mediated by muscarinic synapses.

IV. GASTROINTESTINAL FUNCTION

Visceral functions are intimately related to the general autonomic state of the animal. As early as 1935, Kabat *et al.* (1935) showed that electrical stimulation of the hypothalamus altered gastrointestinal motility; Hess, Gellhorn and many other investigators have confirmed these findings. Only in recent years, however, has attention been given to the difficult problem of whether gastric function and intestinal activity have some independent representation in terms of the regulatory mechanism in the brain that operates through neurohumoral factors. Even though only a limited number of researchers have dealt with this question, many fruitful ideas have emerged from these investigations.

The synthetic glucose analogue, 2-deoxy-D-glucose (2-DG), stimulates gastric acid secretion when given systemically, presumably because the amount of glucose available for metabolism is diminished. It now appears that a CNS chemo-

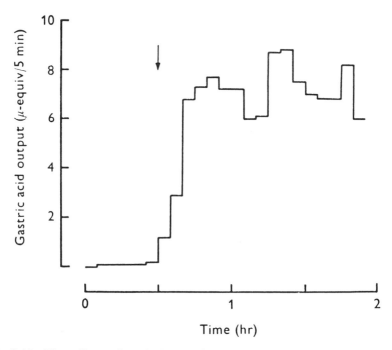

Fig. 3-13   The effect of a single intrahypothalamic injection of 2-deoxy-D-glucose (at arrow, 0.25 mg in 5 μl) upon the gastric acid output. (From Colin-Jones and Himsworth, 1970)

receptor also may modulate gastric secretion. When 2-DG was injected into the lateral hypothalamus, secretion of gastric acid was stimulated at a rate similar to that following insulin-induced hypoglycemia (Colin-Jones and Himsworth, 1970). This response illustrated in Fig. 3-13 occurred, however, in only half of the experiments, perhaps because the lateral hypothalamus was subjected to an overdose of 2-DG or because of the extremely small area of tissue that was stimulated. No dose response analysis was undertaken, and the large 3 to 5 μl volume could also account for the inconsistency in these findings. As shown in Fig. 3-14, lignocaine and phenol, injected also in the lateral hypothalamus, reduced considerably the gastric secretion produced by intravenous 3-O-methylglucose. This supports the notion of some sort of chemospecificity of this diencephalic area. It is not unlikely, therefore, that the gastric effects of hypothalamic inhibition of local glucose metabolism by 2-DG reflects the existence of a glucose chemoreceptor in the hypothalamus.

To determine whether a synergism exists between serotonin and the antidepressant, imipramine, Vahing *et al.* (1968) infused 5-HT in a large dose and volume into the hypothalamus, septum or amygdala of the conscious cat. After the animal was pretreated with imipramine given intramuscularly, 5-HT injected into the hypothalamus evoked intense vomiting in 5 of 11 experiments and

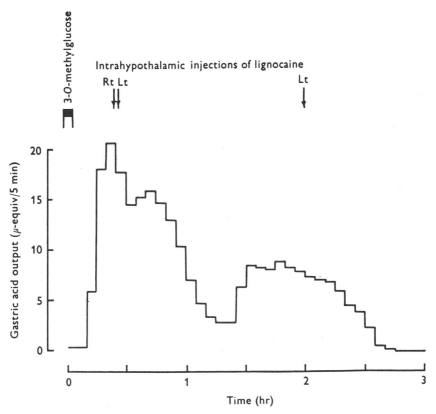

Fig. 3-14 The effect of injections of 3 μl lignocaine into the lateral hypo-thalamic area on each side upon the gastric acid output caused by the intra-venous infusion of 300 mg 3-O-methylglucose. During the course of the experi-ment a further 450 mg 3-O-methylglucose was given to maintain the plasma concentration of this substance.   After the initial diminution, acid secretion increased suggesting some escape from the effects of the lignocaine. A single further injection of the same dose of lignocaine into the left side only finally abolished the gastric acid secretion. (From Colin-Jones and Himsworth, 1970)

other symptoms including motor excitation, salivation, mouth spasms, and tachypnea. Emesis was also observed in 4 of 6 experiments when 5-HT was in-jected into the septum and in 1 of 8 when the amine was injected in the amyg-dala. Unfortunately, vomiting is a symptom that is probably secondary to the overall generalized arousal of the autonomic system. According to the percent-ages of the experimental observations, vomiting represents one of the most ex-treme responses on the continuum of sympathetic activity. Nevertheless, the strong potentiation by 5-HT of the systemic action of imipramine suggests an indole-aminergic interaction with the mechanism by which this anti-depressant works.

Cholinergic excitatory and inhibitory circuits in the hypothalamus may also selectively modify colonic motility. By recording intestinal activity with transducers inside polyethylene catheters that were placed in both proximal and distal segments of the colon, Boom *et al.* (1965) found that crystals of ACh or carbachol placed in the posterior or medial anterior hypothalamus reduced or abolished the spontaneous waves of motor activity in the colon. As portrayed in Fig. 3-15, an implant of ACh deposited similarly in the lateral portion of the rostral hypothalamus enhanced colonic motility. Noradrenaline had no effect on motility of the intestine when deposited at any of these hypothalamic loci. Since carbachol applied to the medial forebrain bundle can induce defecation, which is considered to be a fully integrated autonomic response (Hernández-Peón *et al.*, 1963), it is conceivable that a cholinergic link subserves separate pathways passing through the hypothalamus for individual visceral activities.

Another interesting observation was made by Plekss and Margolin (1968) on one of the central effects of morphine. After the alkaloid was injected "intracerebrally" into the rat, gastrointestinal motility was suppressed as measured by the reduced distance of a charcoal marker placed in the small intestine. Unfortunately, there was no indication given by the authors of the site at which the injection was given in the brain. However, the constipating effects of morphine

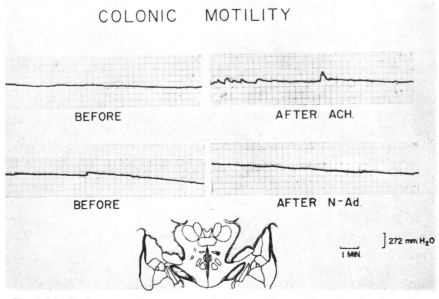

Fig. 3-15 Excitatory effects upon colonic motility produced by local application of acetylcholine in the dorsolateral hypothalamic region shown in the lower part of the figure. (From Boom R. *et al.*, 1965. Changes of colonic motility induced by electrical and chemical stimulation of the forebrain and hypothalamus in cats. *Int. J. Neuropharmacology.* 4: 169–175. Pergamon Press, New York)

may be due to its central action, since the intravenous dose must be 11 times greater for an equivalent reduction in intestinal propulsion.

V. MIXED AUTONOMIC EFFECTS

Many experimenters have been unable to make an incisive distinction between the myriad autonomic effects produced by an individual chemical injected at a single site. In a way, this circumstance is reminiscent of some of the observations of Hess and others who found that electrical stimulation produced simultaneous changes, usually of the same trend for both cardiac and respiratory activity. By using two chemical substances of opposing action, the complex of responses are often conjoined, but in an opposite direction.

Perhaps the first demonstration of a functional opposition of two cations in the CNS was in a study completed by Demole in 1927 in Switzerland. Potassium ions injected at the base of the diencephalon, i.e., hypothalamus, of the conscious rabbit or cat evoked tachycardia and tachypnea in addition to other autonomic effects. On the other hand, calcium ions produced bradycardia and a fall in the respiratory rate concomitant with sleep and other changes. At that time, it was impossible for Demole to attach any physiological significance to these interesting observations.

In another early study, the Swiss workers Clöetta and Fischer (1930) also examined the effect of six cations on respiration and other vital functions of the rat, rabbit or cat, all of which were unanesthetized. The large 12 to 50 μl volumes that were injected, usually bilaterally and mainly at the base of the brain, were believed to be in the region of the infundibulum; undoubtedly each solution diffused immediately into the ventricular cavity and, thus, the results paralleled those obtained with ventricular injections. Calcium evoked sleep, atonia and respiratory depression; magnesium had somewhat similar effects but only when injected in much higher doses. Although both strontium and barium ions injected at the base of the diencephalon impaired the animal's motor movements, barium also caused disorientation, tremor and intense convulsions.

In a much later but nevertheless exploratory study, Rech and Domino (1959) infused chloride salts and a variety of drugs, all in large 2 to 50 μl volumes, into the medulla, caudate nucleus and hypothalamus of the anesthetized cat. They then compared the effects of the salts at each site with those elicited by electrical stimulation. One reproducible response was the distinct pressor effect of potassium ions and the simultaneous inhibition of patellar and linguomandibular reflexes produced when a solution of KCl was injected into the medullary reticular formation. Some of the other responses, which were not obtained consistently, were attributed to a local lesion produced by the injection volume of 10 μl or larger. A 50 μl volume usually caused a large lesion which erupted into the cerebrospinal fluid.

The rise in blood pressure, tachypnea and tremor seen when tubocurarine is injected or perfused in the cerebral ventricles (Salama and Wright, 1950) can be duplicated by giving a small fraction of the intraventricular dose. Upon infusing tubocurarine in a large volume into the posterior or ventromedial hypothalamus of the anesthetized cat, Fletcher and Pradhan (1969) observed the typical hypertensive response, increase in respiratory rate, tremor and knee jerks. These combined effects are shown in Fig. 3-16. The local electrical activity of the hypothalamus also showed the high voltage waves and spike discharges (Baker and Benedict, 1967) characteristic of localized tubocurarine stimulation (see Chapter 10). A prior injection of the anticholinesterase, neostigmine, into the same hypothalamic locus counteracted only slightly the tubocurarine-induced autonomic reaction, which is very different from the nicotinic antagonism clearly demonstrable at peripheral sites. These data illustrate further the convergence of autonomic outflow at the level of the hypothalamus, which can be stimulated with the curare analogue.

In an early attempt to elucidate the actions of a barbiturate on vital signs, Masserman (1937) found that sodium amytal caused a fall in blood pressure, heart rate and respiration when injected into the hypothalamus. However, the infused doses of 20 to 40 mg were so high and the volumes of up to 300 μl were so large that some systemic effect could not be ruled out. Interestingly, Coramine, a potent central stimulant, raised the cat's blood pressure and increased the respiratory rate. The material undoubtedly flowed through much of the ventricular cavity rendering localization impossible.

Another study was done in the same era by Masserman (1938a) to find out whether sodium amytal, which was used in the 1930s for psychiatric purposes, had any influence on the emotional response produced by electrical stimulation of the hypothalamus. Using the anesthetized cat, he injected 10 to 50 mg of sodium amytal in a volume of 50 μl into the hypothalamus through one of the first "chemitrode" devices, an insulated hypodermic needle which could be used to electrically stimulate the same site at which the solution was injected. Blood pressure and respiratory rate fell, and if the site was stimulated electrically, the intrahypothalamic amytal attenuated the enhanced vasomotor and respiratory responses. Once again in the high doses and large volumes used, the drug surely could have acted via the ventricles or even partially by way of the blood stream.

When ethyl alcohol was injected into the hypothalamus of the cat, Masserman and Jacobson (1940) found that during electrical stimulation of the hypothalamus the current threshold required to elicit so-called vegetative responses often shifted. For example, 0.02% ethanol injected into the cat's hypothalamus in a volume of 100 to 200 μl acted to stimulate the structure, whereas solutions greater than 0.06% appeared to be toxic to diencephalic tissue and subsequently to depress hypothalamic function. Ethanol at these concentrations evoked a concomitant decline in blood pressure and respiratory rate.

Recounting his vast number of experiments on well over 100 cats, Masserman (1940a) concluded that CNS stimulants such as Metrazol, picrotoxin or nikethiamide act via the hypothalamus to evoke a simultaneous hypertensive response

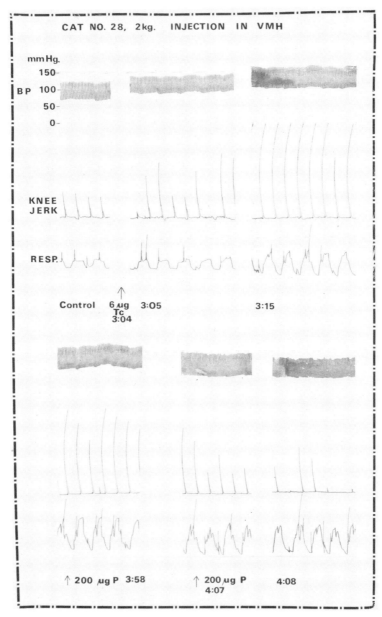

Fig. 3-16 Effects of an intrahypothalamic dose (6 μg) of d-tubocurarine chloride (Tc) on blood pressure, knee jerk and respiration in a cat. To counteract the effects of Tc, Prostigmin (P; 200 μg) was injected twice into the same site. (From Fletcher, A. and S. N. Pradhan. 1969. Responses to microinjections of d-tubocurarine into the hypothalamus of cats. *Int. J. Neuropharmacol.* 8: 373–377. Pergamon Press, New York)

and tachypnea, while barbiturates or morphine given via this route reduce blood pressure and respiratory rate.

VI. CONCLUDING CONSIDERATIONS

In a number of studies described in the preceding sections, mammoth doses of a given compound were often used. As a result, there exists a considerable danger of a clouded interpretation regarding the cerebral action of a specific drug, primarily because the agent may be entering into the circulation and thereby exert its effect on a peripheral organ system. A self-evident control is the administration of a matched dose given by the systemic route.

In the case of the pressor effect evoked by angiotensin II injected into hypothalamic tissue, another physiological factor renders an accurate interpretation of a local hypertensive mechanism somewhat difficult. If a high dose of angiotensin II constricts the blood vessels, specifically arterioles, in the immediate vicinity of the micro-injection, the critical neurons that mediate pressor activity could alter their discharge characteristics with a net effect of elevating blood pressure. The use of appropriate pharmacological blocking agents given centrally and peripherally would factor out the complicated problem of peptide sensors, receptors or detectors in the CNS.

In addition to the urgent need for dose response information, the use of much smaller volumes to provide a punctate distribution of anatomical sites would serve to separate from one another the chemically sensitive areas that evoke a generalized autonomic response. Experiments are thus needed that parallel the classical studies employing the methods of ablation and electrical stimulation. As a result, anatomical reconstructions and maps of chemosensitive sites could be produced.

Finally, the recent studies of Philippu et al. (1971) point unerringly to certain informative bends on the research road. For example, the superfusion of the cat's hypothalamus with a catecholamine causes a release of labelled amines from the diencephalon and a concomitant sharp rise in arterial pressure. Przuntek et al. (1971) have subsequently shown that the rise in blood pressure evoked by the electrical stimulation of the posterior hypothalamus is: (a) diminished by simultaneous superfusion of the hypothalamus with 6-hydroxytryptamine, which destroys catecholaminergic nerve endings; (b) impaired by small amounts of bretylium, an adrenergic blocking agent; and (c) enhanced by desipramine, which blocks norepinephrine re-uptake and thereby elevates the local concentration of the catecholamine.

Although these findings would seem to conflict with the observation of bradycardia when norepinephrine or epinephrine is injected directly into the hypothalamus or cerebral ventricles, they do, when taken together, point to the involvement, albeit ill-defined, of this humoral system. Further, the necessity of combining the approach of chemical stimulation, the release of the endogenous amine and pharmacological manipulation of the receptor complex is readily apparent.

VII. Master Summary Table

Chemicals That Exerted an Effect When Given at a Specific Site in the Brain

Chemical	Dose	Volume	Site	Species	State*	Response	Reference
Acetylcholine (ACh)	?	crystal	Anterior hypothalamus	Cat	U	Inhibited colonic motility (medial). Enhanced colonic motility (lateral).	Boom et al. (1965)
	?	crystal	Posterior hypothalamus	Cat	U	Inhibited colonic motility.	Boom et al. (1965)
	1–50 μg	1 μl (and crystals)	Hypothalamus (all areas)	Cat	U	Increased heart and respiratory rates.	Myers (1964a)
	50–400 μg	5–10 μl	Amygdala	Cat	U	Autonomic responses, emotional behavior, aggression, sleep, seizures.	Allikmets et al. (1969)
	150–1000 μg	100–150 μl	Hypothalamus	Dog	A	Biphasic action on intestinal motility.	Koval (1969)
ACh + Physostigmine	2 μg + .5 μg	1 μl	Posterior hypothalamus	Rat	A	Fall in arterial blood pressure; bradycardia.	Brezenoff and Jenden (1969)
Aconitine	?	?	Hypothalamus	Rat	A	Severe pulmonary edema and focal hemorrhage.	Lazaris et al. (1967)
	.2–4 μg	20 μl	Anterior hypothalamus	Rabbit	A	Fatal pulmonary edema.	Seager and Wood (1962)
				Rat	A		
	.02 μg	20 μl	Hypothalamus	Rat	A	Pulmonary edema attenuated by adrenergic blockade.	Wood et al. (1964)
Alcohol	10–1250 μg	100–200 μl	Hypothalamus	Cat	A, U	Decreased vasomotor and respiratory responses; altered threshold of electrically elicited vegetative responses.	Masserman and Jacobson (1940)

*U = unanesthetized and unrestrained; C = constrained, confined or curarized; A = anesthetized.

VII. Master Summary Table (Continued)

Chemical	Dose	Volume	Site	Species	State*	Response	Reference
Angiotensin II	?	crystal	Anterior hypothalamus	Rat	U	Drinking and rise in blood pressure.	Hendler and Blake (1969)
	100 ng	10 µl	Mesencephalic tegmentum	Cat	A	No pressor response.	Deuben and Buckley (1970)
	.1–.5 µg	25–50 µl	Posterior hypothalamus	Cat	A	Failed to affect blood pressure.	Severs et al. (1966)
	10 ng – 10 µg	10 µl	Ventromedial hypothalamus	Cat	A	Increase in blood pressure and depth of respiration.	Dutta et al. (1971)
Atropine	5 µg	1 µl	Posterior hypothalamus	Rat	A	Blocked fall in blood pressure produced by muscarinic agents.	Brezenoff and Wirecki (1970)
	400 µg	10 µl	Lateral preoptic area	Rat Rabbit	U U	Severe pulmonary hemorrhage, edema, circling, salivation, convulsions, death.	Reynolds and Simpson (1969a)
Calcium (Ca^{2+})	.05–.5 mg	12.5–25 µl	Infundibulum region	Rat Cat Rabbit	U U U	Sleep, decrease in respiration, atonia.	Clöetta and Fischer (1930)
Calcium chloride (CaCl$_2$)	250 µg – 2 mg	25–50 µl	Hypothalamus	Rabbit Cat	U U	Anesthetic-like sleep; depressed respirations; pupillary constriction, bradycardia.	Demole (1927)
Carbachol	.44–3.94 µg	1 µl	Preoptic area	Rat	U	EEG and behavioral arousal and decline in heart rate.	Macphail (1968)
	.44–3.94 µg	1 µl	Hypothalamic areas, ventral thalamic N.	Rat	U	Drinking without simultaneous EEG seizure activity in hippocampus but increase in theta.	Macphail (1968)

Drug	Dose	Volume	Site	Species	A/U	Effect	Reference
	.05–5 µg	1 µl	Dorsal medulla	Rat	A	Biphasic hypotensive/hypertensive response.	Brezenoff and Jenden (1970)
	1–2 µg	1 µl	Posterior hypothalamus	Rat	A	Fall in arterial blood pressure; bradycardia.	Brezenoff and Jenden (1969)
	3 µg	1 µl	Premammillary area	Rat	A	Fall in blood pressure.	Brezenoff (1972)
	3 µg	1 µl	Ventromedial and posterior hypothalamus	Rat	A	Rise in blood pressure.	Brezenoff (1972)
	3 µg	1 µl	Dorsomedial nucleus	Rat	A	Fall in blood pressure.	Brezenoff (1972)
	8.8–75 µg	1.5–10.5 µl	Lateral preoptic area	Rat Rabbit	U U	Severe pulmonary hemorrhage, edema, circling, salivation, convulsions, death.	Reynolds and Simpson (1969a)
	?	crystal	Posterior hypothalamus	Cat	U	Inhibited colonic motility.	Boom et al. (1965)
	?	crystal	Anterior hypothalamus	Cat	U	Inhibited colonic motility (medial). Enhanced colonic motility (lateral).	Boom et al. (1965)
	4–10 µg	1–4 µl	Thalamus, caudate nucleus, other limbic structures	Cat	U	Autonomic effects, rage, hypothermia.	Hull et al. (1967)
Clonidine	1–50 µg	1 µl (and crystal)	Hypothalamus (all areas)	Cat	U	Increased heart and respiratory rates.	Myers (1964a)
	1–10 µg	1 µl	Posterior hypothalamus	Rat	A	Reduced heart rate and blood pressure.	Struyker Boudier and van Rossum (1972)
Chloralose	7–32 µg	1–2 µl	Anterior hypothalamus	Cat	A	Decline in respiration.	Feldberg and Myers (1965b)
Coramine	25–50 mg	100–200 µl	Hypothalamus	Cat	A	Increased blood pressure and respiration.	Masserman (1937)
Cyclopropane	?	5 µl	Medulla	Dog	A	Inhibited vasodepressor response.	Price et al. (1965)

VII. Master Summary Table (Continued)

Chemical	Dose	Volume	Site	Species	State*	Response	Reference
2-Deoxy-D-glucose	250 µg	3–5 µl	Lateral hypothalamus	Rat	A	Increased stomach acid secretion.	Colin-Jones and Himsworth (1970)
Desoxyn	≃20 µg	40 µl	Posterior hypothalamus	Cat	A	Reduced hypotensive action of ACh and caused pressor response.	Gellhorn and Redgate (1955)
Edrophonium	20–30 µg	1 µl	Hypothalamus	Rat	A	Rise in blood pressure.	Brezenoff (1972)
Epinephrine	150–1000 µg	100–150 µl	Hypothalamus	Dog	A	Biphasic action on intestinal motility.	Koval (1969)
Absolute ethanol	?	?	Basal diencephalon	Dog	C	Reduction in metabolism, convulsions, death.	Grafe and Grünthal (1929)
Halothane	?	5 µl	Medulla	Dog	A	Inhibited vasopressor and depressor responses.	Price et al. (1965)
Histamine	1–2 µg	1 µl	Posterior hypothalamus	Rat	A	Rise in blood pressure.	Brezenoff and Jenden (1969)
Isoprenaline	14–28 µg	.5 µl	Hypothalamus	Chicken	U	Hypotensive responses.	Marley and Stephenson (1970)
Lignocaine	60 µg	3 µl	Lateral hypothalamus	Rat	A	Inhibited gastric secretion.	Colin-Jones and Himsworth (1970)
Magnesium (Mg²⁺)	400 µg – 2.5 mg	20–25 µl	Infundibulum region	Rat Cat	U U	Respiratory depression.	Ciöetta and Fischer (1930)
Methacholine	10–100 µg	1 µl	Posterior hypothalamus	Rat	A	Hypotensive response.	Brezenoff and Wirecki (1970)
3-O-Methylglucose	250 µg	.5 µl	Lateral hypothalamus	Rat	A	Increased stomach acid secretion.	Colin-Jones and Himsworth (1970)
Metrazol	≃4000 µg	40 µl	Posterior hypothalamus	Cat	A	Reduced hypotensive action of ACh and caused pressor response.	Gellhorn and Redgate (1955)
Morphine	50 µg	1 µl	Rostral hypothalamus	Rat	C	Decreased oxygen consumption.	Lotti et al. (1966b)

Drug	Dose	Volume	Site	Species	A/C/U	Response	Reference
Morphine SO$_4$	3.5-60 µg	20 µl	?	Rat	C	Suppressed gastrointestinal motility.	Plekss and Margolin (1968)
Muscarine	3-10 µg	1 µl	Posterior hypothalamus	Rat	A	Hypotensive response.	Brezenoff and Wirecki (1970)
Nembutal	?	?	Rostral hypothalamus	Cat	A	Reversed the bradycardia following I.V. noradrenaline.	Redgate and Gellhorn (1956b)
	2400 µg	40 µl	Posterior hypothalamus	Cat	A	Rapid fall in blood pressure and decline in pulse rate.	Redgate and Gellhorn (1956a)
Neostigmine	3 µg	1 µl	Dorsomedial nucleus; pre-mammillary area	Rat	A	Rise in blood pressure.	Brezenoff (1972)
	150-200 µg	10 µl	Posterior hypothalamus	Cat	A	Slight reduction of local tubocurarine action.	Fletcher and Pradhan (1969)
Norepinephrine (NE)	4.2-6.3 µg	.5 µl	Hypothalamus	Chicken	U	Hypotensive response.	Marley and Stephenson (1970)
	1-200 µg	?	Anterior hypothalamus	Rabbit	C	Decrease in hypothalamic blood flow.	Rosendorff and Cranston (1971)
	15-30 µg	15-30 µl	Rostral hypothalamus	Baboon	C	Hypotension; bradycardia.	Toivola and Gale (1970)
Ouabain	≃10-100 µg	crystal	Hypothalamus	Rat	U	Death.	Bergmann et al. (1967)
	5-20 µg	10 µl	Medulla (dorsal nucleus of the vagus; nucleus of tractus solitaris)	Cat	A	Cardiac arrhythmias, respiratory depression.	Basu-Ray et al. (1972a)
	20 µg	10 µl	Ventromedial hypothalamus	Cat	A	Cardiac arrhythmias, hypotensive response.	Basu-Ray et al. (1972b)
Oxotremorine	?	1 µl	Posterior hypothalamus	Rat	A	Fall in arterial blood pressure; bradycardia.	Brezenoff and Jenden (1969)
	3-30 µg	1 µl	Posterior hypothalamus	Rat	A	Hypotensive response.	Brezenoff and Wirecki (1970)

VII. Master Summary Table (Continued)

Chemical	Dose	Volume	Site	Species	State*	Response	Reference
Pentothal	?	?	Rostral hypothalamus	Cat	A	Reversed the bradycardia following I.V. noradrenaline.	Redgate and Gellhorn (1956b)
	≈1600 µg	40 µl	Posterior hypothalamus	Cat	A	Increased hypotensive action of ACh and reduced the sympathetic responses to electrical stimulation of hypothalamus.	Gellhorn and Redgate (1955)
	1600 µg	40 µl	Posterior hypothalamus	Cat	A	Rapid fall in blood pressure and decline in pulse rate.	Redgate and Gellhorn (1956a)
Phenol	150 µg	3 µl	Lateral hypothalamus	Rat	A	Inhibited gastric secretion.	Colin-Jones and Himsworth (1970)
Physostigmine	10–30 µg	1 µl	Hypothalamus	Rat	A	Rise in blood pressure.	Brezenoff (1972)
Potassium chloride (KCl)	.75–2.3 mg	3–6.5 µl	Hippocampus	Rat	U	Blocked bradycardia during classical conditioning.	Avis (1972)
	200–800 µg	20 µl	Infundibulum region	Rat	U	Increased respiration and muscle tone.	Clöetta and Fischer (1930)
	2.3 µg	2–50 µl	Medulla	Cat	A	Pressor response; suppression of reflexes.	Rech and Domino (1959)
	.5–1 mg	33–50 µl	Infundibulum region	Cat	U	Increased respiration and muscle tone.	Clöetta and Fischer (1930)
	.25–2 mg	25–50 µl	Hypothalamus	Rabbit Cat	U U	Stupor, muscle spasms and tachycardia, tremor, tachypnea.	Demole (1927)
Procaine	10–20 µg	5 µl	Medulla	Dog	A	Inhibited vasopressor and depressor response.	Price et al. (1965)

Drug	Dose	Volume	Site	Species	Response	Effect	Reference
	≈400 μg	40 μl	Posterior hypothalamus	Cat	A	Increased hypotensive action of ACh and reduced the sympathetic responses to electrical stimulation of hypothalamus.	Gellhorn and Redgate (1955)
	400 μg	40 μl	Posterior hypothalamus	Cat	A	Rapid fall in blood pressure and decline in pulse rate.	Redgate and Gellhorn (1956a)
Propranolol	≈250–1000 μg	crystal	Anterior hypothalamus, cerebellum, MRF, hippocampus, cortex	Rat	A	Bradycardia.	Lavy and Stern (1970)
Serotonin (5-HT)	20–80 μg	?	Anterior hypothalamus	Rabbit	C	Increased hypothalamic blood flow.	Rosendorff and Cranston (1971)
	100 μg	5 μl	Hypothalamus, septum, amygdala	Cat	U	Vomiting and autonomic effects after systemic imipramine.	Vahing et al. (1968)
	50–400 μg	5–10 μl	Amygdala	Cat	U	Salivation; exploration.	Allikmets et al. (1969)
	15 μg	15 μl	Rostral hypothalamus	Baboon	C	Mixed effects.	Toivola and Gale (1970)
Silver nitrate	?	?	Basal diencephalon	Dog	C	Reduction in metabolism, convulsions, death.	Grafe and Grünthal (1929)
Sodium amytal	20–40 mg	100–300 μl	Hypothalamus	Cat	A	Fall in blood pressure and respiration, tachycardia.	Masserman (1937)
	10–50 mg	50 μl	Hypothalamus	Cat	A	Fall in blood pressure and respiratory rate; decreased vasomotor and respiratory response when site was stimulated electrically.	Masserman (1938a)
Sodium citrate	45–90 μg	3 μl	Medullary reticular formation	Cat	A	Ventilatory arrest; rise in blood pressure and other autonomic effects.	Kim and Carpenter (1961)

VII. Master Summary Table (Continued)

Chemical	Dose	Volume	Site	Species	State*	Response	Reference
Sodium bicarbonate (NaHCO₃)	13–65 µg	1–5 µl	Medulla (obex), pons, upper spinal cord	Cat	A	Increase in rate and depth of respiration.	Comroe (1943)
	39 µg	3 µl	Medullary reticular formation	Cat	A	Ventilatory arrest; rise in blood pressure and other autonomic effects.	Kim and Carpenter (1961)
Sodium phosphate (NaHPO₄)	39 µg	3–5 µl	Medulla	Cat	A	Excitation of respiration.	Liljestrand (1953)
	108 µg	3 µl	Medullary reticular formation	Cat	A	Ventilatory arrest; rise in blood pressure and other autonomic effects.	Kim and Carpenter (1961)
Strychnine	≈400 µg	40 µl	Posterior hypothalamus	Cat	A	Reduced hypotensive action of ACh and caused pressor response.	Gellhorn and Redgate (1955)
d-Tubocurarine	3–6 µg	10 µl	Posterior hypothalamus	Cat	A	Rise in blood pressure; increased respiration; tremor.	Fletcher and Pradhan (1969)
133Xenon	12.5–50 µc	2.5–10 µl	Hypothalamus	Rabbit	U, A	Rise in hypothalamic blood flow after increase in pCO_2.	Cranston and Rosendorff (1971)

4 Adrenal, Thyroid and Other Hormonal Systems

I. INTRODUCTION

Viewed from an anatomical perspective alone, it is difficult to imagine that the brain does not influence directly, by way of the pituitary gland and autonomic connections, the activity of hormonal systems throughout the body. Yet, strong disagreements in all quarters continue to flare about (1) the sites at which a hormone may act on cerebral tissue and (2) mechanisms by which a steroid can modify neuronal function.

Even without extensive knowledge of the physiology of a system such as the adrenal, one could logically assume that a consanguineous pathway has evolved to link the brain to each target gland. For example, an internalized psychological stressor of moderate intensity would ordinarily evoke an adrenal response. Therefore, it would not be at all surprising to find that an externalized physiological stressor such as cold, hemorrhage, rotation or pain is perceived as such and, by virtue of at least a partial impact on the nervous system, is also translated into a full-blown glandular reaction. In this chapter, we will examine the question of how different steroids affect diverse parts of the nervous system in such a way as to alter thyroid activity, the pituitary-adrenal axis and growth function.

A. Neuroendocrine Relationships

The intricate relationship between the brain and the endocrine system has become recognized as a well-established one only in the last 25 years. Traditionally, the management of nearly every endocrine event was originally conceived of as based on the servo-systems principle of negative feedback. Essentially, the pituitary dispatches a chemical "message" in the form of a trophic hormone such as adrenocorticotrophic (ACTH) or thyroid-stimulating hormone (TSH) to the proper target gland. In turn, the cellular production of the gland's hormone increases, and the trophic substance would then be secreted into the blood stream. The pituitary, sensing the elevation in the respective hormone level, would shut down the production of the trophic substance or continue to elaborate more if its level were insufficient. Many proofs of this feedback relationship have been advanced. For example, if a drug such as thiouracil is given which blocks the thyroid gland's production of thyroxine, then TSH production abounds; if thyroxine itself is administered systemically, then TSH output slackens.

A staggering number of experiments in this field have been undertaken from every biological sector—anatomical, chemical and physiological. Although these investigations have dealt with each aspect of pituitary-target organ function, it is certain now that circumscribed parts of the central nervous system are media-tors, in many instances of equal importance, in the endocrine control process. This duality of regulatory action is probably not due to Nature's intent of building in a certain amount of redundancy in the glandular network. Nor is the hormonal-neural interaction immutable in spite of a Sherringtonian-type pathway "of excitation or inhibition" common to both systems. For example, one must always recall either one of two points that: (1) an ocular graft of anterior pituitary can maintain almost normal gonadal function; or (2) the adrenal gland functions perfectly well in animals with vast lesions of the central nervous system (Greep, 1963). Instead, the brain seems to participate actively in the regulation of hormone release, not as a separate control system but in harmony with the pituitary and the specialized autonomic pathways which subserve this control, e.g., vagus and splanchnic nerves.

Undoubtedly, in all circumstances in which a neural element is an integral part of the response mechanism, as in the case of stress or the arousal of sexual behavior, a collective or combined action ensues. Even with respect to thyroid function, neural processes governing feeding, body temperature and other aspects of metabolism would necessarily have to be locked into thyrotrophic conse-quences. Otherwise, energy balance within the body would be erratic and difficult to maintain.

1. *Anatomical Connections*

Figure 4-1 serves to outline the major kinds of neural pathways postulated by Scharrer, to mediate the discharges of humoral factors from both the anterior and posterior pituitary (Scharrer, 1965).

Distinct morphological connections exist between the hypothalamus and the posterior pituitary, also termed pars nervosa or neural lobe. Neurons with cell bodies present in the supraoptic and paraventricular nuclei of the hypothalamus extend their axonal processes to pituitary capillary beds (Bargmann, 1960). Into these vascular depots, oxytocin is secreted by the nerve endings in response to suckling or genital stimulation. Similarly, vasopressin is secreted following a change in plasma osmolality or volume of extracellular fluid (Scharrer, 1965).

A second major class of neuroendocrine control is exerted by neurons which end in the median eminence but whose endings, unlike those terminating in the

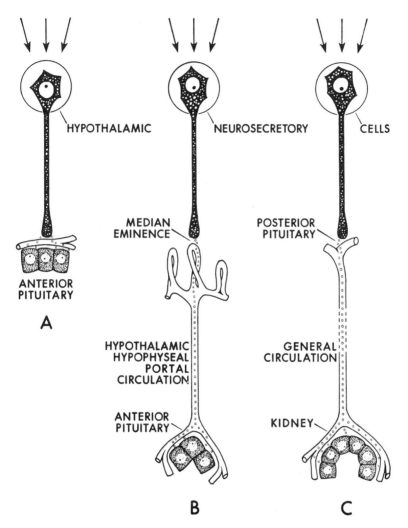

Fig. 4-1 The most common mode of distribution of neurohormones is via vascular channels. A. These may require only a short distance from the site of release to the site of effect, namely anterior pituitary cells in teleosts. B. In vertebrates other than fishes a portal system of vessels occurs which carries neurohormones from axon terminals in the median eminence of the neurohypophysis to the anterior pituitary. C. Neurohormones are in many cases discharged into the general circulation, e.g., chromatophorotropins of neural origin, vasopressin, oxytocin. (From Scharrer, E. 1965. *Arch. Anat. Microscop.* 54:359–370. Masson & Cie, Paris)

posterior pituitary, do not contain granules of neurosecretory material that can be visualized with the Gomori stain. On the contrary, these endings influence the function of the pituitary by releasing specific factors into the hypophyseal portal vessels. These substances are then transported via the blood supply to the anterior pituitary (Harris, 1964).

The chemical extraction from the tissue of the ventral hypothalamus of factors that stimulate the release of the trophic hormones from the anterior pituitary of the mammal has provided compelling evidence for a direct neuroendocrine regulation. Some of these mammalian factors are designated as follows: GHRF (growth hormone releasing factor); GIF (growth hormone release inhibiting factor); LHRF (luteinizing hormone releasing factor); FSHRF (follicle-stimulating hormone releasing factor); CRF (corticotrophic releasing factor); TRF (thyrotropin releasing factor); PRF (prolactin releasing factor); and one substance that retards the output of prolactin, PIF (prolactin inhibitory factor). Although not including melanocyte stimulating (MSF) or other factors, Fig. 4-2 presents the hypothetical schema of the relationship envisaged by Ganong (1966) between each of these hypothalamic factors and the respective trophic hormone which is liberated from the anterior pituitary of the mammal.

Other specialized cases have been documented of the neural innervation of the pituitary either directly or by way of its portal vasculature or systemic circulation. However, the caution expressed by Bern and Knowles (1966) is noteworthy in that the evidence for neurosecretory neurons has been primarily based on

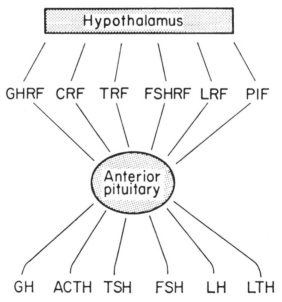

Fig. 4-2 Anterior pituitary hormones and the hypothalamic factors known to affect their secretion. (From Ganong, 1966)

cytological findings rather than on more rigid electrophysiological criteria involving the transmission of action potentials. Although a unitary concept that emphasizes the morphological and biochemical similarities among all neurons is always attractive from a parsimonious viewpoint, the neuroendocrine cells are not only distinct in terms of their secretory properties but perhaps represent a unique feature of the more primitive aspects of the nervous system.

During the 1960s many investigations were designed to find out whether neural tissue is sensitive to a given molecule in a hormone. Specifically, the purpose was to determine whether (a) distinct anatomical regions are responsive to steroids that correspond to those implicated in hormonal function as a result of lesioning or electrical stimulation; (b) the steroid acts locally to inhibit or augment hormone production within the target gland; (c) a given area is activated by a specific steroid; or (d) a biogenic amine could participate as the linking mechanism in the final common pathway between the brain-stem and the pituitary.

Crucial to these questions are a number of observations made over the last five years or so. A number of researchers have successfully established, beyond a doubt, that radio-labelled gonadal hormones, corticoids and other steroids pass into the brain from the systemic circulation. For example, Kato and Villee (1967) have even demonstrated that the entry of estrogen into the cortex, hypothalamus or cerebellum increases in direct proportion to the quantity of hormone injected systemically.

II. ACTH RELEASE: THE HYPOTHALAMUS

On the basis of a variety of studies, the median eminence is considered to be the final common pathway involved in the release of ACTH. As reviewed by Mangili et al. (1966), a discrete lesion in the hypothalamus can reduce the stress-induced stimulation of the adrenal gland as reflected by serum corticosteroid level, can lower the weight of the pituitary, or can block ACTH secretion. A chemical lesion to the ventromedial hypothalamus-arcuate complex produced by gold thioglucose given systemically enhances the adrenal response to stress and increases the excretion of 17-hydroxycorticosteroids (Deter and Liebelt, 1964). Further, when the anterior pituitary is transplanted to the anterior chamber of the eye or to other sites remote from the median eminence, the characteristic features of the adrenal response to stress are reduced or absent (Greer et al., 1963).

Electrical stimulation of several regions of the hypothalamus of the cat, dog, rabbit and other species can also evoke ACTH release. Unfortunately, the most sensitive site is not agreed upon. Cooling of the preoptic area with thermodes also evokes a rise in plasma cortisol in the dog (Chowers et al., 1964).

Although the hypothalamus may act both as a funnel and a processor of the afferent signals which activate the pituitary-adrenal axis, structures throughout the limbic-forebrain-midbrain system also seem to participate in the adrenal regulatory mechanism. For example, following the electrical stimulation of the amygdala, pre-pyriform region, hippocampus and mesencephalon, striking changes occur in the corticosteroid concentration in serum, the output of ACTH and other adrenal responses. Lesions of the spinal cord or cerebral cortex often produce the same sort of disturbance.

A. Hypothalamic Regulation of the Pituitary-Adrenal Axis

Chemical extraction of the rat's hypothalamus and pituitary before and after stress shows convincingly that the corticotropin-releasing activity is focused within the median eminence (Vernikos-Danellis, 1964). Of equal significance is the observation that ^{3}H-corticosterone given systemically to the adrenalectomized male rat is not only bound by brain tissue, but accumulated differentially in different structures (McEwen et al., 1969). The hippocampus, for instance, takes up even more corticosteroid than the pituitary itself. Moreover, the septum, amygdala, and hypothalamus also bind a considerable amount of the steroid. The corticosteroid molecule seems to be bound principally to the nuclear protein of the hippocampal neurons (McEwen et al., 1970). When these studies are considered in the light of the following experiments involving implantation of the steroid, the fascinating concept of ACTH feedback control becomes more clear.

In an early study of the direct central action of cortisone, large volumes of cortisone were infused by Endröczi et al. (1961) into the anterior or posterior hypothalamus, mesencephalic reticular formation, or thalamus of the rat and cat. Corticosteroid levels in adrenal venous blood declined only in those animals in which the steroid was infused into the caudal hypothalamus or MRF. Thus, Endröczi and his colleagues concluded that the secretion of ACTH was blocked by the feedback action of cortisone on the hypothalamus. Unfortunately, the large volumes given did not preclude the possibility that the steroid could have diffused directly to the pituitary.

The first study to show that there is a pathway within the hypothalamus for "feedback" regulation of ACTH secretion from the pituitary was carried out by Davidson and Feldman (1962). After the rat was adrenalectomized unilaterally, a crystalline implant of hydrocortisone (cortisol) blocked the usual compensatory hypertrophy in the remaining adrenal gland and even caused some atrophy. This is a very unusual finding that is characteristic of an abatement of ACTH output. An implant in the pituitary failed to produce these effects, and thus the results of Endröczi et al. (1961) which could have been due to the diffusion of the steroid to the hypophysis seem to have been interpreted in a valid manner.

If a rabbit is stressed by the immobilization of tight restraint, the level of plasma corticosteroids rises. This adrenal response is inhibited when hydrocortisone is implanted in parts of the basal hypothalamus of the rabbit, including the median eminence and antero-medial area (Smelik and Sawyer, 1962). This inhibition, which persisted for 5 weeks, did not occur if the implants were placed in the posterior hypothalamus, reticular formation, interpeduncular region and most important in the hypophysis itself. The latter finding provides strong evidence that the inhibition of corticotropin synthesis is mediated by the cells in a very circumscribed area of the hypothalamus.

Chowers and his colleagues (1963) examined the effects of cortisol implanted in the rat's hypothalamus on adrenal weight and on the level of adrenal ascorbic acid, which is depleted following a unilateral adrenalectomy. Both values are an accepted index of ACTH secretion. The local action of the corticosteroid on the hypothalamus prevented the usual adrenal ascorbic acid depletion within 5 to 6 days and caused a subsequent adrenal atrophy after 10 days. The ascorbic acid response returned to normal after 21 days but adrenal weight continued to decline. Similar control implants of crystalline testosterone or of cortisol in the pituitary failed to cause these effects. These results support the concept that the brain-stem is the locus of action of corticosteroids in the feedback inhibition of ACTH secretion following the surgical trauma of adrenalectomy. Again there is a dissociation between the maintenance of adrenal weight and the adrenal ascorbic acid level.

When crystalline hydrocortisone is deposited in the posterior median eminence or the more anterior but medial portion of the hypothalamus of the male rat, as illustrated in Fig. 4-3, the contralateral adrenal gland does not exhibit the typical

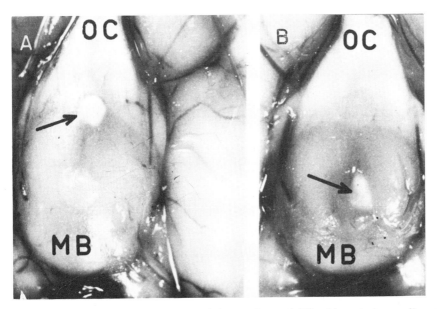

Fig. 4-3 Hydrocortisone implants in (A) anterior and (B) mid-posterior median eminence, respectively, which resulted in adrenal atrophy. Arrows indicate implant. OC: optic chiasm; MB: mammillary body. (From Davidson and Feldman, 1963)

compensatory hypertrophy after a unilateral adrenalectomy has been performed (Davidson and Feldman, 1963). Single or double implants in the pituitary or at sites in the midbrain, forebrain, cerebellum or posterior diencephalon are almost entirely ineffective in blocking the usual hypertrophy. Furthermore, the cytological features of the thyroid and gonads remain normal. These results thus reinforce the idea that the basal hypothalamus is a main part of the final common pathway in the feedback inhibition of ACTH secretion by corticosteroids.

The function of the adrenal is likewise inhibited by a corticosteroid feedback mechanism in other areas of the rat's brain-stem (Bohus and Endröczi, 1964). After a unilateral adrenalectomy was carried out, an implant of hydrocortisone in either the mesencephalon or hypothalamus reduced the secretion of corticosterone from the contralateral adrenal for 8 days after implantation. In contrast to the report of Davidson and Feldman (1963), the degree of compensatory hypertrophy of the remaining adrenal was relatively unchanged. This suggests that the feedback mechanism, which seems to have a representation in the mesencephalon may be a dual one which regulates in an independent fashion both corticosteroid synthesis and the proliferation of adrenal tissue. The dose may be an important consideration here in the dual response to the implant because hypertrophy of the adrenal did occur in the control non-adrenalectomized animal. Other implants of cortisol in the cortex, thalamus or preoptic area had no effect.

The blood chemistry of the rabbit shifts during immobilization stress. When hydrocortisone was implanted in the median eminence-arcuate region, the stress response as reflected by the level of blood lymphocytes was reduced (Kawakami et al., 1966). The corticosteroid did not prevent the changes due to stress when it was implanted in other regions including the septum, central gray matter and the reticular formation. Again the basal hypothalamus would appear to be a focal point for the negative feedback control of ACTH secretion.

A careful comparison of the usual elevation in plasma corticosterone in response to the stress of ether vapor was made in the male rat for the two steroids, cortisol and corticosterone (Grimm and Kendall, 1968). Following their implantation into the median eminence, both steroids inhibited the stress response after 2 to 4 days; however, as shown in Fig. 4-4, cortisol acetate had a much longer-lasting suppressive action that persisted for 21 days. The cortisol implant, which also produced adrenal atrophy, was also visible at the site of its deposition in the hypothalamus after 3 weeks. Apparently, it is absorbed from the tissue much more slowly than corticosterone or its acetate salt.

An implant of cortisol in the median eminence of the rat inhibits the usual rise in plasma corticosterone values in the presence of a whole host of stressors including a loud alarm bell, a bright flashing light in a darkened room, immobilization by binding the rat's feet, hemorrhage under ether anesthesia or ether alone (Feldman et al., 1969). Corticosterone implants exerted the same inhibitory effect on the photic and sound stressors but less of an effect on the ether stress and no change in adrenal activity following immobilization or bleeding. These local ef-

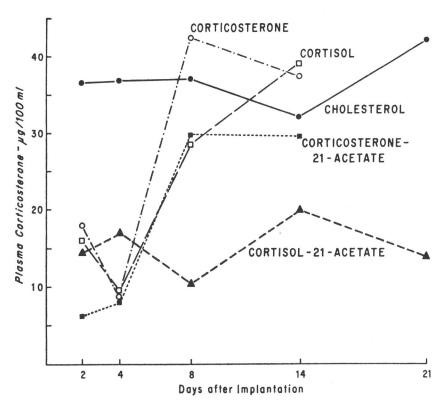

Fig. 4-4   The effect of cholesterol and glucocorticoid implants in the median eminence on the ether-induced plasma-corticosterone response. Mean values of 4 to 6 animals per group are depicted. (From Grimm, Y. and J. W. Kendall. 1968. *Neuroendocrinology*. 3:55–63. S. Karger, Basel, Switzerland)

fects of corticosterone on the median eminence are different from those observed by Davidson *et al.* (1967). The immediacy of testing within 24 to 48 hours after implantation can account for the effects. Further, it would appear that the neurogenic stressing properties of light and sound stimuli are qualitatively different and perhaps more sensitive to the steroid's action on the cells of the hypothalamus.

The long-term effect of corticosteroids on the hypothalamus has also been demonstrated by Feldman *et al.* (1967). A steady decline in the weight of the adrenal glands persisted for up to 70 days after implantation of cortisol or dexamethasone crystals in the median eminence of the rat. However, the compensatory adrenal hypertrophy, following unilateral adrenalectomy, returned to normal after only 21 days had elapsed after implantation. Although this rapid differential recovery of the adrenal response in contrast to the prolonged action on the normal atrophic reaction cannot be explained readily, the feedback signals to the hypothalamus and pituitary are in some way modified.

1. *Dexamethasone—Suppression of the ACTH Pathway*

Complementing the foregoing investigations are studies with dexamethasone, a powerful synthetic corticosteroid which inhibits ACTH release. They have revealed that the hypothalamus is an important neurological site for the feedback suppression of ACTH secretion in the rat. Since the mesencephalon may also be involved in this inhibition, Corbin *et al*. (1965) deposited steroids that possess ACTH inhibiting properties there and in the hypothalamus. Although dexamethasone implanted in the hypothalamus reduced serum and adrenal corticosterone levels as well as adrenal weight, cortisol affected only the corticosterone levels in blood and in the gland. A cortisol implant in the midbrain had no effect, but the more potent dexamethasone deposited there did lower serum and adrenal corticosterone levels. Implants in the pituitary or frontal cerebral cortex were ineffective. Thus, it would appear that adrenal function as reflected by its secretory activity may change independently of the weight of the gland. Receptors in both the hypothalamus and mesencephalon are sensitive to ACTH suppressing steroids. In addition, the mesencephalon may play an important role in the negative feedback action of adrenal steroids.

Attempting once more to answer the question of whether there is a direct action of ACTH inhibitors on the hypothalamus, Feldman *et al*. (1966) implanted cortisol and dexamethasone into the median eminence of the rat. Neither adrenal atrophy nor the compensatory hypertrophy of a single adrenal gland following the removal of its opposite number occurred. An implant of the more potent dexamethasone directly into the pituitary had very little inhibitory effect on the adrenal activity. Similarly, reserpine which acts peripherally to cause adrenal hypertrophy had no significant effect when it was implanted bilaterally in the median eminence or other structures. Supplementary evidence was also presented against the notion that an implant in the median eminence diffuses through the circulation to the pituitary. Double implants of the steroids into the intraperitoneal cavity, where absorption into systemic circulation is excellent, were relatively ineffective.

In the anesthetized rat, dexamethasone micro-injected in a small 0.5 μl volume into the anterior pituitary as well as the median eminence or septum does block the acute release of ACTH (Russell *et al*., 1969). This finding raises the possibility that the pituitary also may be a site subserving the feedback inhibition of the adrenocortical system. However, the total volume of steroid injected could have reached the median eminence, since the spread of dexamethasone was found to be very rapid. The high degree of site specificity found with tissue implants of dexamethasone would nevertheless suggest a dual site of action in brain and pituitary (Kendall *et al*., 1969). The amount of stored corticotropin releasing factor (CRF) within the median eminence as well as ACTH in the anterior pituitary decreased after dexamethasone was placed in the median eminence of the rat (Chowers *et al*., 1967). A most important observation made subsequently was the fact that CRF stores in the hypothalamic tissue increased after dexamethasone was implanted in the pituitary. This shows that CRF synthesis or release may be regulated by the level of circulating corticosteroids or even by the amount of ACTH which reaches the hypothalamus (Motta *et al.*, 1965).

When deposited in the median eminence of the rat, both cortisol and dexamethasone in low doses suppress the basal level of ACTH secretion and reduce the usual increase of ACTH in response to two kinds of stressor: ether anesthesia or 15-second bursts of electric shock to the paws (Davidson *et al.*, 1968). ACTH or corticosterone as well as cholesterol implants had essentially no effect on adrenal weight or on the measures of plasma corticosterone. An important point here is that the inhibition could not be explained simply on the basis of a loss in adrenal sensitivity, since cortisol did exert its effect within 4 hours after its implantation in the hypothalamus, and in doses many times below those that are effective systemically.

The acute effect of dexamethasone deposited in the hypothalamus is also manifest in the suppression of the diurnal peak in the plasma corticosterone level of the rat (Zimmerman and Critchlow, 1969). In only 8 hours after crystals of dexamethasone were implanted in either the posterior or anterior hypothalamic areas, the adrenal rhythm was markedly affected. However, the elevation in plasma corticosterone seen following the stress of ether inhalation plus double bleeding was not altered. The doses were too small to have a systemic action and control implants at other cerebral sites including the amygdala did not interfere with the usual diurnal rise in steroid levels that occurs in the normal non-stressed animal. The failure of the steroid to attenuate the acute stress response is probably explicable on the basis of the low dose of the compound implanted.

That dexamethasone implanted in the anterior border of the median eminence of the rat blocks the stress-induced release of ACTH has been further confirmed by Smelik (1969). The sensitivity of the adrenal is not a factor in the implanted animal, since peripherally given ACTH produces the usual rise in the corticosteroid production in the gland. Of all the agents tested including histamine, vasopressin and other ACTH releasing substances, CRF extract given intravenously was the only compound that stimulated the pituitary-adrenal axis after dexamethasone blockade of the median eminence. This critical finding emphasizes the fact that the function of the pituitary-adrenal axis itself is not abolished by the presence of hypothalamic dexamethasone. Furthermore, the content of pituitary ACTH was not altered by the dexamethasone implant, which exerts its suppressive action within 10 hours after its implantation.

Within 2 to 11 days after implantation of dexamethasone into the median eminence of the male rat, the stress-induced release of ACTH was suppressed for 12 days; control implants of the steroid in the cortex had no effect (Strashimirov *et al.*, 1969). Quite surprisingly, pituitary-thyroid function, as reflected by ^{131}I uptake, was not influenced in spite of prolonged inhibition of ACTH secretion. Thus, the preservation of the normal function of the pituitary-thyroid axis would reflect the remarkable specificity of dexamethasone on the release or stimulation of ACTH activity.

Using the stress of ether vapor to evoke the release of ACTH as indicated by an elevation in the *in vivo* production of adrenal corticosteroid, Bohus and Strashimirov (1970) probed further into the question of whether the site of action of a steroid exists in the anterior pituitary or median eminence of the rat. When crystals of dexamethasone, cortisol, and three corticosterone compounds were placed in the anterior median eminence, the production of adrenal steroid was blocked when the rat was stressed. When deposited in the anterior pituitary or in the infundibular stalk, the corticosteroids were without effect. This suggests two alternatives: (1) the solubility of the crystals in neural tissue could influence the response; or (2) there are, in fact, two or more anatomically distinct sets of receptors that are sensitive to various steroid molecules which differ in chemical structure. Certainly, a conclusion based on lesion studies that the only site of the blocking action of dexamethasone is the anterior pituitary (de Wied, 1964) does not seem to be warranted.

2. *Short-Feedback Control Loop*

Hormones produced by the anterior pituitary are believed to be capable of influencing their own rate of secretion by way of a short or internal feedback mechanism. The primary target of the feedback signals is the hypothalamus, whereas the route of retrograde transport is the hypophyseal-portal blood supply which carries the hormone back to the median eminence (Motta *et al.*, 1969). The purpose for such a short-feedback loop would seem to be the auto-regulation of each trophic principle by the respective hypothalamic releasing factor. Different kinds of evidence exist for short-feedback control over the release of corticotropin releasing factor (CRF), melanocyte stimulating hormone (MSH), luteinizing hormone releasing factor (LHRF), growth hormone releasing factor (GHRF), thyrotropin releasing factor (TRF) and prolactin inhibitory factor (PIF).

The suppression of the amount of circulating corticosterone in the rat can be brought about by an implant of as little as 5 units of crystalline synthetic ACTH (β-corticotrophin) in the median eminence (Motta *et al.*, 1965). In this instance, the weight of the pituitary also declined but the adrenal weight was unchanged. Luteinizing hormone implanted in the same way at homologous sites failed to cause any changes. Thus, it would appear that brain tissue in the region of the median eminence contains receptors sensitive to ACTH. These receptors respond to the trophic hormone, seemingly by way of a "short" negative feedback loop coursing from the pituitary to the hypothalamus. The bidirectional supply of blood flowing between the structures via the hypophyseal portal system is the likely anatomical route by which the feedback loop is connected.

With regard to the localization of action of ACTH in the CNS, Ferrari *et al.* (1966) contend that the anterior hypothalamus and mammillary bodies are the most sensitive areas in terms of the latency and magnitude of the adrenal response. The reticular formation, putamen, globus pallidus and other structures are either insensitive or minimally sensitive to the local injection of ACTH. Results somewhat different from that of Motta *et al.* and Ferrari *et al.* have been obtained by Davidson *et al.* (1967) who deposited crystals of ACTH again in the median eminence of the rat. They found no reliable decline in plasma corticosterone levels during the 15 days after ACTH implantation. The reason for the discrepancy could rest in strain differences or in the way the hormone was implanted, since Motta *et al.* (1965) used cocoa butter as a carrier vehicle in which the ACTH was prepared (see Chapter 2).

3. *Steroid Sensitivity of Single Neurons*

By using an array of three microelectrodes, the discharge rate of individual neurons in the posterior hypothalamus and midbrain was recorded simultaneously following the infusion of hydrocortisone on the contralateral side (Slusher *et al.*, 1966). The hypothalamic injection of hydrocortisone altered the firing patterns in many single units in the mesencephalon with some increasing and others decreasing their discharge frequency. When the steroid was infused into the midbrain, units in the hypothalamus either accelerated or did not change their firing rate. Examples of these changes are presented in Figs. 4-5 and 4-6. In view of the shorter latency in the change in the pattern of potentials following the hypothalamically injected cortisone, Slusher *et al.* agree with Endröczi *et al.* (1961) and Corbin *et al.* (1965) that neurons in the midbrain are probably less sensitive to adrenal cortical steroids than the cells of the hypothalamus.

In a study on the steroid-sensitivity of cerebral neurons, Ruf and Steiner (1967) found that the synthetic corticosteroid, dexamethasone, either totally blocked or suppressed almost immediately the firing rate of 15 out of 115 single neurons in the rat's hypothalamus at recording sites located close to the third ventricle. At the cellular level, the adrenocortical end-product could control directly, by negative feedback, the activity of the neurons that are ostensibly involved in the release of CRF. Alternatively, each of these cells could be a monitor for blood concentration of circulating steroids (Steiner *et al.*, 1969). In relation to this idea, van Delft and Kitay (1972) have found that intravenous ACTH evokes a very rapid increase in the firing rate of a small proportion of anterior hypothalamic neurons, although the morphological distribution of responsive cells is rather diffuse.

Interestingly, the injection of epinephrine into the third ventricle sometimes causes an increase or decrease in the discharge rate of single neurons in the median eminence complex (Weiner *et al.*, 1971). Usually, however, the change in the firing pattern is biphasic. The consistency of these localized changes suggests that this catecholamine is involved in the release of anterior pituitary hormones.

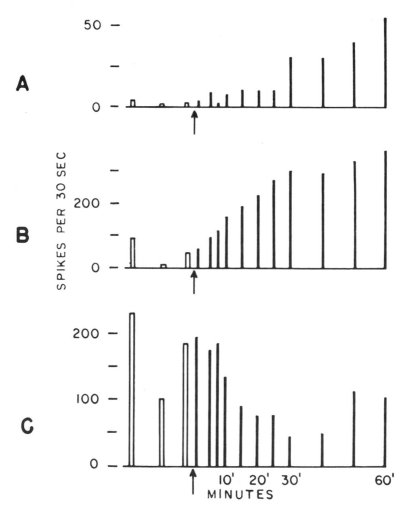

Fig. 4-5 Effect of intracerebral (midbrain) hydrocortisone on spontaneous firing rate of three units at dorsal hypothalamic site of cat 18. Ordinate: number of spikes in 30 seconds. Abscissa: time in minutes; arrow denotes time of injection of 250 μg of hydrocortisone into contralateral midbrain. A. amplitude > 135 μV; B. amplitude range 100 to 130 μV; C. amplitude range 80 to 100 μV. (From Slusher *et al.*, 1966)

B. Extra-Hypothalamic Sites of Corticoid Action

The intimate relationship of the limbic system to certain aspects of emotional behavior and stress is well known. Because of the rich anatomical connections between the structures comprising the limbic system and the ventral hypothalamus, it is probable that an adrenal principle does modify the local function of

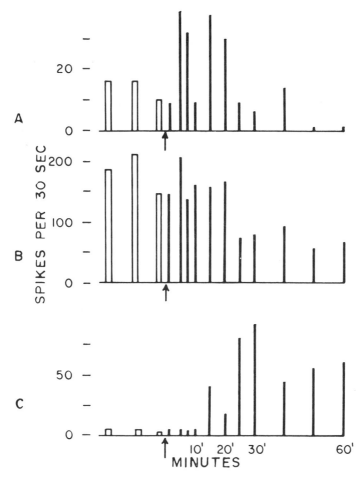

Fig. 4-6 Effect of hypothalamic hydrocortisone on spontaneous firing rate of three midbrain units in cat 13. Ordinate: number of spikes in 30 seconds. Abscissa: time in minutes; arrow denotes time of injection of 250 μg of hydrocortisone into contralateral hypothalamus. A. unit from anterodorsal midbrain tegmentum, amplitude range 90 to 110 μV; B. unit from same site, amplitude range 65 to 80 μV; C. unit from posteroventral midbrain tegmentum, amplitude > 65μV. (From Slusher et al., 1966)

more than one subcortical region at any given time. In this regard, a rather diffuse pathway with multiple synapses arises in the hippocampus which follows a branching trajectory to the anterior thalamus, septum and arcuate nucleus. This pathway terminates in the mammillary complex.

To determine whether the hippocampus itself is sensitive to an adrenal steroid, Slusher (1966) deposited crystalline cortisol in the ventral part of the hippocampus, as illustrated in Fig. 4-7. Plasma corticosteroids dropped when the measures

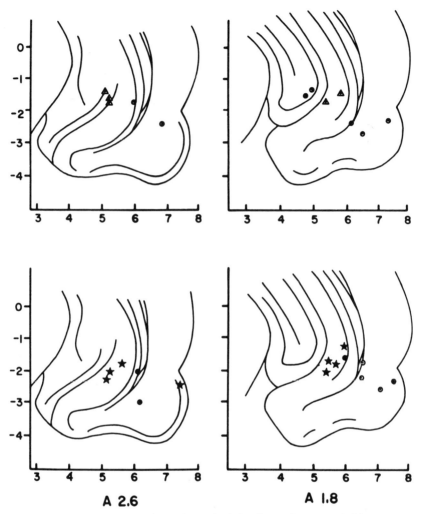

A 2.6   A 1.8

Fig. 4-7 Anatomical location of cortisol implants in ventral hippocampus, plotted on sections of the lateral cortex at the level of the dentate gyrus and ventral hippocampus. Upper sections: implant sites in rats decapitated in A.M.; lower sections: sites in rats decapitated in P.M. Responses are indicated as follows: *dotted circles:* normal; *dotted triangles:* high plasma corticosteroids; *solid circles:* low plasma corticosteroids; *stars:* low adrenal and plasma corticosteroids. (From Slusher, 1966)

were taken during the afternoon hours, a finding also obtained when cortisol was placed in the arcuate-median eminence complex, or in the midbrain reticular formation. Of special import is the fact that an implant in the hypothalamus was the only one that caused an effective reduction in adrenal weight. Nevertheless,

Mason's (1958) belief is upheld that the hippocampus is intimately related to the hypothalamus and mesencephalic reticular formation in the modulation of ACTH release. The influence of the midbrain on ACTH release could be exerted through the hippocampus. Alternatively, the ventral hippocampus itself could contain one of the primary collections of receptor sites which help to monitor plasma corticosteroids.

Additional support for the participation of the limbic system structures in ACTH control has been obtained under different experimental conditions. When stress was induced in the rat by handling or by transfer to a new cage, an implant of crystalline cortisol placed in the amygdala, basal septum, midline thalamic nuclei or mesencephalic reticular formation caused a diminution of ACTH release (Bohus and Lissák, 1967; Bohus et al., 1968). The resting level of ACTH release was unaffected by the steroid deposited at any of these sites. On the contrary, a similar implant of cortisol in the ventral hippocampus increased the activity of the pituitary-adrenal axis and enhanced the basal release of ACTH as well. The specificity of the site of feedback action was again substantiated since cortisol was not effective when deposited in the dorsal hippocampus or rostral septum.

When the rat is adrenalectomized unilaterally, the usual compensatory hypertrophy in the remaining adrenal is prevented by dexamethasone crystals deposited in widespread areas of the limbic system outside of the hypothalamus (Davidson and Feldman, 1967). The most effective sites of this blockade were found in the septum, anterior hypothalamus and thalamic nuclei. A partial inhibition of the usual increase in adrenal weight also occurred when the steroid was placed in the hippocampus. Since sites close, but posterior, to the median eminence were insensitive to dexamethasone, these findings could not be due to simple diffusion of dexamethasone to this structure or to the pituitary. However, Kendall et al. (1969) have presented evidence contrary to this interpretation.

The direct involvement of different parts of the hippocampus in adrenocortical activity has been further clarified by the important finding of Kawakami et al. (1968). After corticosterone crystals were deposited in Ammons horn in the hippocampus, the adrenal increased its synthesis of corticosterone. On the other hand, after corticosterone was deposited in the amygdala, the production of the adrenal steroid was reduced. These responses, represented anatomically in Fig. 4-8, correspond precisely with those produced by electrical stimulation at the same areas, and point to a reciprocal functional relationship between the amygdala and hippocampus. The pathways in either case apparently terminate at the hypothalamic level.

The undeniable sensitivity of the median eminence in regulating ACTH secretion was illustrated by Dallman and Yates (1968) who showed that only 10 ng (nanograms) of dexamethasone placed in this area suppressed the usual rise in plasma corticosterone when the foot of the anesthetized rat was scalded by placing the limb in water heated up to $90°C$. Even more impressive was the observation that dexamethasone injected in the same 10 ng dose into the anterior thalamic-

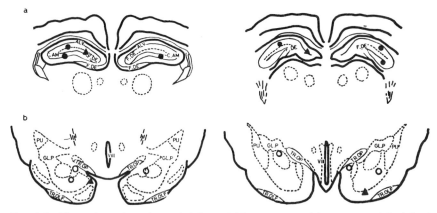

Fig. 4-8 Frontal section through bilateral hippocampus (a) and amygdala (b) of rabbit. Location of corticosterone implants and their effects on incorporation of acetate-1-^{14}C in adrenal. *Solid circle* = increased incorporation of acetate-1-^{14}C; *open circle* = no effect; *triangle* = decreased incorporation of acetate-1-^{14}C. (From Kawakami, M. *et al.*, 1968. *Neuroendocrinology*. 3:349–354. S. Karger, Basel, Switzerland)

septal region had an even greater inhibitory effect on the so-called ACTH-stress pathway when the scalding stimulus was applied. Vasopressin-induced secretion of CRF was also inhibited by dexamethasone injected into the thalamic-septal sites but not into the median eminence. It is therefore possible that the CRF-secreting neurons in the hypothalamus are closer in a functional sense to the septum and rostral thalamus than the steroid sensitive elements of the median eminence (Dallman and Yates, 1968).

C. Interaction with Other Hormonal Mechanisms

As one would expect, the activity of the adrenal gland affects rather profoundly other endocrine functions, in part by way of the hypothalamus. The converse of this interaction also holds since many hormone principles are able to alter the CRF mechanism in the diencephalon and perhaps other parts of the limbic system (Hedge, 1971 and 1972; Tallian *et al.*, 1972).

When cortisol is implanted in the medial portion of the basal hypothalamus in either 30-day-old male or female rats, the development of the reproductive system is effectively prevented (Smith *et al.*, 1971). The magnitude of atrophy of the organs of reproduction, which reflects a suppression of gonadotropin secretion, is shown in Figs. 4-9 and 4-10. In contrast, adrenalectomy does not produce these effects, and ACTH replacement therapy fails to attenuate the dramatic atrophic effects of hypothalamic cortisol. A comparison of cortisol implanted similarly in the adrenalectomized rat showed that hypoadrenalism was not the cause of arrested reproductive development. Since thyroid function was also

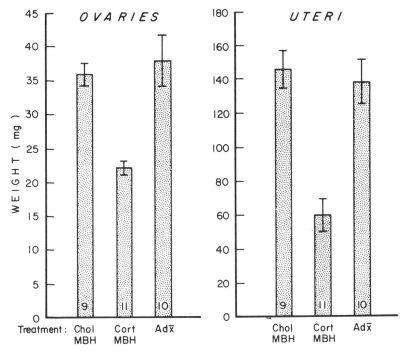

Fig. 4-9   Ovarian and uterine weight 3 weeks following cortisol acetate (Cort) or cholesterol (Chol) implantation in the medial basal hypothalamus (MBH) of prepubertal rats. Results are expressed as mean ± standard error and numbers of rats are shown at the bottom of the bars, here and in Fig. 4-10. (From Smith, E. R. *et al.*, 1971.   *Neuroendocrinology*.   8:94–106.   S. Karger, Basel, Switzerland)

impaired, as reflected by the reduction of ^{125}I uptake in cortisol-implanted rats, the adrenal steroid thus has a direct action on the hypothalamic mechanism involved in the secretion by the pituitary of both gonadotropin and TSH.

After ovulation was induced in infantile female rats by pregnant mare serum (PMS) given intraperitoneally, dexamethasone micro-injected in a small 4 μg amount into the preoptic area blocked ovulation when given the day before (Hagino *et al.*, 1969).   When the steroid was injected into the ventromedial hypothalamus-arcuate complex, the percent of rats that ovulated was much higher. After injection into the mammillary bodies, dexamethasone did not inhibit the ovulatory pattern.   Propylene glycol control injections at the same sites had no effect, so even with the large 1 μl volume used by Hagino *et al.*, the preoptic area seems to be the principal locus of the neural regulation of gonadotropin release (see Chapter 5).

Estrogens implanted in low doses into the supraoptic region of the male rat caused, in 8 to 10 days, an increase in corticosterone secretion with a concomitant

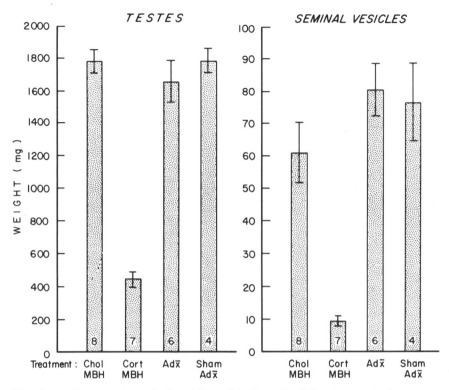

Fig. 4-10 Testes and seminal vesicle weight 3 weeks following cortisol acetate (Cort) or cholesterol (Chol) implantation in the medial basal hypothalamus (MBH) of immature rats. (From Smith, E. R. *et al.*, 1971. *Neuroendocrinology*. 8:94–106. S. Karger, Basel, Switzerland)

decrease in adrenal weight (Telegdy *et al.*, 1964). This response did not appear if the crystals of estrogen were deposited in the posterior hypothalamus. Although the dose and sex of the animal are probably significant factors, the local mechanism of action of the female hormone is in all likelihood mediated through the anterior hypothalamic-pituitary-adrenocortical system.

A thorough mapping of the basal hypothalamus of the anesthetized rat by Hedge *et al.* (1966) showed that a minute 0.5 μl volume of vasopressin injected into the median eminence increased levels of plasma corticosterone through the release of pituitary corticotropin. In this careful and well-controlled study, pituitary extract also caused the same effect; however, when both vasopressin and the extract were injected into the adenohypophysis, only the pituitary extract evoked a release of ACTH. Thus, vasopressin seems to act directly on sites in the ventral hypothalamus, illustrated in Fig. 4-11, to liberate endogenous

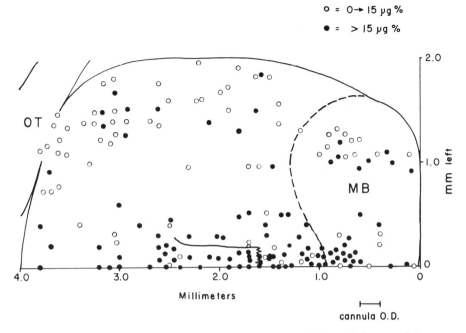

Fig. 4-11   Distribution of injection sites in the ventral hypothalamus of dexamethasone-pretreated female rats, at which lysine vasopressin (2 to 8 mU/100 g body weight) caused ACTH release. Plasma corticosterone concentrations 15 minutes following the injection that were greater than 15 μg/100 ml were considered definite evidence of ACTH release. The ordinate scale gives the lateral coordinates of the injection sites from the midline. The optic tract (OT), the mammillary body (MB) and half of the pituitary stalk are indicated. The diameter of the cannula through which each injection was made is shown to scale. The dots represent the centers of the injection sites, as determined by the dye marker. (From Hedge et al., 1966)

corticotropin releasing factor (CRF). What is exceptionally important is Hedge's demonstration that the effective intrahypothalamic dose represents only 10 to 15% of the amount naturally present in the tuberal region of the rat.

In conjunction with the study of Hedge et al. (1966), Hiroshige et al. (1968) showed that when vasopressin was injected into the neurohypophysis but not the adenohypophysis, a significant amount of ACTH was released. This suggests that vasopressin is not the corticotropin releasing factor, but rather that it mobilizes neurohypophyseal CRF. Neither norepinephrine nor 5-hydroxytryptamine possesses CRF activity when injected similarly into the pituitary gland, but the injection of epinephrine and histamine did evoke a significant release of ACTH.

The implantation of 5 to 15 μg of crystalline thyroxine into the posterior

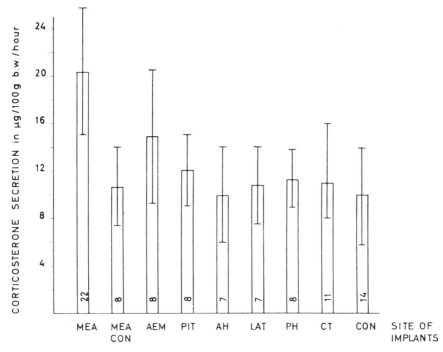

Fig. 4-12 The effect of thyroxine implantation in hypothalamic structures and in the anterior pituitary on the pituitary-adrenal system. MEA: mid-posterior median eminence including the posterior part of the arcuate nucleus; AEM: anterior median eminence; MEA CON: agar-agar implants in MEA; PIT: anterior pituitary; AH: anterior hypothalamus; PH: posterior hypothalamus; CT: cerebral cortex and thalamus; CON: agar-agar implants in hypothalamic structures except MEA. (From Bohus, B. *et al.*, 1965. *Neuroendocrinology*. 1:15–22. S. Karger, Basel, Switzerland)

median eminence and arcuate nucleus of the rat causes a sharp increase in the adrenal venous concentration of corticosterone (Bohus *et al.*, 1965). Implants in the thalamus, cortex, other parts of the hypothalamus, or into the anterior pituitary did not have a significant effect on pituitary-adrenocortical activity. These responses are portrayed in Fig. 4-12. The stimulation of the median eminence with thyroxine also produced a substantial decline in the weight of the thyroid gland. Thus, thyroxine can activate the pituitary release of ACTH at the same time that TSH release is reduced.

D. Putative Transmitters in the Hypothalamic Pathway

A major issue now resting before the entire field of neuroendocrinology is the characterization of the humoral mediation or transmission of specific signals along the final common pathway which comprises the limbic-hypothalamic-pituitary axis. Although the monoamines have been implicated in this mechanism as in so many other functional processes, it is far from clear how the effects of a steroid on a neuron or one of its elements within the hypothalamus is translated into an enhanced or attenuated production of a releasing factor. Because of the clear-cut circadian fluctuations in adrenal activity and other variables, investigations using a peripheral approach are difficult to interpret (Scapagnini et al., 1970).

A preliminary study by Endröczi et al. (1963a) examined the relationship between biogenic amines and the adrenal response of the conscious cat. They found that cholinergic stimulation of the rostral hypothalamus and septum caused a decrease in the elaboration of serum corticosteroids. Following cholinergic or adrenergic stimulation of the posterior hypothalamus and mesencephalic tegmentum, the steroid level increased. Only a tentative indication of an action of an amine can be surmised because of the lack of a dose-response analysis, the use of large volumes which always precludes localization of the effects, and the absence of any correlation between the level of corticosteroid in adrenal blood and the behavioral arousal and rage observed in the cat.

After the implantation into the median eminence of an amount of reserpine sufficient to deplete monoamines in the hypothalamus, as measured by fluorescence microscopy, corticosteroid production nevertheless continued to increase following various treatments known to evoke corticotropin activity, including such stimuli as the stress of handling, intravenous vasopressin, skin incision, loud noise and an injection of chlorpromazine intraperitoneally (Smelik, 1967). These results could be viewed as refuting the hypothesis of Westermann et al. (1962) that the monoamines present in the hypothalamus play an essential role in the control of ACTH secretion. On the contrary, the amines do not seem to alter whatever the mechanism of action is of systemically administered reserpine on ACTH secretion. Unfortunately, the use of reserpine alone, without comparison with the amines deposited in the same way, vitiates this interpretation. In fact, the effective moiety of reserpine may not have been acting directly on the neurons since this drug may exert its central action only after it enters the bloodstream.

Acute implantation of crystals of the cholinomimetic, carbachol, as well as norepinephrine or GABA into the median eminence or mammillary bodies of the cat activates the pituitary-adrenal axis (Krieger and Krieger, 1964). Repeated measures of the increase in plasma 17-hydroxycorticosteroids (17-OHCS) for over 6-hour periods showed, however, that carbachol evoked an early rise in 17-OHCS, whereas GABA caused a much later elevation in the steroid level. Although the relationship is unclear, it would seem that some sort of chemospecificity does exist in the hypothalamus for the adrenal activation. Systemically administered dexamethasone, which blocks ACTH release in response to a wide variety of stimuli, failed in 9 out of 12 cats to have any effect on the release of corticosterone induced by carbachol implanted in crystalline form in the hypothalamus (Krieger and Krieger, 1970a). Thus, a neurotransmitter such as acetylcholine could act on the postsynaptic membrane of a neurosecretory cell which in itself may be insensitive to the presence of a steroid.

In an extensive study of 428 histological sites in 148 cats, Krieger and Krieger (1970b; 1971) showed that the pituitary-adrenal axis can be activated selectively by different substances deposited in different regions of the limbic system. The

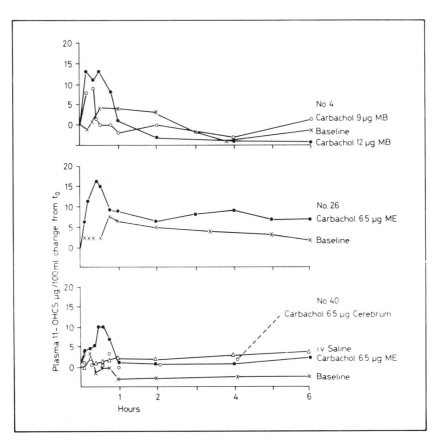

Fig. 4-13 Plasma 11-OHCS response to carbachol in three cats. Upper section: positive response with mammillary body (MB) implantation compared to baseline variation. Middle section: positive response following median-eminence (ME) implantation. Lower section: positive response from median-eminence implantation and lack of response to intracerebral implantation and intravenous saline. Plasma 11-OHCS levels in this and subsequent graphs indicated as change from level at t_o, time at onset of study. (From Krieger, H. P. and D. T. Krieger. 1971. *In: Influence of Hormones on the Nervous System*, pp. 98–106. S. Karger, Basel, Switzerland)

typical excitatory effects of carbachol and norepinephrine are illustrated in Figs. 4-13 and 4-14, respectively. Four excitatory pathways delegated to adrenal stimulation seem to be present: (1) a cholinergic one in the anterior amygdala; (2) a GABA pathway originating in the lateral amygdala; (3) a 5-HT system that utilizes the septum; and (4) an adrenergic pathway that follows the septum, amygdala and hippocampus. Krieger and Krieger postulate that all of these pathways converge upon the basal portion of the hypothalamus, because only at the level of the median eminence did all compounds cause an elevation in 11-hydroxycorticosteroid (11-OHCS) levels in plasma. The pretreatment of the cat with systemic dexamethasone failed to block the increase in 11-OHCS when carbachol or NE was implanted in the median eminence. Thus, the presumed

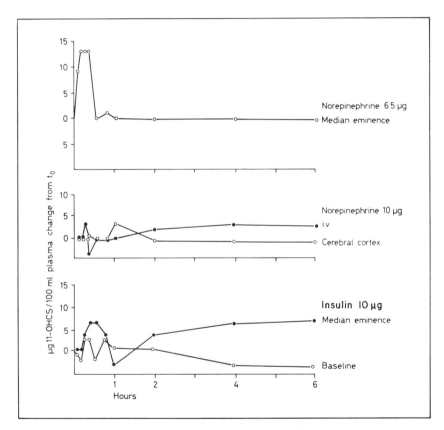

Fig. 4-14   Upper section: positive 11-OHCS response to norepinephrine implantation into median eminence. Middle section: lack of response to intracerebral implantation and to intravenous injection of norepinephrine. Lower section: lack of response to median eminence implantation of insulin, similar to base-line variation. All studies performed on one animal. (From Krieger, H. P. and D. T. Krieger. 1971. *In: Influence of Hormones on the Nervous System.* pp. 98–106. S. Karger, Basel, Switzerland)

terminal secretory neurons in the hypothalamic-pituitary pathway are triggered by synaptically active agents within different structures of the CNS. Further verification was given once again that specific substances do act differentially when applied at different sites. However, it is difficult to understand how all of the substances tested, even those that are as divergent chemically and functionally as an amino acid and a monoamine, can produce an equal rise in serum 11-OHCS, particularly when they are deposited in the so-called "final common pathway," the neurons in the median eminence. In any event, Krieger and Krieger concluded from these results that the CNS control mechanism for the adrenal is chemically "coded" in a manner analogous to that proposed for temperature regulation, feeding behavior, thirst and other functions. A most important possibility is that different physiological conditions which augment the actual release of ACTH, including various stressors or the intrinsic circadian rhythm, may be modulated by the activity of different neurohumoral factors. Obviously, it is essential to know whether ACh is released during these conditions from structures implicated in the ACTH excitatory pathway in the brain.

1. *Cholinergic Link of Hypothalamic-Hypophyseal Pathways*

When deposited in the anterior hypothalamus of the rat, crystalline atropine inhibits the *in vivo* production of corticosteroids in the adrenal gland and reduces simultaneously the level of plasma corticosterone when the animal is stressed by surgery, ether or intravenous injection of vasopressin (Hedge and Smelik, 1968). As illustrated in Fig. 4-15, a similar implant of atropine either in the septum or posterior hypothalamus exerts no effect on this adrenal response. Thus, there may be a cholinergic component in the rostral hypothalamus that is involved in the activation of the adrenocortical activity engendered by stress.

Other rather convincing evidence has recently come to light for a cholinergic link in the hypothalamus underlying the adrenocortical response to a stressful stimulus. When atropine is implanted in the anterior hypothalamus of the rat, the typical rise in the concentration of plasma corticosterone fails to ensue even after a variety of noxious stressors is applied (Kaplanski and Smelik, 1973). Acetylcholine may be released from hypothalamic neurons onto muscarinic receptors, which in turn activate the final pathway to the pituitary that is responsible for ACTH secretion. Thus, cholinergic synapses for the release of CRF may be common to all stressful stimuli.

2. *Serotonin and the Adrenal Axis*

A dramatic illustration of the central effect of serotonin (5-HT) on the pituitary-adrenal system was presented by the Russian workers, Naumenko *et al.* (1967). A rise in plasma corticosteroids in the guinea pig followed the injection of 5-HT into the cerebral ventricles. However, the key point is that these animals had undergone transcollicular section or other deafferentation of the

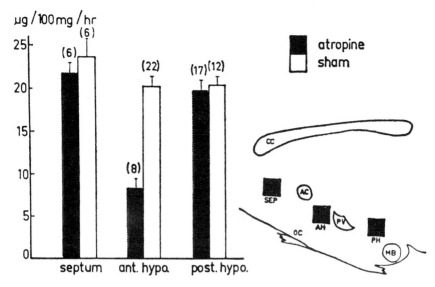

Fig. 4-15 Effective site of implantation. The histogram indicates corticoid productions *in vitro* 60 minutes after implantations were made in the three brain areas depicted in the accompanying mid-sagittal section of the rat brain. Abbreviations: CC, corpus callosum; SEP, septum; AC, anterior commissure; OC, optic chiasm; AH, anterior hypothalamus; PV, paraventricular nucleus; PH, posterior hypothalamus; MB, mammillary body. (From Hedge, G. A. and P. G. Smelik. 1968. *Science*. **159**:891–892. Copyright, 1968 by the American Association for the Advancement of Science)

neuraxis rostral to the medulla. This, of course, rules out any possibility of a peripheral effect of the indoleamine. In another study by the Russian group in which the hypothalamus of the rat was deafferented by knife-cut (Popova *et al.*, 1972), 5-HTP given systemically still stimulated the hypothalamic-pituitary-adrenal pathway even though this precursor of serotonin exerts no direct effect on the adrenal gland itself. Thus, a serotonergic system in the "hypophyseotrophic" region of the rat's hypothalamus is seemingly related to CRF secretion.

Recent contradictory findings have been reported by Vermes and Telegdy (1972) who found that stress-induced corticosterone production is inhibited by crystalline serotonin deposited in the medial hypothalamus. The persistent effect of this inhibition for 10 days would, however, militate against a direct effect of serotonin because of its rapidity of degradation.

In an exceptionally important report, Naumenko (1968) studied the local effect of carbachol, norepinephrine or 5-HT injected in a 1 μl volume into the hypothalamus of the unanesthetized guinea pig. Each substance given in only one dose had a virtually undifferentiated and nonspecific action in elevating plasma corticosteroids when it was injected in widespread areas of the hypothalamus. However, after total mesencephalic transection, only 5-HT injected intrahypothalamically exerted this effect. Therefore, Naumenko concluded that the cholinergic or noradrenergic activation of the adrenal axis could only occur via the stimulation of direct efferent pathways that traverse the spinal cord and link up with "chemoreactive structures" in the adrenal gland. Thus, adrenoceptive and cholinoceptive neurons are *not* involved in the central hypothalamic release of CRF. Since 5-HT did activate the CRF-ACTH system, whether the brain-stem was sectioned or intact, Naumenko suggests that serotonergic elements mediate directly the local pathway for the pituitary-adrenal function, and that serotonin-containing terminal neurons stimulate the release of CRF. The conceptual schema illustrating the differential effects of serotonin in contrast to those of norepinephrine is presented in Figs. 4-16 and 4-17, respectively.

In attempting to localize the stimulating effect on the pituitary-adrenal axis of 5-HT (Naumenko and Ilyutchenok, 1967) given intraventricularly, Naumenko (1969) found that 5-HT injected into the ventral hippocampus, septum, mesencephalic reticular formation or ventral tegmentum evoked a sharp elevation in the level of plasma 17-OH corticosteroid in the guinea pig. However, a fall in the steroid concentration occurred when 5-HT was injected into the dorsal hippocampus and at some sites in the amygdala, as portrayed in Figs. 4-18 A and B. Thus, serotonergic receptors in restricted parts of several structures in the limbic system seem to participate in both the excitation and inhibition of the hypophyseal-adrenal function. The connections to the mammillary bodies via the fornix in the Nauta circuit (1960; 1963) could, of course, account for these intriguing anatomical results. In accord with the findings of Endröczi *et al.* (1963a), the internal connecting pathway may also be linked by cholinergic synapses.

3. *Drug Interactions*

The secretion of epinephrine from the adrenal medulla may also be mediated partially by a chemoreceptor in the lateral hypothalamus of the rat (Himsworth, 1970). When 3-0-methylglucose is given systemically, epinephrine release is augmented and a hyperglycemia is produced. However, the nerve blocker, lignocaine, inactivates these actions when it is injected into the rat's lateral hypothalamus. Presumably, this blockade of hyperglycemia occurs as a result of lignocaine's ability to chemically paralyze the hypothalamus. Sufficient anatomical controls are required before this view can be accepted, and the extent of diffusion of the large 3 μl volume given is not known.

The activity of the pituitary-adrenal system can also be modified by the local hypothalamic action of morphine (Lotti *et al.*, 1969). When injected into the rostral, dorsal or ventromedial regions in the unanesthetized rat, morphine reduces the level of adrenal ascorbic acid which reflects the pituitary-adrenal activity. These morphine-sensitive sites are designated on the sagittal section

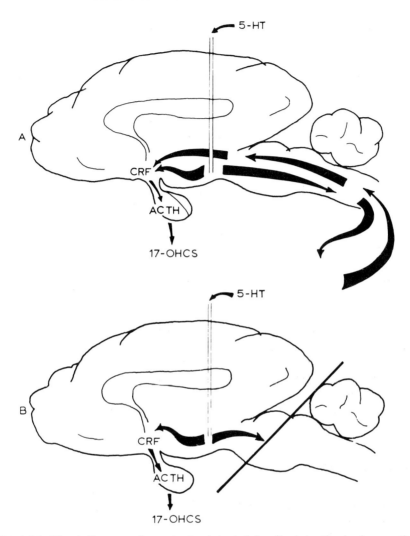

Fig. 4-16 The influence of serotonin, injected locally into the brain, on the hypothalamic-pituitary-adrenal system. The effect is stimulatory not only when efferent neurons are intact (A), but also after the blocking of descending nervous pathways by transection (B). In the latter case the effective mechanism must involve ascending pathways. (From Naumenko, E. V. 1968. *Brain Research*. 11:1–10. S. Karger, Basel, Switzerland)

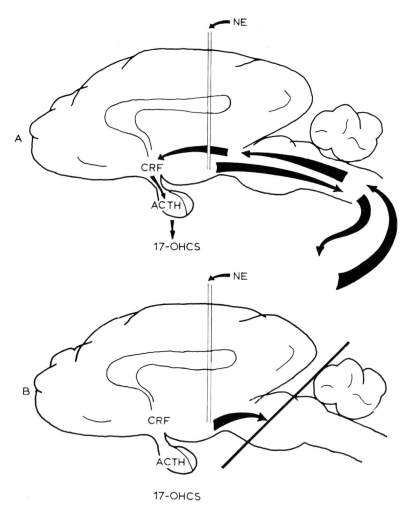

Fig. 4-17 The influence of norepinephrine, injected locally into the brain, on the hypothalamic-pituitary-adrenal system. Norepinephrine stimulates the pituitary-adrenal system only if the efferent neurons from the hypothalamus are intact (A), but it does not intensify the corticosteroid secretion in guinea pigs with midbrain transection despite the existence of unimpaired ascending pathways to CRF producing area (B). (From Naumenko, E. V. 1968. *Brain Research*. 11:1–10. S. Karger, Basel, Switzerland)

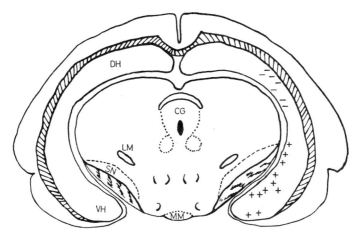

Fig. 4-18A Influence of 5-HT, injected locally into the hippocampus. VH = hippocampus ventralis; DH = hippocampus dorsalis; + = stimulating effect; − = inhibiting effect. (From Naumenko, E. V. 1969. *Neuroendocrinology*. 5:81–88. S. Karger, Basel, Switzerland)

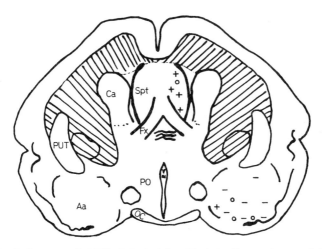

Fig. 4-18B Influence of 5-HT, injected locally into the septum and the amygdala. Spt = septum; Aa = amygdala; + = stimulating effect; − = inhibiting effect; o = no effect. (From Naumenko, E. V. 1969. *Neuroendocrinology*. 5:81–88. S. Karger, Basel, Switzerland)

portrayed in Fig. 4-19. At the same time, intrahypothalamic morphine increases the plasma concentration of corticosterone. These findings correspond with the results of local lesions which implicate the hypothalamus in the effects of morphine within the CNS-pituitary-adrenal pathway.

Another significant observation was made by Naumenko (1967) who sectioned the midbrain of the guinea pig at the pre-trigeminal level so that all sensory input to the hypothalamic-pituitary-adrenal axis was destroyed. Surprisingly, drugs such as amphetamine and neostigmine given peripherally failed to activate the adrenal response even though the enhanced activity of the EEG showed unequivocally that the blood supply rostral to the lesion was intact. Thus, the activation of a peripheral rather than central receptor mechanism is probably responsible for some of the potent effects of these compounds given

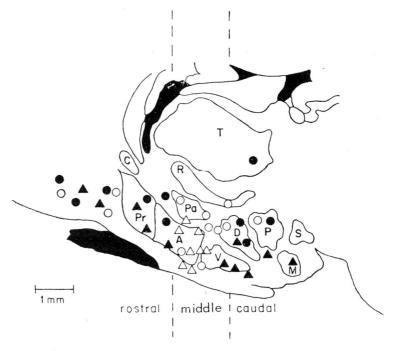

Fig. 4-19 Sagittal view of the rat brain (240 μ lateral to midline) showing effective and ineffective sites of morphine concerning adrenal activation. O = sites producing adrenal ascorbic acid depletion; ● = sites producing no effect on adrenal ascorbic acid; △ = sites elevating plasma corticosterone level; ▲ = sites having no effect on plasma corticosterone level. Abbreviations: A = Anterior hypothalamic nucleus; C = Anterior commissure; D = Dorsomedial nucleus; M = Mammillary nucleus; P = Posterior hypothalamic nucleus; Pa = Paraventricular nucleus; Pr = Preoptic nucleus; R = Reuniens nucleus; S = Supramammillary nucleus: T = Thalamus; V = Ventromedial nucleus. (From Lotti, V. J. et al., 1969. Neuroendocrinology. 4:326–332. S. Karger, Basel, Switzerland)

systemically, since they could still reach the diencephalon via its unimpaired blood supply.

III. GROWTH HORMONE RELEASE

The regulation of the release of growth hormone (GH) is believed by most neuroendocrinologists to be under the direct physiological influence of the nervous system (Schally *et al.*, 1968). The probable locus of such a control is the hypothalamus. Even though the amount of research dealing with this question is considerably less than that concerning other endocrine systems, there is some distinct evidence for the concept of the neural control of the cyclic secretion of growth hormone.

When using growth rate as the primary measure, a number of investigators have found that massive lesions to the hypothalamus seriously disturb the secretion of growth hormone (Pecile and Müller, 1966). Although precise localization through the isolated ablation of tissue has not been accomplished, the anterior part of the hypothalamus and the paraventricular nucleus always seem to be involved in the deficiency of growth hormone production. Among the stimuli which have been described as those that evoke the release of growth hormone are: a shortage of carbohydrate substrate as seen during an insulin or other hypoglycemia; deep sleep; emotional deprivation in children; protein deprivation; and falling or aberrant levels of free fatty acid (Glick, 1969).

As in other systems, a GHRF is apparently present in the hypothalamus. The release of a GHRF would subsequently influence the release of growth hormone from the pituitary (Glick, 1969). In fact, insulin may deplete hypothalamic GHRF (Katz *et al.*, 1967) as well as the content of growth hormone in the pituitary gland (Müller *et al.*, 1967). Starvation and several varieties of stressor may similarly reduce the stores of both GHRF and the trophic hormone. The existence of a growth hormone inhibitory factor (GIF) in the hypothalamus has been suggested by workers in McCann's laboratory but its isolation, chemical structure and route of synthesis remain unconfirmed at this writing.

A. Hypothalamus and Growth Hormone

When bovine growth hormone (GH-B8) is implanted in a range of 16 to 160 μg doses in the basal hypothalamus of the rat, the overall weight of the pituitary is reduced significantly within 7 to 14 days (Katz *et al.*, 1969). During this interval, the rat's growth rate decelerates and the GH content of the pituitary also declines. That growth hormone must act centrally to moderate its own secretion is indicated by the important fact that there is no systemic absorption of the implanted hormone. Unfortunately, Katz *et al.* were unable to identify precisely any localized region that was more sensitive to growth hormone than another. Furthermore, it is not known whether growth hormone acts on a specific complex of receptors to alter the synthesis or release of GHRF or GIF.

In monkeys sedated with Sernylan, a single large dose of 250 μg of 2-deoxy-D-glucose (2-DG) given in a large volume caused an immediate rise in plasma growth hormone (Himsworth *et al.*, 1972). Although a much needed pharmacological control for the specificity of the 2-DG response was not undertaken and no dose-response curve was presented, it is possible that the local depletion of metabolizable glucose in the lateral hypothalamus stimulates the elaboration of the growth hormone from the anterior pituitary. This conclusion was reached by Himsworth *et al.* since injections in other hypothalamic areas did not cause this effect. However, this is probably an oversimplification since norepinephrine and other compounds injected at homologous sites in the hypothalamus may also cause the same response (Toivola and Gale, 1972a and b).

The release of growth hormone may be mediated by an adrenergic mechanism. After norepinephrine was injected in a single dose into the hypothalamus of the restrained baboon, the level of serum growth hormone was significantly elevated 25 to 40 minutes later (Toivola and Gale, 1972a). Although a very large volume of catecholamine was infused into the hypothalamus, the site of noradrenergic sensitivity was found to be the ventromedial region, which corresponds to the lack of effect on growth hormone concentration when norepinephrine is infused into the rostral hypothalamus (Toivola and Gale, 1970). Although no signs of stress or sedation appeared as measured by blood pressure, heart rate, serum glucose, glycerol and motor activity, Toivola and Gale surprisingly found that the plasma levels of 17-hydroxycorticosteroids were also elevated following an injection of norepinephrine.

The receptors in the proposed adrenergic pathway mediating the release of growth hormone may be in the alpha classification (Toivola *et al.*, 1972). An infusion of a large dose of phentolamine at a rate of 10 μl/minute for 25 to 30 minutes into the anterior hypothalamus produces a fall in the serum concentration of growth hormone. At the same time the level of plasma insulin, glucose and 17-OH corticosteroids rises sharply. Unfortunately, propranolol injections and other obvious controls, both pharmacological and anatomical, are required before receptor specificity can be considered. This is especially important in view of the report of Toivola and Gale (1970) that 30 to 150 μg of dopamine infused into the hypothalamus of the monkey also cause a sharp and significant fall in serum growth hormone.

The hypothetical model devised by Toivola and Gale (1972b) to describe the adrenergic regulation of the release of growth hormone is shown in Fig. 4-20. Here, the ventromedial nucleus is viewed as an integrator which monitors afferent neural input and blood-borne information. This input is converted to a "chemically coded" output in the form of norepinephrine release from nerve terminals in the VMH. The output in turn releases GHRF at the level of the median eminence. The transport of GHRF to the adenohypophysis stimulates the secretion of growth hormone there. Toivola and Gale postulate that alpha

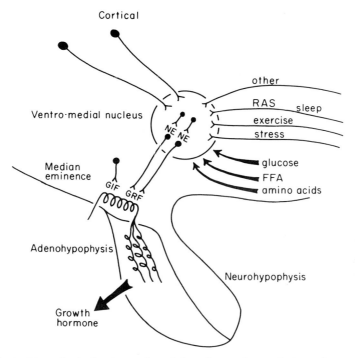

Fig. 4-20 Hypothetical schema for alpha adrenergic regulation of growth hormone in the hypothalamus. The ventromedial nucleus acts as an integrator which monitors afferent neural and blood borne information and converts input to a chemically coded output in the form of norepinephrine which then releases GHRF. GHRF conveyed in the hypophyseal portal vessels stimulates growth hormone secretion in the adenohypophysis. (From Toivola and Gale, 1972b)

receptors mediate the integrator mechanism, since 10 μg norepinephrine infused in a large volume into the VMH of the conscious baboon augments rather markedly the level of plasma growth hormone. On the other hand, the infusion of phentolamine, not in the VMH but in the anterior hypothalamic region, lowers the basal level of circulating growth hormone. This latter somewhat confusing anatomical datum can be explained by the fact that 250 μl of the alpha blocker were infused. Although the receptors in the VMH are reached, presumably as a result of the extensive diffusion, additional research will go far to strengthen the validity of this interesting model.

IV. THYROTROPHIC HORMONE RELEASE:
THE HYPOTHALAMUS

Considerable controversy has surrounded the idea that a portion of the thyroxine that is secreted by the thyroid gland feeds back to the hypothalamus, which is over and above that affecting the accepted target tissue in the pituitary. As late as 1966, Reichlin diagrammed the major "servo-link" in the thyroid axis as being positioned between the thyroid and anterior hypophysis with a question mark on the pathway between the thyroid and the so-called thyrotrophic area (Reichlin, 1966). Today, overwhelming evidence exists that thyrotropin releasing factor (TRF) is present in the hypothalamus. The local content of this releasing factor can vary according to the level of thyroid stimulating hormone (TSH) and possibly thyroxine in the hypothalamus. The concentration may change also after lesions to widespread areas of the hypothalamus (Motta *et al.*, 1969).

A. Anatomical Localization of Thyrotrophic Area

Most investigators pinpoint the cerebral thyrotrophic region as situated in the anterior hypothalamus between the preoptic area and the median eminence. Findings based on lesions and electrical stimulation indicate that the area or components of it might be somewhat more diffuse. This latter position would not be difficult to accept in view of the complex interplay of the thyroid gland with a myriad of functions including the control of body temperature, feeding behavior, metabolism and the severe psychological changes that are associated with the diseases of cretinism, myxedema and thyrotoxicosis. For example, the learning process of the rat may be altered straightforwardly by interfering with the animal's thyroid function (Denenberg and Myers, 1958).

1. *Hypothalamic Lesions*

The symmetrical destruction bilaterally of a region between the paraventricular nucleus and the median eminence of the rat prevents the typical goiter from developing upon feeding thiouracil (Greer, 1957), a drug which blocks thyroid function. Because goiter formation is caused by thyroxine deficiency, this part of the hypothalamus is ostensibly involved in the pituitary regulation of TSH output. Lesions placed in other parts of the hypothalamus are very effective in reducing ^{131}I uptake and release, the weight of the thyroid gland, and the serum levels of TSH (see Reichlin, 1966). Although the lesions are not nearly so devastating to thyroid function as a hypophysectomy, it is possible that the thyrotrophic area within the hypothalamus may establish some sort of baseline or even a "set-point" for TSH release. On the other hand, the pituitary is responsive autonomously, or partially so, to the local concentration of thyroxine in the circulating plasma.

2. *Electrical Stimulation*

Experiments utilizing electrical stimulation show that thyroid activity can be activated when areas corresponding to those implicated by ablation are excited. Using rabbits, Harris and his co-workers showed that the release of ^{131}I from the thyroid is accelerated when the electrode tip is located in the anterior median eminence. Although vasopressin may also be released by such stimulation, the change in thyroid activity is probably due to an increased release of TSH from the pituitary (Harris, 1964). In another important set of studies, D'Angelo discovered that electrical stimulation of several rostral hypothalamic sites depleted TSH stores in the pituitary. At the same time, serum TSH levels increased and, quite remarkably, microscopic changes were observed in the pituitary gland (D'Angelo et al., 1964).

In an overall sense, these observations taken together with the results based on lesions point clearly to a diencephalic mechanism in the control of TSH release. This is now thought to be the local manufacture and liberation of the releasing factor, TRF. The recent isolation and chemical identification of TRF in hypothalamic extracts is concordant with such a view (e.g., Bøler et al., 1969).

B. Action of Thyroxine on Hypothalamic Tissue

At the heart of the disagreement about the presence of a thyroxine receptor zone in the hypothalamus has been the question of localizing the effect of a hormone injection. In discussing the regulation of TSH release, Rose et al. in 1960 put it succinctly as follows:

> "Since drugs injected into the anterior hypothalamus can diffuse into the portal circulation and be carried down to the entire pars distalis, it is conceivable that a drug acting only at the pituitary is more effective when injected into the anterior hypothalamus than when injected directly into the pituitary; from the latter site the drug might have a variable and less efficient spread through the gland."

Until recently, this telling criticism has not been resolved.

The search for the thyrotrophic zone was begun by Kollros in a pioneering study in 1943. Kollros showed that thyroxine acted directly on the central nervous system of the tadpole to enhance its development. When an agar pellet soaked in a dilute thyroxine solution was inserted into the fourth ventricle so as to rest on the surface of the developing frog's medulla, the corneal lid-closure reflex appeared, in some instances, overnight, instead of in the usual period of up to weeks later. If thyroxine was added to the water in which the anuran lived, the total metamorphosis was generally advanced but the corneal reflex did not appear earlier. Thus, the thyroid hormone is capable of accelerating the regional development of neural tissue, at least in the frog and for a very primitive reflex (Kollross, 1943).

Are thyroxine receptors located in the mammalian brain-stem which possess similar functional features as those in the anterior pituitary in the regulation of TSH elaboration? In another early paper, von Euler and Holmgren (1956) demonstrated that the release of thyroxine from the thyroid gland is inhibited by the injection of thyroxine directly into the anterior lobe of the pituitary of the rabbit. However, an injection of thyroxine in a large 2 to 5 μl volume in the same dose into the median eminence and other hypothalamic areas failed to alter thyroxine output. This would pinpoint the site of thyrotrophic feedback activity to the hypophysis rather than to neural tissue. Interestingly, however, von Euler and Holmgren (1956) found that epinephrine inhibited thyroxine liberation when the amine was injected into the mammillary region, a response linked perhaps to the effect which adrenaline has on ACTH release.

In contradiction to these findings was a dramatic demonstration of thyroxine's central action shown by Yamada (1959a) who produced thyroid hypertrophy and a goiter by systemic administration of propyl thiouracil. When thyroxine was injected in a volume of 20 μl into the anterior hypothalamus in a dose that was ineffective systemically, the formation of the goiter was entirely blocked. Even though most of the thyroxine solution probably passed into the third cerebral ventricle because of the large volume, a rather larger area of rostral hypothalamic tissue was apparently inundated by the steroid. This would explain the discrepancy between this account and the earlier results of von Euler and Holmgren (1956) who made their injections of thyroxine at sites located far more caudally. Nevertheless, the action of thyroxine on the pituitary by means of diffusion or transport could not be ruled out at that time.

A complementary study of the action of the thyroid principle also did not help to resolve the issue. The action of L-thyroxine on the pituitary revealed again the inhibition of thyrotropin (TSH) release from the pituitary of an unanesthetized rabbit. However, thyroxine failed to exert this effect when the hormone was micro-injected again in a large 2 to 3 μl volume into the mammillary body, ventromedial hypothalamus or amygdala (Harrison, 1961). Either epinephrine or substance P blocked the release of TSH when injected into the mammillary region or ventromedial region of the hypothalamus, but both failed to do this when injected directly into the pituitary or amygdala. Although ACh, GABA and serotonin injected similarly into brain tissue were without effect on TSH release, the work of von Euler and Holmgren was confirmed that a thyroxine sensitive "receptor" is located in the pituitary. The notion of a hypothalamic "thyrotrophic zone" as described earlier by Yamada (1959a) was rejected by Harrison, since Yamada's injections of L-thyroxine were in a volume which may have diffused into the pituitary as portrayed so graphically in Fig. 4-21. Unfortunately, Harrison neglected to inject thyroxine in all the areas of the hypothalamus.

1. *Local Feedback Inhibition of Thyroxine*

The first description of a feedback inhibitory effect on thyrotropin release of centrally administered thyroxine was presented by Yamada and Greer (1959). In spite of the use of an enormous volume of 20 μl, thyroxine injected into the

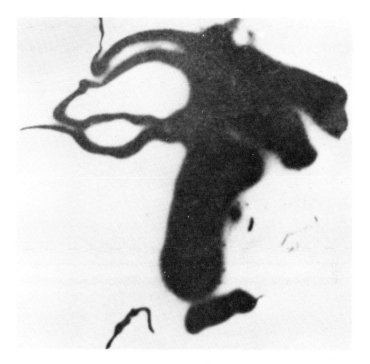

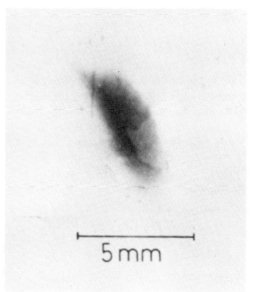

Fig. 4-21 Radioautographs obtained from the rabbit brain after injection of .02 ml, top and .003 ml bottom, of radiothyroxine into the hypothalamus. Magnification of both pictures is the same, X 6. (From Harrison, 1961)

anterior part of the rat's hypothalamus reduced ^{131}I thyroid secretion usually 6 to 9 hours after injection. This inhibition lasted for up to 20 hours on the average. Although the thyrotrophic inhibition did not occur when the thyroxine solution was injected purportedly into the preoptic area or posterior hypothalamus, almost immediately thyroid output lessened when thyroxine was injected directly into the pituitary. The duration of inhibition was identical to that seen when the steroid was injected into hypothalamic tissue. In analyzing these results, it is possible that: (a) thyroxine has an indirect feedback action on the anterior hypothalamic cells; or (b) it simply takes 6 to 9 hours for the steroid to diffuse or to be transported via the hypophyseal portal vessels to the pituitary gland, believed of course by von Euler and Holmgren (1956) to be the primary site of action.

A follow-up study in which graded doses of 0.05 to .25 µg of L-thyroxine were injected into the rostral hypothalamus also demonstrated the dose-dependent nature of the suppression of thyroid secretion as reflected by the shift in ^{131}I activity (Yamada, 1959b). The same sort of inhibition was likewise observed when the doses were injected directly into the anterior pituitary. However, to rule out the possibility of portal transport, Yamada also injected 0.25 µg of radioactive thyroxine into the hypothalamus. Measured 30 minutes or 4 hours later, less than 1% of the radioactivity was present in the pituitary, which demonstrated that even though some transport of the hormone occurred, the amount was below the minimal dose required to exert an inhibitory effect on the cells of the anterior hypophysis.

Using a 1 µl agar medium implant containing 0.25 µg of hormone, Kovács and Vértes (1961) also found that when thyroxine was placed in the hypothalamus of the rat, ^{131}I level in the plasma declined and ^{131}I uptake in the thyroid gland was suppressed. The site of the maximum inhibitory effect of thyroxine was found to be just caudal to the preoptic area and dorsal to the ventromedial nucleus, but certainly not in the lateral or posterior regions of the hypothalamus. Control implants in the cerebral cortex were without effect.

Arguing strongly against Yamada's concept of a "dual receptor site" for thyroid feedback, Bogdanove and Crabill (1961) demonstrated that thyroid tissue grafted to the pituitary of the rat suppressed thyroid activity far more than a thyroid fragment transplanted to the animal's anterior hypothalamus. They, therefore, attributed Yamada's findings, based on direct micro-injections, to a rapid flushing away of the thyroxine solution by the blood supply to the pituitary. Moreover, a hypothalamic injection of thyroxine could simply reach the hypophysis in a manner equivalent to a slowly diffusing infusion. Thus, the controversy flared again and left the matter unresolved until much later.

2. Anatomical Localization of Thyroxine's Action

In 1969, Kajihara and Kendall presented incontrovertible evidence that the anterior hypothalamus is indeed a site of paramount importance in thyroid function. First, they hypophysectomized the rat and grafted the pituitary under the kidney, then thyroxine was deposited bilaterally in the anterior hypothalamus in the region of the paraventricular nuclei; they found that the uptake as well as release from the thyroid gland of ^{131}I was suppressed significantly (Kajihara and Kendall, 1969).   Clearly, TSH activity in a remotely placed pituitary can be inhibited by the local feedback action of thyroxine on hypothalamic neurons. Nevertheless, the whole question of why there should be two thyroxine sensitive sites—hypothalamic and anterior pituitary—in the control of TSH secretion remains a baffling one (Strashimirov, 1971).

Recently, additional compelling evidence for a hypothalamic "thyrotrophic zone" was presented by Knigge and Joseph (1971). Pellets of thyroxine mixed with cholesterol were implanted in the preoptic area of the cat that had a prior hemi-thyroidectomy. The compensatory hypertrophy of the remaining portion of the gland was substantially retarded. Further, if the basal hypothalamus was deafferented by a horizontal knife-cut following the Halasz technique, similar deposits of thyroxine in the cat did not prevent the expected compensatory increase in the size of the animal's remaining thyroid. Thus, an inhibitory neural pathway seems to extend from the preoptic area to the region of the median eminence of the cat in the negative feedback action of thyroxine on the diencephalon.

Of critical importance to the question of the local action of thyroxine in hypothalamic tissue is the nagging question of the magnitude as well as the rate at which the hormone may be transported directly to the hypophysis or into the general circulation (e.g., Bogdanove, 1963b; Averill, 1970). Convincing observations by Chambers and Sobel (1971) have helped to answer this question. When thyroxine was deposited in the hypothalamus of the rat, a reduction ensued in the ^{131}I epithyroid disappearance rate, reflecting the activity of the thyroid.   Since this response, illustrated in Fig. 4-22, occurred only when thyroxine was deposited in the vicinity of the paraventricular nucleus, TSH elaboration from the pituitary is inhibited by the local presence of thyroxine in this highly restricted region of the hypothalamus. The most significant result was that after ^{131}I-thyroxine had been placed in the paraventricular nucleus, absolutely no radioactivity appeared in the pituitary gland. Hence, the thyroid principle must exert its feedback effect directly on the hypothalamus and independently of the pituitary. The position of the paraventricular nucleus also explains why Yamada found such clear suppression of thyroid activity even with such large injection volumes.

A significant observation pertains to the hypothesis of the possible transport of hypophyseotrophic hormones to the pituitary by way of the CSF instead of the blood supply. The injection of 10 to 50 μg of thyrotropin releasing hormone (TRH) into the median eminence was found to be far more potent in elevating plasma TSH levels than a similar injection into the third ventricle (Gordon et al., 1972). However, as one would expect, TRH injected into the anterior

TRF Centers of Hypothalamus

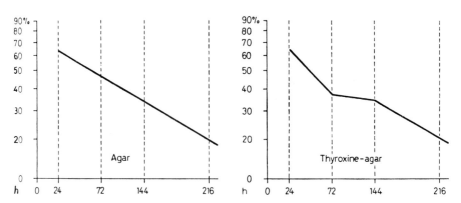

Fig. 4-22 Results of counts made over the thyroid expressed as a percentage of the total dose of ^{131}I administered. Counting started 24 hours after the administration of ^{131}I. The curve on the right is with a thyroxine-agar tube in the nucleus paraventricularis area from the 22nd to the 144th hour, and the curve on the left is with a plain agar tube in the same animal during the same period. (From Chambers, W. F. and R. J. Sobel. 1971. *Neuroendocrinology*. 7:37–45. S. Karger, Basel, Switzerland)

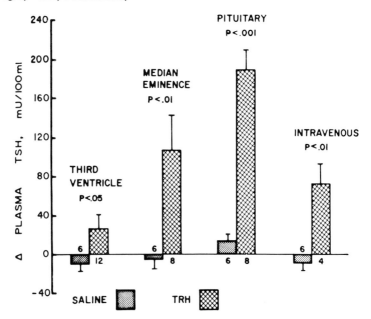

Fig. 4-23 Maximum change in plasma TSH after injection of 50 ng of TRH into the third ventricle, median eminence, anterior pituitary, and intravenous compared to saline controls similarly injected. The significance of the change, *p* value, is noted on the figure; vertical bar shows SE. Number of rats used is indicated. (From Gordon *et al.*, 1972)

pituitary exerted the greatest effect on plasma TSH as shown in Fig. 4-23. Thus, the third ventricle is the least effective route by which TRH reaches the anterior pituitary.

Other kinds of evidence support the view of a neural mechanism in the control of thyroid function.   For instance, ^{131}I release rates from the thyroid, as illustrated in Fig. 4-24, are suppressed when morphine is micro-injected in the hypothalamus in either the supramammillary or supraoptic regions (Lomax *et al.*, 1970). Because of the lack of anatomical specificity, a direct effect of morphine on the pituitary gland cannot be ruled out. Nevertheless, morphine could have a dual action on the basal diencephalon by (1) stimulating caudal neurons that inhibit TSH release, and (2) depressing rostral neurons that activate the pituitary-thyroid axis.

In the neonatal rat, the local injection of thyroxine in the arcuate region or its deposition at the same site in crystalline form causes protracted and delayed effects on both thyroid and gonadal functions.   When Bakke *et al.* (1972) either

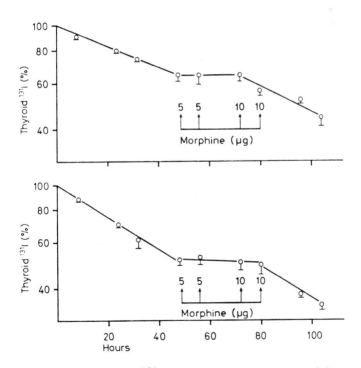

Fig. 4-24   (Top) Mean thyroid ^{131}I release curve from a group of six rats receiving bilateral injections of morphine sulphate into the supraoptic region. Vertical bars represent standard errors of the means. (Bottom) Mean thyroid ^{131}I release curve from a group of 8 rats receiving bilateral injections of morphine sulfate into the supramammillary region. Vertical bars represent standard errors of the means. (From Lomax, P. *et al.*, 1970. *Neuroendocrinology*. 6:146–152. S. Karger, Basel, Switzerland)

injected or implanted thyroxine in rats 3 days of age, the pup's body weight as well as the weights of the pituitary and thyroid were reduced at 4 months of age. Serum thyroxine and TSH levels were similarly lower. In several rats, the onset of puberty was delayed, ovarian weight was reduced and the estrous cycle was also prolonged. Because of the concentrations used, the involvement of the pituitary could not be excluded; however it is indeed possible that the developing brain is exceptionally sensitive, as Kollros proposed over 30 years ago, to the presence of thyroxine in relation to the profound functional modifications which occur if the concentration of the hormone is irregular.

V. CONCLUDING CONSIDERATIONS

If the findings presented in the previous sections of this chapter are scrutinized in the context of the important role of the trophic releasing factors manufactured in the hypothalamus, it is apparent that the feedback action of a hormone does take place at two major target sites—the hypothalamus and the anterior pituitary. What is especially significant is the discrete regional sensitivity of the brain to adrenal steroids, growth hormone and the thyroid principle.

In the case of the adrenal axis, the neural structures for which evidence of hormone receptors is confirmed are the: median eminence, ventral hippocampus, anterior thalamus, septum and perhaps the mesencephalic reticular formation. In this connection, the specific site of corticosterone action has been made unclear by the findings of Knizley (1972). As shown earlier by McEwen et al. (1969), the septum and hippocampus of the rat have the capacity to concentrate the steroid selectively. The differential uptake of corticosterone in these structures and the simultaneous failure of the hypothalamus to show hormonal uptake indicate that the hypothalamus may be a secondary rather than primary target of the glucocorticoids. As was intimated by Knizley (1972), this conclusion is in stark contrast with all of the pharmacological findings based on the direct implantation of corticoids into the hypothalamus. Interestingly, Knizley found that even the pituitary is second to the hippocampus in the capacity to concentrate corticosterone; further, the cerebral cortex also showed some uptake of the hormone.

How these results can be reconciled with the preponderance of evidence provided by the implantation studies that do suggest a unique chemosensitivity to corticosteroids will await further research. Perhaps the uptake measure itself is misleading in that the steroid may exert feedback effects or participate in functional control by a mechanism that does not require binding to tissue. At any rate, some caution in interpretation should accompany each observation as it is viewed in the perspective of the entire body of data on the sensitivity of CNS structures to individual hormones.

Of special significance are the critical anatomical loci of each set of postulated receptors for individual hormones. In each instance, important functions related to the activity of the hormone are associated with the morphological region. For example, the TSH release mechanism has been localized by Kajihara and Kendall (1969) to the anterior hypothalamus where the neurons are delegated to detecting changes in thermal input or are sensitive to monoamines, pyrogens and other substances; in fact, the anterior region is the main site of origin of the heat production pathway (see Chapter 6). Taken together, these studies indicate that this part of the hypothalamus serves as a master integrator for a variety of homeostatic processes concerned with energy metabolism with all of its facets—both long-term and short-term.

Not far remote from this area are the cellular elements within the ventromedial and lateral hypothalamus that are implicated in the stimulation of GHRF and the ultimate regulation of growth hormone secretion. These regions are also those which subserve one or more aspects of the act of feeding or the inhibition of eating behavior (see Chapter 7). Thus, the neurons in this part of the hypothalamus mediate the long-term as well as short-term regulation of ingestive functions. Sensory impulses signalling the state of hunger in a food deprived animal may not be entirely divorced from the afferent signals calling for heat production in an animal exposed to the cold. Undoubtedly, a crucial functional interaction occurs between the secretion of growth hormone and thyroid activity. The integrated triggering of both GHRF and TRF release would constitute an ideal mechanism for such a relationship.

A. Feedback Loops

As more and more releasing factors and their inhibitory counterparts are isolated from hypothalamic tissue and chemically identified, it will be possible to determine the precise nature of the feedback system of each hormone. For example, ACTH released from the anterior lobe acts back upon the median eminence or other parts of the basal brain. As yet, the possibility that CRF may have a self-regulating capacity has not been tested. Thus far, the only factor that exhibits a potent local action on hypothalamic tissue is TRH (Gordon *et al.*, 1972).

If the speculation is borne out that each releasing hormone could possess a rate-limiting control over its own release, then the concept of an "ultra-short" feedback loop will have to be considered seriously. To carry further the example of a thyroid factor in relation to the acknowledged short and regular feedback mechanisms, three substances would provide their respective information to the specific cell groups in the hypothalamus: (1) the hormone (thyroxine) secreted systemically (regular feedback loop); (2) the trophic hormone (TSH) secreted by the anterior pituitary (short-feedback loop); and (3) the releasing factor (TRH) elaborated by the anterior hypothalamus (ultra-short feedback loop).

Several points should not be overlooked in considering some of the problematical issues in respect to feedback mechanisms. First, the molecular characteristics and specificity of the neuronal receptors and receptor sites are virtually unknown. A great deal of prodigious research will be required to characterize the hypothalamic receptors for each systemic hormone and its trophic substance. Another profound question centers on the matter of inter-species variability. An examination of the response of each releasing factor throughout the phylogenetic scale may help to resolve some of the strange discrepancies in observations which may not be due wholly to procedural differences at the laboratory bench. To illustrate this point, several of the species commonly used for endocrine experiments, including the rat, are nocturnal creatures. In their natural underground habitat, the rodent never witnesses daylight since it emerges from cover only during the night. The 12-hour light-dark cycle which the scientist artificially imposes upon the animal in the laboratory setting undoubtedly disturbs many aspects of endocrine balance to which a certain physiological adaptation *per se* may never really occur (Reiter and Fraschini, 1969). The relationship between photoperiodicity and reproductive hormones is especially critical.

Internal factors released within the brain itself may also modify secondarily the hypothalamic neurosecretory activity. For example, the release of factors from the supraoptic and paraventricular nuclei are apparently influenced by the output of the pineal gland. Recently, de Vries (1972) found that in the pinealectomized rat, the hypothalamic implantation of a fragment of pineal gland, obtained from a littermate donor, prevents the decline in neurosecretory activity in both nuclei. This illustrates the concept that the pineal gland can operate as an endocrine gland: the effect of its removal is reversible by its re-implantation into diencephalic tissue.

B. Biogenic Amines

That the transmission of afferent impulses along a pathway is chemically mediated is not disputed; however, the substances responsible for this mediation are unknown. The important experiments of the Kriegers, Smelik and others are indicative of a cholinergic or adrenergic link in the hypothalamic-hypophyseal pathway. In the model portrayed in Fig. 4-25, the point of synaptic junction rests between a neuronal element and a hypothalamic secretory cell. In this model, a transmitter is postulated to act on the postsynaptic membrane of a terminal secretory neuron which, in this example, releases CRF into the portal blood supply to the pituitary.

From the experiments of Naumenko in which the neuraxis was lesioned at different coronal levels, it would appear that serotonin is the modulator (Chapter 13) within the local hypothalamic-hypophyseal pathway. This monoamine when applied locally is the only one that retains the capacity to augment the plasma level of corticosteroids. As in other studies of this nature,

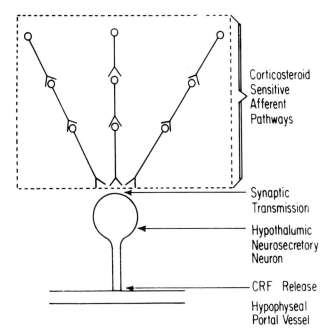

Fig. 4-25   Possible localization of steroid feedback. Synaptically active neuro-transmitter agents are postulated to act on the synaptic membrane of the terminal hypothalamic neurosecretory neuron. Such action is not blocked by steroids. Steroid feedback may act instead on any of the links in the various afferent pathways which ultimately impinge upon the hypothalamic neurosecretory neuron. (From Krieger and Krieger, 1970a)

a dose-response relationship must be specified and a demonstration of pharmacological antagonism would be desirable. However, should the release of 5-HT occur presynaptically within the neurosecretory area at the same time that CRF is liberated from the terminal ending of the secretory neuron, then the first clear-cut relationship between a hormonal process and amine function will finally be established.

VI. Master Summary Table
Chemicals that Exerted an Effect when Given at a Specific Site in the Brain

Chemical	Dose	Volume	Site	Species	State*	Response	Reference
Adrenocorticotrophic hormone (ACTH)	≃ 5 units	crystal	Median eminence	Rat	U	Lower serum corticosterone.	Motta et al. (1965)
	20 µg	?	Hypothalamus	Rat	U	Adrenal activation.	Ferrari et al. (1966)
	≃ 53–130 µg	crystal	Median eminence	Rat	U	No change in plasma corticosterone.	Davidson et al. (1967)
Atropine	≃ 200–250 µg	crystal	Anterior hypothalamus	Rat	U	Blocks adrenocortical response to stress.	Hedge and Smelik (1968)
Carbachol	5 µg	1 µl	Hypothalamus	Guinea pig	U	Increase in plasma corticosteroids; but not after brain-stem section.	Naumenko (1968)
	5 µg	10 µl	Mesencephalon	Cat	U	Autonomic reaction, rage, motor activity, fear, escape, and lower corticosteroids, plus increase corticosteroids (ACTH).	Endröczi et al. (1963)
	6.5 µg	?	Median eminence	Cat	U	Rise in plasma corticosterone after pretreatment with dexamethasone.	Krieger and Krieger (1970a)
	≃ 6.5–10 µg	crystal	Median eminence, mammillary body	Cat	U	Elevated 17-hydroxycortico-steroids (17-OHCS).	Krieger and Krieger (1964)
	≃ 4–24 µg	crystal	Hypothalamus, amygdala, hippocampus, septum, fornix, thalamus	Cat	U	Rise in plasma corticosteroids; sham rage.	Krieger and Krieger (1970b)
	≃ 4–24 µg	crystal	Median eminence, amygdala, mammillary body	Cat	U	Rise in plasma 11-hydroxycortico-steroids.	Krieger and Krieger (1971)

*U = unanesthetized and unrestrained; C = constrained, confined or curarized; A = anesthetized.

	Dose	Form	Site	Animal		Response	Reference
Corticosterone	≈ 200 µg	crystal	Median eminence	Rat	U	Suppressed steroid response to stress.	Grimm and Kendall (1968)
	≈ 200 µg	crystal	Median eminence	Rat	U	Inhibited adrenocortical response to auditory or photic stressors.	Feldman et al. (1969)
	≈ 50–80 µg	crystal	Amygdala	Rabbit	U	Decreased adrenal synthesis of corticosterone.	Kawakami et al. (1968)
	≈ 50–80 µg	crystal	Hippocampus (Ammons horn)	Rabbit	U	Increased adrenal synthesis of corticosterone.	Kawakami et al. (1968)
Cortisol (Hydrocortisone)	?	crystal	Amygdala, basal septum, midline thalamus	Rat	U	Diminution of stress-induced ACTH.	Bohus and Lissak (1967)
	?	crystal	Ventral hippocampus	Rat	U	Increase of pituitary adrenocortical activation.	Bohus and Lissak (1967)
	≈ 5 µg	crystal	Median eminence	Rat	U	Suppressed ACTH release (corticosteroid production) due to ether stress.	Bohus (1968), Bohus and Strashimirov (1970)
	≈ 5 µg	crystal	Hippocampus	Rat	U	Enhanced stress-induced release of ACTH.	Bohus et al. (1968)
	≈ 5 µg	crystal	Amygdala, septum, medial thalamus, mesencephalic reticular formation	Rat	U	Suppressed stress-induced release of ACTH.	Bohus (1968), Bohus et al. (1968)
	10–20 µg	1 µl (agar)	Baso-medial hypothalamus, rostral MRF	Rat	U	Decrease in adrenal corticosterone secretion.	Bohus and Endröczi (1964)
	≈ 35–70 µg	crystal	Median eminence	Rat	U	Lowered serum and adrenal corticosterone.	Corbin et al. (1965)
	≈ 35–70 µg	crystal	Mesencephalic reticular formation	Rat	A	No effect.	Corbin et al. (1965)

VI. Master Summary Table (Continued)

Chemical	Dose	Volume	Site	Species	State[*]	Response	Reference
Cortisol (Hydrocortisone)	≃ 20–200 µg	crystal	Arcuate, median eminence, midbrain, ventral hippocampus	Rat	A	Decline in plasma corticosteroid levels.	Slusher (1966)
	≃ 30–240 µg	crystal	Median eminence	Rat	U	Suppressed basal level of ACTH and reduced ACTH increase caused by stress.	Davidson et al. (1968)
	≃ 60–200 µg	crystal	Median eminence	Rat	U	Inhibited adrenocortical response to auditory or photic stressors.	Feldman et al. (1969)
	≃ 200 µg	crystal	Hypothalamus (Basal), median eminence	Rat	U	Blockade of compensatory adrenal hypertrophy following unilateral adrenalectomy.	Davidson and Feldman (1962)
	≃ 200 µg	crystal	Median eminence and centero-medial hypothalamus	Rat	U	Abolished compensatory adrenal hypertrophy in adrenalectomized rat.	Davidson and Feldman (1963)
	≃ 200 µg	crystal	Median eminence	Rat	U	Adrenal atrophy and lack of ascorbic acid depletion in adrenal.	Chowers et al. (1963)
	≃ 200 µg	crystal	Median eminence	Rat	U	Suppressed steroid response to stress.	Grimm and Kendall (1968)
	≃ 200 µg	crystal	Median eminence	Rat	U	Adrenal atrophy, prevents adrenal hypertrophy after unilateral adrenalectomy.	Feldman et al. (1966)
	≃ 200 µg	crystal	Medial basal hypothalamus	Rat	U	Blocks development of gonads in accessory organs in immature rat, and TSH production.	Smith et al. (1971)
	?	crystal	Ventral hypothalamus	Rabbit	C	Reduced stress response.	Kawakami et al. (1966)

Compound	Dose	Form	Site	Species		Effect	Reference
	≈ 200 µg	crystal	Median eminence, antero-medial hypothalamus	Rabbit	C	Blockade of stress-induced rise in plasma corticosteroid.	Smelik and Sawyer (1962)
	250 µg	11.7 µl	Hypothalamus midbrain	Cat	A	Increase and decrease of neuron firing rate.	Slusher et al. (1966)
Cortisone	10–50 µg	10–50 µl	Posterior hypothalamus, mesencephalic reticular formation	Rat / Cat	U / U	Reduced corticosteroid level in blood.	Endröczi et al. (1961)
11-Dehydrocorticosterone	≈ 5 µg	crystal	Median eminence	Rat	U	Suppressed ACTH release (corticosteroid production) due to ether stress.	Bohus and Strashimirov (1970)
Cyclic AMP	49 µg	1–10 µl	Median eminence	Rat	A	ACTH release.	Hedge (1971)
2-Deoxy-D-glucose	250 µg	5 µl	Lateral hypothalamus	Monkey	A	Increased plasma-growth hormone.	Himsworth et al. (1972)
Dexamethasone	?	crystal	Median eminence	Rat	U	Reduced CRF in median eminence and ACTH in pituitary.	Chowers et al. (1967)
	?	crystal	Septum, preoptic area	Rat	U	Blocked compensatory adrenal hypertrophy.	Davidson and Feldman (1967)
	≈ 5 µg	crystal	Median eminence	Rat	U	Suppressed ACTH release (corticosteroid production) due to ether stress.	Bohus and Strashimirov (1970)
	≈ 5 µg	crystal	Median eminence	Rat	U	Suppressed stress-induced ACTH release.	Strashimirov et al. (1969)
	≈ 20 µg	crystal	Basal hypothalamus	Rat	U	Blocked stress-induced ACTH release.	Smelik (1969)
	≈ 35–70 µg	crystal	Mesencephalic reticular formation	Rat	U	No change in adrenal weight.	Corbin et al. (1965)
	≈ 35–70 µg	crystal	Median eminence	Rat	U	Lowered adrenal weight and reduced plasma and adrenal corticosteroid levels.	Corbin et al. (1965)
	≈ 200 µg	crystal	Median eminence	Rat	U	Suppressed basal and stress-induced secretion of ACTH.	Davidson et al. (1968)
	≈ 200 µg	crystal	Median eminence	Rat	U	Adrenal atrophy, prevents adrenal hypertrophy after unilateral adrenalectomy.	Feldman et al. (1966)

VI. Master Summary Table *(Continued)*

Chemical	Dose	Volume	Site	Species	State*	Response	Reference
Dexamethasone	.01–2 µg	.5 µl	Median eminence, anterior thalamic septal region	Rat	A	Reduced corticosterone production after stress.	Dallman and Yates (1968)
	.1–2 µg	.5 µl	Anterior pituitary, median eminence, septum	Rat	A	Inhibited ACTH release.	Russell *et al.* (1969)
	4 µg	1 µl	Preoptic area	Rat	U	Blockade of ovulation; suppression of ACTH release.	Hagino *et al.* (1969)
	4 µg	1 µl	Ventromedial hypothalamic-arcuate complex	Rat	U	Suppression of ACTH release.	Hagino *et al.* (1969)
Dopamine	30–150 µg	30 µl	Rostral hypothalamus	Baboon	C	Fall in growth hormone.	Toivola and Gale (1970)
Ephedrine	.5 µg	?	Posterior hypothalamus, ventral tegmentum	Cat	U	Increased corticosteroids.	Endröczi *et al.* (1963a)
Epinephrine	.7 µg	2–3 µl	Hypothalamus	Rabbit	C	Blocked TSH (thyroid stimulating hormone) release.	Harrison (1961)
	2 µg	2–5 µl	Mammillary bodies	Rabbit	U	Inhibited thyroxine release.	von Euler and Holmgren (1956)
	2 µg	10 µl	Posterior hypothalamus, ventral tegmentum	Cat	U	Increased corticosteroids.	Endröczi *et al.* (1963a)
Eserine	5–10 µg	10 µl	Medial and posterior hypothalamus	Cat	U	Autonomic reaction, rage, motor activity, fear, escape, and lower corticosteroids plus increase in corticosteroids (ACTH)	Endröczi *et al.* (1963a)
	5–10 µg	10 µl	Septum, anterior hypothalamus	Cat	U	Autonomic reaction, rage, motor activity, fear, escape, lower corticosteroids.	Endröczi *et al.* (1963a)

Substance	Dose	Volume	Site	Species	U/A	Effect	Reference
Estradiol or Estradiol + Hydrocortisone	≈ 4.5–15 μg	crystal	Median eminence	Rat	U	Compensatory adrenal hypertrophy.	Tallian et al. (1972)
GABA (γ-amino-butyric acid)	≈ 6.5 μg	crystal	Amygdala, median eminence	Cat	U	Rise in plasma 11-hydroxycorticosteroids.	Krieger and Krieger (1970b; 1971)
	≈ 6.5–50 μg	crystal	Median eminence, mammillary body	Cat	U	Elevated 17-hydroxycortico-steroids (17-OHCS).	Krieger and Krieger (1964)
Growth hormone (GH-B8)	≈ 16–160 μg	crystal	Basal hypothalamus	Rat	U	Decline in pituitary weight and GH concentration.	Katz et al. (1969)
^{14}C Histamine	126 μg	3 μl	Paraventricular nucleus, supraoptic nucleus	Cat	A	Failure of transport to hypophysis.	Lippert and Waton (1969)
Lignocaine	60 μg	3 μl	Lateral hypothalamus	Rat	A	Prevents glycemic response to systemic 3-O-methylglucose.	Himsworth (1970)
Luteinizing hormone (LH)	≈ 5 units	crystal	Median eminence	Rat	U	Lower serum corticosterone.	Motta et al. (1965)
Morphine	5–10 μg	1 μl	Posterior hypothalamus, supraoptic region	Rat	U	Reduced thyroid release rates.	Lomax et al. (1970)
	50 μg	1 μl	Rostral and medial hypothalamus	Rat	U	Reduced adrenal ascorbic acid, elevated plasma corticosterone.	Lotti et al. (1969)
Norepinephrine (NE)	1 μg	1 μl	Hypothalamus	Guinea pig	U	Increase in plasma corticosteroids, but not after brain-stem section.	Naumenko (1968)
	2 μg	10 μl	Posterior hypothalamus, ventral tegmentum	Cat	U	Increased corticosteroids.	Endróczi et al. (1963a)
	≈ 10 μg	crystal	Median eminence, mammillary body	Cat	U	Elevated 17-hydroxycorti-costeroids (17-OHCS).	Krieger and Krieger (1964)
	≈ 4–19 μg	crystal	Median eminence, amygdala, dorsal septum, hippocampus, mammillary body	Cat	U	Rise in plasma 11-hydroxy-corticosteroids.	Krieger and Krieger (1970b; 1971)

VI. Master Summary Table (Continued)

Chemical	Dose	Volume	Site	Species	State*	Response	Reference
Norepinephrine (NE)	10 μg	10 μl	Ventromedial hypothalamus	Baboon	C	Increased plasma growth hormone	Toivola and Gale (1972b)
	10 μg	10 μl	Ventromedial hypothalamus	Baboon	U	Elevated serum growth hormone (GH) and 17-OH corticosteroids.	Toivola and Gale (1972a)
Phentolamine	25 μg	250 μl	Anterior hypothalamus	Baboon	C	Reduced plasma growth hormone.	Toivola and Gale (1972b)
	25–150 μg	250–300 μl	Anterior hypothalamus	Baboon	U	Decline in serum growth hormone (GH), insulin, glucose and 17-OH corticosteroids.	Toivola et al. (1972)
Prostaglandin E_1	.5–1 μg	.1 μl	Median eminence	Rat	A	Enhanced ACTH secretion.	Hedge (1972)
Reserpine	2 μg	gelatin pellet	Median eminence	Rat	U	No effect on ACTH release.	Smelik (1967)
	$\simeq$ 200 μg	crystal	Median eminence	Rat	U	No adrenal atrophy.	Feldman et al. (1966)
Serotonin (5-HT)	$\simeq$ 10 ± 3 μg	crystal	Medial hypothalamus	Rat	U	Inhibited stress-induced corticosterone output.	Vermes and Telegdy (1972)
	4.3 μg	1 μl	Ventral hippocampus, septum, mesencephalon	Guinea pig	U	Increased plasma 17-hydroxycorticosteroid.	Naumenko (1969)
	4.3 μg	1 μl	Dorsal hippocampus, amygdala	Guinea pig	U	Fall in plasma 17-hydroxycorticosteroid.	Naumenko (1969)
	5–32 μg	1 μl	Median eminence, septum	Cat	U	Rise in plasma 11-hydroxycorticosteroids.	Krieger and Krieger (1970b; 1971)
Substance-P	.3 μg	2–3 μl	Hypothalamus	Rabbit	C	Blocked TSH release.	Harrison (1961)
Theophylline	1.80 μg	1–10 μl	Median eminence	Rat	A	ACTH release.	Hedge (1971)

Substance	Dose	Volume	Site	Species		Effect	Reference
Thyrotropin releasing hormone (TRH)	10–50 ng	2.5 μl	Median eminence	Rat	U	Elevated plasma TSH levels.	Gordon et al. (1972)
Thyroxine	?	crystal	Paraventricular nucleus	Rat	U	Decreased TSH secretion.	Chambers and Sobel (1971)
	≃ .4 μg	crystal	Anterior hypothalamus, paraventricular nucleus	Rat	U	Suppressed thyroidal ^{131}I uptake and release.	Kajihara and Kendall (1969)
	≃ 3 μg	crystal	Median eminence	Rat	U	Inhibited thyroid iodine release.	Strashimirov (1971)
	≃ 66 μg	crystal	Arcuate nucleus	Rat	U	Reduced pituitary, thyroid, gonadal and body weights.	Bakke et al. (1972)
	.25 μg	20 μl	Anterior hypothalamus	Rat	U	Blocked goiter formation after thiouracil treatment; increase in adrenal weight. Dose dependent suppression of thyrotropin secretion.	Yamada (1959a and b)
	.25 μg	20 μl	Hypothalamus	Rat	U	Inhibition of thyrotropin secretion.	Yamada and Greer (1959)
	5–15 μg	5 μl	Median eminence, arcuate nucleus	Rat	U	Elevated venous corticosterone.	Bohus et al. (1965)
	20–200 μg	2–5 μl	Arcuate nucleus	Rat	U	Reduced pituitary, thyroid, gonadal and body weights.	Bakke et al. (1972)
	2 μg	2–3 μl	Hypothalamus, amygdala	Rabbit	C	Failed to inhibit TSH release.	Harrison (1961)
	2 μg	2–5 μl	Mammillary bodies	Rabbit	U	No effect on thyroxine output.	von Euler and Holmgren (1956)
	10–25 μg	25 μl	Posterior hypothalamus	Cat	A	Desynchronization followed by hypersynchronization of cortical EEG.	Amiragova and Svirskaia (1968)
^{131}I-thyroxine	≃ 6.4 μg	crystal	Anterior hypothalamus	Rat	U	Rapid entry into systemic circulation.	Averill (1970)
Vasopressin	5 mU	.5 μl	Median eminence	Rat	A	Evoked ACTH release (elevated plasma corticosterone).	Hedge et al. (1966)

5 Reproductive Functions and Sexual Behavior

I. INTRODUCTION

Even though the Freudian kind of urge and other personal aspects of sexual expression are readily acknowledged to be psychological in nature, an organic, anatomical basis for the cerebral control over the reproductive function is only now becoming firmly established. This short history is somewhat surprising in view of the widely known symptoms following specific neurological injury. For example, in the Klüver-Bucy syndrome, a male monkey attempts to mount indiscriminately and copulate compulsively because its amygdala is simply ablated bilaterally. Granting that it would probably be going too far to accept the notion of von Hohlweg and Junkmann, set forth over 40 years ago, of the existence of a sex "center" at the base of the brain (von Hohlweg and Junkmann, 1932), we shall nevertheless see in this chapter that several distinct regions of the diencephalon are implicated in a remarkable way in the variety of gonadal and behavioral activities of both male and female.

A. Sex Hormones-Brain Interaction

The divergent nature of the sexual process in its broadest spectrum reflects almost *a priori* the necessity for an intact pathway integrated at three levels: brain, pituitary and the organs of reproduction. As in the case of adrenal and thyroid mechanisms, the clear involvement of neural systems in certain facets of reproduction is virtually proven. These include the dependence on light of the development and function of the testes in hamsters, estrous cyclicity in rodents and egg laying in birds, as well as the fact that ovulation can be triggered by coitus in the rabbit and other species (Davidson and Smith, 1966; Davidson and Bloch, 1969). Even feeding behavior and perhaps weight regulation may be severely altered by the level of female hormone present in the system (Wade, 1972).

Aside from these isolated examples, a vast number of experiments have provided major scientific breakthroughs along four principal lines of investigation: (1) brain tissue is selectively sensitive to gonadal steroids and gonadotrophic hormones; (2) the subcortical regions involved in the control of gonadotropin release in the pituitary are anatomically separate from those mediating specific patterns of sexual behavior; (3) a short-feedback loop enables gonadotropin released from the anterior pituitary to be monitored by cells in the hypothalamus, which in turn controls the output of releasing factor; and (4) biogenic amines present endogenously in the brain influence the hypothalamic activity of trophic releasing factors, gonadotropins or both.

In the early 1930s, the idea was put forward by Moore and Price that the reproductive hormone secreted by male or female gonads exerts a feedback action on the pituitary which "results in a diminished amount of the sex-stimulating factor available to the organism" (Moore and Price, 1932). Perhaps the first clear statement of the role of the CNS in the feedback control of pituitary secretion was postulated in 1932 by von Hohlweg and Junkmann. On the basis of injections into the pituitary of the rat that had been treated with atropine, they hypothesized that gonadal secretions affected CNS activity which in turn influenced the output of hormone from the anterior lobe of the pituitary via a "nervös" pathway. At the time, this initial concept of a brain center for the production of a sexual hormone was indeed revolutionary.

B. Anatomical Relationships

Although all aspects of reproduction can transpire in the female mammal in the absence of the cerebral cortex, this is not the case for the male. Both sensory and motor regions seem to be required for copulatory activity generally. Sexual drive and the attendant frequency of copulation seem to depend upon the integrity of structures in the temporal lobe including the amygdala and pyriform cortex (Schreiner and Kling, 1953; Green et al., 1957). However, experiments in which a part of the diencephalon is lesioned or stimulated electrically have revealed that individual sites are delegated to a specific sexual response.

1. Hypothalamic Lesions

In the female, several characteristic gonadal syndromes follow a discrete lesion placed in diencephalic tissue (Flerkó, 1966; Lisk, 1968). Destruction of the median eminence of the rat and other animals causes ovarian and uterine atrophy as well as anestrus, presumably by the prevention of the production and release of follicle stimulating hormone (FSH) and luteinizing hormone (LH); replacement therapy with exogenous hormone does not restore normal estrus. A lesion placed in the anterior hypothalamus can produce a persistent vaginal estrus and the continual production of FSH. At the same time, mating behavior is suppressed or it completely disappears. In the rabbit, the ablation of the premammillary area also attenuates the frequency of copulation, whereas the electrolytic

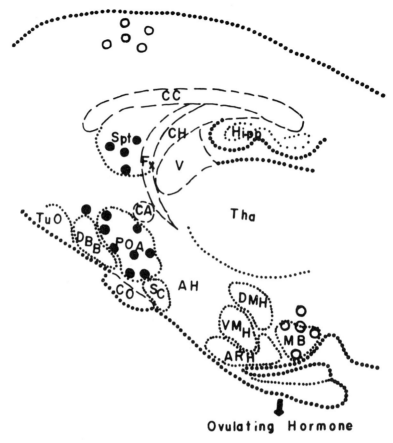

Fig. 5-1 Midsagittal diagram of rat brain indicating effect of Nembutal in blocking PMS-induced precocious ovulation. (● Blocked ovulation, O Ovulation). AH: Anterior Hypothalamus, ARH: Arcuate nucleus, CA: Anterior Commissure, CO: Optic Chiasma, DBB: Diagonal Band of Broca, DMH: Dorsomedial Hypothalamus, Fx: Fornix, Hipp: Hippocampus, MB: Mammillary Body, POA: Preoptic area, SC: Suprachiasmatic Nucleus, Spt: Septum, Tha: Thalamus, TuO: Tuberculum Olfactorium, V: Ventricle, VMH: Ventromedial Hypothalamus. (From Hagino, 1967)

destruction of the preoptic area interferes with the normal estrous cycling of the female and may block ovulation entirely.

Of historical relevance is the paper of Westman and Jacobsohn (1942), the Swedish workers who found that in the female rabbit, an injection of a high dose of Novocaine into the base of the brain inhibited the usual ovulation following copulation. Even though a large 40 μl volume was given in the region of the optic chiasm, these results were taken to support the idea that a "nervous impulse transmitted through the pituitary stalk" stimulates the gonadotropin necessary for ovulation.

If the rostral hypothalamus of the immature female rat is subjected to a local chemical blockade, the ovulation ordinarily induced by pregnant mare's serum is delayed (Hagino, 1967). Sodium pentobarbital injected in a large dose and volume, purportedly in the preoptic area or lateral septum, blocked ovulation but had no effect when injected into other areas including the mammillary region. The direct anesthetization of the preoptic area depicted in Fig. 5-1, which would have the same result as a reversible lesion, thus could block a septal-preoptic pathway mediating the feedback of the ovarian hormones.

In the male, innumerable studies dating back to 1912 show that lesions of the hypothalamus produce dysfunction of the testes, aspermatogenesis and atrophy of accessory structures (see the reviews of Davidson, 1966a; 1969). The region comprising the arcuate nucleus-median eminence has been implicated in many species although the area encompassing the mammillary bodies is also an anatomical site of equal importance for maintaining androgen activity in other species. Large doses of testosterone usually fail to restore normal testicular function in the lesioned animal. Apparently, an ablation of the lateral or anterior hypothalamus does not affect male sexual behavior, but rather astounding hypersexuality is produced not only by lesions in the temporal lobe but also by those placed along the border of the mesencephalon and diencephalon (Davidson, 1966a).

2. *Electrical Stimulation*

The research on the female by Harris, Markee, Everett, Sawyer and others has shown that the release of LH, ovulation and pseudopregnancy can be elicited by electrical stimulation of the anterior hypothalamus, preoptic area, tuber cinereum and other adjacent regions (see reviews of Lisk, 1968; Gorski, 1966; Gorski, 1971). Ovulation can also be induced in the rat in which pentobarbitone has been used to block ovulation. A fascinating observation is that while stimulation of the amygdala induces ovulation, the current applied simultaneously to the hippocampus inhibits the release of gonadotropin.

In the male animal, electrical stimulation of the anterior hypothalamus can evoke the complete pattern of copulation. In the mammillary area of the rat, electrical current will produce ejaculation or stimulus-bound copulation. The anatomical pathway for penile erection has also been described by MacLean (1962).

3. *Steroid Uptake in Brain Tissue*

The preferential accumulation of estrogen in the hypothalamus is indicative of the presence of specific receptors or binding sites. These receptors could be those which sense, so to speak, and thereby monitor the steroid titre in the blood. McGuire and Lisk (1968; 1969) and others have found that ^{3}H estradiol is taken up and bound specifically in the cells of the anterior hypothalamus and/or preoptic area as well as the median eminence. Thus, rostral receptors may play a key role in the estrous cycle. McEwen and his colleagues (see review of McEwen *et al.*, 1972) have shown that ^{3}H testosterone also binds to the preoptic area and hypothalamus in the same manner as estradiol. In the following sections, the striking concordance between these sites of uptake and those sensitive to a local increase in the concentration of gonadal steroid is at once apprehensible.

II. CENTRAL ESTROGEN RECEPTORS

That estrogen has a direct effect on the pituitary insofar as the production of gonadotropin was clearly demonstrated by Rose and Nelson (1957) who infused estradiol continuously into the hypophyseal fossa. They observed that estrogen inhibited the local gonadotrophic activity as measured by the cellular changes within the pituitary. The question then revolves about the validity of von Hohlweg's so-called "sex center." Although this center was postulated to exist in a part of the nervous system that was relatively unknown, its nature was equally uncertain. In 1957, the search to find the answers to these difficult questions began.

In their classical study, Flerkó and Szentágothai (1957) found that a small fragment of about 1 mm^3 of ovarian tissue implanted in the region of the paraventricular nucleus of the rat succeeded in reducing the weight of the rat's ovary. The usual increase in uterine weight during estrus was also prevented. When grafted to the anterior lobe of the pituitary, the ovarian tissue had no effect. This was the first major piece of evidence to show that an estrogen could affect the function of the pituitary by means of a direct nervous mechanism located somewhere near the midline of the hypothalamus in the region of the paraventricular nucleus. As we shall see in Section VI of this chapter, Harris and his colleagues began at the same time their studies on the sensitivity of this region to estrogen using behavioral end-points as well as physiological ones.

In another major study, Lisk (1960) discovered that crystalline estradiol deposited in the arcuate nucleus of a rat of either sex or in the mammillary body of the female caused a functional condition after 30 days identical to that following hypophysectomy. Thus, estradiol seemed to act on areas of hypothalamic tissue, illustrated in Fig. 5-2, to retard severely the output from the pituitary of

Fig. 5-2   Female rats: Cross-sectional diagrams of hypothalamus showing a plot of estradiol and blank needle implants. Diagrams 1 to 3 show the anterior hypothalamus, 4 and 5 the medial hypothalamus while 6 and 7 show the posterior hypothalamus. Estradiol implants which resulted in a significant change in weight of the reproductive tract are shown as black rectangles. Abbreviations: ANT, anterior nucleus; ARC, arcuate nucleus; DMD, dorsomedial nucleus, dorsal part; DM, dorsomedial nucleus; DMV, dorsomedial nucleus, ventral part; FIL, filiform nucleus; FX, column of fornix; LAT, lateral nucleus; ML, lateral mammillary nucleus; MML, medial mammillary nucleus, lateral part; MMM, medial mammillary nucleus; MT, mammillo-thalamic tract; OT, optic tract; PA, periventricular nucleus; PD, premammillary dorsalis nucleus; PV, premammillary ventral nucleus; REU, reuniens thalamic nucleus; SCH, suprachiasmatic nucleus; SO, supraoptic nucleus; VM, ventromedial nucleus; VMP, ventromedial nucleus, posterior part. (From Lisk, 1960)

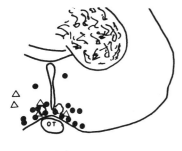

DIAG. 1

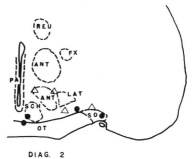

DIAG. 2

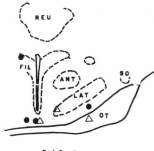

DIAG. 3

FEMALE RATS

▮	●	estradiol needle implants
	△	blank needle implants

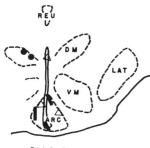

DIAG. 4

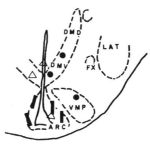

DIAG. 5

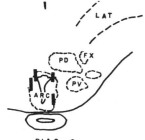

DIAG. 6

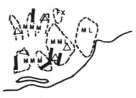

DIAG. 7

both FSH and LH. Although blank control needles had no effect, steroid controls were not carried out. Interestingly, Lisk found that the condition of the genital tract and gonads following implants of estradiol in the arcuate region resembled an atrophy of the same magnitude as that seen after hypophysectomy. Lisk then advanced the supposition that a neural mechanism governs the secretion of LH and FSH, probably through the concentration-dependent activation of cells by estrogen in the local blood supply.

A related experiment of Lisk also showed that when estradiol is implanted only in the arcuate nucleus or in the immediate surroundings of the median eminence, the normal pituitary weight and cytological characteristics are maintained in the castrated rat (Lisk, 1963). An implant of estradiol in the mammillary body failed to prevent the changes in pituitary tissue attendant to castration. These findings emphasize further the likelihood of a direct action of estrogen, probably in very low titre, on hypothalamic neurons, which in turn play a vital role in the normal functioning and structural integrity of the adenohypophysis. Since the size of a nucleolus may be an index of hormonal influence on the neuron, the diameter of the nucleoli in the arcuate nucleus was also determined (Lisk and Newlon, 1963). When estradiol was implanted in the baso-medial hypothalamus, a profound reduction was seen in the size of the arcuate nucleoli. This structure presumably mediates the amount of estrogen liberated in the circulation, by virtue of a feedback mechanism which limits the rate of release of gonadotropin.

A. Anatomical Localization

An equally important set of investigations on the rabbit was contributed by Sawyer and his co-workers beginning in the 1960s. By implanting crystalline estrogen in the tuberal region of the hypothalamus of the female rabbit, ovulation was prevented and the gonads of the animal atrophied (Davidson and Sawyer, 1961a). Nevertheless, the hormone-implanted animals mated and ovulated readily within a few days, which suggests an initial facilitatory effect of centrally acting estrogen. Implants of estrogen into other sites failed to produce similar results. This evidence favors the view that circulating estrogen acts at the level of a "gonadotropin center" in the hypothalamus to inhibit gonadotropin secretion in a negative feedback manner. The region postulated by Flerkó and Szentágothai (1957) was thought to exist in the rostral hypothalamus.

One of the first major investigations of a neural intervention in the feedback control loop for gonadal function was done on the rabbit by Kanematsu and Sawyer (1963a). They found that crystals of estradiol placed in the posterior median eminence caused an almost complete disappearance of LH from the pituitary. Subsequently, the ovarian tissue atrophied and the weight of the rabbit's uterus declined significantly. Inasmuch as estrogen implants in the anterior median eminence, pituitary stalk, or antero-dorsal part of the pars distalis failed to alter the LH levels significantly and in fact had an opposite effect on prolactin activity when the hormone was implanted into the hypothalamus or pituitary, it is not likely that estrogen exerts its effect as a result of transport to the rabbit's pituitary. Each one of these structures has an equally rich contact with the portal blood supply to the hypophysis.

Another significant observation by Kanematsu and Sawyer (1964) was the inhibition in the usual rise of LH in the plasma which follows castration 8 weeks after the local implant of estrogen in the posterior median eminence of the rabbit. The magnitude of this blockade is portrayed in Fig. 5-3. Surprisingly, when estradiol was placed in the anterior pituitary of the castrated rabbit, the LH content in plasma was even higher than the normal castrated control. As illustrated in Fig. 5-4, the implants of estrogen in the median eminence also caused a doubling in the weight of the pituitary but the steroid, as shown also in Fig. 5-4, did not have this effect when deposited either in the hypophysis itself or in other areas of the hypothalamus. In this connection, Babichev and Telegdy (1968) demonstrated that a more rostral implant of estrogen reduced progestin secretion, whereas estrogen in the medial hypothalamus enhanced its secretion. When acting on neuronal tissue, estrogen thus seems to inhibit the synthesis of

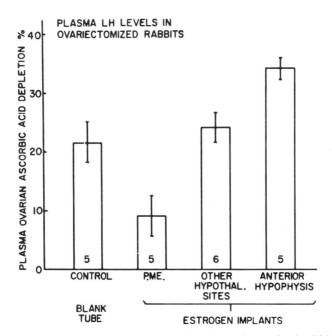

Fig. 5-3   Plasma LH levels in estrogen-implanted ovariectomized rabbits. Numbers at the bases of broad bars indicate number of rabbits on which individual plasma LH determinations were made. Narrow bars depict standard errors of the means. The PME group is significantly lower than the control group ($p < 0.05$), the other hypothalamic sites group ($p < 0.01$) or the anterior hypophysis group ($p < 0.001$). The anterior hypophysis group is significantly higher than the controls or the other hypothalamic sites group ($p < 0.02$). (From Kanematsu and Sawyer, 1964)

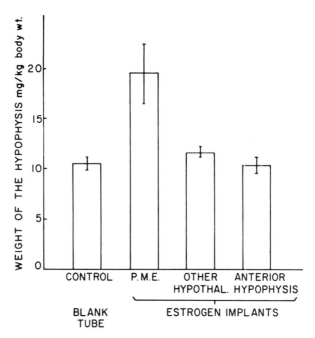

Fig. 5-4 Weight of the hypophysis relative to sites of implantation of estrogen. (From Kanematsu and Sawyer, 1964)

pituitary LH which serves to prevent an elevation of plasma LH after ovariectomy. These findings illustrated for the first time the clear-cut differences between the action of the gonadal steroid at different anatomical sites.

In the ovariectomized rat, the implantation of a mixture of crystalline estradiol-cholesterol in either the median eminence or anterior pituitary abolishes the rise in plasma LH which occurs after castration (Ramírez *et al.*, 1964). The content of LH in the rat's pituitary was similarly reduced when the steroid was placed in the hypothalamus but not in the hypophysis. In both cases, the anterior lobe was also enlarged. As depicted in Fig. 5-5, implants of the cholesterol alone or of the estrogen mixture in other parts of the brain, including the mammillary region and the nucleus suprachiasmaticus, were without effect. Thus, it would appear that two sites of action exist for the negative feedback regulation of LH synthesis and/or release.

1. *Pseudopregnancy*

A pseudopregnancy-like condition can also be induced by an implant of estrogen in the median eminence, but in an amount only a fraction of that required via the systemic route (Ramírez and McCann, 1964). The striking results of estradiol crystals placed either in the basal hypothalamus or anterior pituitary itself were: persistent diestrus; lobuloalveolar development of the mammary

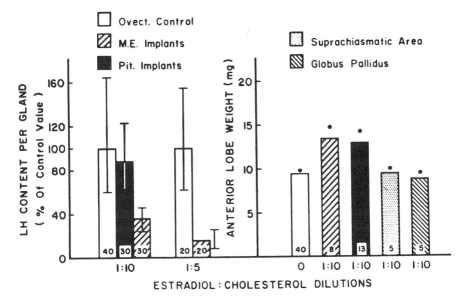

Fig. 5-5   Pituitary LH content and hypophyseal size in rats with implants of a 1:10 dilution of estradiol in cholesterol in various loci. Values for pituitary LH at the 1:10 dilution are the pooled results of two assays. Vertical lines give the 95% confidence limits. Ovect. = ovariectomized; M.E. = median eminence; Pit. = anterior pituitary; numbers = number of test rats; dots = standard error (SEM). (From Ramírez *et al.*, 1964)

glands; enlargement of the corpora lutea; an increase in the weight of the anterior lobe; and a concomitant elevation in the amount of prolactin. Control placements of a blank tube or one containing the cholesterol carrier salt had no consistent effect on the estrous response. Prolactin secretion can therefore be evoked by the direct stimulating properties of estrogen on either the hypothalamus or hypophysis.

Confirming this earlier study, Chowers and McCann (1967) again observed a pseudopregnancy after they implanted crystalline estrogen in the median eminence of the rat. Further, they confirmed Lisk's (1962a) finding that an androgen deposited in an homologous region of the rat's brain resulted in a reduction in the ovarian and uterine weights of the animal. A systemic involvement was similarly ruled out since uterine enlargement followed the subcutaneous administration of estradiol.

B. Differential Effects of Central Estrogen

After a rat has been ovariectomized unilaterally, crystalline estradiol implanted in only a 5 μg pellet in the anterior median eminence retards the compensatory hypertrophy usually witnessed in the remaining gonad (Fendler and Endröczi,

1966). A similar implantation of cortisone had a slight enhancing effect on the size of the remaining ovary. The sites of action are portrayed in Fig. 5-6. Estradiol deposited in the lateral or posterior parts of the hypothalamus (Fig. 5-6) failed to prevent the compensatory hypertrophy. These data clearly show that the estrogen inhibition of pituitary gonadotropin hypersecretion can be blocked by the action of cortisone on the basal hypothalamus. In all probability, some sort of competitive antagonism exists between the steroids.

Substantial increases in plasma corticosteroid levels occur two weeks following the deposition of estrogen in the arcuate nucleus, mammillary region or ventral tegmentum of the ovariectomized rat (Richard, 1966). If the hormone is implanted in the anterior pituitary, the adrenal steroid level is elevated as well. Both adrenal and uterine weights remain unchanged, indicating that the action of estrogen on the hypothalamic-pituitary-adrenal axis is independent of any anatomical change in the target gland. This result corresponds to those of Ramírez and McCann (1963) in that there is a possible direct effect of estrogen on the hypothalamic activation of the ACTH release from the pituitary.

Neurosecretory material (NSM) in the median eminence of the bird or rat fluctuates according to the period of exposure to light and dark. After NSM was identified histologically by a differential staining technique, Lisk (1965) observed that an implant of estrogen in the mammillary-arcuate complex augmented the amount of NSM in the median eminence of the female rat. When the animal was gonadectomized, estradiol implanted similarly prevented the typical, immediate decline in the NSM value. These changes in the amount of NSM appear to be related to the titre of estrogen circulating within the hypothalamus. Thus, a photic-induced change in NSM in the bird or rat may be the primary consequence of an altered estrogen level rather than the direct effect of light as such.

Another effect that estrogen exerts on the hypothalamus occurs during the interval of sexual development. After estradiol is implanted acutely in the anterior hypothalamic, preoptic area of the 26-day-old rat, precocious vaginal opening occurs with no notable change in either the ovarian-uterine development or in cyclicity (Smith and Davidson, 1968). On the other hand, the chronic implantation of estrogen in the median eminence of the prepubertal female impairs the normal development of the ovaries and uterus. Moreover, the period of vaginal opening is advanced by one week probably as a result of dif-

---

Fig. 5-6   Sites of action of cortisone and estradiol. AH = anterior hypothalamus; CM = mammillary body; F = fornix; OC = chiasma optici; Pa = nucleus paraventricularis; PH = posterior hypothalamus; PO = preoptic area; TC = tractus chiasmaticus; VM = ventromedial region; $\circ$ = 17-β-estradiol implants, without action; $\bullet$ = 17-β-estradiol implants, with action; $\square$ = implants of Δ^1-cortisone; $\blacklozenge$ = double implants of the two steroids, with action; $\diamondsuit$ = double implants of the two steroids, without action. (From Fendler, K. and E. Endröczi. 1966. *Neuroendocrinology.* 1:129–137. S. Karger, Basel, Switzerland)

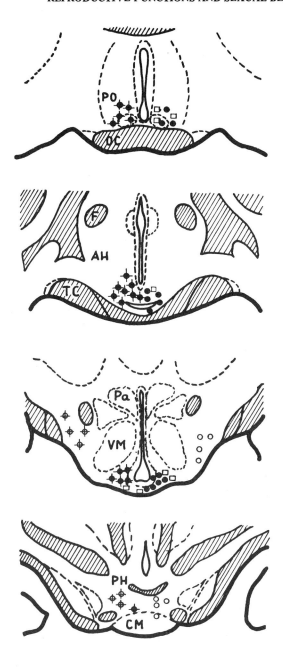

fusion to the anterior region. Thus, two localized actions of the hormone can be distinguished: (1) the acute positive estrogenic stimulation of the rostral hypothalamic cells that causes precocious puberty; and (2) the prolonged negative feedback of the female hormone on the median eminence which acts to inhibit puberty. These relationships are represented diagrammatically in Fig. 5-7 which shows the role of estrogen at three stages of puberty.

I: EARLY PRE-PUBERTY

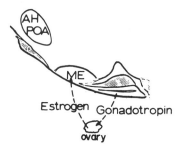

ME threshold low.
low circulating estrogen.

II: LATE PRE-PUBERTY

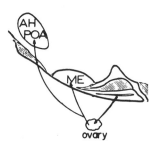

ME threshold rising.
↑ Estrogen level acts on
    anterior region.

III: PUBERTY

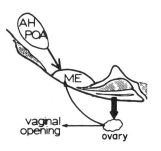

Anterior region triggered
    to activate ME
↑ Gonadotropin release

Fig. 5-7 Diagrammatic representation of hypothesis to explain the role of estrogen in the onset of puberty in the female rat. (From Smith and Davidson, 1968)

In agreement with previous reports, Motta *et al.* (1968) have also concluded that the hypothalamic implant of estrogen in the 26-day-old rat induces or advances precocious puberty and causes ovulation.   Further, the influence of estradiol on the median eminence generally is to reduce the synthesis of LH in the pituitary but in some instances increase its release into the bloodstream. When estradiol was deposited in the habenular nuclei, pituitary LH increased, whereas the weights of the uteri and ovaries declined.   The close anatomical relationship to the pineal gland could explain the negative feedback role that may be played by the habenula. The individual sites of action of estradiol within the hypothalamus probably contribute to the differences observed between the pubertal and prepubertal animal.

A diffuse system of cells traversing the hypothalamus seems to be sensitive to estrogen in relation to behavior that is not entirely sexual. For example, when crystals of estradiol are deposited in the basal anterior, posterior and even lateral areas of the hypothalamus, a sudden onset in running activity ensues in females that were relatively indolent following prior ovariectomy (Colvin and Sawyer, 1969). Wade and Zucker (1970) confirmed these findings again in the ovariectomized rat, although the anatomical sites in the two studies that were sensitive to estrogen do not correspond precisely. Of some note is the fact that the basal anterior hypothalamus is the same area in which Lisk (1962b) induced the lordosis response in the rat with estrogen. Thus, the motor components of the hypothalamic efferent outflow may be modified by female hormones.

C. Hypothalamic Versus Pituitary Receptors

The inhibitory effect on male gonads of an estrogen injected in the anterior hypothalamus was reported by von Hohlweg and Daume in 1959 to be over a 100-fold more potent than when the hormone was given by the subcutaneous route. This report was taken as further evidence of the feedback action on neural structures that are highly sensitive to the presence of a hormone. However, Bogdanove (1963a) questioned the efficacy of intrahypothalamic estrogen and reported that estrogen pellets deposited intracranially were no more effective than a subcutaneous implant of the hormone.

Estrogen implanted into the hypothalamus retards the development, histologically speaking, of castration cells within the pituitary of the rat following removal of its gonads (Bogdanove, 1963b).   The direct implantation in the pituitary of estrogen had a much more localized effect which meant that an insufficient amount of the glandular tissue was influenced for an effect to be detected systemically. From these data arose the famous "implantation paradox" of Bogdanove (see Chapter 2). In essence, Bogdanove proposed that the action of the steroid on the hypothalamus is due solely to its local uptake into the hypophyseal-portal blood supply. After the hormone enters the capillary network or other small blood vessels, it is then distributed evenly throughout the pituitary where it exerts a direct, primary action. Bogdanove implied that hypothalamic tissue may not contain steroid receptors after all but instead a convenient route of entry into the local circulation. The implications of the paradox hypothesis are discussed fully in Chapter 2 in the broader context of transport hypotheses.

1. *Dual Target Sites*

That a critical region for estrogen suppression of gonadotropin function in the rat may be in the mammillary-arcuate complex has nevertheless been argued by many scientists. For example, Lisk (1965b) demonstrated that estrogen crystals deposited in the anterior hypothalamus or directly in the adenohypophysis in equal quantity evoked pseudopregnancy in a large number of cases. These findings taken together with others do not support the hypotheses of Flerkó and Szentágothai (1957) or Bogdanove (1963a). On the contrary, they show that there are probably at least three regions of estrogenic receptivity: (a) one located in the anterior hypothalamus which when stimulated initiates and maintains mating behavior; (b) a second more posterior area that is a key neural link in the feedback inhibition of the hypophyseal-gonadal axis; and (c) a conglomerate of trophic-hormone releasing cells in the anterior pituitary. An inexplicable finding is the deleterious effects on parturition produced by testosterone or progesterone implanted in the same regions. Prolonged and often lethal labor ensued and at parturition, although the rats carried the litter to term, some of the young were not viable. In other cases, the mothers ate the newborn pups at once.

Another crucial experiment to test the Bogdanove hypothesis was conducted by Palka *et al.* (1966) who used tritium-labelled estradiol or the acetate salt in order to trace the activity of the steroid both in the brain and hypophysis. As in the report of Michael (1966), a sharp gradient in the distribution of estrogen radioactivity was found in the area surrounding the implant 4 to 5 days after its placement in the median eminence. As shown in Fig. 5-8, only small amounts of estrogen were detected beyond 1.0 mm of the site. Unexpectedly, greater radioactivity was found in the ipsilateral pituitary than when ^{3}H estradiol was placed directly into the hypophysis itself, which would lend partial support to a portal vessel transport hypothesis. Physiologically, the rats with the hypothalamic estrogen implant showed an elevation in plasma LH, but those animals containing a pituitary implant did not; hence, estrogen crystals implanted in the pituitary seem to be carried away at a faster rate than those deposited in the median eminence. The latter animals did, however, show ipsilateral pituitary hypertrophy which again shows that estrogen does exert separate actions on neural and glandular tissue. Palka *et al.* concluded that estrogen stimulates LH release when acting on the median eminence of the hypothalamus, and also causes cytological changes in the pituitary by its direct action on the hypophyseal cells.

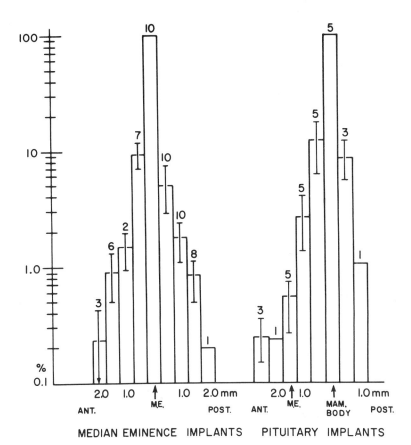

Fig. 5-8 Spread of radioactivity within the brain around site of implantation. Activity at implantation site is expressed as 100%; radioactivity at other sites is expressed as a percentage of this value. Values on the abscissa indicate distance in millimeters from the implantation site. Vertical lines indicate standard error of the mean and numbers above each column indicate number of determinations performed. In the case of pituitary implants, greatest activity was in implantation track in mammillary region. (From Palka *et al.*, 1966)

III. PROGESTERONE RECEPTORS

Even though theirs was one of the first definitive anatomical investigations in this field, Ralph and Fraps (1960) nevertheless showed convincingly that 5 μg of progesterone injected in only a 1 μl volume into the brain of the female chicken induces premature ovulation. The sites sensitive to progesterone were located mainly in the rostral and caudal portions of the hen's hypothalamus as well as in the caudal neostriatum. When injected into the pituitary of the chicken, progesterone exerted no effect. This result corresponds with the finding that a lesion in a similar part of the hen's brain also blocks ovulation (Ralph and Fraps, 1959).

A. Anatomical Localization

The site at which progesterone acts to suppress the ovulatory surge of LH release in the mammal again is the basal portion of the hypothalamus (Labhsetwar and Bainbridge, 1971). About 400 μg crystalline progesterone deposited in the median eminence of the prepubertal rat reduces the weight of the uterus and suppresses estrous cycling (Smith *et al.*, 1969). In the pubertal rat, so designated by the day of vaginal opening, progesterone implanted similarly also eliminated the luteinization of the ovaries and lowered the weight of the gonads, as shown in Fig. 5-9. A critical aspect of these findings is the absence of any major effect when the steroid was placed in the pituitary, anterior hypothalamus or mesencephalon. When implanted chronically in the median eminence of the adult rat, there were no changes in sexual function except for the disruptive effect on vaginal cycling which appeared only to be transitory. Although the negative feedback property of progesterone that is characteristic of androgen and estrogen was demonstrated, a very high 400 μg dose was required to produce this effect. This could account for the relative lack of gonadotropin suppression reported by Lisk (1965b) and Kanematsu and Sawyer (1965) following the implantation of much lower doses of progesterone at an homologous site.

When crystals of progesterone are implanted in the ventromedial hypothalamic arcuate region in an amount one-hundredth of the effective systemic dose, ovulation occurs in rats that have been treated earlier with systemic progesterone during metestrus (Döcke and Dörner, 1969). When progesterone is deposited in the anterior pituitary or in the anterior or posterior parts of the hypothalamus depicted in Fig. 5-10, the ovulatory response advances in relatively few cases. Bilateral implants of progesterone in the anterior pituitary do not induce ovulation, thus minimizing the possibility that the steroid is acting on the hypophysis rather than on the relatively circumscribed, basal area of neural tissue. Progesterone could facilitate ovulation by lowering the activation threshold for the releasing factors in the ventromedial hypothalamic-arcuate complex. This activation is initiated by the neural impulses emanating from the anterior, preoptic region, a supposition derived from experiments utilizing lesions and electrical stimulation.

Further anatomical delimitation of the ovulatory mechanism has been provided by experiments with copper salts which, when given intravenously, can evoke ovulation in the rabbit. When Hiroi *et al.* (1965) implanted copper sulfate in the posterior median eminence of the rabbit, ovulation, as determined by postmortem examination, occurred in every animal within 24 to 48 hours. In all rabbits in which the copper was deposited in the anterior pituitary, copper failed to evoke the ovulatory response. Even so, the local mechanism of action

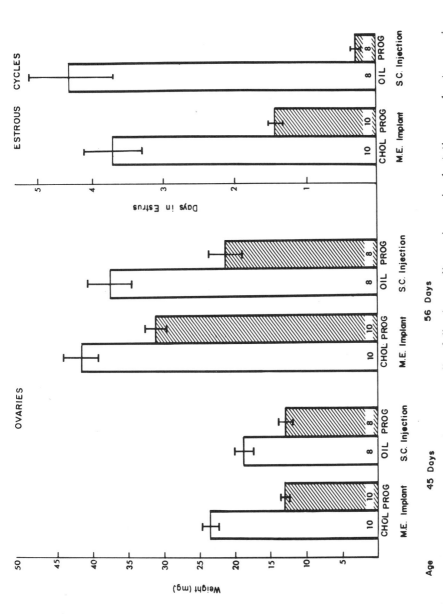

Fig. 5-9   Ovarian weight and estrous cycling following median eminence implantation or subcutaneous injection (5 mg/day) of progesterone.   Treatments commenced at 30 days of age.   (From Smith *et al.*, 1969)

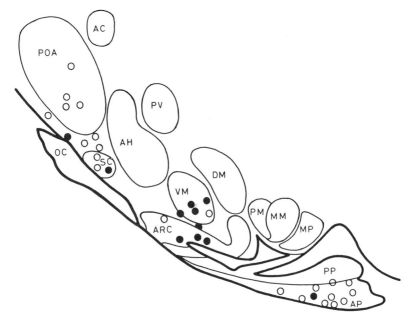

Fig. 5-10   Parasagittal diagram of rat hypothalamus (de Groot, 1959) illustrating localizations of bilateral progesterone implants in cyclic progesterone-pretreated female rats.   Solid circles represent bilateral implants that advanced ovulation; open circles indicate implants that did not advance ovulation. Abbreviations: AC = anterior commissure; AH = anterior hypothalamic area; AP = anterior pituitary; ARC = arcuate nucleus; DM = dorsomedial nucleus; MM = medial mammillary nucleus; MP = posterior mammillary nucleus; OC = optic chiasma; PM = dorsal premammillary nucleus; POA = preoptic area; PP = posterior pituitary; PV = paraventricular nucleus; SC = suprachiasmatic nucleus; VM = ventromedial nucleus. (From Döcke, F. and G. Dörner. 1969. *Neuroendocrinology.* 4:139–149. S. Karger, Basel, Switzerland)

of the metal on the cells of the tuberal region remains obscure. It should be mentioned that the same Japanese workers were able to determine the effective dose of copper sulfate on the cells of the median eminence. By infusing a solution rather than implanting crystals, they found that 0.76 μg/kg of copper, which was only $\frac{1}{4000}$ of the effective intravenous dose, induced ovulation (Suzuki *et al.*, 1965). This reflects the extreme sensitivity of the basal hypothalamus to the copper salt.

B. Induced Functional Changes

It is possible to introduce an alteration in the diestrous interval of the rat if estrogen is administered on the second or third day of diestrus. In this case, the 5-day cycle is advanced and the rat ovulates 1 day early (Weick and Davidson,

1970). The locus of this estrogenic effect is apparently in the pituitary, since an implant of estradiol in the rostral hypothalamus or median eminence is not effective. However, if estradiol is placed in the anterior pituitary of 5-day "cyclers," ovulation is advanced by 1 day and vaginal cornification appears. Thus, the steroid acts on the rat's hypophysis to precipitate the release of gonadotropin. In addition, the estrogen may sensitize the pituitary cells to gonadotropin-releasing factor elaborated from the hypothalamus as proposed by Döcke and Dörner (1969).

By varying the size of the progesterone or estrogen implant in 27 or 30 gauge tubing, Lisk (1969a) has been able to show that localized implants of estrogen in the basal hypothalamus can augment the pituitary weight probably by a direct action on the gland itself. The distance of the implant site from the region of the sella turcica determines the size of the increase. On the other hand, a similar implant of progesterone has no effect on the pituitary although the usual diminution in uterine weight and ovarian weight does occur.

The extent to which anatomical sites of the hypothalamus and limbic system are sensitive to ovarian steroids has been examined extensively by Kawakami et al. (1969). In terms of the localized action of female hormones deposited in brain tissue in mediating the biosynthesis of ovarian steroids including progesterone, estrogen and their analogues, the structures delimited in order of their sensitivity to crystalline implants of estrogen are: arcuate nucleus > amygdala > anterior hypothalamus > supraoptic nucleus > preoptic area > ventromedial hypothalamus. Somewhat different is the order of the sensitivity of structures stimulated with crystals of progesterone, again with the biosynthesis of ovarian steroids as the index of action: hippocampus > ventromedial hypothalamus > preoptic area > arcuate nucleus > supraoptic nucleus > anterior hypothalamus > amygdala. Based on these morphological considerations, unusually complicated anatomical interrelationships exist within these subcortical structures. In terms of either the acceleration or inhibition of the ovarian synthesis of both progesterone and estrogen, some of the pathways are reciprocal while others are probably strictly facilitory. With this morphological analysis, Kawakami et al. make a strong case that multiple cerebral foci for feedback control must be recognized instead of only those presumed to be present in the hypothalamus. This view is currently being upheld with some certitude by the studies on the binding by the brain of labelled gonadal steroids.

IV. ANDROGEN RECEPTORS

In the 1960s, a series of experiments similar to that undertaken with the female steroids were begun in an attempt to find out whether androgen-sensitivity is also a property of neural elements in the brain-stem. For example, Knigge (1962) implanted a whole pituitary of a rat into the anterior hypothalamic, preoptic area and ventromedial hypothalamus of the male rat after it had been hypophysectomized. Although gonadotrophic activity seemed to be maintained, no other trophic influences were noted. However, earlier experiments with the dog had revealed that testosterone implanted in the hypothalamus had very unique physiological effects (Davidson and Sawyer, 1961b). When the locus of the crystalline implant is the median eminence, gonadotropin secretion is held in check by the presence of the androgen in this region. The testes and prostate glands become atrophied, the sperm count is reduced and motility of sperm declines sharply. These observations of Davidson and Sawyer (1961b) provided the first direct evidence for the role of the hypothalamus in a negative feedback mechanism involving androgen in the release of male gonadotropin from the pituitary.

A. Anatomical Localization

The implantation of crystals of testosterone in the arcuate nucleus or rostral mammillary region of either the female or male rat causes ovarian atrophy as well as atrophic responses in the testes and accessory male organs when these tissues are examined 50 days later (Lisk, 1962a). However, the tuberal region of the female rat is far more sensitive to an implant of crystalline testosterone than the same area in the male. It would appear that the tuberal area-median eminence serves possibly as the final common pathway for the negative feedback control of the gonadotropin secretion from the pituitary.

In a similar study, an implant of either crystalline testosterone or estrogen in the median eminence or mammillary bodies of the male rat again reduced the size of the accessory organs, the ventral prostate and seminal vesicles (Chowers and McCann, 1963). When deposited directly into the anterior pituitary or in the lateral or anterior hypothalamus, the hormones were without effect. Similarly, peripherally administered testosterone produced the typical opposite change, thus demonstrating a clear-cut central action. In addition to confirming the earlier results of Lisk with the rat (1960, 1962a) and Sawyer and his colleagues with the dog and rabbit (Davidson and Sawyer, 1961b; Kanematsu and Sawyer, 1963a), the negative results with implants of crystalline cholesterol demonstrated again the hypothalamic sensitivity to gonadal steroids.

When testosterone pellets are implanted in the median eminence of immature 30-day-old rats, the subsequent development of the testes and accessory glands, on examination 3 weeks later, is severely impeded (Smith and Davidson, 1967). This retardation fails to occur in the young adult that is 70 days of age or older. Cholesterol implants in control rats also produced no developmental anomalies. These striking differences in testicular growth are illustrated in Fig. 5-11. In the young rat, probably FSH and LH secretion from the pituitary is inhibited by the presence of androgen in the hypothalamus in an artificially high concentration.

In the normal or castrated male rat, a bilateral implant of testosterone in the pituitary increases the concentration of FSH as well as the absolute content of

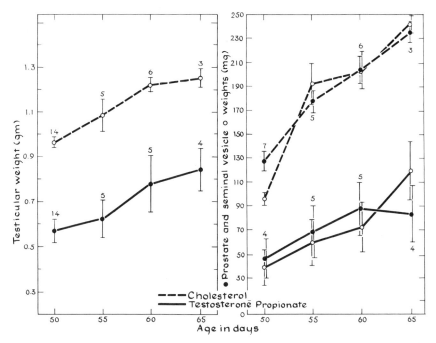

Fig. 5-11   Growth of right testis, ventral prostate (●), and seminal vesicle (○) with increasing time after implantation of cholesterol or testosterone in median eminence. All implants were placed at 30 days of age, and left testis was removed at 50 days in all cases. (From Smith and Davidson, 1967)

FSH in pituitary tissue (Kamberi and McCann, 1972). A unilateral implant in the median eminence, however, causes only a slight augmentation in FSH levels in the pituitary which is not statistically significant. Thus, the androgen acts on the pituitary directly in a feedback manner to diminish the release of FSH from the pituitary which would naturally elevate its content. On the other hand, the concentration of testosterone in the median eminence may not have been sufficiently high to produce an effect on FSH. It is possible, furthermore, that testosterone's effect on neural tissue may be somewhat greater than that on the pituitary.

B. Seasonal Factors

The nervous systems of certain seasonal breeders such as the duck and lizard also possess a remarkable sensitivity to sex steroids. When either testosterone or estradiol is implanted in the median eminence of the desert iguana shortly after its emergence from hibernation in the spring, the seasonal maturation of gonadal elements is retarded or totally abolished (Lisk, 1967a). Spermatogenesis ceases in the male lizard, whereas ovarian weight and egg size are reduced in the female. An implant of hormone outside of this region is not effective.

That seasonal development of the gonads depends on a hypothalamic stimulus in this poikilotherm is comparable to the situation in a homeothermic bird. Kordon and Gogan (1964) found that testosterone deposited in the ventromedial portion of the hypothalamus of the Pekin duck maintains the regression of the testicles that was induced earlier by keeping the birds in total darkness. It is particularly interesting that the median eminence of the duck does not appear to be sensitive to the presence of excess androgen.

Later, Gogan (1968) delimited two regions of the Pekin duck's hypothalamus that are reactive to androgen. Testicular development is inhibited and the content of pituitary gonadotropin is reduced after testosterone is deposited in the anterior region. The effect is much more potent, however, when the androgen is implanted in the ventromedial area. Then the duck's testes undergo complete regression and the gonadotropin in the pituitary is depleted.

The Japanese quail possesses an identical anatomical organization in terms of androgen receptivity. Deposited in the ventromedial part of the hypothalamus, testosterone crystals act to regress the quail's testes and cloacal gland and to lower the concentration of pituitary gonadotropins (Stetson, 1972). Although these effects are transitory in the adult breeder, the control implants in the preoptic, supraoptic, infundibular and other regions, all of which have no effect, confirm the morphological specificity of androgen's effect on the bird's hypothalamus. Since testicular and cloacal regression also follow the placement of testosterone in the adenohypophysis, the quail, just as in the rodent, could have dual target sites for the androgen feedback control mechanism.

V. MECHANISM OF GONADOTROPIN RELEASE

As a corollary to the hypothesis of a short-feedback loop described in Chapter 4 for the hypothalamic control of ACTH release, suprisingly good support has likewise evolved for a similar sort of mechanism underlying gonadotropin secretion. To illustrate, part of the volume of FSH secreted from the pituitary, for example, would reach the cells in the hypothalamic hypophysiotrophic area that liberate the corresponding releasing factor, FSH-RF. The possibility has been raised by many investigators that a distinct neural locus for this feedback activity has developed in the mammal. For example, Gorski and Barraclough (1962) showed that a small lesion placed in the anterior hypothalamus curtails rather markedly the secretion of FSH from the adenohypophysis with a subsequent imbalance in the release of LH as well.

A related study of Ramírez and McCann (1963) has revealed that the content of LH in the blood following gonadectomy nevertheless increases in both the immature and adult rat. Based on the evidence that the small amount of estrogen released by the immature ovary could act to prevent LH secretion, the notion has arisen logically that puberty could be dependent upon a resetting of a hypothalamic "gonadostat." Consequently, the loss in the hypothalamic sensitivity of this negative feedback effect of estrogen, as the animal grows, signals the onset of full sexual development.

A. Luteinizing Hormone (LH)

When luteinizing hormone (LH) is implanted directly in the median eminence of the intact rat, the pituitary stores of the hormone are reduced. In the castrated female, the plasma LH levels are also lower after an LH implant indicating that an accelerated release of LH from the pituitary is not the prime cause (David *et al.*, 1966). FSH implanted similarly or LH crystals placed in the cerebral cortex or pituitary itself have no effect. Therefore, LH receptors which are part of a short-feedback mechanism seem to be present in the neural tissue of the basal hypothalamus. A summary of the distinct feedback loops that are believed to control LH secretion is presented in Fig. 5-12. An excess of hormone upon

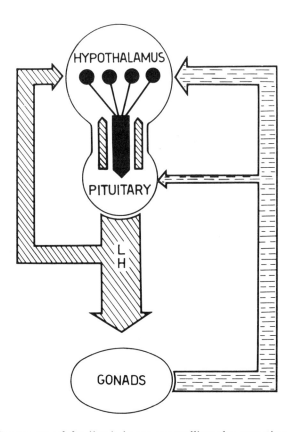

Fig. 5-12 Summary of feedback loops controlling the secretion of LH. The black arrow which connects the hypothalamus with the pituitary is a schematic representation of the main portal vessels, into which hypothalamic neurosecretion cells and fibers release their stimulating peptides (LH-RF, CRF, etc.). Interrupted lines = gonadal steroids feeding back on the hypothalamus and/or on the pituitary. Diagonal lines = LH feeding back on the hypothalamus either through the general circulation or through the blood of the portal vessels. (From David *et al.*, 1966)

reaching these receptors would inhibit further production of LH. These findings correspond well with the related fact that there is a high concentration of LH in the median eminence as well as a portal system for bi-directional transport of the hormonal factor.

The implantation of LH in the median eminence of the intact 50-day-old female rat lowers the content of LH in the pituitary (Corbin and Cohen, 1966). A true inhibition of LH synthesis is inferred from these results, and the mechanism would seem to involve a direct negative feedback effect on the mobilization of LH releasing factor (LHRF). Together with gonadal steroids, LH could play a role in impinging upon the neural controller in the basal hypothalamus. Repeating the study with 50-day-old ovariectomized instead of intact rats, Corbin (1966) saw the same sort of reduction in pituitary stores of LH following its implantation in the median eminence. Once again, a significant decline in plasma LH was not found.

To obtain additional insight into the question of a short-feedback loop of endogenous LH, Makino et al. (1972) implanted a specific rabbit anti-sheep LH serum into the median eminence of the ovariectomized rat. Using the technique of radio-immunoassay, they found that the content of LH in the pituitary is lower 6 days later but the serum level remains unchanged. Since the specific antiserum is able to neutralize rat LH, Makino et al. concluded that endogenous LH within the hypothalamus is involved in the control of LH synthesis in the hypophysis. However, it is possible that the neutralizing effect may have been on the anterior pituitary, since LH itself possesses the same action in lowering pituitary LH.

B. Follicle Stimulating Hormone (FSH)

Contrary to the report by David et al. (1966) that FSH has little effect on the cells of the median eminence, Corbin and Story (1967) provided the initial positive result to support the belief that this pituitary gonadotropin could feed back directly to the hypothalamic control mechanism via the so-called "short" route. By chemically extracting the cells of the pituitary stalk-median eminence and using a bioassay to detect a releasing factor, Corbin and Story showed that the content of hypothalamic FSH-RF is markedly lower in the intact female rat with a median eminence implant of crystalline FSH. The amount of pituitary FSH is likewise lower in these animals. These results parallel quite distinctly those in which LH has the same internal feedback property of trophic inhibition of neural tissue.

The surprisingly specific action of FSH in contrast to other trophic hormones was demonstrated by Arai and Gorski (1968). Following the removal of one ovary, an implant in the basal medial hypothalamus of the rat of either FSH or pregnant mare's serum gonadotropin blocks very effectively the typical compensatory hypertrophy of the remaining ovary. A similar implant of LH, ACTH,

TSH or human chorionic gonadotropin does not interfere with the ovarian hypertrophy. Thus, it would seem that FSH acts to selectively inhibit the hypothalamic FSH-releasing factor system, presumably by the internal, short-feedback mechanism.

After crystalline LH is deposited within the median eminence of the 30-day-old-rat, the ovaries atrophy and the formation of corpora lutea is almost entirely absent (Ojeda and Ramírez, 1969). A rat that receives a similar implant in the pituitary itself is identical to a cholesterol implanted control. On the other hand, FSH deposited again in the median eminence surprisingly does not reduce the size of the uterus; instead, these rats presented a high incidence of corpora lutea, shown in Fig. 5-13, and clear evidence of luteinization and large follicles. In the immature rat, LH apparently regulates its own local secretion by acting back directly on the cells of the stalk-median eminence region. This clearly supports the idea of a short-feedback mechanism for this hormone. However,

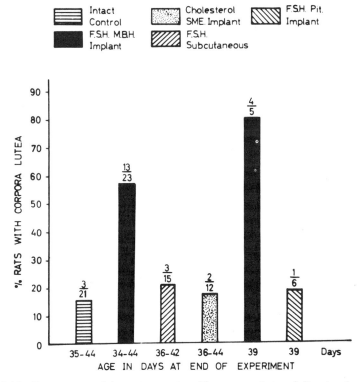

Fig. 5-13 Percentage of immature rats with corpora lutea following implantation of FSH and cholesterol in different loci. The bars indicate the percentage value of corpora lutea present in each group. Figures above bars refer to ratio of number of rats with corpora lutea to the total number of animals. (From Ojeda and Ramírez, 1969)

FSH deposited in the young animal seems to cause a greater release of FSH from the pituitary which may differ from the local hypothalamic action of FSH in the adult rat (Corbin and Story, 1967).

In the immature male rat with one testis surgically removed, an FSH implant in the medial-basal portion of the hypothalamus has little effect on the compensatory hypertrophy ordinarily seen in the remaining testicle (Ojeda and Ramírez, 1972). In the adult male, however, FSH deposited at homologous sites did diminish significantly the compensatory testicular growth in males that had retained the implant for 20 days. Similarly, in the immature female rat subjected to hemi-ovariectomy at 30 days of age, an implant of FSH in the ventromedial hypothalamus could not block the compensatory hypertrophy of the remaining ovary (Ojeda and Ramírez, 1970). Even estrogen injected subcutaneously in the implanted prepubertal female fails to prevent the gonad's development. The factor of age seems critical since the negative feedback mechanism for FSH in the adult is absent in the sexually immature rat.

Using a bioassay technique for FSH, Hirono et al. (1970) further tested the hypothesis of the short-feedback control of gonadotropin release. After FSH was deposited in the median eminence of an ovariectomized or normal adult rat, the plasma level and pituitary content of FSH declined significantly; the latter reduction of pituitary FSH has also been observed in the adult male rat after an implant of FSH in the hypothalamus (Ojeda and Ramírez, 1972). In both instances, the plasma and pituitary concentration of LH remained unaltered. These data supplement those of Corbin and Story (1967) and further support the idea of a "short negative feedback" pathway taken by FSH in inhibiting both the synthesis of the gonadotropin in the pituitary and its subsequent release into the bloodstream.

C. Prolactin

An important observation of Clemens and Meites (1968) has helped to clarify the central participation in the control of prolactin secretion. When they deposited crystalline prolactin in the median eminence of either the intact or ovariectomized mature rat, the mammary glands regressed rapidly in relation to the simultaneous decline in the content of prolactin in the pituitary. Of special significance was the elevated concentration of prolactin-inhibitory factor (PIF) within the hypothalamus observed by Clemens and Meites in the prolactin implanted rat. This, of course, reflects a sharp increase in PIF synthesis.

The concept that the basal tuberal region of the hypothalamus produces a prolactin-inhibitory factor (PIF) to control prolactin release from the pituitary was further explored by Mishkinsky et al. (1968). Perphenazine, a tranquilizer which induces copious lactation, presumably by blocking the CNS inhibitory mechanism, was implanted in the median eminence or other sites in the brain of the rabbit. After 14 days had elapsed, the mammary glands were fully developed. This indicates the lack of release of the inhibitory factor (PIF) from the hypothalamus which in turn stops the secretion of prolactin from the anterior pituitary. A specificity of action was shown by the controls consisting of an implant of aminopromazine in the tuberal region or perphenazine crystals deposited in other parts of the brain, both of which were without effect. Fluphenazine has a similar mammotrophic action (Mishkinsky et al., 1969).

Although a single implant of FSH or LH in the median eminence of the pseudopregnant rat has no effect on the duration of pseudopregnancy, prolactin deposited at the same site shortens the period of pseudopregnancy. In addition, prolactin inhibits the formation of deciduomata by acting in a negative feedback manner (Chen et al., 1968). Prolactin, therefore, appears to be an integral if not essential factor in the maintenance of this artificial condition. Apparently, the presence of prolactin in the hypothalamus in an elevated quantity can depress its subsequent synthesis and release from the pituitary which seems to be requisite for normal luteal function.

In the 21-day-old rat, prolactin placed in the median eminence of the female causes a release of hypophyseal FSH as indicated by the fall in the level of the trophic hormone in the pituitary (Voogt et al., 1969). Acting directly on the immature ovaries, FSH stimulated the growth of follicles and enhanced estrogen secretion with a resultant development of the uterus. The local hypothalamic action of prolactin corresponds to earlier results obtained with mature rats (Clemens and Meites, 1968) as well as to the effect of terminating pregnancy or pseudopregnancy (Chen et al., 1968). A complex interaction between prolactin and gonadotropin secretion seems to exist at the level of the basal hypothalamus (Welsch et al., 1968).

An interesting series of experiments has been performed by Tindal and his co-workers using what they term an "oestrode," a cannula containing fused estrogen at its tip. When an "oestrode" was implanted in amygdaloid nuclei or in the rostral or lateral hypothalamus of the rabbit made pseudopregnant with human gonadotropin, lactogenesis occurred in only 8 out of 48 rabbits studied (Tindal and Knaggs, 1966). In each case, the "oestrode" tip was found to be in the basomedial part of the amygdala. Thus, prolactin or prolactin-ACTH release may be triggered by estrogen-sensitive neurons in the amygdala which act via the stria medullaris on the hypophysiotrophic area of the hypothalamus. Other sites in the limbic system are also sensitive to estrogen since lactogenesis, resulting ostensibly from pituitary prolactin secretion, occurred in pseudopregnant rabbits after estradiol was implanted in the medial amygdaloid nucleus or the stria terminalis (Tindal et al., 1967). Negative sites were found in the more anterior part of the amygdaloid complex as well as in many parts of the limbic system including the lateral hypothalamus and hippocampus. Thus, a fine-control mechanism of the hypothalamic-hypophyseal final common pathway for the lactogenic response may be mediated by the amygdala via the stria medullaris.

VI. CENTRAL ENDOCRINE EFFECTS ON SEXUAL BEHAVIOR

Among the neuroendocrinologists there is a widespread concurrence that gonadal hormones are necessary for the distinctive expression of mammalian sexual behavior. Historically, the significance of specific areas of the central nervous system was examined experimentally in the 1930s by Ranson and his colleagues (Fisher *et al.*, 1938; Dey *et al.*, 1940; Brookhart *et al.*, 1941). Generally, they found that a lesion of the rostral hypothalamus halted all aspects of mating behavior. Moreover, these remarkable deficits could not be reinstated by the so-called replacement therapy of giving estrogen systemically. What was such a telling point was the absence of ovarian or uterine atrophy. This is opposite to the atrophy of the gonads and pituitary hyperfunction following a lesion to the median eminence (Bogdanove, 1957; Sawyer, 1959); the decline in estrous behavior in these latter animals is usually reversible if exogenous hormone is administered.

A. Mating in the Female

The original observation in 1958 of Harris and Michael on the estrogen-induced mating behavior in the castrated cat led to an entirely new approach to the experimental analysis of hypothalamic function (Harris and Michael, 1958; Harris *et al.*, 1958). When the dibutyrate form of stilbestrol was applied locally to the posterior hypothalamus, 13 of 17 ovariectomized cats exhibited persistent mating behavior even though 9 of the 13 animals showed all of the signs of an anestrous genital tract. Harris *et al.* (1958) concluded that these sexual responses were due to a local action of the hormone on neurons in the caudal hypothalamus.

In an unusually detailed study with a large number of cats and carefully prepared histology, Harris and Michael (1964) found that stilbestrol, which was fused to a needle tip implanted in the region of the mammillary body of the ovariectomized cat, produced a sustained sexual receptivity even in the absence of a developed genital tract. The latency of onset of mating after the stilbestrol implant ranged from 4 to 106 days—the latter of which is difficult to explain. An implant in other sites including the amygdala, thalamus and cerebellum failed to evoke mating behavior in that only 1 out of 21 females developed estrous reflexes and accepted a tomcat. These anatomical controls and the control implants with cholesterol, progesterone and paraffin wax that were all ineffective would rule out any systemic influence of the steroid. Harris and Michael concluded that an estrogen sensitive mechanism exists in the hypothalamus since the hormone seems to act directly on neural tissue.

Later, Michael found that the deposition of a large amount of stilbestrol at individual sites extending from the preoptic area to the caudal mammillary region could evoke the full pattern of mating behavior in an ovariectomized cat (Michael, 1965). The active implant sites, however, were always situated in

TABLE 5-1   Calculation of Approximate Concentration of Stilbestrol di-*n*-butyrate ^{14}C in Tissue Adjacent to the Site of 0.2 mg Implant (from Michael, 1961)

Cat killed after 41 consecutive days of mating
Incubation time t = 305 days

Distance in μ	50	150	250	350	450	
Average grain count per $(10\,\mu)^2$ above background	146	26	9	4	3	
Stilbestrol di-*n*-butyrate concentration in γ per 1000 μ^3	64	11.6	4.1	1.8	1.4	$\times 10^{-9}$
Concentration in moles per 1000 μ^3	9.6	1.7	0.6	0.3	0.2	$\times 10^{7}$

Not significant
above
background

the very basal portion of this diencephalic region, indicating that specific neural receptors for estrogens can trigger the complete sexual response.

The release rate of estrogen crystals placed in the hypothalamus is not necessarily correlated with the manifestation of mating behavior in the female cat (Michael, 1961). Further, absorption curves for each implant can show a differential rate of release of estrogen from the needle tip regardless of the neuroanatomical site of implantation. After radio-labelled estrogen (^{14}C diethyl-stilbestrol di-*n*-butyrate) was placed in the hypothalamus of the female cat, the spread of the steroid as assessed by autoradiography was negligible within 250 μ from the site of the implant. As shown in Table 5-1, such a steep concentration gradient of the hormone in the neural tissue in the immediate vicinity of the implant is probably sufficient for maintaining sexual behavior in the animal for many weeks or even months.

In cats which had been ovariectomized 6 months before stilbestrol di-*n*-butyrate was implanted, a minute quantity of the hormone again evoked mating behavior if the crystals were placed in the medial-basal hypothalamus at sites extending from the anterior to posterior hypothalamus (Michael, 1966). The sensitive loci are portrayed in Fig. 5-14. Sexual responses never occurred when the estrogen crystal was deposited in the ventricle. Even with a completely atrophied genital tract, the female cat exhibited the entire pattern of mating behavior. As soon as the implant was removed from the hypothalamus, the mating behavior disappeared, which demonstrates the entire dependence of the sexual response on the presence of the estrogen in the hypothalamus.

1. *Species Continuity*

An implant of 10% estrogen in crystalline cholesterol in a circumscribed area in the medial hypothalamus of the rabbit just rostral to the mammillary complex

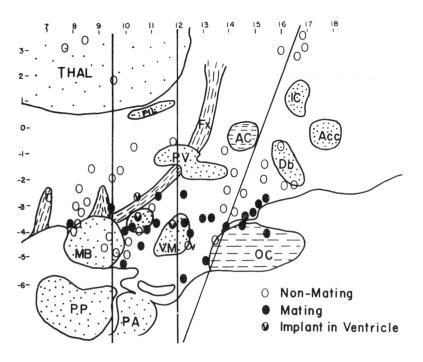

Fig. 5-14 Distribution of stilbestrol di-*n*-butyrate implants on a lateral projection of the cat hypothalamus and the effects upon mating behavior (results from 65 experiments). The sexual "system" extends from the mammillary region to the preoptic region. Sagittal plane: 1.0 mm lateral (millimeter scales give anterior and vertical stereotaxic coordinates). Abbreviations: AC, anterior commissure; Acc, nucleus accumbens; Db, diagonal band; FIL, nucleus filiformis; Fx, fornix; IC, island of Calleja; MB, mammillary body; OC, optic chiasm; PA, pars anterior; PP, pars posterior; PV, paraventricular nucleus; THAL, thalamus; VM, ventromedial nucleus. (From Michael, R. P. 1966. *In: Brain and Behavior, Vol. III.* R. A. Gorski and R. E. Whalen (eds.), pp. 81–98. Originally published by the University of California Press; reprinted by permission of the Regents of the University of California)

evoked estrous behavior including a marked lordosis within 1 to 2 days. As indicated in Fig. 5-15, this did not happen when the steroid was placed in other hypothalamic regions (Palka and Sawyer, 1966a). The morphological features of the rabbit's uterus in each instance were identical to the anestrous castrate control. When crystals of undiluted estradiol were implanted again at sites throughout the hypothalamus, the same mating pattern was evoked within 3 to 4 days which would reflect the probable spread of the concentrated steroid to the ventromedial region. Progesterone implants in the VMH tended to reduce the mating response in the ovariectomized rabbit brought into heat by systemic estrogen.

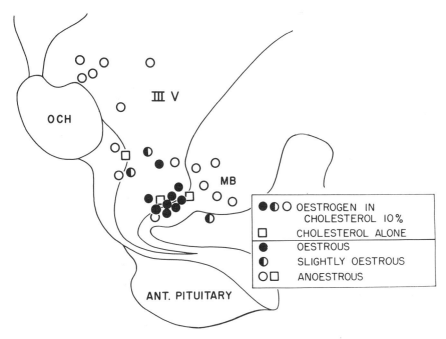

Fig. 5-15 Midsagittal diagram of the rabbit hypothalamus indicating the location of bilateral implants of 10% estrogen in cholesterol and the effects of these implants on estrous behavior. Note that rabbits which became estrous had implants in the posterior ventromedial-premammillary region. MB: mammillary body, OCH: optic chiasm, III V: third ventricle. (From Palka and Sawyer, 1966a)

A very elegant behavioral demonstration of a powerful physiological mechanism has been presented by Michael (1968) who showed that estrogen implanted in the hypothalamus of the ovariectomized female rhesus monkey not only increased the mounting frequency of her male partner but also the number of his ejaculations. These responses are plotted for the male monkey in Fig. 5-16. When the implant in the female was located in sites outside the hypothalamus including the dorsomedial thalamic nucleus, caudate nucleus, or cortical fiber pathways, there was a slight influence on the male monkey's sexual activity. However, "to those observing the behavior, the enhancement of the male's ejaculatory performance was dramatic" only following a hypothalamic implant of estrogen. The net result of estrogen on the neurons of the monkey's diencephalon in an overall increase in the number of sexual "invitations" by the female, to which the male responded vigorously.

In an extension of the 1968 study, Zumpe and Michael (1970) found that in an ovariectomized rhesus monkey, the hypothalamic implantation of estrogen elevated the frequency of the "threatening-away" responses as well as those of

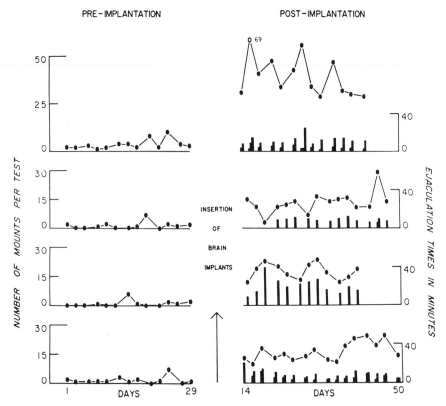

Fig. 5-16   The effects upon the sexual activity of male rhesus monkeys when bilateral implants of stilbestrol di-*n*-butyrate were introduced into the brains of their female (ovariectomized) partners (4 pairs). (From Michael, 1968)

her male sexual partner. When progesterone was given subcutaneously to the female, her threat behavior declined whereas the male's remained essentially the same. The condition of the female's sexual receptivity influenced the willingness to join in the threatening-away behavior.

2. Anatomical Differences in the Rat

After estradiol is implanted in the anterior hypothalamic preoptic area of the spayed female rat, the animal becomes sexually receptive within 3 to 5 days (Lisk, 1962b). The lordosis reflex which also appears at the same time is evoked by implants at sites shown in Fig. 5-17. Surprisingly, estradiol positioned at other more posterior sites, also illustrated in Fig. 5-17, causes either ovarian atrophy or no effect. Although a clear anatomical differentiation of estrogen sensitive sites was demonstrated in the rat, even more important is the possibility that a species difference exists between the rat and the cat in terms of the anatomical location of estrogen receptors involved in copulatory activity (Harris and Michael, 1958).

A finding inconsistent with these reports has been summarized by Dörner *et al.* (1968a). They found that estradiol implanted also in the anterior preoptic region of a spayed female rat evoked male mating behavior characterized by mounting of other female rats in estrus. They did, however, find that 1 μg of the estrogen deposited in the ventromedial hypothalamus produced the complete display of lordosis described by Lisk. Although the source of this anatomical discrepancy is unclear, the dose of estrogen, the size of the implanting tube or other technical matters could account for the differences.

When a crystalline mixture of estrogen plus progesterone or estrogen alone is placed in the anterior preoptic area of the castrated female rat, the lordosis response is displayed eventually, but the combination of the two steroids reduces the latency interval to one week (Lisk and Suydam, 1967). When these steroids are deposited similarly in the prepubertally castrated male rat, the lordosis response can be elicited within 3 to 12 days after implantation. Then 34 to 60 days later, male sexual behavior including mounting, pelvic thrusts and the ejaculatory reflex appears. In testing every other day, a bisexual pattern is overtly manifest in the male that depends solely on the sex of the rat partner with which the implanted male is placed. This pattern may last for up to 8 weeks but fails to emerge if the crystals are placed in the mammillary body or other area. One critical variable that determines the male's sexual response is the period when the gonadectomy is performed; this factor does not seem to be as important to the female. Proof seems to be forthcoming now of some sort of masculinization of the nervous system which takes place very soon after birth. In any event, a physiological trigger for estrous behavior apparently depends on the synergistic activity of progesterone and estrogen at the hypothalamic level.

If an ovariectomized rat is given progesterone systemically after estrogen is implanted in the anterior hypothalamic, preoptic area, lordosis occurs in most rats about 3 hours later (Lisk, 1969b). Since this response wanes quickly, progesterone has a very limited facilitatory action which quickly becomes refractory for the mechanism underlying lordosis behavior. Of special interest was Lisk's finding that the male or female rat when castrated neonatally also displays the lordosis response following estrogen priming of the rostral hypothalamus. Estrogen also has some priming effect on lordosis when deposited in the medial or posterior hypothalamus, which supports the view based on radioactive tracer studies that estrogen sensitive cells may be dispersed throughout the hypothalamus.

The ovariectomized rat primed with estradiol given systemically also displays lordosis behavior after progesterone is implanted in the mesencephalic reticular formation (Ross *et al.*, 1971). Progesterone receptors possibly exist in the midbrain that operate in conjunction with estrogen sensitive cells in the hypothalamus to facilitate female sexual behavior. Powers (1972) has found that

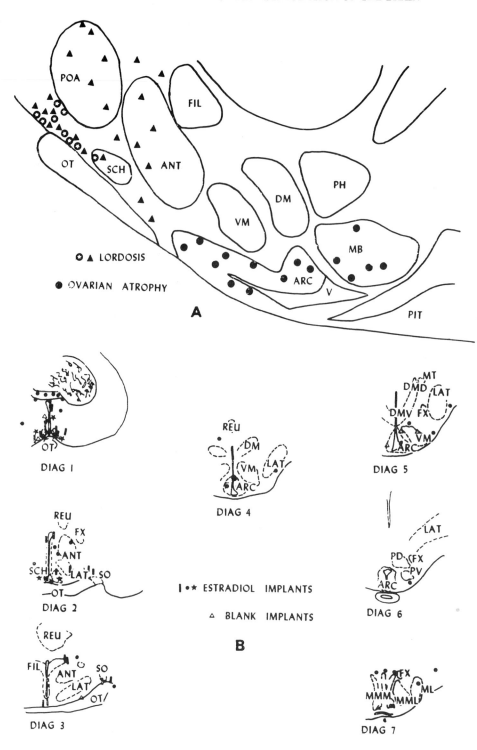

progesterone also evokes lordosis when the hormone is deposited in the ventro-medial hypothalamus, although the rat was given progesterone subcutaneously.

B. Mating in the Male

In a brief anecdotal account of the responses of a few rats, Fisher reported that after testosterone was injected into sites identified tentatively as the preoptic area, the male rat would retrieve a female in heat, build a nest, or attempt copulation while taking a rat pup to its nest (Fisher, 1956). Although the report was incomplete, the surprising aspect was that androgen placed in the hypo-thalamus independently evoked maternal behavior as well as sexual responses, which would reflect a dual property of the hormone.

In an informal discussion ten years later, Fisher (1966) again described the dual effect of androgen in eliciting both sexual and maternal behavior in the male rat, but only when testosterone was placed in the preoptic region. These responses occur in less than 10% of the animals if one "is lucky." Interestingly, testosterone implanted in one female rat resulted in male copulatory responses including mounting of another rat and pelvic thrusting. One difficulty en-countered in the interpretation of the data is the reason for the short latency of the response following the testosterone infusion. Such a rapid action of a steroid on nervous tissue is difficult to understand in view of the long period of even four or five days required for the same hormone to act when given systemically.

1. Behavioral Specificity of Androgen Action

Sexual behavior in the male rat is independent of androgen sensitive tissue in the periphery but is influenced by a direct action of testosterone on the brain-stem. To confirm this, Davidson (1966b) castrated the rat and then placed testosterone in one of several areas of the hypothalamus, thalamus, cortex, hippocampus and brain stem. Except for the occasional positive sexual responses arising from stimulation of the hippocampus or other subcortical implantation sites, the crystals of androgen deposited in the medial part of the preoptic area restored full-blown sexual behavior. In fact, the castrated male would mount a female in

---

Fig. 5-17 Location of implants of estradiol in the hypothalamus of the female rat. Diagram A shows in sagittal view the regions involved in behavioral recep-tivity or ovarian atrophy as a result of estradiol implants in 27 gauge tubing (triangles) and 30 gauge tubing (stars). In B, a series of seven transverse diagrams through the hypothalamus indicates the location of estradiol implants resulting in behavioral receptivity; black bars and stars indicate positive points found with implants in 27 gauge and 30 gauge tubing respectively; black circles: negative responses; triangles: blank tubing implanted as control. (From Lisk, R. D. 1966a. *In: Brain and Behavior, Vol. III.* R. A. Gorski and R. E. Whalen (eds.), pp. 98–117. Originally published by the University of California Press; reprinted by permission of the Regents of the University of California)

estrus and appear to ejaculate. The sexual response required on the average of 8 days to appear after the testosterone was implanted in the hypothalamus, although great variability was recorded in latency, frequency and other indices of the sexual act.

In an identical study, Lisk (1967b) implanted testosterone in the anterior hypothalamic, preoptic area in a castrated male, after which the complete pattern of copulatory responses was restored. The latency averaged about 10 days for mounting behavior and the ejaculatory reflex, the latter being manifest in 50% of the rats. Since animals with a testosterone implant positioned either in the arcuate or mammillary region did not show signs of copulatory behavior, the anatomical specificity of androgen potency is validated. Lisk postulated that some aspect of sexual excitability may be mediated through the posterior mammillary region, since a testosterone implant there evoked a striking arousal of the male within 6 to 12 days when it was presented with a receptive female in heat. However, Johnston and Davidson (1972) have recently confirmed the fact that the androgen sensitive elements are far more concentrated in the rostral hypothalamus.

In the adult female rabbit that is ovariectomized, androgen acting on the hypothalamus exerts the same effect as estrogen (Palka and Sawyer, 1966b). Testosterone deposited in the ventromedial part of the hypothalamus evoked lordosis within 3 days. Most rabbits exhibited the complete pattern of mating, and they also became somewhat aggressive toward the anestrous female but did not attempt to mount the female. Since the control implants as well as testosterone deposited at other sites had no effect, the gonadal steroids acting on the adult hypothalamus tend to stimulate sexual activity rather than to organize a specific pattern of male or female behavior.

A fascinating account of the effect of androgen on mating behavior in the bird has been given by Hutchison (1967). Testosterone implanted in the male dove's rostral hypothalamus evokes courting behavior that is characterized by chasing of females, nest soliciting and some bowing responses. This activity which disappeared within 8 to 12 days following implantation was less frequent or even absent when the steroid was placed in another region of the bird's limbic system. Thus, the androgen sensitive area that mediates courtship behavior in the dove is rather circumscribed and corresponds anatomically to that of the mammal (Davidson, 1966b; Fisher, 1966; Lisk, 1966; Yahr and Thiessen, 1972).

After the male Barbary dove is castrated and shows no sexual interest in other birds, testosterone deposited again in the anterior hypothalamic, preoptic area evokes the chasing behavior, soliciting and bowing (Hutchison, 1969). However, the effectiveness of androgen in eliciting courtship activity declines sharply in birds that are implanted 30 days after castration, and is entirely lost 90 days after castration. Clearly, the hypothalamic androgen receptors lose their sensitivity possibly because of the absence of testicular hormones or other functional changes brought about by an androgen deficit. Anatomically, the efficacy of the implant was directly correlated with the proximity to the rostral sites (Hutchison, 1971) as measured by the number of courtship responses, the peak duration of activity and the latency which was usually 2 to 5 days.

When testosterone is implanted in the rostral hypothalamus of a 4-week-old male chick, the mating response as reflected by previously obtained copulatory scores doubles over that seen prior to the implant when testing was carried out over the next 3 weeks (Gardner and Fisher, 1968). Testosterone does not cause this effect if it is implanted in other areas of the brain, nor does mating behavior arise when blank cannulae are positioned in the same locus. Comb growth is not different in any of the chicks, which would rule out a systemic effect. Thus, in the bird as well as in the mammal, an androgen sensitive region apparently exists in a small area of the hypothalamus which stimulates sexual behavior.

Even if the chicken is castrated at 6 to 8 weeks of age prior to the implantation of androgen in the preoptic area, the complete copulatory response occurs in most birds in response to the hypothalamic action of testosterone (Barfield, 1969); however, none of the capons will show aggressive behavior, waltzing or other aspects of the normal courtship activity when confronted with a receptive hen. Contrary to the finding of Gardner and Fisher (1968), Barfield saw a slight increase in the capon's comb growth, but the difference was significant only in capons with bilateral implants of testosterone. The site of this action of testosterone is highly localized in the chicken.

2. *Androgen Masculinization of the Female*

The age at which gonadal activity can affect the hypothalamic regulation of gonadotropin secretion is a critical factor. For example, testosterone given systemically to the newborn female or male masculinizes the neonatal rat of either sex, thus interfering with the normal process of sexual differentiation (Gorski and Wagner, 1965). The duration is not known of the so-called "critical period" of development during which time the brain of the newborn animal is highly sensitive to androgens. However, total physiological masculinization of a male or female rat as a result of testosterone injection takes place probably after the fourth day postpartum but before 21 days of age (Swanson and van der Werff ten Bosch, 1964).

The placement of testosterone crystals in the basal hypothalamus of a 4-day-old female rat advances the age at which vaginal opening occurs (Wagner *et al.*, 1966). Further, testosterone causes persistent vaginal estrus in those animals in which the implant is in the antero-ventral hypothalamus. In comparison to the efficacy of the steroid given subcutaneously, a relatively small amount of testosterone reproduces the chief features of androgen sterilization in the neonatal female. Such results are consistent with the belief that this type of hormonal sterilization results from a dysfunction of essential hypothalamic activity.

So-called homosexuality in the female rat is evoked by androgen acting on the diencephalon. After 200 μg of testosterone crystals were implanted in the anterior hypothalamus of a postpubertally spayed rat, each female mounted an estrous female (Dörner *et al.*, 1968b). Similar mounting behavior can be elicited in the castrated male by similar implants of testosterone. However, when the androgen is deposited in the medial region of the hypothalamus, the spayed female exhibits normal lordosis, whereas the castrate male shows no response. Dörner *et al.* offer the hypothesis that two independent mating "centers" in the hypothalamus are organized during a critical period of androgen-dependent differentiation.

To determine whether complete masculinization of the neonatal female can be attained by treating the brain with androgen, Nadler (1968) deposited

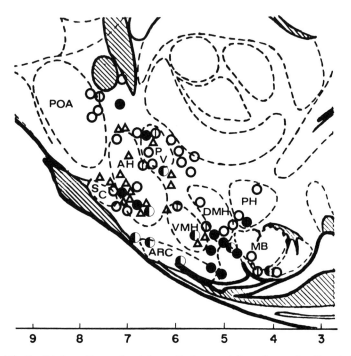

Fig. 5-18 Sagittal section of rat hypothalamus taken from de Groot (1959), illustrating the loci of implants in neonatal female rats associated with development of different patterns of vaginal cyclicity. Implants with 2% TP-paraffin: dark circle = acyclic; open circle = cyclic. Implants with 1% TP-paraffin: half-dark circle = acyclic; divided open circle = cyclic. Implants of paraffin or cholesterol alone: open triangle = cyclic. Abbreviations: AH = area anterior hypothalami; ARC = nucleus arcuatus hypothalami; DMH = nucleus dorsomedialis hypothalami; MB = nuclei mammillaris; PH = nucleus posterior hypothalami; POA = area preoptica; PV = nucleus paraventricularis hypothalami; SC = nucleus suprachiasmaticus; VMH = nucleus ventromedialis hypothalami. (From Nadler, R. D., 1972. *Neuroendocrinology.* 9:349–357. S. Karger, Basel, Switzerland)

pellets of testosterone in the amygdala or hypothalamus. When the implant was in the basal portion of the brain, a number of changes occurred that depended on the site and quantity of crystal given. For example, the time of vaginal opening was advanced; persistent vaginal estrus arose; ovulation was inhibited regardless of the dose of the implant; female sexual behavior was inhibited; and there were some indications of an augmentation of mounting and general male sexual behavior patterns. The hypothesis is thus supported that androgen, coming in contact in a sufficient concentration with the developing brain of a female, can alter its sexual pattern remarkably and indeed induce masculinization.

When the brain of a female is exposed to androgen stimulation very early in life, a pattern of persistent vaginal estrus and an acyclic, anovulatory condition evolves. Such a set of responses is produced when testosterone is placed at sites shown in Fig. 5-18 in the ventromedial-arcuate nucleus complex in the 5-day-old rat (Nadler, 1972a). The earliest age of onset is associated with the implantation of androgen in this region of the hypothalamus. Although testosterone may exert the same effect if deposited in other areas, the latency is significantly longer. These data further implicate these nuclei in the negative feedback system in the pituitary-ovarian axis (Beyer *et al.*, 1971).

Nadler (1972b) has provided yet another outlook on the site of action of androgen in the female rat. An implant of testosterone in the arcuate-VMH complex but not in the anterior preoptic or posterior hypothalamic area of the newborn female retards the development of the ovulatory cycle as well as inhibits the lordosis reflex and receptivity to a male rat. This developmental retardation lasts long after the female has reached maturity over 100 days later. Nadler concluded that the anatomical regions involved in the endocrine system as well as behavioral responses to normal estrogen influence are probably overlapping and undifferentiated at least at birth. Of course, this supposition must be held in light of a relatively gross implant in a tiny brain of a neonate.

VII. INHIBITION OF SEXUAL FUNCTION

The entire concern with population control in the world today has certain well-defined roots in the scientific understanding of the mechanism responsible for a direct blockade of sexual function. Obviously, reproductive processes can be inhibited either by the removal of peripheral glandular tissue or by circumscribed lesions to structures in the brain, the surgical intricacies of which render this latter approach clinically impractical. Therefore, the anti-fertility drugs which have been developed rapidly over the past two decades seem to provide a sociological recourse of immense desirability and with utilitarian importance for the greatest number of people. During the last few years, interest has grown steadily in the question of whether specific regions of the central nervous system are involved in the chemical blockade of sexual activity.

A. Blockade of Female Responses

That a major locus of action of the powerful anti-fertility compounds could be the hypothalamus is not problematical (Bainbridge and Labhsetwar, 1971). Kanematsu and Sawyer (1965) showed that a contraceptive progestational steroid used by women, norethindrone (17-ethinyl-9-nortestosterone) implanted in the posterior median eminence successfully blocks ovulation in the multiparous rabbit. Furthermore, copulation-induced ovulation is also inhibited. In 5 out of 7 rabbits, norethindrone deposited in the median eminence also prevents ovulation even after coital stimulation following estrogen priming. An implant in other areas shown in Fig. 5-19, including the anterior pituitary, fails to affect the ovulatory response. Another fascinating aspect of these findings is the unwillingness of the norethindrone-implanted rabbit to accept the mounting behavior of a vigorous buck. Although the locus of action of an anti-fertility progesterone has been assumed to be on the efferent side of the pituitary, it is clear that a chemical may interrupt the "reflex arc" subserving ovulation at the level of the hypothalamus.

Chlormadinone, another potent anti-ovulatory compound, exerts its effect both on neural tissue and on the cells of the anterior pituitary (Döcke et al., 1968). When the adult rat in diestrus or prepubertal female is given systemic estradiol simultaneously, only 7.5 µg of chlormadinone acetate, which is one-

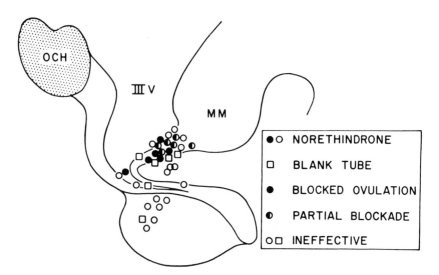

Fig. 5-19 Location of norethindrone implants and blockade of ovulation. OCH = the optic chiasma; III V = the third ventricle; MM = the mammillary body; "partial blockade" signifies that ovulation was blocked in 1 of 2 tests (10 to 12 days, 34 to 39 days, or 57 days) but was not blocked in the other. (From Kanematsu and Sawyer, 1965)

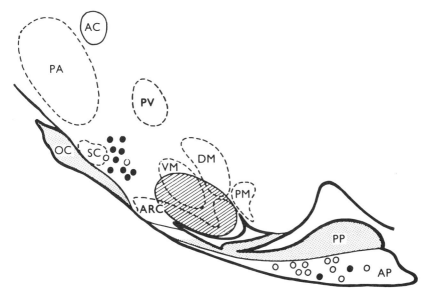

Fig. 5-20 Parasagittal diagram of rat hypothalamus (de Groot, 1959) illustrating localization of bilateral chlormadinone implants (3.8 µg) and electrode tips. Solid circles represent bilateral implants that did not influence ovulation; open circles indicate implants that prevented the electrically induced ovulation. The position of electrode tips is indicated by the shaded area. Abbreviations: AC, anterior commissure; AP, anterior pituitary; ARC, arcuate nucleus; DM, dorso-medial nucleus; OC, optic chiasma; PA, preoptic area; PM, dorsal premammillary nucleus; PP, posterior pituitary; PV, paraventricular nucleus; SC, suprachiasmatic nucleus; VM, ventromedial nucleus. (From Döcke et al., 1968)

hundredth of the effective subcutaneous dose, implanted in the region of the median eminence posterior to the optic chiasm, prevents spontaneous ovulation as well as the formation of a corpus luteum. The area of maximum sensitivity is portrayed in Fig. 5-20. However, since the same dose was equally effective when the drug was deposited in the pituitary, an intrahypophyseal action of the compound is also likely. The reason for this view is that the design of the portal system favors the vascular transport of the hormone in the direction from the hypothalamus to the pituitary (Bogdanove, 1963b) rather than the reverse. Thus, the position of Palka et al. (1966) and Bainbridge and Labhsetwar (1971) on a dual site of action of substances affecting anti-gonadal function is reasonable in this instance.

A somewhat different approach to analyzing the inhibition of sexual behavior has been taken by Quadagno et al. (1971). To test the possibility that estradiol acts by centrally stimulating the synthesis of RNA or protein, crystals of actinomycin D, an inhibitor of RNA synthesis, were deposited in the preoptic area of the female rat. The lordosis response induced by systemic estradiol was blocked 12 hours later by the actinomycin, in a dose-dependent fashion. Although the integrity of the mechanism for RNA synthesis may be a factor in the steroid-induced sexual behavior, the extreme toxicity of actinomycin D is always a worrisome factor even in spite of the dose-response relationship of the lordosis or its inhibition.

B. Blockade of Male Responses

Cyproterone is a drug which when given systemically antagonizes the action of androgens on the male sex organs and also suppresses the development of male characteristics during the growth of the fetus. When cyproterone is implanted in the hypothalamus it also stimulates gonadotropin secretion (Bloch and Davidson, 1967). Crystals of cyproterone deposited in the median eminence of the immature male rat cause an increase in the weight of the testes, seminal vesicles and prostate after a 2-week interval. The site of action was the area of the median eminence. Thus, the local action of cyproterone is probably the prevention of the acknowledged inhibitory action that testosterone exerts on the basal part of the hypothalamus.

The potency of cyproterone has been demonstrated dramatically in terms of the mating behavior of the male rat. When the anti-androgenic compound is implanted bilaterally in high doses in both the anterior and posterior parts of the hypothalamus, the sexual response of the male is totally abolished (Bloch and Davidson, 1971). However, if testosterone is administered subcutaneously for 14 days to the implanted rats, they mount females and ejaculate significantly more often than the control males in which cholesterol had been implanted at corresponding hypothalamic sites. This evidence plus that obtained from the results of systemic injections suggests that the compound may under certain circumstances possess a weak androgenic effect. Probably, the dose is a critical factor in determining the action of the drug on androgen receptor sites in the hypothalamus, particularly when appropriate steroid-dependent responses are under study.

In summarizing the evidence available at the present time on the efficacy of cyproterone, Davidson et al. (1970) have drawn a significant conclusion insofar as the properties of receptor recognition for the drug are concerned. The hypothalamic receptors involved in the pathway for stimulating male sexual behavior are probably different than the receptors concerned with the gonadotrophic feedback regulator. Thus, within the diencephalon, an anatomical separation of the receptor-effector systems would seem to exist.

1. Inhibition by Female Hormones

Endogenous female hormones can also exert an inhibitory action on male sexual function. For example, an injection of estradiol into the median eminence blocks the copulatory activity of the male rabbit (Hartmann et al., 1966). Crystals of progesterone, androsterone or control injections of saline did not prevent the mating response, nor did estrogen when infused into the preoptic area or mammillary bodies. Because of the immense volume injected into the basal hypothalamus, it is difficult to understand how the hormone could have exerted such a localized effect.

A purely behavioral analysis of the central effect of progesterone has revealed that the hormone profoundly influences the reproductive activity of the ring dove. Although steroid controls were not utilized, Komisaruk (1966) found that progesterone crystals deposited at sites scattered widely including the rostral hypothalamus and lateral forebrain evoke egg-sitting or incubation behavior in both the male and female dove. However, bowing and cooing responses, which are characteristic of pigeon courtship, were partially or totally suppressed in the males by progesterone implanted at sites scattered throughout the brain. Crystals of the hormone placed in the ventricle had no effect, a finding which served to rule out any nonspecific transport by this route to a specially sensitive but unknown site. The anatomical diffuseness of these effects are still a matter of some perplexity.

Following the observations of Komisaruk (1967), Meyer (1972) showed that precocial copulation in the 14-day-old male chick primed with androgen is blocked by progesterone deposited in the medial preoptic area. The copulatory behavior is ordinarily characterized by grasping and mounting, posterior contact of the cloaca, treading of feet, the waggle of the chick's posterior from side to side, and pecking behavior. Sexual responses were not suppressed by similar implants of cholesterol when progesterone was implanted in other areas of the brain. Support for the hypothesis is thus given that progesterone can act as a powerful anti-androgenic agent.

VIII. BIOGENIC AMINES IN THE HYPOTHALAMUS

Whether or not there is a specialized neurohumoral link between the cells that secrete a trophic hormone and the local action of a gonadal steroid on neurons that elaborate a specific trophic releasing factor is still uncertain. Studies in which certain classes of drug are administered systemically in order to alter the content of biogenic amines in nervous tissue favor indirectly some sort of relationship. For example, the drug-induced depletion of monoamines in the brain can prevent ovulation and cause pseudopregnancy (see Martini and Meites, 1970). A logical question arising from this type of study is the central locus of action of a drug that affects the estrous cycle, lactation or other reproductive functions.

A. Monoamines

To test the hypothesis that reserpine given systemically activates lactation by blocking the hypothalamic control over prolactin release, Kanematsu and Sawyer (1963b) implanted reserpine in the hypothalamus and pituitary. They found that reserpine activates lactation only when acting on the hypothalamus in the region of the posterior median eminence. Crystals deposited in the hypophysis fail to produce much of an effect on mammary function. Furthermore, the local pharmacological action of reserpine does not seem to be due to a lesion in that the time course was very different than that seen when the site was ablated electrolytically.

To explore the notion of a monoaminergic pathway in the inhibition of pro-lactin function, the regional stores of amines were reduced centrally (van Maanen and Smelik, 1968). Reserpine in a gelatine medium was implanted in the basal hypothalamus rostral to the median eminence in female rats on the day of proestrus or estrus. Each implant depleted monoamines in the brain-stem as detected by the absence of local fluorescence when the brain was examined histologically. Of 29 rats tested, the estrous cycles in 22 were markedly disturbed as shown by vaginal smears. About half of the rats showed formation of deciduomata in the uterine horn which had been earlier traumatized when the MAO inhibitor, iproniazid, was given systemically. These responses are presented in Fig. 5-21. Thus, a monoaminergic system of neurons in the median eminence could be involved in the regulation of prolactin secretion, particularly in the inhibition of its release, since reserpine in other areas of the brain-stem did not produce these effects. More direct pharmacological controls including that of the dose are required for such a supposition. Nevertheless, these data support the idea of a hypothalamic prolactin-inhibitory factor (PIF) which would act on the pituitary to prevent the persistent functioning of the corpus luteum.

An implant of norepinephrine, serotonin, dopamine (DA) or melatonin in the median eminence of the lactating, nursing rabbit reduces, in a seemingly non-specific manner, the volume of milk secreted from the mammary during the peak output of the milk-yield curve (Shani et al., 1971). None of the endogenously occurring compounds blocks prolactin secretion completely and the effect on milk yield could be secondary to a suppression of appetite, feeding or other physiological processes. Although the question of the role of a putative neurotransmitter on the lactogenic response still remains unanswered, a variation of the dose of a monoamine applied to neural tissue, particularly in the lower range, is essential (see Chapter 13).

In the female rat pretreated with gonadotropin, the ovulatory response is severely retarded when α-methyl-dopa, which reduces endogenous dopamine available for release, is micro-injected in a very small volume and dose (Kordon and Glowinski, 1970). Since this "false transmitter" has the capability of reducing transmitter levels at the synapse, it would seem reasonable that the attenuated release of dopamine affects ovulation during a critical period. Interestingly, this observation corresponds well with the histochemical demonstration that the arcuate-median eminence complex is comprised chiefly of dopamine-containing nerve endings and that the fluorescence in this region changes during estrus or after castration (e.g., Lichtensteiger, 1970).

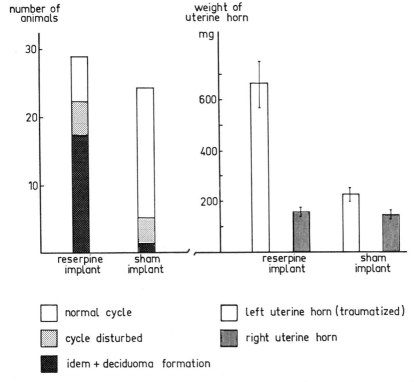

Fig. 5-21 Effect of hypothalamic reserpine or sham implants on estrous cycle and occurrence of pseudopregnancy in rats. Left: number of animals in which vaginal smears and deciduomata formation indicate absence of estrous cycle and occurrence of pseudopregnancy. Right: weight of uterine horns, after traumatization of left uterine horn. Standard error of the mean indicated by vertical line. (From van Maanen, J. H. and P. G. Smelik. 1968. *Neuroendocrinology.* 3:177–186. S. Karger, Basel, Switzerland)

The involvement of a catecholamine in the secretion of LH from the pituitary, proposed on the basis of studies of peripheral administration of different drugs, probably revolves about the release of dopamine rather than norepinephrine from the CNS. Kordon (1971) verified this supposition quite clearly. When α-methyl-dopa is micro-injected in a small volume in a concentration as low as 80 ng in the arcuate nucleus of the rat, the frequency of ovulation decreases sharply. Quite significantly, the micro-injection of α-methyl-dopa into the pituitary or into other sites in the basal hypothalamus, shown in Fig. 5-22, failed to affect the ovulatory sequence. In contrast to the similarity in the blocking effect of the drug given systemically, the intra-arcuate potency of α-methyl-dopa was estimated by Kordon to be about 250,000 times greater and in the physiological range.

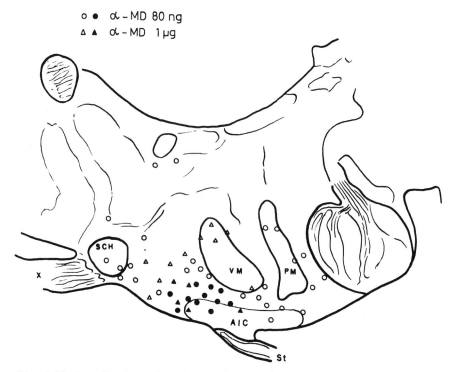

Fig. 5-22 Localization of ovulating-blocking (black symbols) and ineffective (open symbols) micro-injections of α-methyl-dopa (α-MD) into the hypothalamus. All effective micro-injection sites are located within 0.8 mm from the midline. AIC = arcuate nucleus; PM = premammillary area; SCH = suprachiasmatic nucleus; St = pituitary stalk; VM = ventromedial nucleus; X = optic chiasm. (From Kordon, C. 1971. *Neuroendocrinology.* 7:202–209. S. Karger, Basel, Switzerland)

A puzzling contradiction to these rather substantial findings has erupted from the careful experiment of Craven and McDonald (1971) who have infused DA and NE directly into the median eminence of the mature cycling female rat. After they blocked ovulation by Nembutal on the afternoon of proestrus, the micro-injection of 40 μg of either DA or NE in a volume of 0.4 μl failed to induce ovulation. Even systemic pretreatment with the MAO inhibitor, iproniazid, did not alter the impotency of either catecholamine on the median eminence. Craven and McDonald conclude from their astonishing results that the role of DA in the normal cycling animal may be quite different from that in the gonadotropin-primed immature rat. Moreover, since NE but not DA induced ovulation in MAO-pretreated rats, a noradrenergic rather than dopaminergic component may be part of the mechanism involved in ovulation during the critical period in proestrus.

Related also to the issue of the catecholamines is the substance which cannot be excluded from any of a myriad of functions in the brain—adenosine $3',5'$-monophosphate (cyclic AMP). This compound is thought to be involved in the release of transmitter and other substances from cells in the nervous system. In an exploratory study, Breckenridge and Lisk (1969) describe briefly the relatively long-term action of crystals of cyclic AMP implanted in a high 250 μg concentration into one of several hypothalamic areas of the rat. Deposited in the arcuate nucleus, cyclic AMP lengthened the estrous cycle, but when placed in the anterior hypothalamic area, it caused hyperthermia. After cyclic AMP was implanted in the mammillary region, the rat developed a marked hyperphagia and its weight showed an accelerated gain. These results suggest that cyclic AMP could somehow be significantly involved at the cellular level in each of the homeostatic regulatory systems mediated by the hypothalamus.

1. *Pineal and Indole Factors*

Just as we saw in Chapter 4, there is now some basis for the speculation that the activity of a structure remote from the median eminence may influence its receptors. According to Fraschini (1968), the pineal gland releases melatonin and 5-hydroxytryptophol (5-HTOL) as specific messengers to the median eminence that serve the purpose of inhibiting LH secretion. Similarly, 5-HT and 5-methoxytryptophol (5-MTOL) may act as messengers to inhibit FSH secretion (Fraschini *et al.*, 1970).

The content of luteinizing hormone (LH) in the anterior pituitary of the rat is reduced following the implantation for 5 days of melatonin or 5-HTOL but not 5-HT or 5-MTOL in the median eminence (Fraschini *et al.*, 1968a). The same effect occurred when these two compounds as well as 5-MTOL were placed in the reticular formation. Thus, receptors are perhaps located in each of the areas which are sensitive to the presence of the indole class of compounds. These substances somehow could participate in the regulation of the synthesis and/or the release, of LH with the hypophysis. Although no dose response was obtained for these indoles, a differentiation exists anatomically between the reticular formation and the hypothalamus in terms of the relative sensitivity, or lack thereof, to one of the indole derivatives, 5-MTOL.

To test the role of the pineal indole amine, melatonin, on the reproductive process, Fraschini *et al.* (1968b) deposited crystals of melatonin or fragments of pineal tissue itself in the cerebral cortex, median eminence, midbrain reticular substance or pituitary gland in the castrated male rat. Melatonin requires hydroxy-indole-O-methyl-transferase, found only in the pineal gland, for its synthesis. When either melatonin or pineal tissue is deposited in the median eminence or mesencephalic reticular substance, both plasma LH levels and stores of pituitary LH decline. Most likely, the melatonin that is secreted from the pineal gland participates in the regulation of the output of luteinizing hormone from the pituitary. The hypothalamic-mesencephalic pathway is a likely anatomical route because implants in other areas do not produce these effects.

B. Cholinergic Link

Acetylcholine may serve as the transmitter along each neural pathway that terminates in a secretory cell. An experimental example of this concept is provided by the fact that eserine or diisopropylfluorophosphate (DFP) injected into the supraoptic nucleus causes a rapid increase in the size of spontaneous uterine contractions; DFP has about four times the duration in its effect (Abrahams and Pickford, 1956). The anatomical controls showed that these drugs fail to alter uterine motility when injected into the fornix or posterior hypothalamus, and 0.9% saline was without effect. From these findings, a cholinergic substance may be acting on cells in the supraoptic nucleus to liberate an oxytocic factor. Since the duration of action of eserine and DFP corresponds to the longevity of their anticholinesterase activity, Pickford's view is supported that ACh could be responsible for releasing both oxytocin and ADH from the supraoptic and posterior regions of the hypothalamus, respectively.

From the results of lesions and electrical stimulation, it is clear that the paraventricular nucleus and median eminence are also structures concerned with secretion of oxytocin and the subsequent milk-ejection reflex, the onset of which is provoked by suckling stimuli. The idea of a cholinergic link in this reflex is supported by the investigation of Ôba et al. (1971). When atropine mixed with cholesterol is deposited in the paraventricular nucleus of the lactating mother rat on the seventh day following parturition, the offspring lose weight. Even though each pup suckled vigorously, it was unable to obtain milk from the teats. After the atropine was implanted, the milk yield was significantly reduced for several days; thereafter, almost normal milk production resumed. Control implants and systemic treatment verified the anatomical and chemical specificity of the cholinergic blocking agent in inhibiting the milk-ejection reflex and subsequent milk secretion.

To explore the effect of a cholinergic antagonist on prolactin activity, Gala et al. (1970) implanted large amounts of atropine in the medial hypothalamus of the female rat. Within 8 days, atropine had caused deciduomata formation. After pseudopregnancy was induced by electrical stimulation of the cervix, hypothalamic deposits of crystalline atropine or Dibenamine did not inhibit this induction of deciduomata. Since neither drug affects body or organ weights, except for the adrenal, it is possible that a cholinergic fiber system in the hypothalamus is involved in the diencephalic inhibition of prolactin secretion.

Atropine prolongs diestrus and also inhibits ovulation possibly as a result of its specific antagonistic action on the cells of the anterolateral hypothalamus (Benedetti et al., 1969), as illustrated in Fig. 5-23. Atropine's lack of action on ovulatory function, following the implantation of the blocking agent into the amygdala or the posterior hypothalamus and the re-appearance of the normal estrous cycle after 30 days indicate that a cholinergic pathway in the hypothalamus is only temporarily blocked. In essence, these results seem to implicate

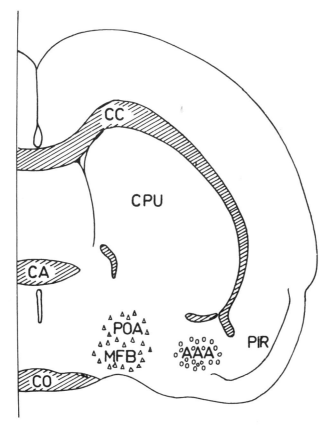

Fig. 5-23 Transverse section of the rat hypothalamus (de Groot, 1969). Δ, area where atropine implants inhibit ovulation; O, area where atropine implants were negative. (From Benedetti *et al.*, 1969)

ACh also in the release of the gonadotrophic factors from the pituitary. (Sala *et al.*, 1971).

Changes in the lordosis reflex have been examined after estrogen, progesterone, carbachol or atropine was applied to the rostral hypothalamus, septum, amygdala or habenula. Lordosis behavior was evoked nonspecifically by all compounds deposited at all sites, but the response depended on the length of time the implanted substance remained in the brain tissue (Rodgers and Law, 1968). Generally, the estrogen crystals were more potent than the other substances, and the hypothalamus and amygdala were the two most sensitive sites in mediating the sexual response. Although the authors conclude that the system mediating lordosis is anatomically widespread, each of the chemicals is given in an unknown dose and volume. This latter variable which has been shown to be such a crucial factor (Lisk, 1962b; Harris and Michael, 1964) renders such a supposition difficult to accept.

IX. CONCLUDING CONSIDERATIONS

Some of the extraordinary observations described in the preceding sections have clarified a great many issues that are concerned with the participation of different structures in the central nervous system in reproduction and sexual behavior. Certainly, no one would now assert that the feedback action of a gonadal steroid is limited to a single locus. Rather, the entire complex of endocrine responses is superbly integrated by way of multiple sites of action in the brain and the pituitary—each one receptive in a special way to a given hormone (Sawyer and Hilliard, 1971). The difficult problem facing research workers in neuroendocrinology today centers on the reason why one restricted region of tissue in the CNS constitutes a sensitive part of a particular feedback mechanism while other regions do not.

One major breakthrough generated by these studies has been the demonstration that separate anatomical regions regulate the pituitary gonadal axis on the one hand and the expression of sexual behavior on the other (Lisk, 1966a and b; 1970). Immediately, one must recognize that these distinct anatomical systems are not unrelated and probably are not functionally independent from one another. However, the insightful observations made in the laboratories of Lisk, depicted in Fig. 5-24, Sawyer and the late Geoffrey Harris have shown unequivocally that the anterior hypothalamus, preoptic area or structures quite remote from the pituitary portal blood supply are reactive to the local action of a gonadal steroid. The full complement of sexual behavior in either male or female can be elicited by an implant of estrogen or testosterone in one of these areas. Although there is some inconsistency across species, sexual arousal, exhibitory display and actual performance are brought about by such diencephalic implants in several varieties of mammals as well as in the domestic and wild fowl.

The anatomical complex comprising the arcuate nucleus, median eminence and rostral mammillary region is one which is more directly concerned with the synthesis and secretion of releasing factors (Fig. 5-24). Thus, the local deposit of a gonadal hormone can exert a wide variety of powerful effects, including the modification of gonadotropin manufacture and release from the pituitary, the atrophy of ovaries or testes and accessory organs, the alteration in ovarian cyclicity, reduction in sperm count and marked cytological disturbances within the pituitary gland itself. As described in the previous sections, the local presence of excess hormone in this most basal and medial portion of the diencephalon can also induce more subtle changes in the concentration of trophic and other hormones circulating in the plasma as well as retard or advance certain stages of gonadal development in the immature animal. Overall then, it is fair to state that a certain specificity exists in the activity of a given hormone in the central nervous system. For example, progesterone, the hormone of pregnancy, acts on specific cells in the rostral hypothalamus of the ring dove to obliterate all forms of court-

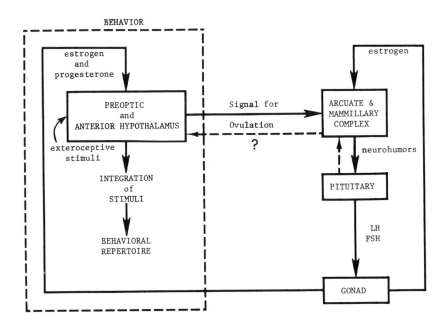

OVULATION AND REPRODUCTIVE RHYTHM

Fig. 5-24 Schematic representation for the female rat indicating the areas of interaction of the gonadal hormones with the brain for regulation of behavioral receptivity and ovulation. (From Lisk, R. D., 1966a. *In: Brain and Behavior, Vol. III.* R. A. Gorski and R. E. Whalen (eds.), pp. 98–117. Originally published by the University of California Press; reprinted by permission of the Regents of the University of California)

ship and sexual behavior, but at the same time progesterone excites maternal or incubation behavior. Estrogen or estrogen plus progesterone impinges on sensitive loci in the diencephalon to trigger the sexual response in the female and stimulate the mechanism which evokes copulatory behavior.

As alluded to earlier, an exceptionally critical factor that should not be overlooked is the age of the animal when a gonadal steroid begins to act on nervous tissue. In the neonate or prepubertal animal, neurons in the central nervous system have unique attributes. In fact, the developing neural elements may be affected quite differently than adult tissue within a corresponding anatomical area. In this regard, the negative feedback effect of estrogen on the content of LH in the pituitary may depend partially on the stage of the estrous cycle itself (McCann and Ramírez, 1964). Thus, the endogenous ratio of estrogen and progesterone, which are in a constant state of flux, will probably influence the reactivity of neurons that are capable of monitoring such changes. Therefore, the entire endocrine history of the animal is always of paramount significance.

In the broadest sense, structures in the diencephalon that are implicated in sexual processes probably are distinct morphologically in the male and female. Lisk has defined the nature of these differences succinctly:

> "What does seem fairly certain at present is that the timing and degree of sexual activity in the male and female are regulated via separate mechanisms. In both sexes the patterning is carried out at the level of the central nervous system. In the female, receptivity or its suppression is the result of interacting and ever changing hormonal titers acting on the neural tissue; while in the male the patterning of the sexual activity is inherent in the nervous tissue with hormone acting only to maintain the integrity of the relevant neural systems." (Lisk, 1970)

Finally, mention should be made of the constantly growing role of the hypothesized intermediary factors, the biogenic amines. These endogenous substances could well be involved to some degree, as yet unknown, with the mechanism of secretion of LH, FSH or prolactin from the adenohypophysis. For example, much indirect evidence has accumulated that endogenous catecholamines are capable of triggering the ovulatory surge of LH secretion from the pituitary; they may even instigate the phasic activity in the brain-stem of the gonadotrophic releasing factors (e.g., Weiner et al., 1972). Schneider and McCann (1970) have gone so far as to specify the pathway in the median eminence delegated to LH-RF and FSH-RF as being part of a dopaminergic system.

Based on other pharmacological studies in which p-chlorophenylalanine is administered peripherally, serotonergic mechanisms have also been held responsible for the hypersexual reaction of both male and female animals; this contention, however, is fraught with experimental disagreement. In evaluating the relationship of 5-HT to sexual behavior, Davidson and Levine (1972) so aptly point out that vigorous scientific methods must be practiced before the inconsistencies can be reconciled in the results obtained with drugs that alter 5-HT metabolism.

In conclusion, before a biogenic amine, or any other compound for that matter, can be considered to function as a putative transmitter, well-designed pharmacological experiments are required. These have yet to be done. Precise anatomical localization of the effect of a monoamine is necessary. The absolute properties of both agonists and antagonists must be quantitated with great care. But the crucial test that awaits future investigation is the demonstration of the in vivo release of a monoamine or other substance from a pool of neurons, a release that is evoked by a gonadal hormone acting via its normal biological route.

As always, dozens of compounds including endogenous substrates which are given by the intracerebral route may suppress or enhance indiscriminately the local liberation of a trophic releasing factor, and yet have nothing whatsoever to do with the natural synaptic mechanism of release. This important aspect of the theory of transmitter and other neurohumoral activity, as discussed in Chapters 1 and 13, also applies to the intricacies of secretion of CRF, TRF and other endocrine releasing factors that have been identified within cellular fractions of the hypothalamus (Chapter 4).

X. Master Summary Table

Chemicals that Exerted an Effect when Given at a Specific Site in the Brain

Chemical	Dose	Volume	Site	Species	State*	Response	Reference
Actinomycin D	≃2–5 µg	crystal	Preoptic area	Rat	U	Blocked lordosis.	Quadagno et al. (1971)
Androstenedione	?	crystal	Anterior hypothalamus and preoptic area	Rat	U	No sexual response in castrate male or female.	Lisk and Suydam (1967)
Anti-LH-serum	—	7–11 µl	Median eminence	Rat	U	Lowered LH content of pituitary but not serum.	Makino et al. (1972)
Atropine	?	crystal	Paraventricular nucleus	Rat	U	Blocked milk-ejection reflex in lactating female.	Ōba et al. (1971)
	?	?	Anterior hypothalamus, septum, amygdala, habenula	Rat	U	Evoked lordosis, independent of site.	Rodgers and Law (1968)
	≃150–250 µg	crystal	Anterior lateral hypothalamus	Rat	U	Disturbed estrous cycles, blocked deciduoma, diminished ovarian weight, prolonged diestrous period.	Benedetti et al. (1969)
	≃250 µg	crystal	Anterior and lateral hypothalamus	Rat	U	Blocked ovulation	Sala et al. (1971)
	≃500 µg	crystal	Dorsomedial nucleus, ventromedial nucleus (hypothalamus)	Rat	U	Stimulated prolactin production as evidenced by deciduomata formation.	Gala et al. (1970)
Carbachol	?	?	Anterior hypothalamus, septum, amygdala, habenula	Rat	U	Evoked lordosis independent of site.	Rodgers and Law (1968)
Chlormadinone acetate	≃3.8–15.0 µg	crystal	Median eminence	Rat	U	Blockade of ovulation and corpus luteum formation.	Döcke et al. (1968)

*U = unanesthetized and unrestrained; C = constrained, confined or curarized; A = anesthetized.

X. Master Summary Table (Continued)

Chemical	Dose	Volume	Site	Species	State*	Response	Reference
Copper SO$_4$	≈50–100 µg	crystal	Median eminence	Rabbit	U	Caused ovulation.	Hiroi et al. (1965)
	.015–250 µg	5 µl	Posterior median eminence	Rabbit	U	Induced ovulation.	Suzuki et al. (1965)
Corticosterone	≈5 µg	crystal	Median eminence	Rat	U	Suppressed ACTH release (corticosteroid production) due to ether stress.	Bohus and Strashimirov (1970)
Cortisone	≈10 µg	crystal	Median eminence	Rat	U	Slight enhancement of ovarian hypertrophy after hemicastration.	Fendler and Endröczi (1966)
Cyclic AMP	≈250 µg	crystal	Arcuate nucleus	Rat	U	Pseudopregnancy.	Breckenridge and Lisk (1969)
Cyproterone	≈53–207 µg	crystal	Median eminence	Rat	U	Increased weight of testes, seminal vesicles, prostates.	Bloch and Davidson (1967)
	≈200–300 µg	crystal	Posterior and anterior hypothalamus	Rat	U	Inhibited sexual behavior reversible by subcutaneous testosterone.	Bloch and Davidson (1971)
Dibenamine	≈500 µg	crystal	Dorsomedial nucleus, ventromedial nucleus (hypothalamus)	Rat	U	No effect observed.	Gala et al. (1970)
Diisopropyl fluorophosphate (DFP)	40–100 µg	2 µl	Supraoptic nucleus	Dog	A	Increased duration of uterine contractions 4 times that of Eserine salicylate.	Abrahams and Pickford and (1956)
α-Methyl-dopa	.08 µg	.2 µl	Arcuate nucleus	Rat	U	Blocked ovulation.	Kordon and Glowinski (1970)
	.08–1 µg	.2 µl	Arcuate nucleus	Rat	U	Blocked ovulation (LH release).	Kordon (1971)

Compound	Dose	Form	Site	Species	A/U	Effect	Reference
ICI 46474 [trans-1-(p-β-dimethylaminoethoxyphenyl)-1,2-diphenylbut-1-ene]	≃5–40 μg	crystal	Median eminence	Rat	A	Blocked ovulation.	Bainbridge and Labhsetwar (1971)
Dopamine (DA)	≃62–156 μg	crystal	Median eminence	Rabbit	U	Reduced lactation.	Shani et al. (1971)
Eserine salicylate	40 μg	2 μl	Supraoptic nucleus	Dog	A	Increased uterine contractions.	Abrahams and Pickford (1956)
Estradiol	?	crystal	Median eminence	Desert iguana	U	Inhibited spermatogenesis, retarded testicular and ovarian development.	Lisk (1967a)
	≃47 μg	crystal	Anterior hypothalamus, preoptic area	Dove	U	Courtship behavior in the castrate animal	Hutchison (1971)
	?	crystal	Arcuate-mammillary complex; ventral tegmentum	Rat	U	Elevated plasma corticosteroids after ovariectomy.	Richard (1966)
	?	crystal	Arcuate nucleus	Rat	U	Reduced nucleoli size of arcuate neurons.	Lisk and Newlon (1963)
	?	crystal	Arcuate nucleus	Rat	U	Sustained normal pituitary characteristics in castrate animals.	Lisk (1963)
	?	crystal	Arcuate nucleus, mammillary bodies	Rat	U	Increased pituitary weight.	Lisk (1969a)
	?	crystal	Basal hypothalamus	Rat	U	Diestrus, enlarged corpora lutea and anterior pituitary.	Ramírez and McCann (1964)
	?	crystal	Habenula	Rat	U	Decrease in uterine and ovarian weight, increased pituitary LH.	Motta et al. (1968)
	?	crystal	Anterior hypothalamus and preoptic area	Rat	U	Advanced the time of vaginal opening.	Smith and Davidson (1968)
	?	crystal	Preoptic area	Rat	U	Lordosis in castrate female treated with progesterone.	Lisk (1969b)
	?	crystal	Anterior hypothalamus, preoptic area, median eminence	Rat	U	Failed to advance ovulation.	Weick and Davidson (1970)

X.   Master Summary Table   (Continued)

Chemical	Dose	Volume	Site	Species	State*	Response	Reference
Estradiol	?	crystal	Anterior hypothalamus and preoptic area	Rat	U	Lordosis in castrate female.	Lisk and Suydam (1967)
	?	crystal	Hypothalamus	Rat	U	Inhibited castration cell development in pituitary.	Bogdanove (1963)
	?	crystal	Hypothalamus	Rat	U	Atrophy of genital track and gonad of male or female.	Lisk (1960)
	?	crystal	Mammillary arcuate complex	Rat	U	Increased neurosecretory material, prevented decline in neurosecretory material after castration.	Lisk (1965a)
	?	crystal	Mammillary bodies	Rat	U	Usual pituitary changes in castrate animal.	Lisk (1963)
	?	crystal	Median eminence	Rat	U	Impaired uterine and ovarian development in immature or adult.	Smith and Davidson (1968)
	?	crystal	Median eminence	Rat	U	Enlarged anterior pituitary; prevented post-ovariectomy rise in plasma LH (luteinizing hormone), lowered hypophyseal LH content.	Ramírez et al. (1964)
	?	crystal	Median eminence	Rat	U	Precocious vaginal opening, reduced pituitary LH, increased plasma LH, increased uterine weight.	Motta et al. (1968)
	?	crystal	Median eminence	Rat	U	Pseudopregnancy, diestrus; mammary development.	Chowers and McCann (1967)
	≃1 μg	crystal	Anterior hypothalamus	Rat	U	Male sexual behavior in the female.	Dörner et al. (1968a)
	≃5 μg	crystal	Median eminence	Rat	U	Prevented compensatory ovarian hypertrophy after hemicastration.	Fendler and Endröczi (1966)

Compound	Dose	Form	Site	Animal		Effect	Reference
	≈2.5–5 µg	crystal	Anterior hypothalamus	Rat	U	Increased plasma corticosterone.	Telegdy et al. (1964)
	≈10–500 µg	crystal	Hypothalamus	Rat	U	Sexual receptivity in spayed females.	Lisk (1962b)
	4–500 µg	20 µl	Anterior hypothalamus	Rat	U	Reduced testes weight.	von Hohlweg and Daume (1959)
	?	crystal	Hypothalamus	Rabbit	U	Mating in female castrate.	Palka and Sawyer (1966a)
	?	crystal	Median eminence	Rabbit	U	Decline of pituitary LH, ovarian atrophy.	Kanematsu and Sawyer (1963a)
	≈<100 µg	crystal	Median eminence	Rabbit	U	Reduced pituitary and plasma LH levels.	Kanematsu and Sawyer (1964)
	≈200 µg	crystal	Median eminence	Rabbit	U	Blockade of copulation, induced ovulation, ovarian atrophy.	Davidson and Sawyer (1961a)
	40 µg	40 µl	Median eminence	Rabbit	U	Reduced copulatory behavior in male.	Hartmann et al. (1966)
	≈50–800 µg	crystal	Hypothalamus	Cat	U	Induced vaginal cornification; mating behavior.	Harris and Michael (1964)
	2–5 µg	0.4–1 µl	Medial hypothalamus	Cat	A	Synchronized the cortical EEG.	Morelli (1968)
Estradiol-6,7-^{3}H-acetate	≈1–2 µg	crystal	Median eminence	Rat	U	Rise in plasma luteinizing hormone, diestrus.	Palka et al. (1966)
^{3}H-Estradiol	≈1–2 µg	crystal	Median eminence	Rat	U	Rise in plasma luteinizing hormone, diestrus.	Palka et al. (1966)
Estradiol and Progesterone	?	crystal	Anterior hypothalamus and preoptic area	Rat	U	Lordosis in castrate female.	Lisk and Suydam (1967)
Estriol	≈2.5–5 µg	crystal	Anterior hypothalamus	Rat	U	Increased plasma corticosterone.	Telegdy et al. (1964)
Estrogen	?	crystal	Median eminence, mammillary body	Rat	U	Reduced prostate and seminal vesicle weight, adrenal enlargement.	Chowers and McCann (1963)
	?	crystal	Mammillary body, arcuate nucleus	Rat	U	Inhibited pregnancy; constant mating of female.	Lisk (1965b)

X. Master Summary Table (Continued)

Chemical	Dose	Volume	Site	Species	State*	Response	Reference
Estrogen	≈5–15 μg	crystal	Preoptic area	Rat	U	Reduced progestin secretion.	Babichev and Telegdy (1968)
	?	crystal	Amygdala, anterior hypothalamus, VMH, periventricular nucleus, arcuate nucleus	Rabbit	U	Inhibited estrogen synthesis.	Kawakami et al. (1969)
	?	crystal	Amygdala	Rabbit	U	Lactogenesis in pseudopregnant females.	Tindal and Knaggs (1966)
	?	crystal	Preoptic area, VMH	Rabbit	U	Facilitated progestin synthesis.	Kawakami et al. (1969)
	≈30–300 μg	crystal	Amygdala	Rabbit	U	Lactogenesis in pseudopregnant female.	Tindal et al. (1967)
	≈80–110 μg	crystal	Hypothalamus	Monkey	U	Sexually related threat behavior increased.	Zumpe and Michael (1970)
Estrone	≈2.5–5 μg	crystal	Anterior hypothalamus	Rat	U	Increased plasma corticosterone.	Telegdy et al. (1964)
Fluphenazine	≈600 μg	crystal	Median eminence	Rat	U	Mammary development; milk ejection.	Mishkinsky et al. (1969)
Follicle stimulating hormone (FSH)	?	crystal	Median eminence	Rat	U	Stimulated luteinization and corpora lutea formation.	Ojeda and Ramirez (1969)
	?	crystal	Median eminence	Rat	U	Reduced plasma and pituitary FSH level, no alteration in plasma LH levels.	Hirono et al. (1970)
	?	crystal	Median eminence	Rat	U	Reduction of pituitary FSH and hypothalamic FSH-RF.	Corbin and Story (1967)
	?	crystal	Medial-basal hypothalamus	Rat	U	Inhibited compensatory ovarian hypertrophy after unilateral ovariectomy.	Arai and Gorski (1968)
	?	crystal	Basal hypothalamus	Rat	U	Diminished compensatory testicular hypertrophy in adult male.	Ojeda and Ramirez (1972)

Compound	Dose	Form	Site	Species		Effect	Reference
Hexestrol	?		Anterior hypothalamus, septum, amygdala, habenula	Rat	U	Evoked lordosis independent of site.	Rodgers and Law (1968)
5-Hydroxytryptophol (5-HTOL)	?		Median eminence, midbrain, reticular formation	Rat	U	Lowered LH in pituitary of castrated male.	Fraschini et al. (1968a)
Luteinizing hormone (LH)	?	crystal	Median eminence	Rat	U	Reduced pituitary LH.	Corbin and Cohen (1966)
	?	crystal	Median eminence	Rat	U	Ovarian atrophy, reduced corpora lutea.	Ojeda and Ramírez (1969)
	?	crystal	Median eminence	Rat	U	Reduction in pituitary LH.	Corbin (1966)
	≈20 μg	crystal	Median eminence	Rat	U	Lowered pituitary LH stores and plasma LH in castrated female.	David et al. (1966)
	≈100–150 μg	crystal	Median eminence	Rat	U	Lowered LH content of pituitary but not serum.	Makino et al. (1972)
Melatonin	?	crystal (solid pellet)	Median eminence, midbrain, reticular substance	Rat	U	Reduced pituitary LH stores and plasma LH levels in castrated males.	Fraschini et al. (1968b)
	?		Median eminence, midbrain, reticular formation.	Rat	U	Lowered LH in pituitary in castrated male.	Fraschini et al. (1968a)
	≈146 μg	crystal	Median eminence	Rabbit	U	Reduced lactation.	Shani et al. (1971)
5-Methoxytryptophol (5-MTOL)	?		Median eminence, midbrain, reticular formation	Rat	U	No significant lowering of LH in the pituitary.	Fraschini et al. (1968a)
Novocaine	20 mg	40 μl	Basal diencephalon	Rabbit	U	Prevented ovulation after mating.	Westman and Jacobsohn (1942)
Norepinephrine (NE)	≈158 μg	crystal	Median eminence	Rabbit	U	Reduced lactation.	Shani et al. (1971)
Norethindrone (17α-ethinyl-9-nortestosterone)	?		Anterior hypothalamus, septum, amygdala, habenula	Rat	U	Evoked lordosis independent of site.	Rodgers and Law (1968)

X. Master Summary Table (Continued)

Chemical	Dose	Volume	Site	Species	State*	Response	Reference
Norethindrone (17α-ethinyl-9-nortestosterone)	≈<100 μg	crystal	Median eminence	Rabbit	U	Blockade of normal or post-coital ovulation after estrogen priming.	Kanematsu and Sawyer (1965)
Pentobarbital sodium	150–250 μg	3–5 μl	Preoptic area, septum	Rat	U	Delayed induced ovulation.	Hagino (1967)
Perphenazine	?	crystal	Median eminence and frontal lobe, thalamus, ant. pituitary, occiptal lobe	Rabbit	U	Increased mammary gland development after ovariectomy.	Mishkinsky et al. (1968)
Pineal tissue	?	crystal (solid pellet)	Median eminence, midbrain, reticular substance	Rat	U	Reduced pituitary LH stores and plasma LH levels in castrated males.	Fraschini et al. (1968)
Potassium chloride (KCl)	447.33 μg	2 μl	Mesencephalic tegmentum	Toad	U	Hypertonus and sexual clasp.	Segura et al. (1971)
PMS (pregnant mare's serum)	?	crystal	Medial-basal hypothalamus	Rat	U	Inhibited compensatory ovarian hypertrophy after unilateral ovariectomy.	Arai and Gorski (1968)
Progesterone	?	crystal	Preoptic area	Chicken	U	Inhibited precocial copulatory behavior.	Meyer (1972)
	5 μg	1 μl	Anterior, preoptic region, posterior hypothalamus, caudal neostriatum	Chicken	U	Premature ovulation.	Ralph and Fraps (1960)
	?	crystal	Hypothalamus, lateral forebrain tracts, preoptic area	Ring dove	U	Induced egg sitting, inhibited male courtship.	Komisaruk (1967)
	?	crystal	Arcuate nucleus, mammillary bodies	Rat	U	Decrease in gonad weight of female.	Lisk (1969a)
	?	crystal	Mammillary bodies, arcuate nucleus	Rat	U	Interference with normal parturition.	Lisk (1965b)

	Dose	Form	Site	Species		Effect	Reference
	?	crystal	Mesencephalic reticular formation	Rat	U	Lordosis of short latency.	Ross et al. (1971)
	≈10 µg	crystal	Ventromedial hypothalamus	Rat	U	Lordosis.	Powers (1972)
	≈10 µg	crystal	Ventromedial hypothalamus, arcuate nucleus	Rat	U	Facilitated ovulation.	Döcke and Dörner (1969)
	50 µg	crystal	Median eminence	Rat	U	Inhibited ovulation.	Labhsetwar and Bainbridge (1971)
	≈200 µg	crystal	Anterior hypothalamus, preoptic area, median eminence	Rat	U	Failed to advance ovulation.	Weick and Davidson (1970)
	≈400 µg	crystal	Median eminence	Rat	U	Reduced uterine weight, suppressed estrous cycling in prepubertal or pubertal rats.	Smith et al. (1969)
	?	crystal	Hypothalamus	Rabbit	U	Only partial block of estrous behavior.	Palka and Sawyer (1966a)
	?	crystal	Hippocampus, arcuate nucleus	Rabbit	U	Increased progestin synthesis.	Kawakami et al. (1969)
	?	crystal	Preoptic area	Rabbit	U	Suppressed estrogen synthesis.	Kawakami et al. (1969)
	?	crystal	VMH	Rabbit	U	Suppressed progestin synthesis.	Kawakami et al. (1969)
Prolactin	≈125–150 µg	crystal	Median eminence	Rat	U	Reduced duration of pseudopregnancy, prevented deciduomata formation.	Chen et al. (1968)
	≈250 µg	crystal	Median eminence	Rat	U	Fall in pituitary FSH concentration; follicular and uterine growth.	Voogt et al. (1969)
	≈250 µg	crystal	Median eminence	Rat	U	Elevated PIF in hypothalamus; reduced pituitary weight and prolactin content, regressed mammary glands.	Clemens and Meites (1968)
	≈300 µg	crystal	Median eminence	Rat	U	Reduced prolactin in anterior pituitary.	Welsch et al. (1968)

X. Master Summary Table (Continued)

Chemical	Dose	Volume	Site	Species	State*	Response	Reference
Reserpine	2 µg	gelatine	Basal hypothalamus	Rat	U	Induced pseudopregnancy; disturbed estrous cycle.	van Maanen and Smelik (1968)
	<100 µg	crystal	Basal hypothalamus	Rabbit	U	Activation of mammary glands.	Kanematsu and Sawyer (1963b)
Serotonin (5-HT)	?	?	Median eminence, mid-brain, reticular formation	Rat	U	No significant lowering of LH in the pituitary.	Fraschini et al. (1968a)
	4.3 µg	1 µl	Hypothalamus	Guinea pig	U	Increase in corticosteroids before and after brain-stem section.	Naumenko (1968)
	≈150 µg	crystal	Median eminence	Rabbit	U	Reduced lactation.	Shani et al. (1971)
Stilbestrol	≈.5–1 µg/day	crystal	Medial hypothalamus	Cat	U	Mating behavior after bilateral ovariectomy.	Michael (1966)
	≈50–150 µg	crystal	Hypothalamus	Cat	U	Mating behavior after ovariectomy.	Michael (1965)
	≈200 µg	crystal	Posterior hypothalamus	Cat	U	Mating after ovariectomy.	Harris and Michael (1958)
	≈50–800 µg	crystal	Hypothalamus	Cat	U	Induced vaginal cornification; mating behavior.	Harris and Michael (1964)
	≈450 µg	crystal	Hypothalamus	Monkey	U	In females, increased sexual performance of male partner.	Michael (1968)
Testosterone	?	crystal	Median eminence	Desert iguana	U	Inhibited spermatogenesis, retarded testicular and ovarian development.	Lisk (1967a)
	?	crystal	Anterior hypothalamus	Chicken	U	Increased mating in males.	Gardner and Fisher (1968)

Dose	Form	Location	Animal	U	Effect	Reference
?	crystal	Preoptic area	Chicken	U	Copulation in the castrate.	Barfield (1969)
≈100 µg	crystal	Anterior hypothalamus	Duck	U	Reduced testicular development and pituitary gonadotropin.	Gogan (1968)
≈100 µg	crystal	Ventromedial hypothalamus	Duck	U	Testicular regression; pituitary gonadotropin depletion.	Gogan (1968)
≈33–41 µg	crystal	Anterior hypothalamus, preoptic area	Dove	U	Courtship behavior in the castrate.	Hutchison (1969, 1971)
≈36–52 µg	crystal	Rostral hypothalamus	Dove	U	Male courtship behavior after castration.	Hutchison (1967)
≈35 µg	crystal	Ventral hypothalamus	Quail	U	Testicular regression.	Stetson (1972)
?	crystal	Anterior hypothalamus	Gerbil	U	Increased territorial scent marking in castrate male.	Yahr and Thiessen (1972)
?	crystal	Anterior hypothalamus and preoptic area	Rat	U	No sexual response in castrate male or female.	Lisk and Suydam (1967)
?	crystal	Mammillary bodies, arcuate nucleus	Rat	U	Interference with normal parturition.	Lisk (1965b)
?	?	Preoptic area	Rat	U	In male, maternal and sexual behavior. In female, male sexual behavior.	Fisher (1966)
?	crystal	Median eminence	Rat	U	Slight increase in pituitary FSH (follicle stimulating hormone) in the castrate animal.	Kamberi and McCann (1972)
?	crystal	Median eminence	Rat	U	Reduction in ovarian and uterine weights.	Chowers and McCann (1967)
?	crystal	Median eminence, mammillary body	Rat	U	Reduced prostate and seminal vesicle weight, adrenal enlargement.	Chowers and McCann (1963)
?	crystal	VMH-arcuate complex	Rat	U	Anovulatory syndrome, persistent vaginal estrus; inhibition of receptivity to male.	Nadler (1972b)
≈1.25–1.67 µg	crystal	Hypothalamus	Rat	U	Inhibited ovulation; persistent vaginal estrus.	Nadler (1968)
≈1–6 µg	crystal	Basal hypothalamus	Rat	U	Advanced vaginal opening, persistent vaginal estrus.	Wagner et al. (1966)

X. Master Summary Table (Continued)

Chemical	Dose	Volume	Site	Species	State*	Response	Reference
Testosterone	≈12.5 μg	crystal	Hypothalamus	Rat	U	Inhibited ovulation and female mating; increased male mating.	Nadler (1968)
	≈25 μg	crystal	Ventromedial-arcuate nucleus	Rat	U	Produced anovulatory condition; persistent vaginal estrus.	Nadler (1972a)
	3–50 μg	?	Preoptic area	Rat	U	Evoked in males: nest building, sexual behavior, grooming and retrieval of pups.	Fisher (1956)
	≈50–100 μg	crystal	Hypothalamus	Rat	U	Atrophy of testes and ovaries.	Lisk (1962a)
	≈200 μg	crystal	Median eminence	Rat	U	Retarded sexual development.	Smith and Davidson (1967)
	≈200 μg	crystal	Anterior hypothalamus	Rat	U	Male sexual behavior in the female.	Dörner et al. (1968b)
	≈200 μg	crystal	Dorsal or medial hypothalamus	Rat	U	Normal female behavior in spayed female.	Dörner et al. (1968b)
	≈220 μg	crystal	Medial preoptic area	Rat	U	Restoration of sexual behavior in castrated male.	Davidson (1966b)
	≈179–320 μg	crystal	Hypothalamus	Rat	U	Restoration of copulation in castrate male.	Lisk (1967b)
	?	crystal	Ventromedial hypothalamus	Rabbit	U	Estrous behavior after ovariectomy.	Palka and Sawyer (1966b)
	≈500 μg	crystal	Median eminence, posterior hypothalamus	Dog	U	Aspermia, testicular and prostatic atrophy.	Davidson and Sawyer (1961b)
Testosterone propionate	≈180–220 μg	crystal	Anterior hypothalamus	Rat	U	Activated male sexual behavior.	Johnston and Davidson (1972)
5-α-Dihydrotestosterone	?	crystal	Medial hypothalamus	Rat	U	Blocked ovarian compensatory hypertrophy after unilateral ovariectomy.	Beyer et al. (1971)

6 Temperature Regulation

I. INTRODUCTION

The daily preoccupation with the vicissitudes of our climatic condition underscores the personal nature with which one's body temperature is contemplated. The very fact that different animals which have large or small areas of body surface can survive and procreate in almost unimaginable extremes of environmental temperature attests to the unusual adaptability of the temperature-sensor-effector system. Perhaps the capability of homeotherms to maintain a set temperature within fairly restricted limits, against all sorts of challenge, is the most intriguiging aspect of the physiological and behavioral mechanisms of thermoregulation. How this is accomplished is a most difficult question. Several approaches to the answer are described in a number of comprehensive reviews including those of Ström, 1960; von Euler, 1961; Hardy, 1961, 1972a; Hammel, 1968; and Benzinger, 1969.

As a result of a number of early studies, the efforts to understand temperature control have converged on the hypothalamus. Historically, a deficit in thermoregulation was evaluated, generally speaking, by the circumscribed destruction of this structure (Isenschmid and Krehl, 1912; Meyer, 1913; Barbour, 1921). The defense against heat seemed to depend on the anterior hypothalamus, whereas the integrity of the posterior hypothalamus was implicated in heat production in defense against the cold (Ranson, 1940). In accord with these lesion studies, Andersson et al. (1956) and Hemingway et al. (1954) found that hypothermia or the suppression of shivering could be brought about by electrical stimulation of the anterior hypothalamus. Conversely, shivering and a rise in temperature occur when the posterior part of this structure is stimulated electrically (Hemingway, 1963). Although we know now that these concepts of an anterior heat loss center and posterior heat maintenance center represent an inordinate oversimplification (Myers, 1971c), the foundations nevertheless were laid down upon which the cellular mechanisms for each anatomical area have been examined.

A. Central Mechanisms

One distinct quirk in the theorizing of the thirties arose when it was demonstrated repeatedly that either warming or cooling of the hypothalamus evoked a compensatory change in core temperature in the opposite direction (e.g., Barbour, 1912; Magoun et al., 1938). Later, Ström (1950), Freeman and Davis (1959), Hardy and his colleagues (Hardy, 1961) and many others (e.g., Jell and Gloor, 1972) have convincingly documented the existence of so-called thermoreceptors or thermosensors in the anterior hypothalamic, preoptic area while abnegating such thermosensitivity in the posterior region. With the classical experiments of von Euler (1950) and of Nakayama et al. (1961; 1963), it became certain that the anterior receptors possessed a rather narrow band of temperature sensitivity. Further painstaking research has revealed that different kinds of thermosensitive neurons can be categorized rather remarkably as warmth detectors, cold detectors and general temperature sensors (e.g., Hardy et al., 1964; Hellon, 1967) some of which either increase or decrease their firing patterns according to a shift in local (brain) or environmental (peripheral) temperature (Hellon, 1969).

How is thermal balance achieved? Presumably, the cold sensitive units trigger an effector pathway for shivering, metabolic heat production and other responses. Warmth sensitive units activate the heat loss mechanism which would include in part the inhibition of heat production. However, the total thermoregulatory response to a sudden or prolonged shift in the environmental temperature is the outcome of physiological reactions and behavioral adjustments to conserve or to dissipate body heat (Hardy, 1972b). In addition to the feedback influence of the temperature of the blood circulating within the hypothalamus (Cooper, 1972a) and possibly other parts of the central nervous system (Kosaka et al., 1969; Cabanac and Hardy, 1969), it is certain that the peripheral input via afferent fibers to the anterior hypothalamus represents an equally critical signal. In fact, Corbit (1969) believes that the temperature input to the brain received from skin receptors may play a far greater role than the factor of hypothalamic temperature, particularly in governing the behavior of avoiding the discomfort of untoward ambient temperatures. This point is emphasized here, since diencephalic monoamines and other substances implicated in the cellular regulation of body temperature may well be linked to the afferent stream of impulses that relay peripheral information rather than to carrying the local depolarizations of thermosensitive neurons in the hypothalamus.

With respect to the central control of temperature as well as to hunger, sleep and other processes discussed in this volume, two scientifically pertinent observations have had a bearing on the direction that the research has taken. One was the presence of monoamines in the diencephalon and mesencephalon in relatively high concentrations (Chapter 1). The other was the tracking by histochemical fluorescence of ascending monoaminergic pathways which terminate in the hypothalamus (Fuxe, 1965; Fuxe et al., 1970; Ungerstedt, 1971). The anatomical correlates of certain neurochemical characteristics provide a basis for understanding the monoamine theory of thermoregulation, which should now be referred to more properly as the amine theory because of the recent inclusion of acetylcholine (Myers, 1970b).

A most surprising facet of the neurochemistry of thermoregulation is the extraordinary sensitivity of certain distinct regions to: 5-HT, ACh, catecholamines, pyrogens, cations, anesthetics and morphine. The distinct "chemosensitivity" of some regions and the selective "chemo-blindness" of others (Myers, 1969c) have enabled scientists to formulate a rather clear picture of a number of central mechanisms of thermoregulation.

B. What are the Main Issues?

The control process for body temperature can be made use of in many ways as a basic model of brain-stem function. One reason for this is that a thermoregulatory response itself is ordinarily unidirectional. As important as the variation in the temperature of the rectum, colon, brain or blood is the pattern of the physiological and behavioral responses that accompany a temperature change. These responses often serve to reinforce the observation of a shift in the temperature measure and may help to disassociate one mechanism from another. Furthermore, the regulatory mechanism can be studied quite readily during a pathological condition such as a fever induced by bacteria or the deep hypothermia resulting from the administration of certain drugs.

A number of technical difficulties may arise in terms of how body temperature is measured. Examples of these are as follows: (1) When a thermistor probe is introduced into the rectum or colon, the animal usually struggles during the insertion and may "fight" the probe for some time thereafter; the result is a rise in temperature. (2) Placing an animal in a harness, stock, sling or other restraining device results in struggling, which again elevates body temperature. In the contrary case of the rabbit, an emotional hypothermia occurs after restraint (Grant, 1950). A period of adaptation may attenuate these artificially induced changes. (3) Most anesthetics usually abolish a part of the temperature regulating mechanism, the degree of impairment depending on the potency of the agent. Usually, the accompanying sharp fall in temperature must be counteracted by external warming, which immediately complicates and confounds the effect of a specific stimulus or variable. (4) Unless ultra-filtration and other standard methods for rendering a fluid pyrogen-free are used, the intracerebral injection of a chemical frequently will elicit a fever with concomitant shivering, vasoconstriction or change in respiratory rate. This is due to the solution which may contain bacteria, spores or other contaminants. These symptoms may be misinterpreted as a direct effect of that drug in the temperature "center" or else on systems involving tremor, cardiovascular tone or pCO_2 receptors. In fact, a dose response curve can even be generated on the basis of the strength of the pyrogen contaminant. (5) Cells such as leucocytes or phagocytic neuroglia that are dislodged from the tip of a guide cannula are also potent pyrogens and may cause a severe hyperpyrexia, presumably by their action within the extracellular fluid of the hypothalamus. (6) The impaling of brain tissue with an injector tube often produces a local hemorrhage in the capillary bed; the presence of whole blood within the calvarium, ventricles or tissue will result in a fierce fever due perhaps to 5-HT in platelets or to the constituents in the lipid fraction (Myers, 1971b). (7) Swamping specific receptor sites in the diencephalon with an overdose of a drug such as carbachol abolishes thermoregulatory activity, and a transitory fall in body temperature toward the ambient end usually ensues; for this reason, dose response plots are vital to the interpretation of any study in which hyper- or hypothermic agents are examined. (8) When an animal's baseline temperature is falling or rising it is fallacious to micro-inject a drug since it is impossible to determine the specific action of the chemical; for example, if the animal's temperature is already rising when a pyrogen is given, that aspect of the hyperthermia produced by the pyrogen cannot be discriminated from that which is already in progress.

In summary, a valid recording of body temperature not only requires an adequate baseline of several hours but also an interval which lasts longer than 30 minutes following an injection. By this procedure, a pyrexic response or other aberration can be ruled out or at least evaluated. To record only an initial rise or fall in the temperature of an animal without specifying the apex or nadir and the termination of the response to the normothermic baseline will preclude any understanding of the total thermoregulatory reaction of the animal to the chemical. Temperature experiments are tedious and each recording requires an abscissa marked off in hours, not minutes.

How many degrees or fraction thereof does the print-out record of body temperature have to deviate to reflect an effect of the stimulus? Although this question can be construed as cumbersome and complicated, generally some sort of arbitrary value must be selected above or below the baseline level of temperature, which falls out of the range of the normal diurnal fluctuation. This value depends on a whole host of important variables including the species examined, the ambient temperature at which the experiments are to be carried out, the feeding regimen, the availability of water, the health and demeanor of the animal, the gonadotropin cycle and the activity of the thyroid axis. In one sense or another, the direction that the temperature curve follows is inextricably bound to the variation of each of these factors; therefore, each one must be carefully scrutinized and controlled to ensure that the response is due to an alteration in the temperature mechanism. For example, if a drug or salt causes an animal to take a long draught of water, the temperature will decline secondarily as a result of the cold water in the stomach, not because the drug affects the hypothalamic "thermostat."

Whether a change in temperature is due to a shift in set-point or is a regulatory response *around* a given set-point is also of great concern. In most mammals the set-point is established *de novo* at parturition at about 37°C. But the set-point concept is often used rather glibly and incorrectly to describe any temperature level which is achieved after a drug has been given.

II. NEUROHUMORAL CONTROL MECHANISMS—AMINES

From all available evidence, it would appear that the anterior hypothalamic, preoptic area contains cells that not only sense differentially the local temperature of the blood but also detect the presence of toxins or drugs. These cells then integrate this localized information with the afferent impulses coming in from receptors in the skin, from deep in the body, and from blood vessels (Bligh, 1966; Hammel, 1968; Lomax, 1970). This complex of information is then translated into a set of efferent impulses that traverse the hypothalamus and pass caudally through the mesencephalon (Benzinger, 1969; Myers and Yaksh, 1969; Myers, 1973).

In this context, the anterior portion of the hypothalamus has been designated as a "chemical thermostat" (e.g., Myers, 1969c) because of three principal reasons: (1) direct injections of specific chemical substances in this region produce remarkably different changes in body temperature; (2) chemical factors, which are opposite to one another in their potent pharmacological properties, are actively released from this region when an animal is exposed to a warm or cold environment; and (3) changes in unit activity that follow local or peripheral warming or cooling also occur in response to the application of a pathogen or other substance. As discussed later, areas of the mesencephalon also have some of these attributes and, therefore, may duplicate certain of the functions of the anterior hypothalamus.

A. Monoamine Theory of Thermoregulation

Two issues are at the vortex of the questions concerning the neurohumoral control of body temperature. First, what are the intrinsic neurochemical processes which establish the temperature set-point? Second, what are the neurochemical mechanisms that mobilize the heat production system in defense against the cold or conversely activate the heat loss system to defend against a hot environment? The problem of the anatomical location of each, if different, is inherent in each question.

In 1963, Feldberg and Myers proposed a new theory to explain how a change in temperature is brought about by the hypothalamic release of three monoamines, 5-HT, norepinephrine and epinephrine. When 5-HT was injected into the cerebral ventricle of the cat, whether conscious or anesthetized, a long-lasting hyperthermia developed (Feldberg and Myers, 1964a;

1965b). On the other hand, norepinephrine or epinephrine injected in the same way lowered normal temperature. A fever induced in the cat by a bacterial pyrogen injected previously into the ventricle was also reduced by the catechol-amines. On the basis of these findings, Feldberg and Myers hypothesized that the balance between the release of 5-HT and the two catecholamines within the hypothalamus was the mechanism whereby temperature was regulated. Summaries of all of the early evidence are given by Feldberg (1968), Myers (1969) and Hellon (1972).

In the first study involving the action on temperature of putative neurotransmitters within tissue, the three monoamines were injected into different parts of the hypothalamus of the conscious cat (Feldberg and Myers, 1965a). When 5-HT was injected in doses of 2 to 10 μg into the anterior hypothalamus, the temperature of the cat rose rapidly after a short latency and remained elevated for several hours. Epinephrine or norepinephrine in corresponding doses caused

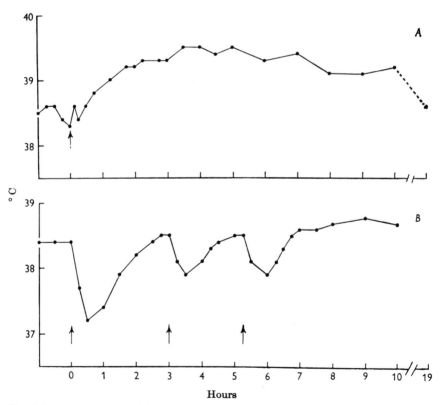

Fig. 6-1a Records of rectal temperature of two unanesthetized cats. The arrows indicate micro-injections (1 μl) into the anterior hypothalamus. In record A of 2 μg 5-HT; in record B of 5 μg adrenaline (1st arrow), of 5 μg noradrenaline (2nd arrow) and of 2.5 μg adrenaline (3rd arrow).

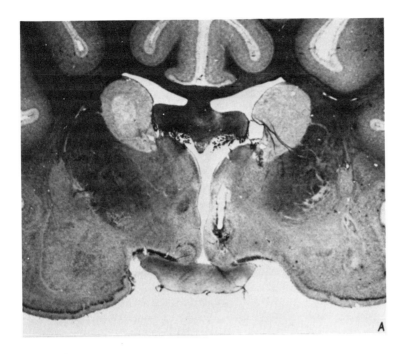

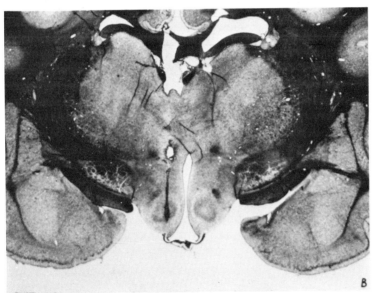

Fig. 6-1b Two coronal sections from two cats' brains with cannula tract ending in anterior (A) and ventromedial (B) hypothalamus. Co-ordinates: A, 13.0; L, 1.5; H, 2.5 (section A); A, 10.0; L, 1.5; H, 5.0 (section B). (From Feldberg and Myers, 1965a)

a profound dose-dependent hypothermia either in the normal cat or in one with a fever induced earlier by typhoid vaccine also injected directly into the anterior hypothalamus. Epinephrine was twice as potent as norepinephrine, an indication that the action on the rostral hypothalamic receptors was more of a beta than alpha adrenergic effect. Basic evidence for an anatomical localization of the monoamine action was thus provided, since the animal's body temperature did not vary if the amines were infused in the ventromedial or posterior hypothalamus. From these experiments, the opposing actions of the amines were localized, as shown in Fig. 6-1a and b, with doses 100 times less than those required to produce an equivalent change in temperature when the compounds were given by the cerebral ventricular route.

1. Anatomical Localization of Monoamine Actions

In a more elaborate anatomical study with the cat, Rudy and Wolf (1971) also confirmed the earlier finding of Feldberg and Myers (1965a) that epinephrine injected into the rostral hypothalamus was more potent than norepinephrine in evoking hypothermia. However, as shown in Fig. 6-2, the relative potencies of

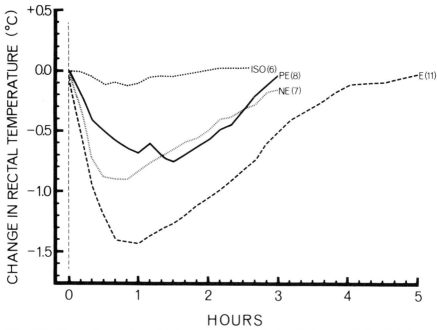

Fig. 6-2 Mean change in rectal temperature elicited by intrahypothalamic injection at time zero of 1 μl of $0.03M$ epinephrine (E), norepinephrine (NE), phenylephrine (PE) and isoproterenol (ISO). Numbers in parentheses refer to the number of animals tested with each agent. (From Rudy, T. A. and H. H. Wolf. 1971. *J. Pharmacol. Exptl. Ther.* **179**:218–235. The Williams and Wilkins Co., Baltimore, Md.)

the alpha and beta adrenergic agonists, phenylephrine and isoproterenol, bore out the notion that alpha receptors are those to which the norepinephrine or epinephrine attach. Pretreatment with phentolamine, an alpha receptor antagonist, effectively blocked the hypothermic effect of intrahypothalamic epinephrine; propranolol, a beta receptor antagonist, exerted only a slight attenuation of the response.

In moving up the phylogenetic scale to the primate, Myers (1968) demonstrated an initial continuity between species with respect to the specific sensitivity of the anterior, preoptic region to the monoamines. When 5 μg of 5-HT were injected in a 1 μl volume in the conscious rhesus monkey, hyperthermia ensued, whereas histamine injected at the same site was without effect. Epinephrine injected similarly at the same site caused a fall in the animal's temperature that had been elevated previously by 5-HT. An important observation was the dose-dependent nature of the 5-HT hyperthermia in that a higher dose of 10 μg injected into the same anterior site caused a fall in temperature.

Later that same year, Myers and Sharpe (1968a) showed that a relatively high dose of 5-HT (12.5 μg) injected into the anterior hypothalamus evoked a sharp increase in the temperature of the monkey which lasted about 45 minutes, in spite of the transitory fall which preceded the rise. This, of course, re-emphasized the necessity of following the time course of a temperature response to an amine rather closely for some hours. In addition, when norepinephrine was injected in the same dose (12.5 μg) as 5-HT and at the same anatomical site, the monkey's normal body temperature declined, then returned to its normal baseline without any pyrexic after-rise. This result not only demonstrated the specificity of the amine response but also abrogated the possibility that the carrier solution for 5-HT or norepinephrine possessed pyrogenicity.

The overlapping locus of action of both 5-HT and norepinephrine in evoking hyper- and hypothermia, respectively, has been mapped in the rhesus monkey (Myers and Yaksh, 1969). In doses of 2 to 10 μg, 5-HT caused a long-lasting elevation in temperature, whereas noradrenaline in doses as low as 1 μg evoked a fall in the animal's normal temperature. The site of action of both amines, as shown in Figs. 6-3 and 6-4, was the region ventral to the anterior commissure and dorsal to the optic chiasm, an area identical to that which Hayward and Baker (1968) found in the same species to be thermosensitive. The dose-dependent nature of the hyper- and hypothermia caused by 5-HT and NE, respectively (Myers, 1970b), when micro-injected into the anterior hypothalamus is shown in Fig. 6-5. Acetylcholine mixed in equal concentration with eserine produced a sharp rise in temperature which was also dose-dependent but different in latency and duration from the more sluggish 5-HT hyperthermia (Fig. 6-5). In the baboon, Toivola and Gale (1970) have also confirmed the hypothermic action of norepinephrine infused into the rostral hypothalamus. In addition, they again showed that a high dose of 5-HT (15 μg) infused into the same region evoked a hypothermic effect.

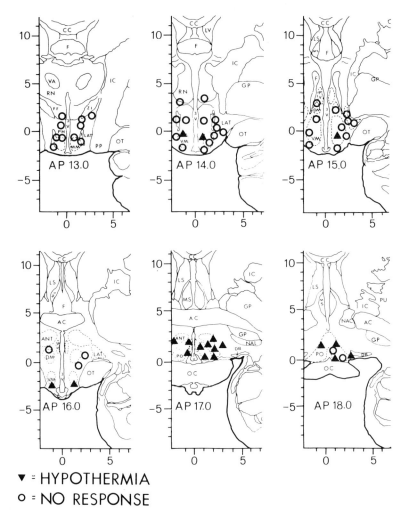

▼ = HYPOTHERMIA
○ = NO RESPONSE

Fig. 6-3 Anatomical 'mapping' at six coronal (AP) levels of sites in the hypothalamus at which micro-injections of 5-HT in doses of 2 to 10 μg produce
hyperthermia (▲). Sites at which 5-HT injections cause no change in temperature are also indicated (○). AC anterior commissure; ANT anterior hypothalamic
area; CC corpus callosum; DB diagonal band of Broca; DM dorsomedial nucleus;
F fornix; FF fields of Forel; GP globus pallidus; IC internal capsule; LAT lateral
hypothalamus; LV lateral ventricle; LS lateral septal nucleus; MM mammillary
body; MS medial septal nucleus; NAC nucleus accumbens; OC optic chiasm;
OT optic tract; PH posterior hypothalamic area; PO preoptic area; PP cerebral
peduncle; PU putamen; PV paraventricular nucleus; RN reticular nucleus of the
thalamus; VA antero-ventral nucleus of the thalamus; ZI zona incerta; 3 V third
ventricle. Horizontal and lateral scales are in millimeters. Vertical zero represents the stereotaxic zero plane 10 mm above the interaural line. (From Myers
and Yaksh, 1969)

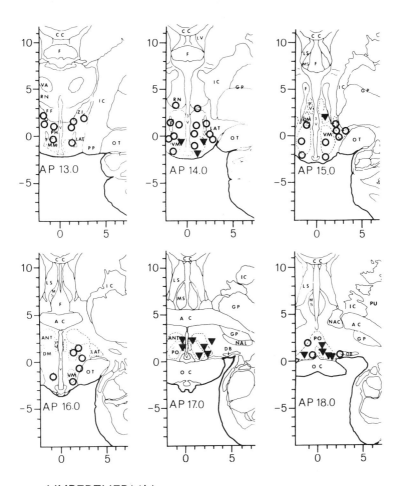

▲ = HYPERTHERMIA
○ = NO RESPONSE

Fig. 6-4   Anatomical 'mapping' at six coronal (AP) levels of sites in the hypothalamus at which micro-injections of noradrenaline or adrenaline in doses of
1 to 12 μg produce hypothermia (▼). Sites at which these catecholamines cause
no change in temperature are also indicated (○). Anatomical abbreviations and
the stereotaxic scales are the same as in Fig. 6-3. (From Myers and Yaksh, 1969)

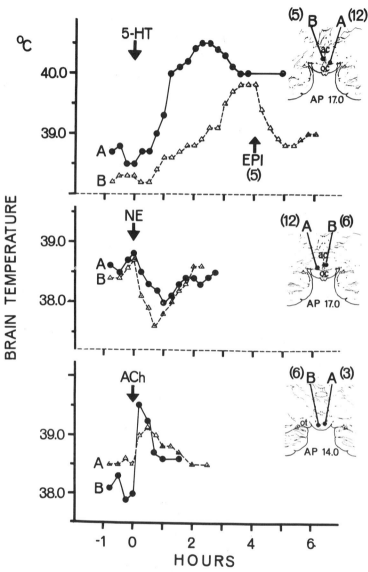

Fig. 6-5 Temperature responses to micro-injections of candidate transmitters in the anterior, preoptic region (AP 17.0) and posterior area (AP 14.0) of the hypo-thalamus. In top panel, 5 and 12 μg 5-HT micro-injected, at first arrow, into sites B and A, respectively; 5 μg epinephrine (EPI) at second arrow, into site B only; in middle panel, 6 and 12 μg norepinephrine (NE), at arrow, into sites B and A, respectively; in bottom panel, 3 and 6 μg acetylcholine (ACh) mixed in equal proportion with physostigmine, micro-injected at arrow, into sites A and B respectively. Brain temperature in °C on the ordinate, time in hours on the abscissa. (From Myers, 1970b)

For the regulation of body temperature around a given level, it would appear that a sustained release of 5-HT from the cells of the anterior region activates the efferent pathway for heat production. Norepinephrine released from the same site seems to function to inhibit the heat production pathway by either competing for 5-HT receptor sites or by interfering in some way with the local action of 5-HT. Alternatively, norepinephrine could block the cholinergic heat production pathway, since the temporal characteristics of the curves of norepinephrine hypothermia and acetylcholine hyperthermia are identical but inversely related.

A relationship between hypothalamic temperature and ingestive behavior is now certain (Hamilton and Ciaccia, 1971). Heating of the anterior hypothalamic, preoptic region to displace its temperature by about 1°C for 24 hours reduces core temperature of the rat as expected, but also evokes a long-term increase in food intake. This result would reflect the need for more energy as the animal's metabolism increases to offset the lowered body temperature. Thus, feeding can be viewed as one kind of thermoregulatory behavior. Of direct bearing on this is the interaction of hypothalamic areas that are reactive to adrenergic stimulation and that mediate either feeding or a fall in body temperature. In an extensive anatomical analysis of each of 179 sites in the diencephalon of the monkey, norepinephrine was micro-injected in doses of 5 to 12.5 µg (Yaksh and Myers, 1972b). At 19 loci, the catecholamine evoked only a fall in temperature of at least 0.4°C; again the region of greatest sensitivity was the anterior hypothalamus. At 27 other sites located in the mid-hypothalamic region in close proximity to the fornix and medial forebrain bundle, only feeding, often accompanied by prandial drinking, was produced by injections of norepinephrine. Interestingly, norepinephrine at 5 sites evoked a simultaneous fall in temperature and spontaneous feeding in the monkey, as illustrated in Fig. 6-6. Even though both of these noradrenergic systems generally exhibited a clear-cut morphological independence, Yaksh and Myers presented evidence in their experiments that the neurohumoral components of the mechanism underlying eating and the loss of body heat are anatomically interconnected.

2. *Species Similarities and Differences*

In a landmark paper, Cooper *et al.* (1965) raised the possibility of species-differences in response to locally applied monoamines. When 5-HT was injected in a large volume into the anterior hypothalamus of the rabbit in a dose of from 2 to 20 µg, there was no effect on body temperature. However, 40 µg of 5-HT caused a pronounced drop in the temperature of a single rabbit with a fever. Injections of 10 µg of norepinephrine in the same sites and in similar volumes caused a hyperthermic response in half of the experiments, but for some unexplained reason had no effect in the other half. Similarly, doses of 2 to 5 µg of the catecholamine, which lowers temperature when injected into the anterior hypothalamus of a cat or monkey had virtually no effect on the rabbit. When

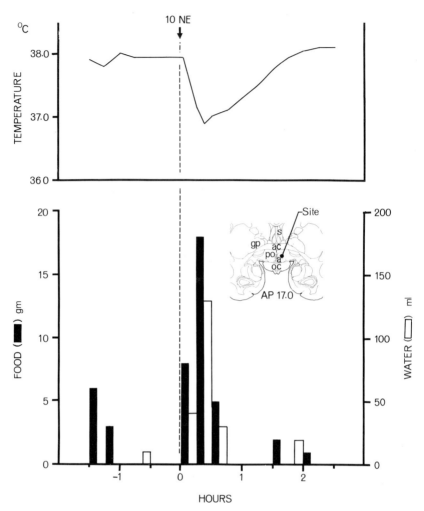

Fig. 6-6 Eating, drinking and temperature responses of an unanesthetized mon-key following injection at the arrow of NE in a dose of 10 μg base into the anterior hypothalamus at AP 17.0 (inset). (From Yaksh and Myers, 1972b)

20 μl of endogenous pyrogen were injected into the same site, fever resulted but such large volumes would be expected to easily affect these sites. Central in-fusions of histamine, acetylcholine and eserine had no effect, although in one rabbit a single infusion of potassium caused a fever. Since the site into which an amine is injected is such a critical factor in the response, it is possible that the crucial pool of neurons in the anterior hypothalamus was actually stimulated. Given the large volumes infused, however, the amines certainly would diffuse into the ventricular cavity where it is possible that the diluted moiety may not have

been sufficiently potent. Obviously, a dose response curve, anatomical mapping of specific sites and a smaller volume are the three requisites that would help to ascertain what effects 5-HT, norepinephrine or acetylcholine have on the anterior hypothalamic, preoptic area in the control of body temperature in the rabbit. Nevertheless, the important possibility was thus first raised by Cooper and his colleagues (1965) that the brain of each and every species may be functionally "wired" in a unique neurochemical manner (Myers and Sharpe, 1968b).

In connection with the inconsistent findings with the rabbit, Peindaries and Jacob (1971) have made an extremely important observation. They found that an intraventricular injection of 5-HT which was contaminated with bacterial pyrogen produced a fall in the temperature of the rabbit; this depended on the dose of the pyrogen. Each rabbit was used only once, and the animals were in restraining cages. With respect to interpreting apparent species differences, un-contaminated, dialyzed 5-HT given intraventricularly to the rabbit evoked a sharp hyperthermia, identical to that seen in the cat, monkey and other species. These results are similar to those of Canal and Ornesi (1961) who found that 5-HTP or 5-HT given intracisternally also caused a fever. The febrile response is believed to be due to the considerable diffusion of the amine to the hypothalamus, which occurs when a compound is injected into the cisterna magna (Banerjee et al., 1970).

Contrary to the hypothermic effect on the rat of 5-HT when given by the intra-ventricular route (Myers and Yaksh, 1968), a rise in temperature is produced when 5-HT is injected directly into the anterior preoptic area in doses of 0.05 to 1.0 μg (Crawshaw, 1972). When a rat that was placed in a cold chamber and pressing a lever for heat lamp reward was given a similar injection of 5-HT, inconsistent changes in bar-pressing were observed. These were probably due to the anatomical differences in the location of the injection needle, although it would probably be difficult to differentiate precisely one locus from another because of the large size of the cannula relative to that of the brain. Nonetheless, these results are among the first to show that there is an important distinction between the intraventricular and intrahypothalamic routes of administration of a monoamine.

Norepinephrine injected into the rostral hypothalamus of the rat in a dose of 2.5 μg in 1 μl caused an average decline in temperature of 0.4°C, whereas 5 μg produced a fall of about twice the magnitude (Lomax et al., 1969). A small rise in temperature was produced by 0.5 μg but, because of the latency, a pyro-genic effect of the solution cannot be ruled out. Surprisingly, an alpha adrenergic antagonist, tolazoline, had no consistent effects but unfortunately only a single dose of 2.5 μg was given.

Using somewhat higher doses than those of Lomax et al. (1969), Avery (1971) found that norepinephrine also evoked a fall in temperature of the rat when the the amine was injected in a volume of 0.5 μl into the anterior hypothalamus. Although Avery showed that 15 μg of norepinephrine produced a hypothermic response ranging from 0.3 to 1.5°C, an injection of either 5 or 25 μg did not evoke a consistent change in temperature, perhaps because of variations in the cannula placement between these two groups or because the small volumes would not reach amine sensitive sites. Even though 5-HT and perhaps other pharmacological controls would be desirable, additional data collected by Avery (1972), again with the rat, correspond well with the 1969 Myers-Yaksh model based on the primate. The respective roles of acetylcholine in heat production and norepinephrine in heat loss were identical for both species. However, the fact that norepinephrine evoked a hyperthermic response when the rat was exposed to an ambient temperature of 5°C led Avery to make an addition to the Myers-Yaksh model (1969), similar to that proposed by Bligh et al. (1971). That is, norepinephrine release in the rostral hypothalamus may inhibit both the heat loss and heat production pathways in the rat, the former at a low environmental temperature.

Using a dose 100 times less than Avery's, Beckman (1970) found that an injection of norepinephrine, again into the anterior hypothalamic preoptic area of the rat, produced an average increase in temperature of 0.7°C as measured by a hypothalamic thermistor. In some experiments, the response to intrahypothalamic norepinephrine was biphasic, with a mean maximum fall in hypothalamic temperature of about 0.3°C occurring first. This was the same response seen by Avery who used a much higher dose but only half of the volume. In some of Beckman's rats, the elevation in hypothalamic temperature was accompanied by an increase in lever pressing for heat lamp reinforcement. This would appear on the surface to be a paradoxical situation, since it is a well-known phenomenon that cooling the hypothalamus is a powerful stimulus which elicits intense behavioral responding to turn on a heat lamp, while hypothalamic warming reduces responding for heat (e.g., Baldwin and Ingram, 1966). However, this result could indicate that in blocking the heat production pathway, norepinephrine evokes or mediates the sensation of cold. It is probably unlikely that the body temperature of the rat itself declined while the hypothalamic temperature was on the increase. Instead, the animal's behavior shows that norepinephrine simply signalled a response to keep warm in the face of heat loss. Clearly, a wider range of doses is required; furthermore, a smaller volume and a record of the core temperature of the rat would aid in a more complete explanation of these fascinating findings.

Preliminary studies with the guinea pig suggest that the rostral hypothalamus of this species is also sensitive to norepinephrine (Zeisberger and Brück, 1971a and b). When a single 2 μg dose of norepinephrine is injected into the anterior hypothalamus of a neonatal or cold-adapted guinea pig, a slight biphasic variation in temperature occurs. Although the hypothermia followed by hyperthermia has a duration of only 30 minutes, O_2 consumption increases by as much as 50%. On the basis of local heating of the hypothalamus and a simultaneous norepinepherine injection, Zeisberger and Brück propose that this catecholamine elevates the "threshold temperature for cold-induced heat production." Without a dose response study and a more detailed explanation of cold adaptation and other methods, it is probably too early to delineate a definite relationship between catecholamines and temperature in the guinea pig.

In the ground squirrel (*Citellus lateralis*), the hypothalamus retains a sensitivity to the monoamines while the animal hibernates (Beckman and Satinoff, 1972) just as the cat's hypothalamus does during anesthesia (Feldberg and Myers, 1964b). Either 5-HT or norepinephrine injected bilaterally into the rostral hypothalamus in a large 1 μl volume aroused the ground squirrel from deep hibernation when the animal's temperature was below 10°C. That this was simply an effect of manipulation was ruled out by control injections of equal volumes of NaCl or the salts of each amine. Although the arousal from torpor was physiologically similar to the spontaneous arousal induced by sensory stimulation, the effect of each monoamine on the normal body temperature of a non-hibernating squirrel was quite different. Generally 5-HT evoked hyperthermia, whereas norepinephrine caused a transient hypothermia or hyperthermia. The latter responses may have been dependent on the temperature of the animal, the site of the micro-injection or the dose of catecholamine. Additional research is required before we can ascertain whether the amines are acting directly on the thermoregulatory pathways, a metabolic mechanism, the sleep system, or on the sensory input to the brainstem.

Other biogenic amines also affect temperature when their levels in the brain are altered. For example, a dose-dependent fall in the body temperature of the rat occurs after the injection of histamine into the rostral hypothalamus (Brezenoff and Lomax, 1970). This hypothermia was prevented by the prior systemic administration of an antihistamine, chlorcyclazine. Since histamine is known to be a powerful releaser of catecholamines, the hypothermic effect could have been indirectly due to such a release. Histamine's local vasodilatory action on the hypothalamic capillaries or blood vessels could also have influenced the temperature neurons. The findings do not correspond with those of Cooper *et al.* (1965), who injected 12 μg of histamine into the anterior hypothalamus of the rabbit, or to those of Myers (1968), who injected 20 μg of histamine in a homologous region of the monkey. In both experiments, histamine was without effect on body temperature.

A study done with the rat by Boros-Farkas and Illei-Donhoffer (1969) would at first glance seem to complicate the picture. Each of nine substances (see Master Summary Table) injected in a single dose into the hypothalamus in a region described as being posterior to the optic chiasm evoked hyperthermia. In many instances a control injection of saline also caused a rise in body temperature of the same magnitude. Furthermore, all of the substances except phenylalanine and GAHBA increased rats' O_2 consumption. Because of a large 20 μl volume and the nonspecific effects alluded to by the authors, in which the simple insertion of a thermocouple through the cannula 0.5 to 1.0 mm into tissue caused a hyperthermia equally as severe as a chemical, a deduction cannot be drawn from this report.

B. Cholinergic Mechanisms

What is the net result of the cellular activity of monoaminergic neurons and what information is thereby provided within the anterior preoptic area? How is such information translated to an effector system and by what route does each message travel? This fundamental conundrum remained following the studies of the localization of action of 5-HT and norepinephrine on body temperature.

1. Heat Production

In 1969, Myers suggested that both 5-HT and norepinephrine present in the hypothalamus somehow "work through the release of acetylcholine" (Myers, 1969c). Although the function of acetylcholine in the anterior region was initially thought to be inconsequential, Myers and Yaksh (1969) showed later that year that acetylcholine or carbachol injected at sites located throughout the hypothalamus including the anterior, preoptic area evoked a sharp increase in temperature. As shown in Fig. 6-5, the characteristics of the temperature rise were very different from those of 5-HT or a pyrogen-induced hyperthermia. Cholinergic thermogenesis is characterized by a short latency, short duration and rapid termination. In fact, the steepness of the rise produced by acetylcholine in the mammillary region is reminiscent of that elicited by electrical stimulation of homologous loci. The sole hypothalamic mapping of cholinoceptive heat-production sites completed at this writing shows that the pathway is not only very diffuse but extends all the way from the preoptic area to the mesencephalon. This ACh map is illustrated in Fig. 6-7. At the diencephalic junction, sites were found at which acetylcholine or carbachol also evoked hypothermia, which has special physiological significance in terms of acetylcholine release as discussed in the concluding section. From this study, several conclusions were reached: (a) acetylcholine acts as the transmitter serving the heat-production pathway which projects caudally from the anterior hypothalamus (Myers, 1970b); (b) a chemically mediated efferent heat-loss pathway, which traverses the hypothalamus, does not exist; and (c) within the posterior hypothalamus, a heat-loss pathway arises, the origin and purpose of which are related possibly to the set-point function (see Section III).

A partial characterization of the cholinergic receptors in heat production was completed by Hall and Myers (1972). In the rhesus monkey, nicotine was injected in 91 sites in the hypothalamus, mesencephalon and contiguous areas. A high degree of localization of action was found in that nicotine evoked a marked fall in temperature only when injected into the anterior hypothalamus (Fig. 6-8) but a rise when injected into more posterior sites in the hypothalamus (Fig. 6-9). Since acetylcholine itself causes a rise in temperature, nicotine probably acts in

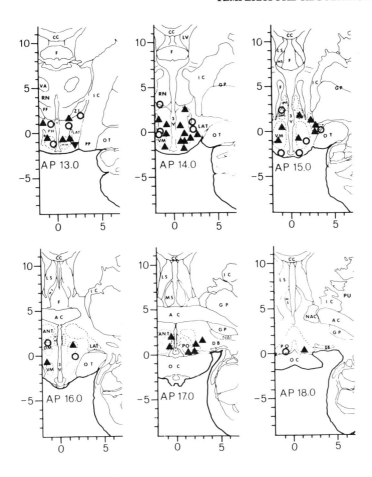

▲ = HYPERTHERMIA

▼ = HYPOTHERMIA

○ = NO RESPONSE

Fig. 6-7 Anatomical 'mapping' at six coronal (AP) levels of sites in the hypothalamus at which micro-injections of acetylcholine, acetylcholine-eserine mixture in doses of 2 to 25 μg, or carbachol in doses of 0.4 to 2.0 μg produce
hyperthermia (▲) or hypothermia (▼). Sites at which these compounds cause no
change in temperature are also indicated (○). Anatomical abbreviations and the
stereotaxic scales are the same as in Fig. 6-3. (From Myers and Yaksh, 1969)

the anterior region to release norepinephrine, thus causing the typical hypothermic response. The main result suggests, however, that the cholinergic pathway for the activation of heat production is a nicotinic one. Additional verification of this view was obtained by further experiments in which the injection of
norepinephrine (Fig. 6-8) or acetylcholine into the anterior or posterior hypothalamus, respectively, altered the temperature of the monkey in the same
manner as nicotine injected into the same sites.

In the rat, a fall in temperature is also produced by nicotine injected into the
anterior hypothalamus (Knox and Lomax, 1972). However, the effects of nicotine on the posterior hypothalamus have not as yet been tested in relation to
temperature.

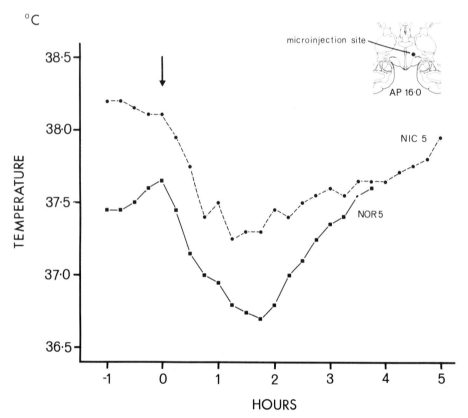

Fig. 6-8 Changes in body temperature of a monkey following the micro-
injection at the arrow of 5 μg of nicotine (NIC) or norepinephrine (NOR) given
in a volume of 1 μl. The anatomical site at which the injection was made at an
interval of 48 to 72 hours is shown on the inset of coronal plane AP 16.0. (From
Hall, G. H. and R. D. Myers. 1972. *Brain Research*. **37**:241–251. Elsevier
Publishing Co., Amsterdam, The Netherlands)

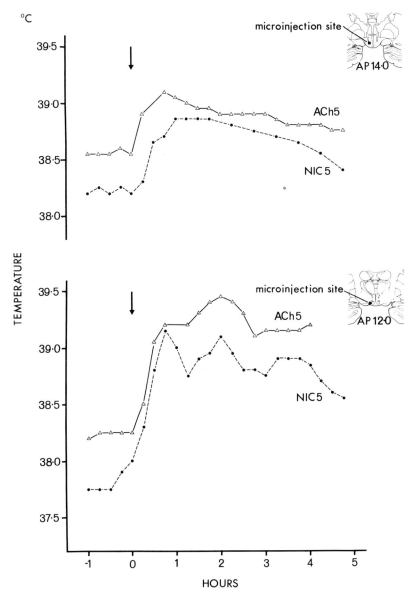

Fig. 6-9 Changes in body temperature of a monkey following the micro-injection at the arrow of 5 μg of acetylcholine (ACh) or nicotine (NIC) given in a volume of 1 μl. The anatomical sites at which the injections were made at an interval of 48 to 72 hours are shown on the insets at coronal planes AP 14.0 (top) or AP 12.0 (bottom) in two different monkeys. (From Hall, G. H. and R. D. Myers. 1972. *Brain Research*. 37:241–251. Elsevier Publishing Co., Amsterdam, The Netherlands)

The function of a cholinergic mechanism in mediating separate heat-production and heat-loss pathways has also been examined in the cat. In structures outside of the diencephalon, cholinergic stimulation ordinarily evokes a rise in temperature that accompanies autonomic and motor responses. When carbachol is injected in doses of 5 to 8 μg into the caudate nucleus, fever occurs along with hind limb tremor or, in some instances, focal EEG seizures (Connor et al., 1966b). Hyperthermia also develops with the injection of a number of other cholinomimetics into the caudate nucleus (Connor et al., 1966a). In this and other structures in the limbic system, including the thalamus, carbachol may cause a rise in temperature in the cat except during severe hyperventilation associated with a gross autonomic discharge. In this case, the animal loses heat readily and its temperature falls sharply for a brief period (Hull et al., 1967).

Using the mapping procedure of Myers and Yaksh (1969) for the monkey, Rudy and Wolf (1972) showed that carbachol could have three separate effects. This cholinomimetic injected in a low dose produced at most hypothalamic loci an increase in temperature, hypothermia followed by hyperthermia at an intermediate dose, and at a high dose, an intense hypothermia. Typical responses are illustrated in Fig. 6-10. Although a mixture of acetylcholine-eserine had much the same pattern of effect, the magnitude and duration of the temperature change were considerably reduced. These data support the view that a cholinergic heat-production system may also exist in the cat, in spite of the fact that hypothermia did not follow cholinergic stimulation of the posterior hypothalamic-mesencephalic junction. The hypothermia caused by carbachol given in a high dose in the anterior hypothalamic area or the slight fall preceding a major rise in temperature may have been due to a partial or total blockade of the cholinergic receptors at the origin of the efferent pathway which is postulated to arise in the anterior thermosensitive zone. Clearly, dose-response curves are always necessary to rule out such a possibility.

2. Cholinergic Hypothermia in the Rat

In a series of experiments with the restrained rat, Lomax and his colleagues have found that temperature falls following the infusion of cholinergic compounds into the hypothalamus. When injected into the preoptic area, oxotremorine or carbachol elicited hypothermia (Lomax and Jenden, 1966). After the antimuscarinic compounds, atropine or trihexyphenidyl, were given in the same area in single high doses, 40 μg and 10 μg, respectively, peripherally administered oxotremorine failed to evoke the typical hypothermic response. Another cholinomimetic, pilocarpine, injected also into the rostral hypothalamus of the rat in a single high dose of 40 μg again blocked heat-production, and hypothermia resulted (Lomax et al., 1969). Using the iontophoretic technique, Kirkpatrick and Lomax (1970) have also validated these earlier findings of a fall in temperature when a high dose of 20 to 100 μg of carbachol or 15 μg of acetylcholine was applied to the rostral hypothalamus of the rat. In these experiments there were

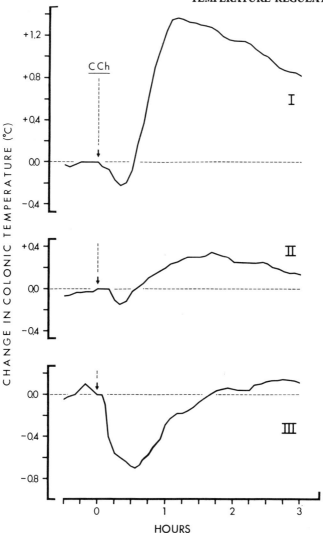

Fig. 6-10 Representative examples of the changes in colonic temperature in response to carbachol (CCh); 0.01 *M* was injected in 1 μl volume at the arrows. (From Rudy, T. A. and H. H. Wolf. 1972. *Brain Research*. 38:117–130, Fig. 1. Elsevier Publishing Co., Amsterdam, The Netherlands)

no anatomical controls in which injections were given more caudally in the posterior or other areas of the hypothalamus; similarly, no dose response measures were obtained. Taken together, however, these data suggest that there could be a cholinoceptive receptor involved in hypothermia.

If atropine is injected into the rostral hypothalamus of the rat, its body temperature rises (Kirkpatrick and Lomax, 1967). Although only a single 5 μg dose was used, atropine may have acted to block the "endogenous cholinergic transmission" of the thermoregulatory pathway. Since a low dose of atropine given peripherally causes hypothermia, whereas a high dose causes hyperthermia, dose response information is certainly required for a more complete interpretation of the central effects of a cholinomimetic or cholinergic blocking agent. Nevertheless, it is interesting that another drug purported to have central muscarinic blocking properties also affects temperature similarly. A single 50 μg dose of DKJ-21 [N-(4-diethylamino-2-butynyl)-succinimide] injected into the anterior hypothalamus also blocks the hypothermia evoked by systemic oxotremorine.

A similar set of experiments has been conducted with the unrestrained rat. At every site tested in the brain including the cerebral ventricles, oxotremorine in doses ranging from 8 to 50 μg evoked a fall in temperature (Staib and Andreas, 1970). In addition to the effect of a high dose is probably the factor of the enormous volume injected, which in the case of the rat's hypothalamus exceeds the entire bilateral dimensions of this structure (Myers and Sharpe, 1968b). When 120 μg/kg oxotremorine was injected intravenously, the hypothermia was attenuated somewhat by the micro-injection of 250 μg atropine, given again in a volume of 10 μl into the anterior hypothalamus or septum. No histology was presented to show the type of lesion produced in the hypothalamic tissue.

Cholinergic stimulation of the rostral hypothalamus of the guinea pig also reduced nonshivering thermogenesis when 1 μl of either carbachol or acetylcholine-eserine solution was injected into the heat sensitive zone (Zeisberger and Brück, 1971c). When given more caudally, these substances had much less of an effect on body temperature of the guinea pig, and oxygen uptake was equally reduced by the more rostral injections. Considering the volume of the injection, it is again possible that the preoptic thermosensitive elements were blocked by the cholinergic compounds applied locally.

3. Cholinergic Hyperthermia in the Rat

In 1967, Hulst and deWied showed that crystals of carbachol deposited in the hypothalamus produced a rise in temperature, or a fall, which was often coordinated with drinking of a fairly large volume of water. A strong hyperthermic response was produced when the cholinomimetic was applied similarly to the areas in the ventral thalamus at which no drinking occurred (Hulst and deWied, 1967). That cholinergic thermogenesis occurs in the rat by a direct action of acetylcholine on the central nervous system was then shown by Myers and Yaksh (1968) who found that acetylcholine or carbachol injected into the cerebral ventricles evoked a sharp rise in temperature.

If carbachol is micro-injected into the anterior hypothalamic area of the rat, hyperthermia is evoked. Although this response was confirmed again with several doses (Avery, 1971), the cholinergically-induced rise in temperature is opposite to that which Lomax and Jenden (1966) had reported. A credible insight of Avery (1970) may provide a clue to a reconciliation of the ostensible species

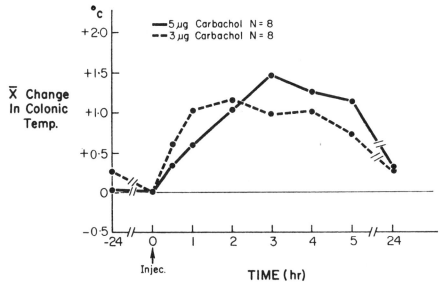

Fig. 6-11 Hyperthermia in both high and low concentration groups, 5 μg or 3 μg of carbachol. The increases in colonic temperature became asymptotic in 2 hours for the low dosage group and in 3 hours for the high dosage group. (From Avery, D. D. 1970. *Neuropharmacology.* 9:175–178. Pergamon Press, New York)

differences in the rodent, since Avery's rats were unrestrained and freely moving. This ought to be a significant experimental variable in view of Grant's observation that restraint and hypothermia are intimately related (Grant, 1950). Most important of all is the 0.5 μl volume used by Avery for the micro-injection of each solution. Logically, a smaller volume of the cholinomimetic would reduce the likelihood of an overall swamping of receptor sites, which does not seem to occur in an animal with a larger diencephalon. In any event, Avery's experiments support the concept of an acetylcholine mechanism arising in the anterior hypothalamus for transmitting signals along the effector pathway for heat production. Although this cholinergic trajectory may extend caudally through the rat's hypothalamus (Myers and Yaksh, 1969; Myers and Waller, 1973), an anatomical mapping of ACh sensitive sites in the rodent's diencephalon is essential.

In an intriguing study, Beckman and Carlisle (1969) examined the function of an acetylcholine mechanism in behavioral thermoregulation. When rats were kept at 5°C, high doses of acetylcholine (20 to 50 μg) injected into the rostral hypothalamus produced a transient fall in hypothalamic temperature. This decline lasted only 10 minutes but was accompanied quite surprisingly by a paradoxical decline in the bar-pressing rate of externally applied heat from a lamp. Ordinarily, when an animal's hypothalamus is cooled (e.g., Baldwin and

Ingram, 1966; Satinoff, 1967), the response rate for heat lamp reinforcement increases sharply. Hence, the results of the ACh injection would appear to be nonphysiological and due perhaps to a paralyzing effect of the high dose. Such an effect wears off very quickly within 10 to 15 minutes and is counteracted by pretreating the site with a micro-injection of a single high dose of 20 μg of atropine. In view of these results, a lower dose of each substance and behavioral tests at three ambient temperatures similar to Avery's (1972) conditions would help to elucidate the mechanisms underlying the reinforcing properties of heat.

Perhaps a cholinergic mechanism within the anterior hypothalamus is involved in the heat-loss mechanism of the rat. More than likely, however, is the possibility that a high dose of a cholinergic substance causes a paralytic antagonism of the hypothalamic neurons involved in heat production, which is similar to the classical blockade of ganglionic transmission seen when a high dose of acetylcholine is applied to sympathetic ganglia. Fitting in with this explanation is the fact that atropine, given systemically, does block the local effect of either acetylcholine or carbachol on the hypothalamus.

From a physiological standpoint, it would seem illogical for such a ubiquitous substance as acetylcholine, which is considered to be almost a universal transmitter in vertebrates and invertebrates, to be used in a biological control system as an inhibitor of heat production, when the rat is ordinarily defending *against* the cold in a thermally hostile environment. Certainly, the release of a rapidly acting transmitter substance such as acetylcholine, which from iontophoretic studies correlates with neuronal firing rate, would more likely be required for heat maintenance. Based on the constant requirement of the heat production mechanism to sustain the life of the mammal, efferent impulses for heat production far outweigh those that signal the need for heat loss.

All in all, an anatomical mapping would always seem to be required to localize the effects of acetylcholine and cholinomimetic substances within thalamic, hypothalamic and mesencephalic structures. In an animal with a relatively small brain, it is essential that a very small volume be used in temperature experiments so that an entire region is not inundated with the chemical solution. Finally, at each cholinoceptive site, several graded doses of each cholinergic substance should be tested.

III. IONIC SET-POINT FUNCTION

The set-point for body temperature established inherently is considered by most physiologists to be a built-in reference temperature around which adjustments are continually made. Inasmuch as the set-point temperature is approximately 37°C in most mammals, it is an interesting intellectual exercise to contemplate why that particular value was assigned by Nature as one so critical for normal physiological activity. Or an extreme position can be adopted that a reference signal or set-point does not really exist at all (Mitchell *et al.*, 1970).

The concept of a temperature set-point is supposed to have originated with von Liebermeister in 1860 (von Liebermiester, 1860; Cremer and Bligh, 1969) but it is still not clear whether this is actually true (Cooper, 1972b). However, the idea itself has developed broadly over the last 20 years (e.g., Hammel, 1965; Hardy, 1965) and even extended to include other physiological set-points, including those for lipids, weight, gonadal function, hunger, sleep and emotion (see Chapters 5, 7, 9 and 11).

A. Ion Balance in the Hypothalamus

A challenge to a subsequent deflection from the set-point temperature of 37°C normally causes the immediate mobilization of the effector pathways for heat gain or loss to hold the temperature to the set level. Thus, following a simple peripheral change in the form of a cold or hot environmental temperature, a deviation from the set-point level is prevented or offset by the excitation of appropriate effector responses.

Up until 1970, the set-point was thought to be integrated anatomically with the thermoreceptors in the same part of the anterior hypothalamus or at some unknown locus in peripheral tissue. A radical departure from conventional theory occurred when Myers and Veale (1970) postulated that the site of the set-point was the posterior hypothalamus which has always been considered to be the "heat maintenance center." They proposed that the local firing rate of the efferent neurons in this region was maintained independently by the inborn ratio of sodium to calcium ions in the extracellular fluid within that region, and that this neuronal activity sustained the set temperature of 37°C.

As early as 1911, it had been known that an alteration in the systemic concentration of calcium or other cations causes abrupt changes in body temperature (Freund, 1911; Schütz, 1916). However, it was not until 1930 that a careful analysis of the diencephalic actions of ions was undertaken.

Hasama (1930) examined the effect on body temperature of the injection of solutions of cations in a volume of 50 μl into the tuber cinerium of the unanesthetized cat. Sodium, potassium and barium had a hyperthermic effect of varying intensity; however, calcium ions caused a fall in temperature. The volumes being so large, the action of the ions could have been on other structures, since the solutions undoubtedly underwent regional diffusion and also passed directly into the ventricular cavity. Nevertheless, the first example of the peripheral antagonism of a centrally acting agent was demonstrated in this work. Hasama found that intravenous calcium blocked the hyperthermic action of intradiencephalic barium; ergotoxin given subcutaneously attenuated the hyperthermia produced by intrahypothalamic potassium.

In 1934, Kym showed that Ca^{2+} ions injected directly into the hypothalamus blocked a pyrogen fever produced by intravenous ergotoxin. This antipyretic effect of calcium ions was not precisely localized because of the large volume injected. An injection of NaCl solution evoked a sharp rise in temperature similar to a pyrogen (Kym, 1934) with both cations having the same short latency. KCl injected similarly in the rabbit had mixed and inconsistent effects; however, in some cases Kym observed a potassium hyperpyrexia. Cooper *et al.* (1965) have also found that potassium infused into the anterior hypothalamus of the rabbit evoked a rise in temperature.

B. Anatomical Localization of the Set-Point

According to Benzinger (1969), the "set-point must be defined as a temperature-dependent property of a definable anatomical or histological substrate with peculiar physiological, molecular characteristics." The announcement of a new anatomical theory of the set-point for body temperature came as the result of experiments in which the balance between essential cations was artificially altered in the extracellular fluid of different parts of the hypothalamus. Push-pull perfusion cannulae (Myers, 1970a) were used to alter the ionic milieu for 30 to 60 minutes during which time a new ionic equilibrium was ostensibly established. The perfusion of the posterior region with Na^+ ions in excess of extracellular fluid evoked a concentration-dependent rise in temperature, whereas a perfusion of excess Ca^{2+} ions caused a deep and prolonged hypothermia (Myers and Veale, 1970). No consistent effects on body temperature were produced when solutions of an equivalent excess in K^+ or Mg^{2+} ions, or of isotonic sucrose, Krebs solution, or a Krebs solution containing double the concentration of ionic constituents were perfused through the same posterior regions. Similarly, no effect on temperature occurred when anatomical areas other than the hypothalamus were perfused with an excess of Na^+ or Ca^{2+} ions.

In a comprehensive anatomical study in which the hypothalamic sites of the cat were mapped, the concentration-dependent hyperthermic effect of sodium and hypothermic action of calcium were localized to the region just dorsal and somewhat lateral to the mammillary bodies (Myers and Veale, 1971a). Again, excess K^+ or Mg^{2+} and other control solutions had virtually no consistent effect at these sites. Na^+ or Ca^{2+} elicited in some instances slight changes in temperature but not nearly of the magnitude following perfusion of the posterior area. Again, it was found that the ratio rather than absolute concentration of Na^+ to Ca^{2+} determined the magnitude of the typical temperature response to these ions as shown in Fig. 6-12.

From these two studies, the conclusion was reached that the set-point mechanism was morphologically specific and based on an ionic ratio between sodium and calcium. The reasons given by Myers (1971b) for this supposition are summarized as follows: (1) the site is different from the regulatory region in the anterior hypothalamus which is both thermosensitive and reactive to amines; (2) the concentrations of each ion are established at birth; (3) calcium levels in the serum fall very briefly during the genesis of an endotoxin fever; (4) isotonic

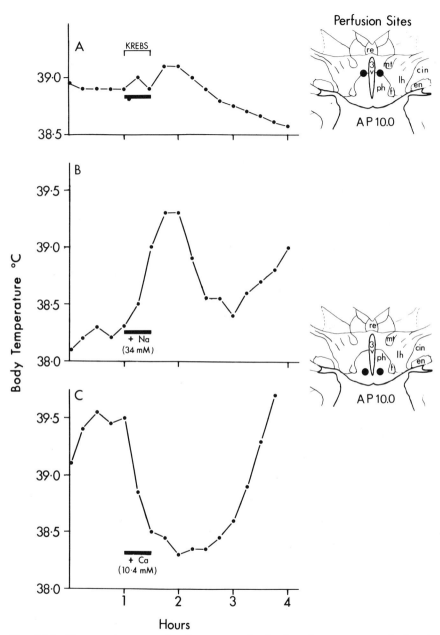

Fig. 6-12 Temperature records of an unanesthetized cat in response to the local perfusions for 30 minutes of: A, Krebs solution alone; B, Krebs solution plus 34 mM excess sodium; and C, Krebs solution plus 10.4 mM excess calcium. The sites of the bilateral perfusions are indicated by the filled circles (●) in the inset. (From Myers and Veale, 1971a)

sucrose has virtually no effect; (5) reducing the endogenous content of 5-HT or norepinephrine in the brain-stem by drugs has little effect on the set-point temperature; and (6) the mechanism is universal for all mammals and possibly lower forms with an inherent set-point temperature.

Evidence for the universality of such a mechanism has already been obtained for four other species in addition to the cat. In a number of experiments in which an injection has been given or the ventricles of a given species have been perfused with a solution containing an excess in ions, sodium elicited hyperthermia and calcium evoked hypothermia. These results are consistent for the monkey (Myers *et al.*, 1971c); rabbit (Feldberg and Saxena, 1970); rat (Myers and Brophy, 1972) and a hibernator, the golden hamster (Myers and Buckman, 1972).

If the artificial changes in temperature induced by a disturbance of the natural balance between sodium and calcium do in fact represent a perturbation in the set-point, then four additional phenomena should be clearly demonstrated: (1) When the balance of the ions is disturbed selectively by removing one of the ions by chelation, then the effect of the other should predominate. (2) It should be possible to reset the set-point at a new level and to keep it there for some time. (3) If it is possible to reset the temperature level, then the animal ought to thermoregulate quite normally around the new set-point level. (4) When the set-point is disturbed pathologically, the actual concentration of sodium and calcium in the hypothalamus ought to change.

With these points in mind, Myers and Yaksh (1971) found that they could reset the temperature set-point of the conscious rhesus monkey for up to half a day to an elevated level by repeatedly perfusing excess Na^+ ions within sites in the mammillary region, which are mapped in Fig. 6-13, or to a deeply hypothermic level by similar perfusions of excess Ca^{2+} ions. Unlike the response to one amine or any other substance, there was no tachyphylaxis to the ions.

Of substantial physiological significance is the fact that at either the high or low abnormal temperature, the animal responded to a hot or cold stimulus. When a volume of either warm or of cold water was given intragastrically, each monkey thermoregulated normally around the new set-point temperature. Thus, by definition, the new temperature established by an imbalance in the ion concentration in the hypothalamus reflects a new physiological set-point around which the animal regulates its body temperature. It is difficult to imagine that a nonspecific depressive or excitatory effect of Ca^{2+} or Na^+ could be responsible for the reset temperature since subsequent regulation would be impaired. For example, if the thermoregulatory pathway was simply depressed by Ca^{2+} ions, the monkey would not be able to shiver and vasoconstrict in response to a cold water stimulus nor vasodilate and lose heat to reduce its temperature in response to hot water. Both sets of responses continued just until the temperature level of the new set-point was attained.

Additional evidence for the $Na^+ - Ca^{2+}$ theory of the set-point was provided

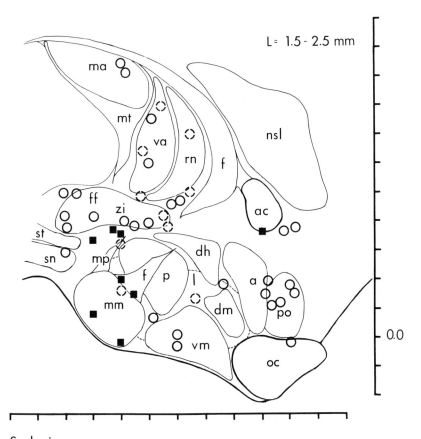

Scale in mm

Fig. 6-13 Sagittal representation of the diencephalic region of the monkey brain portrayed at 1.5 to 2.5 mm off midline. Each square (■) represents a site where the push-pull perfusion of either excess sodium or calcium ions resulted in an immediate change in body temperature of at least 0.8°C. Each open circle (O) indicates a site inactive to the perfusion. A broken circle (◌) indicates an inactive site 3.0 to 5.0 mm off midline. The zero on the vertical scale represents the stereotaxic zero plane 10 mm above the interaural line. a, anterior hypothalamic area; ac, anterior commissure; dh, dorsal hypothalamic area; dm, dorsomedial nucleus; f, fornix; ff, fields of Forel; l, lateral hypothalamus; ma, medial anterior nucleus of the thalamus; mm, mammillary body; mp, mammillary fasciculus princeps; mt, mammillothalamic tract; oc, optic chiasm; p, posterior hypothalamus; po, preoptic area; nsl, lateral nucleus of the septum; rn, reticular nucleus of the thalamus; sn, substantia nigra; st, subthalamic nucleus; va, ventral anterior nucleus of the thalamus; vm, ventromedial nucleus; zi, zona incerta. (From Myers and Yaksh, 1971)

by the first experiments in which Ca^{2+} ions were chelated from the hypothalamus (Myers and Yaksh, 1971). When EGTA (ethylene glycol tetra-acetic acid) was perfused by means of a push-pull cannula positioned in the posterior hypothalamus of the conscious monkey, its temperature rose immediately. The sharp

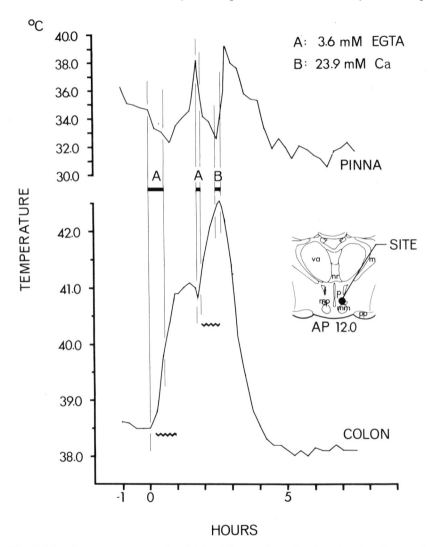

Fig. 6-14 Temperature records obtained from pinna (top) and colon (bottom) of an unanesthetized monkey in response to perfusions at 50 μl/minute (———) at a site (●) in coronal plane AP 12.0 (inset) of 3.6 mM EGTA (A) and 23.9 mM excess calcium (B). The zig-zag lines indicate shivering. Anatomical abbreviations are the same as in Fig. 6-13; also pp, cerebral peduncle. (From Myers and Yaksh, 1971)

perfusion-dependent hyperthermia could be reversed at once simply by reinstating the normal concentration of Ca^{2+} ions in the posterior hypothalamus. These responses are portrayed in Fig. 6-14. What is so striking is that a relative excess of sodium ions following the chelation of Ca^{2+} drives the temperature upwards to an unprecedented and potentially lethal level (Myers and Yaksh, 1971). No other substance which acts physiologically, including endotoxin, leucocyte pyrogen, 5-HT, acetylcholine or other amine has this super-hyperpyrexic capacity.

Finally, parallel evidence has been presented on the endogenous changes of radio-labelled calcium and sodium ions. After a pyrogen is given to a cat, the temperature set-point rises during the course of the incipient fever. As this occurs, the actual efflux from the hypothalamus of the endogenous cations changes in an opposite direction (Myers and Tytell, 1972): $^{22}Na^+$ ions are retained in hypothalamic tissue while $^{45}Ca^{2+}$ ions are extruded. The rates of efflux stabilize at the normal baseline level, once the peak of the fever is achieved. This result reinforces dramatically what one might expect in terms of a direct concordance with the localized perfusion experiments in which Na^+ and Ca^{2+} levels were altered.

Although all four of the major experiments described above have been verified, further research will be required to explain some of the molecular phenomena associated with ionic mechanisms involved in local metabolism, transport and transmitter release.

IV. PYROGENS AND FEVER

Following the illustrious studies of Bennett et al. (1957) and Sheth and Borison (1960) who injected pathogens directly into the cerebral ventricles, there was no doubt that gram-negative bacteria must act in the central nervous system to cause a fever. In spite of the exceptional complexity of the problem of how a pyrogen disrupts normal thermoregulation, scientific advances are now being made along a wide front which are utilizing a number of new techniques, both electrophysiological and pharmacological.

The first account of the direct effect of a pyrogen on brain tissue was a remarkable one by Hashimoto (1915a) who found that whole blood was a potent febrile agent. When horse serum was injected into what Hashimoto termed the temperature centers of the rabbit or guinea pig, an intense hyperthermia developed. The effect was dependent on the concentration and volume of horse serum injected, presumably into the ventral diencephalon, with a rise of as much as $3°C$ occurring 1 to $1\frac{1}{2}$ hours after the injection. Fever did not occur if a previous dose of horse serum had been injected 2 to 3 weeks earlier. Hashimoto believed this to be due to an immunizing reaction that developed. An equally significant fact was that the dose of horse serum required to produce an equivalent effect by the intravenous route had to be much higher than the intracerebral dose.

A. Pyrogen and Disordered Thermoregulation

The search for the specific anatomical site or sites of action of a pyrogen began in the early 1960s. In 1964, Villablanca and Myers published the first report that a bacterial organism acted on the cells of the anterior hypothalamus to produce a fever. Using the unanesthetized cat, a dilution as great as 1:20,000 of *S. typhosa* evoked a pyrexic response which started within 5 to 20 minutes (Villablanca and Myers, 1964; 1965). This concentration of Salmonella was $\frac{1}{320}$ to $\frac{1}{800}$ of the intravenous threshold dose required to produce the same pyrogen effect. Dilutions of 1:8 or 1:10 were the only concentrations that evoked a fever when the pyrogen was injected into the lateral or posterior hypothalamus, but because of the latency of from 2 to 5 hours, the endotoxin in all likelihood diffused to the tissue in the anterior region. That is, the latency of the pyrexic response depended principally on the distance from this region to the injection site. The sensitivity of the anterior hypothalamus to *Sh. dysenteriae* as well as to *S. typhosa* was also confirmed by Feldberg and Myers (1965a).

Because of the 5 to 20 minute latency, Villablanca and Myers suggested that a pyrogen may act on the anterior hypothalamic neurons through the release of 5-HT. Later, however, Myers (1972 b and c) described at least three substances that are released in push-pull perfusates from the rostral hypothalamus of the monkey during fever: (1) a 5-HT like substance; (2) a prostaglandin-like substance; and (3) a substance that relaxes a smooth muscle preparation used for the assays of such contractile substances as 5-HT and prostaglandin.

Raising the question of whether the bacteria itself or a blood-borne pyrogen produced by circulating leucocytes evokes the fever, Cooper *et al.* (1967) found that leucocyte pyrogen injected bilaterally into the rostral hypothalamus in a total volume of 4 μl also caused a pyrexic response. The sites of sensitivity are presented in Fig. 6-15. The latency of this response was on the order of 8 minutes, whereas a bacterial pyrogen (*S. abortus equi*) required an average of 25 minutes to evoke an equivalent rise in temperature when it was micro-injected in the same region. Since norepinephrine injected into the preoptic area of the rabbit can cause a rise in temperature of similar latency, the leucocytes could act to release this catecholamine at the same site. On the basis of these latency data, Cooper *et al.* suggested that to evoke a fever the leucocyte pyrogen rather than bacterial pyrogen passes the blood-brain barrier to act on the anterior cells. But a comparison of the peripheral versus central sensitivity to a bacterial pyrogen indicates, at least in the cat (Villablanca and Myers, 1965), that the anterior hypothalamus could be just as easily affected by bacterial organisms in the circulating plasma.

In the same year that Cooper *et al.* presented their findings, Repin and Kratskin (1967) also reported independently that a bacterial pyrogen (Pyrogenal) or leucocyte pyrogen injected into the medial preoptic region of the rabbit produced an intense fever; both pyrogens had equal latencies of about 30 minutes. In terms of

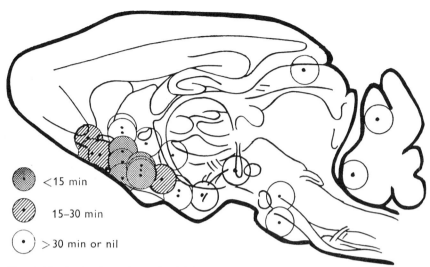

<15 min

15–30 min

> 30 min or nil

Fig. 6-15 Sagittal section of rabbit brain 1.5 mm to the right of the mid-line. Center of circle shows site of injection and circle shows possible limits of spread of leucocyte pyrogen. (From Cooper *et al.*, 1967)

the maximum sensitivity of the hypothalamic tissue, the leucocyte-derived pyrogen was somewhat more potent than the lipopolysaccharide. When an injection of either pyrogen was made in the posterior hypothalamus or midbrain reticular formation, it had no short-term effect, thus confirming the site-specificity documented for a pyrogen by Villablanca and Myers (1965).

Similar fevers of short latency were also produced in the rabbit when a purified leucocyte pyrogen was injected into the rostral half of the hypothalamus in a total volume of 4 μl (Rosendorff and Mooney, 1971). When this pyrogen was infused in other areas, arbitrarily identified as in the brain-stem, a fever was often evoked but with a longer latency and reduced magnitude. The posterior hypothalamus was considered to be an insensitive region. With such a large micro-injection volume, the factor of diffusion could account for a febrile response to leucocyte pyrogen injected in the brain-stem.

In the cat, large volumes (2 to 10 μl) of leucocyte pyrogen injected in the hypothalamus also produce a febrile response (Jackson, 1967). However, the leucocyte pyrogen evoked a fever after a much shorter latency than that caused by dilute typhoid vaccine injected similarly in a large volume into the hypothalamus. The area described by Jackson to be sensitive to leucocyte pyrogen extended from the anterior commissure to the dorsal hypothalamic area. Although a morphological mapping was not presented for the fevers elicited by endotoxin, larger volumes, differences in the batch of organisms or other technical factors such as the repeated usage of the site could explain the discrepancy in latency between this report and those of Villablanca and Myers (1965) and Feldberg and Myers (1965a). They reported that the febrile response to typhoid vaccine given in the anterior hypothalamus occurred in less than 30 minutes. Nevertheless, Jackson provided further confirmation that the anterior hypothalamus of the cat is the area most sensitive to either leucocyte pyrogen or endotoxin since injections into the posterior hypothalamus and other areas had no effect.

Although primates other than the human may have an astoundingly high threshold to bacterial pyrogen (Myers, 1971c), the hypothalamus of the unanesthetized rhesus monkey has also been tested for its relative sensitivity to the presence of a pyrogen. When a dilution of three endotoxins, *Sh. dysenteriae, S. typhosa* or *E. coli* was given in a volume of 1.2 μl or less in the anterior hypothalamic preoptic area, a dose-dependent fever occurred (Myers *et al.*, 1971a). The latency was shortest and the magnitude of pyrexia greatest when the organisms were injected into this region. As shown in Fig. 6-16, if an injection of one of the pyrogens was made in other diencephalic areas including the thalamus, or in the mesencephalic reticular formation, the temperature of the monkey did not change. Especially noteworthy in these experiments is the extreme sensitivity of the monkey's rostral hypothalamus to a small bacterial count. As little as 1000 organisms contained within the microliter that was injected evoked a full-blown fever. This result in itself suggests that bacteria in the blood that courses through the micro-circulation of the hypothalamic capillary beds have a direct action on the thermogenic neurons located in this area. Just as in the cat, there is no tachyphylaxis to endotoxin administered centrally, since *E. coli* injected repeatedly every 72 hours into the hypothalamus, as many as 16 times, always produced a fever of essentially equal characteristics (Myers *et al.*, 1971a).

In searching for another link in the central mechanism of fever, Milton and Wendlandt (1970; 1971) have shown that a marked hyperthermia is evoked by prostaglandin E_1 (PGE$_1$) given by the ventricular route. A similar pyrexia also occurs when PGE$_1$ is injected into the anterior, but not posterior hypothalamus (Feldberg and Saxena, 1971). Norepinephrine given at the same anterior site always reduced the PGE$_1$ fever, which became less and less intense when the micro-injections of PGE$_1$ were repeated on different days. The hypothalamus is extremely responsive to minute amounts of prostaglandin and this reactivity is portrayed in Fig. 6-17, as reflected by the dose-dependent nature of the PGE$_1$ fever.

Even though PGE$_1$ may be present in hypothalamic tissue, nothing is as yet known about its neuronal role in the pathogenesis or production of fever or the cellular mechanism whereby a pyrexic response is elicited. However, it would not be surprising if the prostaglandins act on serotonergic receptor sites in the anterior hypothalamus. Both serotonin and PGE$_1$ affect the receptors of certain smooth muscle tissue in a nearly identical contractile manner and both are released from the hypothalamus of the monkey during a fever (Myers, 1971b). Thus, a PGE$_1$ micro-injection may simply mimic the release of 5-HT or the action of a metabolite of this indolamine (Barofsky and Feldstein, 1970).

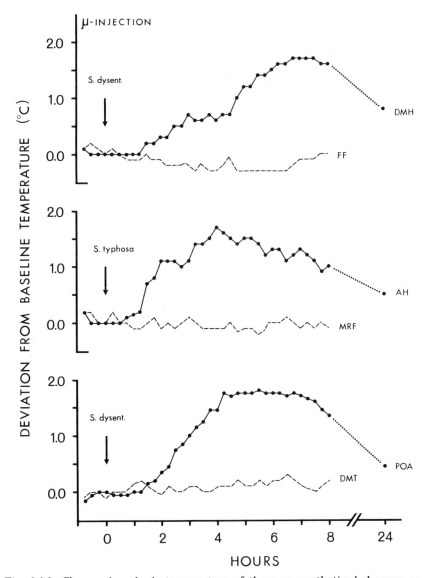

Fig. 6-16 Changes in colonic temperature of three unanesthetized rhesus monkeys in response to injections at zero hour of 1.2 μl of bacterial pyrogen in a 1:2 dilution. Top: *Sh. dysenteriae* was injected into the dorsomedial nucleus of the hypothalamus (DMH) and the fields of Forel (FF). Middle: *S. typhosa* micro-injected in the anterior hypothalamus (AH) and mesencephalic reticular formation (MRF). Bottom: *Sh. dysenteriae* micro-injected into the preoptic area (POA) and dorsomedial nucleus of the thalamus (DMT). (From Myers *et al.*, 1971a)

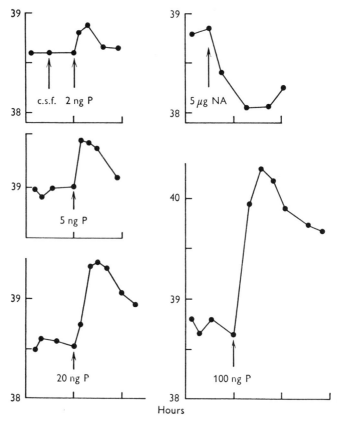

Hours

Fig. 6-17 Records of rectal temperature obtained from two unanesthetized cats, each with an indwelling micro-injection cannula in the left anterior hypothalamus (site of injection: 1.5 mm lateral to midline; 13.5 mm anterior to and 6.5 mm above interaural zero line of Snider and Niemer, 1961). Left records and upper right record were obtained from the same cat on different days. Each arrow indicates a micro-injection of 1 μl fluid of artificial CSF or of artificial CSF containing 2, 5, 10, or 100 ng PGE₁ (P), or 5 μg norepinephrine (NA). (From Feldberg and Saxena, 1971)

Fig. 6-18 The antipyretic effect of sodium salicylate on three fevers induced by micro-injection at zero hour of *Escherichia coli* into the anterior hypothalamus (Ant. Hyp.) of the unanesthetized rhesus monkey. In this animal, 300, 600 and 1200 mg of salicylate were given by the intragastric route at a time indicated by each arrow. The three experiments were carried out at 72-hour intervals. The absence of an effect on temperature of the highest dose of salicylate given in the afebrile monkey is also shown (bottom). (From Myers, R. D. *et al.*, 1971b. *Neuropharmacology.* **10**:775–778. Pergamon Press, New York)

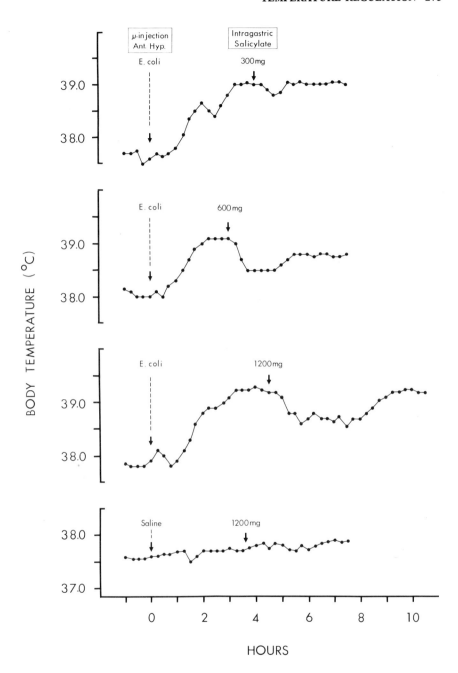

B. Antipyretic Agents

Although it is unknown how an antipyretic drug acts to produce a temporary defervescence, several views are currently held (see Collier, 1969; Myers, 1971 b and c). For example, sodium salicylate may prevent the release of leucocyte pyrogen from host cells or it may block the entry of leucocyte pyrogen into the hypothalamus. Vane (1971) has suggested a third alternative, namely that salicylate may inhibit the synthesis of an enzyme required for the formation of a prostaglandin, which has as one of its properties the capacity to initiate a fever.

In an attempt to resolve the questions inherent in the first two issues, Myers *et al.* (1971b) produced a fever in a monkey by injecting a 1 µl solution of *E. coli* organisms into the anterior hypothalamus. The concentration of bacteria was so small that any peripheral effect of the pyrogen could be ruled out; then, sodium salicylate was given by the intragastric route. The result was an antagonism of the fever which, as shown in Fig. 6-17, was dependent on the dose of salicylate. The highest dose used had no effect on normal temperature. Thus, the antipyretic effect of aspirin cannot be attributed to either the prevention of the manufacture of pyrogen in the blood, since it was present only in the hypothalamus, or to the blockade of the passage of leucocyte pyrogen into the brain.

After fever was induced in the rabbit by *Proteus* endotoxin given intravenously, an antipyretic effect of salicylate was reported to be on the preoptic area and periaqueductal gray (Cranston and Rawlins, 1972). Since the salicylate was injected bilaterally in 10 µl volumes given repeatedly, and in one experiment the volume was 60 µl, it was not surprising that salicylate-sensitive sites were found in the cerebellum and hippocampus, although according to the authors, the latter response may have been an artifact. Further, two anterior commissures were drawn in the sagittal map which would seem to invalidate any precise localization within the subcommissural regions. At any rate, a large dose of salicylate injected in these regions failed to have an effect on the afebrile rabbit. Furthermore, the effective dose was four to ten times less than that required to produce an antipyretic effect when the salicylate was given intraventricularly. These findings correspond with the concept that an antipyretic given systemically exerts an antagonistic effect on a bacterial pyrogen which is acting at least partially on the cells of the anterior hypothalamic, preoptic area (Myers, 1971b and c; Myers *et al.*, 1971).

The fever produced by *Pseudomonas* polysaccharide (Piromen) administered intravenously to the rabbit is partially prevented by a prior injection of 2.5 µg of cortisol into the rostral hypothalamus (Chowers *et al.*, 1968). The exceptionally large volume of 100 µl, the absence of both latency data and pharmacological controls, and no report of the time course of the pyrexic response make the results difficult to interpret. However, when cortisol was injected either intravenously or into the thalamus, caudate nucleus or corpus callosum, the usual fever could be evoked by Piromen. Whether or not cortisol does affect the neural elements related to thermoregulation is unknown since the steroid could have spilled into the pituitary where it influences the activity of a number of trophic hormones (Chapter 4).

V. DRUG EFFECTS

As a side effect, a great many drugs given systemically exert an influence on body temperature. Of special pharmacological interest is the central site of action of these drugs and the way in which they alter temperature. Of course, the action of many compounds is often entirely restricted to a peripheral system; e.g., epinephrine is a potent thermogenic substance responsible for mobilizing heat production in many species, especially those with brown fat depots. Other drugs may act directly on the central nervous system either to impair regulation or to deflect the set-point. Still other compounds such as picrotoxin or aconitine exert simultaneous effects centrally and peripherally (Rosenthal, 1941). How such changes take place has been examined to some degree by a series of micro-injection studies.

A. Sensitivity of the Anterior Hypothalamus

A study of the primary effect of an anesthetic on CNS tissue was among the initial investigations in this field. In cats lightly anesthetized with sodium pentobarbital, chloralose in doses of 7 to 32 μg was micro-injected into the anterior hypothalamus. Chloralose blocked pentobarbitone shivering, retarded respiratory rate and caused a dose-dependent fall in temperature (Feldberg and Myers, 1965b). As illustrated in Fig. 6-19, convincing evidence was thus provided that the well-known hypothermia and the *sequelae* of anesthesia is produced by a direct action of an anesthetic on the cells of the anterior hypothalamus. Moreover, this rostral area seems to be involved also in the neuronal processes that control shivering and respiration.

The expected fall in temperature common to all anesthetics failed to occur when a small dose of sodium pentobarbital was injected into either the anterior or posterior hypothalamus of the rat (Lomax, 1966b). No behavioral effect was noted. The hypothermic effect usually seen when this anesthetic is administered to the rat by the peripheral route could be due to the reduction of oxygen consumption, energy metabolism, and dilatation of the blood vessels. Alternatively, the single 30 μg test dose may have been too low or may not have reached an appropriately sensitive site, particularly since chloralose has a hypothermic action on the hypothalamic control mechanism (Feldberg and Myers, 1965b).

Given peripherally, a phenothiazine and other tranquilizers exert potent effects on temperature, and they may possess a central component as well. With the ambient temperature held at 20°C, chlorpromazine micro-injected in the anterior hypothalamus of the anesthetized rat caused a dose-dependent rise in body tem-

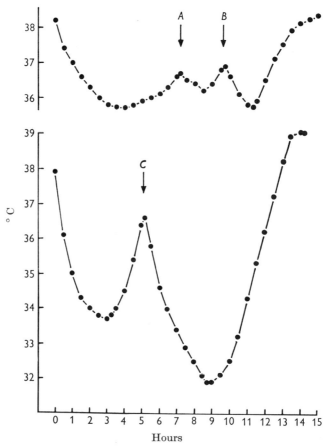

Fig. 6-19 Records of rectal temperature of a cat with a cannula implanted in the left anterior hypothalamus. Both records begin a few minutes after induction of anesthesia with intraperitoneal pentobarbitone sodium 33 mg/kg; the lower record was obtained a week after the upper record. At the arrows micro-injections of chloralose: at A, 7 μg in 1 μl; at B, 14 μg in 2 μl; and at C, 32 μg in 4 μl. Infusion times 46, 92 and 184 seconds, respectively. (From Feldberg and Myers, 1965b)

perature (Rewerski and Jori, 1968a). Similar injections into other structures including the thalamus and frontal lobe had a variable effect on temperature. However, an injection of a low dose of chlorpromazine into the posterior hypothalamus evoked hypothermia, whereas a high dose caused hyperthermia. These findings are difficult to interpret at this time since chlorpromazine did not override the usual hypothermia of reserpine given systemically. A further analysis of the rise in temperature elicited by chlorpromazine applied to the anterior hypothalamus was carried out by Rewerski and Gumulka (1969). They showed that this hyperthermic effect of chlorpromazine infused into the rostral hypothalamus persisted even after the rat was pretreated with systemically given α-methyl-tyrosine, a compound which depletes the hypothalamic stores of norepinephrine. Thus, chlorpromazine does not seem to elicit an increase in temperature through the release of norepinephrine within the anterior preoptic area, which according to Avery (1971) would result in a fall in the rat's temperature.

The fall in the rat's body temperature evoked by systemic chlorpromazine and the hyperthermia caused by chlorpromazine micro-injected into the rostral hypothalamus has been confirmed by Kirkpatrick and Lomax (1971). In addition, 5 μg of the N-methyl quaternary derivative of chlorpromazine also caused an elevation in the temperature of the rat, as shown in Fig. 6-20. The site-specificity was verified since injections at other sites had no other effect. According to the authors, the response could be produced by a local nerve block, perhaps of cholinergic activity, which would correspond to the effects of atropine on the hypothalamus described in the previous section. However, a block-ade of the neural activity within the anterior region should result in an incapacity to thermoregulate and thus a sharp *fall* in temperature. Alternative explanations are that chlorpromazine has a direct pyrogenic action of its own or that it acts locally to release acetylcholine, 5-HT or another substance from nerve terminals which in turn stimulates the heat production pathway.

In the hamster, chlorpromazine has an opposite effect on temperature (Reigle and Wolf, 1971). A dose-dependent hypothermia occurs after 12 to 37 μg chlorpromazine are injected into the anterior hypothalamus, but the crucial variable here is that the experiment was conducted at an ambient temperature of 10°C. Thus, a central component of the disruption of temperature by the phenothiazine probably is the source of the hypothermia seen when the drug is given peripherally. Since atropine given one hour earlier at the same site did not inhibit the chlorpromazine-induced hypothermia, a cholinergic link does not seem to be involved. Differences between the responses of the rat and hamster could be due to species, degree of restraint, the ambient temperature, the use of an anesthetic, the dose injected, or more than one of these.

The effects on temperature of two imidazoline derivatives, both of which are potent sympathomimetic agents, are directly opposite when given intraperito-neally than when injected directly into the hypothalamus. Naphazoline and tetrahydrozoline cause a sharp rise in temperature when injected into the anterior hypothalamic area of the rat, but they evoke hypothermia when administered systemically (Lomax and Foster, 1969). When injected into the hypothalamic sites just before the imidazoline compounds, tolazoline, an alpha adrenergic blocking agent, antagonized the hyperthermia. Although the increase in temperature may be the result of an interference with cholinergic transmission or a local hyperpolarization of the neurons, each compound could be exerting the hyperthermic action by acting as a pyrogenic substance. This conclusion is based on the long latency of 30 minutes before the rise in temperature began; on systemic injection, hypothermia ensues almost immediately.

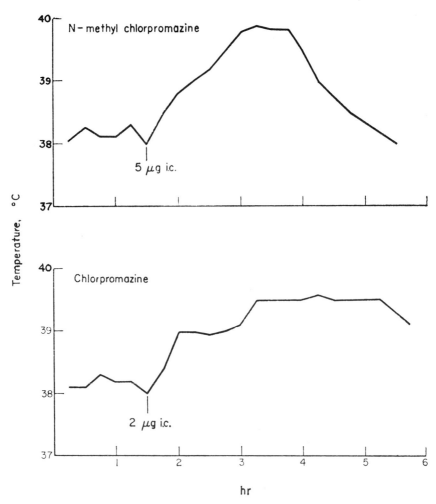

Fig. 6-20 Hyperthermia following injection of chlorpromazine (2 μg) and N-methyl chlorpromazine (5 μg) into the rostral hypothalamic thermoregulatory centers of two rats. The duration of action of the tertiary drug was much longer than that of the quaternary derivative. (From Kirkpatrick, W. E. and P. Lomax. 1971. *Neuropharmacology.* **10**:61–66. Pergamon Press, New York)

In the anesthetized rat, desmethylimipramine (DMI) injected in the anterior or posterior hypothalamus, the rhomboid nucleus of the thalamus, and the third ventricle reversed the hypothermia of anesthesia for some time (Rewerski and Jori, 1968b). An injection of distilled water had little or no effect on the deepening hypothermia. The subsequent hyperthermia evoked by DMI was apparently not dependent on the dose which ranged from 7 to 30 μg. When the anesthetized rat was reserpinized and had a temperature of 28 to 31°C, DMI always elicited a rise in temperature when injected into all sites plus the amygdala and frontal lobe. Thus, it would seem that DMI exerts an anatomically nonspecific effect, perhaps causing a generalized activation and lightening of anesthesia, or acts as a pyrogen rather than by preventing the re-uptake of noradrenaline or serotonin.

Capsaicin is the ingredient responsible for the pungent characteristics of red pepper. In a dose of 0.5 to 50 μg, capsaicin produced a fall in rectal temperature when the substance was injected in a large 5 μl volume into the anterior hypothalamus of the rat (Jancsó-Gábor *et al.*, 1970). The local tachyphylaxis and desensitization to repeated intrahypothalamic injections is portrayed clearly in Fig. 6-21. In subsequent tests, the rat was not able to regulate adequately against peripheral heating. Local heating also failed to evoke a thermoregulatory response, which indicated that this constituent of red pepper permanently impairs the hypothalamic warmth detectors, probably by destroying their mitochondria (Szolcsányi *et al.*, 1971).

Cardiac glycosides given systemically to a primate also produce a protracted hypothermia. When 5 μg of either acetylstrophanthidin or deslanoside is injected into the hypothalamus of the conscious macaque, the temperature falls 1.2 to 3.3°C (Chai *et al.*, 1971). Although the most sensitive locus of action is the preoptic area in terms of the magnitude of hypothermia, the nature and cause of the change in temperature evoked by the glycosides are not known. However, unlike the effect of capsaicin, the rebound hyperthermia following

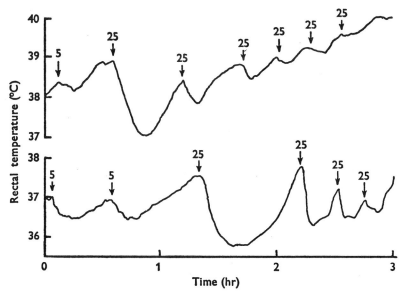

Fig. 6-21 Rectal temperature from two normal rats weighing 300 g in response to repeated intracerebral injections of 5 to 25 μg capsaicin into the preoptic area of the anterior hypothalamus. With repeated applications the effect vanished probably as a result of desensitization. (From Jancsó-Gábor *et al.*, 1970)

the acetylstrophanthidin hypothermia indicates that the thermogenic elements in the hypothalamus remained intact.

B. Morphine

It has been known for some time that morphine has a potent hypothermic action. On the basis of the dose-dependent fall in temperature produced by the opiate, Hashimoto proposed over a half century ago that morphine was acting on the temperature "center" as follows:

> "Durch Morphium in kleinen Dosen wird die Temperaturwirkung der Kälte und Wärme auf das Wärmzentrum stark abgeschwacht, in grossen Dosen völlig aufgehoben" (Hashimoto, 1915b). (The efficacy on temperature of cold or warmth on the heat production center was considerably diminished by small doses of morphine and completely abolished by large doses.)

Using a single high does of 50 μg of morphine, Lotti et al. (1965a) first showed that the opiate produced a marked hypothermia in the rat only when it was injected into the rostral hypothalamus at anatomical loci designated in Fig. 6-22. Although the hypothermia, after morphine is given peripherally, could be due to its action on the anterior thermoregulatory center, hyperthermia and hyperactivity were produced when it was injected into the posterior hypothalamus. When systemic morphine reaches the brain via the bloodstream, the concentration of morphine in anterior and posterior areas presumably would be equal in both structures. Thus, it is difficult to see how one site would predominate over the other, unless the opiate acts on still a third region. Apparently, a functional sensitivity which favors a fall in temperature would have to exist in an additional site.

That morphine-induced hypothermia can be ascribed to a reduction in metabolic heat production is also probable since oxygen consumption also declines as the body temperature of the rat falls (Lotti et al., 1966b). It is interesting that when the rat breathes 100% oxygen, morphine hypothermia is antagonized. In fact, hyperthermia was observed in several rats following the oxygen treatment, although other signs of morphine action including catatonia, exophthalmia and analgesia were still present.

An elegant pharmacological demonstration of drug antagonism within a specific region of the central nervous system was presented by Lotti et al. (1965b). As illustrated in Fig. 6-23, they found that small doses of nalorphine reversed the morphine-induced hypothermia when both of the drugs were injected into the anterior part of the hypothalamus. An injection of either drug into other areas was almost always without effect. Since peripheral nalorphine antagonizes centrally-induced morphine hypothermia, both drugs in all likelihood exert their action on central temperature "centers" (Lomax, 1967). The rebound hyper-

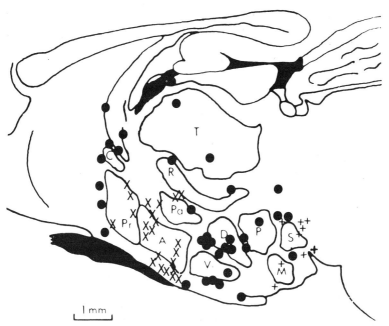

Fig. 6-22   Sagittal section of rat brain 240 μ lateral to midline. X, injection sites resulting in a fall in core temperature; •, injection sites ineffective in lowering temperature; +, injection sites causing hyperactivity.   50 μg morphine sulfate injected at each site.   A. anterior hypothalamic area; C. anterior commissure; D. dorsomedial nucleus; M. mammillary bodies; P. posterior hypothalamic nucleus; Pa. paraventricular nucleus; Pr. preoptic area; R. nucleus reuniens; S. supramammillary nucleus; T. thalamus; V. ventromedial nucleus. (From Lotti, V. J. *et al.*, 1965a. *J. Pharmacol. Exptl. Ther.* **150**:135–139. The Williams and Wilkins Co., Baltimore, Md.)

thermia often seen following the morphine-nalorphine combination of injections (Fig. 6-23) would seem to require further clarification, however, and points to the necessity of using several doses of each substance.

On repeated intrahypothalamic injections of morphine, the characteristic hypothermia of the same magnitude could be obtained only if the doses were increased successively two- to four-fold (Lotti *et al.*, 1966a). This finding shows that within the hypothalamus a local kind of tachyphylaxis or perhaps acute tolerance to morphine occurs. This is characteristic also of the effect on temperature of the monoamines given intracerebrally (Feldberg and Myers, 1965a). Repeated injections of N-methyl morphine into the rostral hypothalamus of the rat evoked a fall in temperature which showed no signs of tolerance (Foster *et al.*, 1967). A marked analgesia, as tested by the rat's response to its feet being placed on a hot plate, was observed in some of the rats after morphine or the N-methyl derivative was injected intrahypothalamically. Thus, even though the derivative

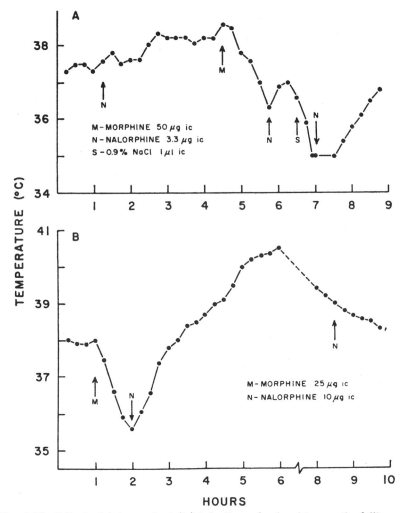

Fig. 6-23   Effect of intracerebral (ic) injection of nalorphine on the falling core temperature of two rats produced by injection of morphine into the same site (anterior hypothalamic nuclei).   In A, nalorphine alone caused a moderate hyperthermia; morphine, 50 μg, 195 minutes later resulted in a fall in temperature which was partially reversed by 3.3 μg of nalorphine after 75 minutes; repeating this dose of nalorphine 75 minutes later led to a rapid return to the resting level.   In B, the effect of 25 μg of morphine was completely antagonized by 10 μg of nalorphine; subsequently a marked hyperthermia occurred; later repetition of the dose of nalorphine was without effect on the temperature. Intracerebral injection of 1 μl of 0.9% NaCl did not affect the falling temperature. (From Lotti, V. J. *et al.*, 1965b. *J. Pharmacol. Exptl. Ther.* **150**:420–425. The Williams and Wilkins Co., Baltimore, Md.)

does not have the same effect when given peripherally, the properties of both compounds are similar when they are applied at the same hypothalamic site.

A serious element of conflicting evidence on the central action of morphine has been introduced by Paolino and Bernard (1968). According to their experiments, morphine in a single high dose of 50 μg has no effect when injected in a volume of 1 μl into the anterior hypothalamus of the unrestrained rat that is kept at 24°C. However, Fig. 6-24 shows that when the experiment is performed at an ambient temperature of 32°C, the same intrahypothalamic injection of morphine produced a rise in temperature of about 1°C. On the other hand, when the environmental temperature was lowered to 5°C, a fall of up to 5°C occurred which is similar to the results of Lotti et al. (1966a and b) who did their experiments at room temperature. Therefore, instead of lowering the hypothalamic set-point, morphine simply may act to depress neurons in the anterior hypothal-

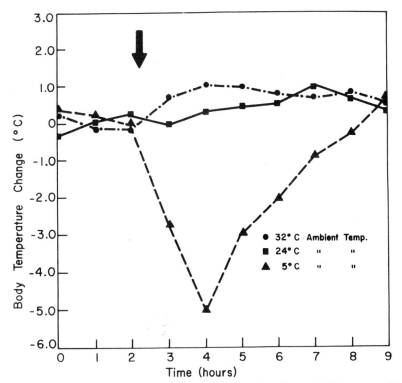

Fig. 6-24 Mean core temperature response to 1 μl volume of 50 μg morphine sulfate injected directly into anterior hypothalamus as a function of environmental temperature. Data are plotted as morphine minus control. Arrow indicates time of injection. (From Paolino, R. M. and B. R. Bernard. 1968. *Life Sciences.* 7:857–863. Pergamon Press, New York)

amus to such an extent that the animal loses all ability to thermoregulate its core temperature. One reason for the discrepancy in the results may be the fact that Lotti *et al.* did restrain their rats. This in itself may have interfered or interacted in some way with the thermoregulatory response to morphine. Again the vital importance of a technique to any experimental interpretation is illustrated. In any case, experiments with the cat and monkey show that the set-point mechanism is located in the posterior hypothalamus. Since the rat responds to Na^+ and Ca^{2+} ions infused intracerebrally in the same way as the cat and monkey, the conclusion of Paolino and Bernard is not illogical.

VI. CONCLUDING CONSIDERATIONS

Just as we have seen in the two chapters on hormones, the selective sensitivity of neurons to biogenic amines, pyrogens and many drugs is most remarkable. The micro-injection experiments carried out in the monkey, cat, rat and other species suggest that two independent neurohumoral systems are located precisely within the anterior hypothalamus. They are specifically activated or reciprocally inhibited when an animal requires heat production to remain warm or it must lose heat to keep cool. On the basis of histochemical fluorescence and additional anatomical findings, the monoamines 5-HT and norepinephrine are the logical candidates which serve these two systems. On the one hand, 5-HT activates heat production, while on the other, norepinephrine causes heat loss in these species.

A third neurochemical system that apparently uses acetylcholine as a synaptic transmitter projects posteriorly in a very diffuse way, extending through the most caudal aspect of the mesencephalon. The first anterior link in the cholinergic pathway seems to be devoted only to heat production. When that pathway reaches the posterior hypothalamus, an additional cholinergic system emerges which subserves the heat loss mechanism. Hence at the junction of the mesencephalon and mammillary bodies, two cholinergic networks exist. Although there was no clue whatsoever as to the functional significance of the second cholinergic system until very recently, it is possible that in addition to transmitting the signals for heat gain from the anterior hypothalamus, acetylcholine has an equally important role in transmitting the set-point impulses from the posterior region (Fig. 6-25).

If we assume that the cells in the caudal part of the hypothalamus are responsible for holding a set-point temperature of 37°C, by virtue of a delicate balance in the ratio between sodium and calcium ions in the extracellular fluid, then the firing rate of these cells and hence their efferent impulses would be constant. Since the output from these cells would have to possess a means of transmission, the reason that acetylcholine, injected into the posterior hypothalamus, evokes either hyper- or hypothermia is that the set-point cells may use acetylcholine in the synaptic propagation of set-point impulses.

A. Biogenic Amines

A beginning has been made toward the pharmacological characterization in the hypothalamus of serotonergic, noradrenergic and cholinergic systems. The adrenergic receptors for heat loss have been elucidated for the cat, and some progress has been made toward the analysis of cholinergic receptors in both the cat and monkey. A nagging question does persist about the role of acetylcholine in the central control of the rat's temperature, primarily because of the unresolved discrepancies in the micro-injection literature. Probably most of these are not the fault of an experimental strategy or technique but rather are due to the anatomical limitations imposed by the size of the brain of this diminutive rodent. Only by using more micromethods, as is now being done by workers in other fields (Swanson et al., 1972; Simpson and Routtenberg, 1972), can a more precise estimate of receptor stimulation be achieved.

Although at least two groups of researchers accept the idea that a catecholamine in the anterior hypothalamus of the rat mediates the function of heat loss, the role of the catechol moiety in this region in the rabbit and other species remains somewhat of a mystery. It is imperative that many more experiments be completed before an unequivocal pronouncement is made that neurochemical circuits have evolved differently in each species, particularly those laid down for the most vital and primitive of bodily functions (Myers and Sharpe, 1968b). In the rabbit, information is requisitive about the dose response to each amine, volume dependence, site-specificity, latency of response, and pharmacological blockade, especially since serotonin causes a rise in temperature when injected into the ventricles or cisterna magna (Canal and Ornesi, 1961; Jacob et al., 1972). Most important, the temperature-evoked release of a neurohumoral factor from the hypothalamus has yet to be shown in any species other than the monkey or cat. Curiously enough, the field of thermoregulation is the only one in which it has been demonstrated that the release of different substances from restricted sites in the brain is evoked by a specific environmental stimulus. The three major types of experimental verification, in which the procedure of push-pull perfusion was used for a localized analysis, coincide anatomically and functionally with the micro-injection experiments as follows.

First, exposing the unanesthetized monkey to a cold environment of 0 to 5°C causes a release of 5-HT only from the anterior hypothalamic, preoptic area; correspondingly, warming has no consistent effect on the hypothalamic output of 5-HT (Myers and Beleslin, 1971). Second, exposure of the conscious cat to a hot but not cold ambient temperature evokes the release of radio-labelled norepinephrine, again from the rostral hypothalamus only. Third, lowering the monkey's ambient temperature to 0 to 5°C enhances the output of acetylcholine from sites scattered widely throughout the anterior, posterior and mid-hypothalamic regions as well as the mesencephalon. On the other hand, warming suppresses the release of acetylcholine at the majority of the rostral sites and enhances its output at only about one-third of the loci within the posterior hypothalamus and mesencephalon.

From these experiments, the most notable fact overall is that two of the principal criteria of Werman (1972), discussed in Chapter 1, for the identification of a transmitter substance are met for 5-HT, norepinephrine and acetylcholine in their proposed role in thermoregulation: (1) identical actions and (2) collectability of the transmitter. Whether or not these criteria alone constitute sufficient proof that the two monoamines could be synaptic transmitters is most uncertain as discussed in the Epilogue.

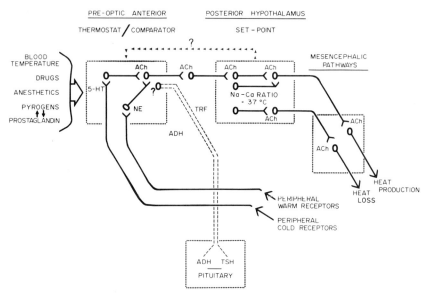

Fig. 6-25 A schematic diagram of a model of thermoregulation based mainly on experimental findings in the monkey and cat. The anterior hypothalamic preoptic area contains neurons which are thermosensitive as well as a comparator mechanism which contrasts the set-point with the local temperature. The region is also sensitive to a number of substances, as indicated, including pyrogens and prostaglandins which may interact functionally. The release of 5-HT acts through a cholinergic pathway to signal heat production, whereas the release of norepinephrine blocks the cholinergic heat production pathway which traverses the posterior hypothalamus. The set-point of $37°C$ depends upon the intrinsic ratio of Na^+ to Ca^{2+} ions, an aberration of which will evoke a shift in the set-point presumably via independent cholinergic pathways. The regulation of body water and thyroid activity may also be partially mediated by synapses arising in the anterior hypothalamus. ACh. acetylcholine, ADH. antidiuretic hormone, NE. norepinephrine, 5-HT. serotonin, TRF. thyrotropin releasing factor, TSH. thyroid stimulating hormone. (Modified after Myers, 1971b)

B. Temperature Control Model

In conclusion, Fig. 6-25 presents an overall summary in schematic form of the anatomical regions at which each class of chemical substance is believed to exert its special effect on distinct pathways or mechanisms. This provisional model takes into account only the morphological data that exist thus far that have been gathered in just ten years. It is based almost solely on the cat and monkey (Myers, 1972), not because most of the initial observations were based on these two species, but because the size of their respective brains provides a more precise anatomical localization and permits the collection of humoral factors.

The preoptic area and anterior hypothalamus contain the nervous elements that are sensitive to a deflection in blood temperature, and to endotoxin or leucocyte pyrogen, anesthetics, opiates and other drugs, and to endogenous humoral factors including biogenic amines, prostaglandins and peptides. The posterior hypothalamus is chemically "blind" to all of these substances, but reacts to a very subtle alteration in the ratio of calcium to sodium ions. Linking these two important areas are cholinergic pathways which carry the signals for thermogenesis. Based on the anatomical analyses contained in the experiments on micro-injection and humoral release, there is at present no evidence of crossed inhibitory axons, as pictured by Maskrey and Bligh (1971) and Bligh (1972). Obviously, however, one would have to expect that some sort of reciprocity in innervation exists that prevents outflowing impulses for heat conservation and heat loss from cancelling each other and thereby counteracting thermoregulation.

Among the plethora of unanswered questions is the special affinity of certain receptors in the anterior hypothalamus for 5-HT, bacteria, leucocytes, prostaglandins, acetylcholine and other factors whose molecular properties have the capacity to elevate temperature. It is not understood whether each substance acts on the same cell groups, let alone the same receptors, nor is it known whether one enhances or inhibits the local synthesis or release of another.

Another profound enigma centers on the relationship between the posterior hypothalamus and the anterior region. Although it is conceivable that the postulated set-point neurons operate independently of the regulatory signals that are superimposed upon a reference temperature, some feedback interaction could certainly exist between the two disparate regions. These and other intriguing issues will be resolved ultimately by neurochemical experiments that are directed toward an analysis of each independent anatomical site rather than by an approach using the systemic or ventricular route.

VII. Master Summary Table

Chemicals that Exerted an Effect when Given at a Specific Site in the Brain

Chemical	Dose	Volume	Site	Species	State*	Response	Reference
Acetylcholine (ACh)	15 µg/30 min	?	Rostral hypothalamus	Rat	C	Hypothermia.	Kirkpatrick and Lomax (1970)
	20–50 µg	1 µl	Anterior hypothalamus, preoptic area	Rat	U	Decreased rate of responding for heat and a brief hypothermia.	Beckman and Carlisle (1969)
	300–500 µg	1–10 µl	Caudate nucleus	Cat	C	Hyperthermia.	Connor et al. (1966a)
ACh and Eserine	5 µg + 6.25 µg	1 µl	Rostral hypothalamus	Guinea pig	U	Reduced non-shivering thermogenesis.	Zeisburger and Brück (1971c)
	5.45–18.17 µg	1 µl	Hypothalamus	Cat	U	Biphasic temperature change.	Rudy and Wolf (1972)
	5 µg	1 µl	Lateral and posterior hypothalamus	Monkey	C	Hyperthermia.	Hall and Myers (1972)
	1.5–5 µg	.5–1 µl	Anterior hypothalamus	Monkey	C	Hyperthermia.	Myers (1970b)
	2–25 µg	.5–1 µl	Anterior, mid- and posterior hypothalamus	Monkey	C	Hyperthermia.	Myers and Yaksh (1969)
Acetylstrophanthidin	5 µg	10 µl	Preoptic area	Monkey	C	Hypothermia.	Chai et al. (1971)
Aconitine	.03 µg	50 µl	Infundibular region	Rabbit	C	Hypothermia.	(Rosenthal, 1941)
Alanine	10 µg	20 µl	Hypothalamus	Rat	U	Hyperthermia.	Boros-Farkas and Illei-Don-hoffer (1969)

*U = unanesthetized and unrestrained; C = constrained, confined or curarized; A = anesthetized.

Drug	Dose	Volume	Site	Species	C/U	Effect	Reference
Arecoline	85–125 µg	1–10 µl	Caudate nucleus	Cat	C	Hyperthermia.	Connor et al. (1966a)
Atropine	5 µg	1 µl	Anterior hypothalamus	Rat	C	Hyperthermia.	Kirkpatrick and Lomax (1967)
	20 µg	1 µl	Anterior hypothalamus, preoptic area	Rat	U	Blocked the effect of acetylcholine.	Beckman and Carlisle (1969)
	40 µg	1 µl	Preoptic area	Rat	C	Antagonized systemic oxotremorine; hypothermia.	Lomax and Jenden (1966)
	250 µg	10 µl	Anterior hypothalamus, septum	Rat	U	Blocked intravenous oxotremorine; hypothermia.	Staib and Andreas (1970)
	2 µg	1–4 µl	Thalamus, caudate nucleus, other limbic structures	Cat	U	Hyperthermia.	Hull et al. (1967)
Barium (Ba^{2+})	5 mg	50 µl	Tuber cinerium	Cat	U	Hyperthermia (intense).	Hasama (1930)
Bethanecol	25–38 µg	1–10 µl	Caudate nucleus	Cat	C	Hyperthermia.	Connor et al. (1966a)
Calcium (Ca^{2+})	.5–2 mg	50 µl	Tuber cinerium	Cat	U	Hypothermia.	Hasama (1930)
	4.01–26.05 µg/min	perfusion 50 µl/min	Posterior hypothalamus	Cat	U	Hypothermia.	Myers and Veale (1970)
	5.21–20.04 µg/min	perfusion 50 µl/min	Hypothalamus	Cat	U	Hypothermia.	Myers and Veale (1971a)
	22.65–95.99 µg/min	perfusion 50 µl/min	Posterior hypothalamus	Monkey	C	Hypothermia.	Myers and Yaksh (1971)
	1 mg	50 µl	Infundibular region	Rabbit	C	Hypothermia.	Rosenthal (1941)
Capsaicin	1.25 mg	50 µl	Hypothalamus	Rabbit	C	Attenuates pyrogen fever.	Kym (1934)
	.5–50 µg	5 µl	Anterior hypothalamus	Rat	U	Hypothermia.	Jancsó-Gábor et al. (1970)

VII. Master Summary Table (Continued)

Chemical	Dose	Volume	Site	Species	State*	Response	Reference
Carbachol	≈ 5 µg	crystal	Red nucleus, septum, preoptic area	Rat	U	Hypothermia.	Hulst and deWied (1967)
	≈ 5 µg	crystal	Anterior hypothalamus	Rat	U	Hyper- or hypothermia.	Hulst and deWied (1967)
	≈ 5 µg	crystal	Ventral thalamus	Rat	U	Hyperthermia.	Hulst and deWied (1967)
	≈ 5 µg	crystal	Limbic system (17 structures)	Rat	U	Hypo- or hyperthermia.	Hulst (1972)
	1 µg	1 µl	Preoptic area	Rat	C	Hypothermia.	Lomax and Jenden (1966)
	3 µg	.5 µl	Anterior hypothalamus, preoptic area	Rat	U	At 5°C, slight hyperthermia. At 35°C, does not attenuate hyperthermia.	Avery (1972)
	3–5 µg	.5 µl	Anterior hypothalamus, preoptic area	Rat	U	Hyperthermia.	Avery (1970)
	3–8 µg	.5 µl	Anterior hypothalamus	Rat	U	Hyperthermia.	Avery (1971)
	20–100 µg/ 5–20 min	?	Rostral hypothalamus	Rat	C	Hypothermia.	Kirkpatrick and Lomax (1970)
	.25 µg	1 µl	Rostral hypothalamus	Guinea pig	U	Reduced non-shivering thermogenesis.	Zeisburger and Brück (1971c)
	5–8 µg	1–10 µl	Caudate nucleus	Cat	C	Hyperthermia.	Connor et al. (1966, a and b)
	.55–18.27 µg	1 µl	Hypothalamus	Cat	U	Hyperthermia, hypothermia.	Rudy and Wolf (1972)
	4–10 µg	1–4 µl	Thalamus, caudate	Cat	U	Rage, autonomic effects, hypothermia.	Hull et al. (1967)

nucleus, other limbic structures

Drug	Dose	Volume	Site	Animal		Effect	Reference
	.4–6 µg	.5–1 µl	Anterior, mid and posterior hypothalamus	Monkey	C	Hyperthermia.	Myers and Yaksh (1969)
Chloralose	7–32 µg	1–2 µl	Anterior hypothalamus	Cat	A	Hypothermia.	Feldberg and Myers (1965b)
Chlorpromazine (CPZ)	2 µg	1 µl	Anterior hypothalamus	Rat	C	Hyperthermia.	Kirkpatrick and Lomax (1971)
	30 µg	1 µl	Anterior hypothalamus	Rat	A	Hyperthermia after α-MT treatment.	Rewerski and Gumulka (1969)
	.5–60 µg	1 µl	Anterior hypothalamus	Rat	A	Hyperthermia.	Rewerski and Jori (1968a)
	12–37 µg	1 µl	Anterior hypothalamus	Hamster	C	Hypothermia.	Reigle and Wolf (1971)
N-Methyl-chlorpromazine	5 µg	1 µl	Anterior hypothalamus	Rat	C	Hyperthermia.	Kirkpatrick and Lomax (1971)
Cortisol	2.5–5 µg	100 µl	Preoptic and other areas	Rabbit	U	Partially attenuated pyrogen induced fever.	Chowers et al. (1968)
Cyclic AMP	≃ 250 µg	crystal	Anterior hypothalamic area	Rat	U	Hyperthermia.	Breckenridge and Lisk (1969)
Deslanoside	5 µg	10 µl	Preoptic area	Monkey	C	Hypothermia.	Chai et al. (1971)
Desmethylimipramine	7.5–30 µg	1 µl	Anterior and posterior hypothalamus, thalamus, ventricle	Rat	A	Long-lasting hyperthermia.	Rewerski and Jori (1968b)
Dextrose	50–150 µg	1 µl	Lateral and ventromedial hypothalamus	Monkey	C	No temperature change. Failed to block feeding in fasted animal.	Myers and Sharpe (1968b)

VII. Master Summary Table (Continued)

Chemical	Dose	Volume	Site	Species*	State*	Response	Reference
N-(4-Diethylamino-2-butynyl)-succinimide (DKJ-21)	50 µg	?	Anterior hypothalamus	Rat	C	Reversed oxotremorine hypothermia.	Kirkpatrick et al. (1967)
Dopamine (DA)	1-12 µg	.5-1 µl	Anterior hypothalamus	Monkey	C	Little hypothermia.	Myers and Yaksh (1969)
EGTA	22.80-68.43 µg/min	perfusion 50 µl/min	Posterior hypothalamus	Monkey	C	Hyperthermia.	Myers and Yaksh (1971)
Epinephrine	.5-10 µg	.5-1 µl	Anterior hypothalamus	Cat	U	Hypothermia.	Feldberg and Myers (1965a)
	.5-18 µg	1 µl	Anterior hypothalamus	Cat	U	Hypothermia.	Rudy and Wolf (1971)
	10 µg	1 µl	Anterior hypothalamus	Monkey	C	Hypothermia.	Myers (1968)
	1-12 µg	.5-1 µl	Anterior hypothalamus	Monkey	C	Hyperthermia.	Myers and Yaksh (1969)
E. coli	.04 µg	20 µl	Hypothalamus	Rat	U	Hyperthermia.	Boros-Farkas and Illei-Donhoffer (1969)
	$1-3 \times 10^9$ organisms/ml	1.2 µl	Anterior hypothalamus	Monkey	C	Fever antagonized by peripheral salicylate.	Myers et al. (1971b)
	2.5×10^9 organisms/ml	.8-1.2 µl	Hypothalamus	Monkey	C	Fever, shivering.	Myers et al. (1971a)
GAHBA DL γ-amino-β-hydroxy-butyric acid	10 µg	20 µl	Hypothalamus	Rat	U	Hyperthermia.	Boros-Farkas and Illei-Donhoffer (1969)
Histamine	1-5 µg	1 µl	Anterior hypothalamus	Rat	U	Hypothermia.	Brezenoff and Lomax (1970)
	20 µg	1 µl	Anterior hypothalamus	Monkey	C	Variable effect on temperature.	Myers (1968)

Substance	Amount	Volume	Site	Species	U/C	Effect	Reference
Horse serum	?	.5–200 μl	"Temperature center"	Rabbit Guinea pig	U U	Hyperthermia–fever.	Hashimoto (1915a)
Isoprenaline	13.9–27.9 μg	.5 μl	Hypothalamus	Chicken	U	Hypothermia.	Marley and Stephenson (1970)
Isoproterenol	2–21 μg	1 μl	Anterior hypothalamus	Cat	U	Hypothermia.	Rudy and Wolf (1971)
Leucocyte pyrogen (L.P.)	?	2 μl bilateral	Hypothalamus, brain-stem	Rabbit	C	Fever.	Rosendorff and Mooney (1971)
	4×10^5 cells/ml	2 μl	Anterior hypothalamus	Rabbit	C	Fever within 8 minutes.	Cooper et al. (1967)
	10^7 cells/ml	2 μl	Rostral hypothalamus	Rabbit	?	Fever with 30 minute latency.	Repin and Kratskin (1967)
	?	2–10 μl	Rostral hypothalamus	Cat	U	Hyperthermia.	Jackson (1967)
Magnesium (Mg^{2+})	1.5–2 mg	50 μl	Tuber cinerium	Cat	U	No effect.	Hasama (1930)
Methacholine	90–110 μg	1–10 μl	Caudate nucleus	Cat	C	Hyperthermia.	Connor et al. (1966a)
Morphine	22–45 μg	1 μl	Rostral hypothalamus	Rat	C	Hypothermia and variable amount of analgesia.	Foster et al. (1967)
	25–50 μg	1 μl	Rostral hypothalamus	Rat	C	Hypothermia.	Lotti et al. (1965a and b)
	50 μg	1 μl	Anterior hypothalamus	Rat	U	Hyperthermia or hypothermia depending upon ambient temperature.	Paolino and Bernard (1968)
	50 μg	1 μl	Rostral hypothalamus	Rat	C	Hypothermia.	Lotti et al. (1966b)
	50 μg	1 μl	Anterior hypothalamus, preoptic area	Rat	C	Hypothermia.	Lomax (1967)

VII. Master Summary Table *(Continued)*

Chemical	Dose	Volume	Site	Species	State*	Response	Reference
Morphine	50 µg	1 µl	Anterior hypothalamus	Rat	U	Hypothermia.	Lomax (1966b)
	10–100 µg	1 µl	Rostral hypothalamus	Rat	C	Tachyphylaxis to morphine.	Lotti et al. (1966a)
Nalorphine	3.3–10 µg	1 µl	Anterior hypothalamus, preoptic area	Rat	C	Blocks hypothermia of systemic morphine.	Lomax (1967)
	3.3–10 µg	1 µl	Rostral hypothalamus	Rat	C	Reversed morphine hypothermia.	Lotti et al. (1965b)
Naphazoline	5 µg	1 µl	Rostral hypothalamus	Rat	C	Hyperthermia.	Lomax and Foster (1969)
Nicotine	4 µg	?	Rostral hypothalamus	Rat	?	Hypothermia.	Knox and Lomax (1972)
	2–10 µg	1 µl	Anterior hypothalamus	Monkey	C	Hypothermia.	Hall and Myers (1972)
	2–10 µg	1 µl	Posterior hypothalamus	Monkey	C	Hyperthermia.	Hall and Myers (1972)
Norepinephrine (NE)	.02–.15 µg	1 µl	Anterior hypothalamus, preoptic area	Rat	U	Rise or fall in temperature. Increase in responding for heat reinforcement.	Beckman (1970)
	.5 µg	20 µl	Hypothalamus	Rat	U	Hyperthermia.	Boros-Farkas and Illei-Donhoffer (1969)
	.5–5 µg	1 µl	Rostral hypothalamus	Rat	C	Variable response but usually fall in temperature with 2.5 µg.	Lomax et al. (1969)
	15 µg	.5 µl	Anterior hypothalamus, preoptic area	Rat	U	At 5°C, great hyperthermia. At 35°C, attenuates hyperthermia.	Avery (1972)

Dose	Volume	Site	Animal	U/C	Effect	Reference
5–25 µg	.5 µl	Anterior hypothalamus	Rat	U	Hypothermia.	Avery (1971)
1 µg	1 µl	Rostral hypothalamus	Guinea pig	U	Hyperthermia, increased O₂.	Zeisburger and Brück (1971a)
2 µg	1 µl	Anterior hypothalamus	Guinea pig	C	Hypo- or hyperthermia of about 0.5°C, increase in O₂ consumption.	Zeisburger and Brück (1971b)
.05–4 µg	1 µl	Rostral hypothalamus	Ground squirrel	U	Arousal from hibernation, hypothermia, hyperthermia.	Beckman and Satinoff (1972)
2 µg	2 µl	Anterior hypothalamus	Rabbit	C	Hyperthermia.	Cooper et al. (1967)
2–10 µg	10 µl	Hypothalamus	Rabbit	C	Rise in temperature (50%) or no effect (50%).	Cooper et al. (1965)
4.2–6.34 µg	.5 µl	Hypothalamus	Chicken	U	Hypothermia.	Marley and Stephenson (1970)
5 µg	1 µl	Anterior hypothalamus	Cat	U	Reduces PGE₁ fever.	Feldberg and Saxena (1971)
5 µg	.5–1 µl	Anterior hypothalamus	Cat	U	Hypothermia.	Feldberg and Myers (1965a)
2–17 µg	1 µl	Anterior hypothalamus	Cat	U	Hypothermia.	Rudy and Wolf (1971)
5 µg	1 µl	Anterior hypothalamus	Monkey	C	Hypothermia.	Hall and Myers (1972)
1–12 µg	.5–1 µl	Anterior hypothalamus	Monkey	C	Hypothermia.	Myers and Yaksh (1969)
1–12 µg	.5–1 µl	Anterior hypothalamus	Monkey	C	Hypothermia.	Myers (1970b)
5–12.5 µg	1–1.2 µl	Hypothalamus	Monkey	C	Hypothermia.	Yaksh and Myers (1972b)
12.5 µg	.5–1 µl	Anterior hypothalamus	Monkey	C	Hypothermia.	Myers and Sharpe (1968a)
15–30 µg	15–30 µl	Rostral hypothalamus	Baboon	C	Hypothermia.	Toivola and Gale (1970)

VII.   Master Summary Table *(Continued)*

Chemical	Dose	Volume	Site	Species	State*	Response	Reference
Oxotremorine	2 μg	1 μl	Preoptic area	Rat	C	Hypothermia.	Lomax and Jenden (1966)
	8–50 μg	10 μl	Anterior hypothalamus, septum, caudate nucleus	Rat	U	Hypothermia.	Staib and Andreas (1970)
	12–18 μg	1–10 μl	Caudate nucleus	Cat	C	Hyperthermia.	Connor et al. (1966a)
Phenoxybenzamine	68 μg	2 μg	Hypothalamus	Chicken	U	Prevented noradrenaline hypothermia.	Marley and Stephenson (1970)
Phenylalanine	10 μg	20 μl	Hypothalamus	Rat	U	Hyperthermia.	Boros-Farkas and Illei-Donhoffer (1969)
Phenylephrine	2–17 μg	1 μl	Anterior hypothalamus	Cat	U	Hypothermia.	Rudy and Wolf (1971)
Physostigmine	70–100 μg	1–10 μl	Caudate nucleus	Cat	C	Hyperthermia.	Connor et al. (1966a)
Picrotoxin	1 μg	50 μl	Infundibular region	Rabbit	C	Hypothermia.	Rosenthal (1941)
Pilocarpine	40 μg	1 μl	Rostral hypothalamus	Rat	C	Hypothermia.	Lomax et al. (1969)
Potassium (K^+)	.2–2 mg	50 μl	Tuber cinerium	Cat	U	Hyperthermia (ta 17–19°C) slight.	Hasama (1930)
Propranolol	.9 mg	50 μl	Hypothalamus	Rabbit	C	Delayed fever.	Kym (1934)
	56 μg	2 μl	Hypothalamus	Chicken	U	Attenuated noradrenaline hypothermia.	Marley and Stephenson (1970)

	Dose	Volume	Site	Species		Effect	Reference
Prostaglandin E_1	.002–1 µg	1 µl	Anterior hypothalamus	Cat	U	Fever.	Feldberg and Saxena (1971)
Pyrexal (*S. abortus equi*)	.025–.050 µg	20 µl	Hypothalamus	Rabbit	C	Fever.	Cooper et al. (1965)
	10–200 µg	2 µl	Anterior hypothalamus	Rabbit	C	Fever within 25 minutes.	Cooper et al. (1967)
Pyrogenal	.001–1 µg	2 µl	Rostral hypothalamus	Rabbit	?	Fever with 30 minute latency.	Repin and Kratskin (1967)
Salmonella typhosa	10^8 organisms/ml	1–2.5 µl	Anterior hypothalamus	Cat	U	Fever.	Villablanca and Myers (1965)
	1:500, 1:1000 dilution	.5–1 µl	Anterior hypothalamus	Cat	U	Fever.	Feldberg and Myers (1965a)
	1:20, 1:100 dilution	4–6 µl	Rostral hypothalamus	Cat	U	Fever.	Jackson (1967)
	2.5×10^9 organisms/ml	.8–1.2 µl	Hypothalamus	Monkey	C	Fever, shivering.	Myers et al. (1971a)
Serotonin (5-HT)	.05–1 µg	1 µl	Anterior hypothalamus, preoptic area	Rat	U	Hyperthermia.	Crawshaw (1972)
	5 µg	20 µl	Hypothalamus	Rat	U	Hyperthermia.	Boros-Farkas and Illei-Donhoffer (1969)
	2–40 µg	10 µl	Hypothalamus	Rabbit	C	No consistent temperature effect	Cooper et al. (1965)
	.8–1.6 µg	1 µl	Rostral hypothalamus	Ground squirrel	U	Arousal from hibernation; hyperthermia.	Beckman and Satinoff (1972)
	2–10 µg	.5–1 µl	Anterior hypothalamus	Cat	U	Hypothermia, shivering.	Feldberg and Myers (1965a)
	5 µg	1 µl	Anterior hypothalamus	Monkey	C	Hyperthermia.	Myers (1968)
	2–10 µg	.5–1	Anterior hypothalamus	Monkey	C	Hyperthermia.	Myers and Yaksh (1969) Myers (1970b)

VII. Master Summary Table (Continued)

Chemical	Dose	Volume	Site	Species	State*	Response	Reference
Serotonin (5-HT)	10 µg	1 µl	Anterior hypothalamus	Monkey	C	Hypothermia.	Myers (1968)
	12.5 µg	.5–1 µl	Anterior hypothalamus	Monkey	C	Hypo- or hyperthermia.	Myers and Sharpe (1968a)
	15 µg	15 µl	Rostral hypothalamus	Baboon	C	Mixed temperature effects.	Toivola and Gale (1970)
Shigella dysenteriae	2.5×10^9 organisms/ml	.8–1.2 µl	Hypothalamus	Monkey	C	Fever, shivering.	Myers et al. (1971a)
Sodium (Na^+)	14.94–39.07 µg/min	perfusion 50 µl/min	Posterior hypothalamus	Cat	U	Hyperthermia.	Myers and Veale (1970)
	14.94–78.13 µg/min	perfusion 50 µl/min	Hypothalamus	Cat	U	Hyperthermia.	Myers and Veale (1971a)
	20–60 mg	50 µl	Tuber cinerium	Cat	U	Hyperthermia (intense).	Hasama (1930)
	22.65–95.99 µg/min	perfusion 50 µl/min	Posterior hypothalamus	Monkey	C	Hyperthermia.	Myers and Yaksh (1971)
	1 mg	50 µl	Hypothalamus	Rabbit	C	Fever.	Kym (1934)
	42–50 µg	50 µl	Tuber cinerium	Cat	U	Hyperthermia (slight).	Hasama (1930)
Sodium pentobarbital	30 µg	1 µl	Anterior and posterior hypothalamus	Rat	U	No effect.	Lomax (1966b)
Sodium salicylate	6–30 µg	10 µl	Rostral hypothalamus, mesencephalon	Rabbit	C	Reduced fever.	Cranston and Rawlins (1972)
Tetrahydrozoline	5 µg	1 µl	Rostral hypothalamus	Rat	C	Hyperthermia.	Lomax and Foster (1969)

Drug	Dose	Volume	Site	Species	C/U	Effect	Reference
Tolazoline	2.5 μg	1 μl	Rostral hypothalamus	Rat	C	Attenuated naphazoline hyperthermia.	Lomax and Foster (1969)
	2.5 μg	1 μl	Rostral hypothalamus	Rat	C	No consistent effect on temperature.	Lomax et al. (1969)
Trihexyphenidyl	10 μg	1 μl	Preoptic area	Rat	C	Antagonized systemic oxotremorine hypothermia.	Lomax and Jenden (1966)
Triiodothyronine	1 μg	20 μl	Hypothalamus	Rat	U	Hyperthermia.	Boros-Farkas and Illei-Don-hoffer (1969)

7 Hunger and Feeding

I. INTRODUCTION

In the everyday life of a human, the word "hunger" or a phrase associated with this uncomfortable state crops up three or four times every day.[1] In the animal kingdom, the search for food and the act of feeding often dominate the whole behavioral style of a given species. These simple facts attest to the importance which a number of physiologists and psychologists have attached to a scientific understanding of the ingestion of food. The classical information about the mechanisms of energy balance, caloric utilization, the role of central nervous influences in the perception of hunger, and feeding behavior itself, have been reviewed comprehensively by Stevenson (1969), Morgane and Jacobs (1969) and Andersson (1971a). Further, these topics are among those that are the subject matter of an entire volume in Section 6 of the *Handbook of Physiology* (Code, 1967).

The actual state of hunger is the first functional condition dealt with in this volume that is almost wholly subjective in nature. Keeping in mind that the concept of hunger is largely an inference in terms of its measurement in an animal, its determinants in experimental investigations are ordinarily expressed quantitatively in relation to the number of hours of deprivation, the quantity of food eaten under one set of circumstances, the selection of a specific nutrient, or some other measure. As we shall see momentarily, these definitions are often the source of consternation and disagreement, particularly with respect to what constitutes a food substance.

It is generally acknowledged that a subtle variation in the constituents of the plasma including carbohydrates, lipids and amino acids plays a crucial part in the complex feedback regulation of energy balance. A state of balance in energy metabolism is, of course, reached when the intake of calories is equilibrated with the expenditure of energy, both in terms of metabolic heat production and muscular energy. A disequilibrium in either direction has important

[1] At least for some of us.

physiological consequences. For example, an accumulation of lipids following the intake of calories in excess of an individual's specific energy requirement will result eventually in a marked obesity.

A primary mechanism delegated to the relatively short-term daily pattern of food intake is thought to involve sensors that monitor the values of circulating carbohydrates in plasma. Quite remarkably, a normal animal is also able to regulate or balance intrinsically the long-term input of nutrients with the output of energy. Such control is manifest even if the animal is forced to eat, is tube fed, temporarily starved, or offered free access to high energy foods. Therefore, a second mechanism operates for the long-term regulation of food intake which could be independent from the more immediate short-term mechanism. For its input signals, this long-term mechanism may depend principally on a blood-borne factor emanating from fat depots (Andersson, 1971a). As described below, an imperious search is on for the chemical factors or complex of factors in the serum, hypothalamus or other structures in the brain, which could monitor and govern one's intake of food or could underlie the psychological phenomenon of hunger in all of its varied aspects (Davis *et al.*, 1967a; Yaksh and Myers, 1972a).

A. Hunger and Satiety Receptors

If factors contained in the serum do operate in some sort of feedback fashion to inform certain elements in the brain that at a critical moment energy replenishment is necessary, then obviously a receptor complex uniquely sensitive to such factors must lie within a part of the brain. Already, the existence of glucose receptors in the liver has been clearly documented by Russek *et al.* (1967). Because of the results of lesion studies, much speculation now centers on the ventromedial and lateral hypothalamus as the two crucial regions which could possess these unique receptors. One factor that has been postulated to trigger the receptors is glucose itself, and, in fact, the so-called "glucostatic theory" has been widely popularized by Jean Mayer (1953). Briefly, the glucostatic theory proposes that glucoreceptors in the ventromedial hypothalamus increase their firing rate as their uptake of glucose increases. An elevation in circulating glucose levels would thus cause an intense discharge of the receptors and thus activate the satiety pathway. The net effect is satiation and the ultimate inhibition of feeding.

Several observations favor such a glucostatic theory. To illustrate, an intravenous injection of either insulin or 2-deoxy-D-glucose (2-DG), a glucose analogue which inhibits glucose utilization, reduces the activity of neurons in the ventromedial hypothalamus (Anand *et al.*, 1964; Desiraju *et al.*, 1968). Moreover, glucogen, which elevates glucose concentration and its utilization systemically has been reported to attenuate the hunger sensation in man following its systemic injection (Stunkard *et al.*, 1955). Finally, gold thioglucose given systemically produces localized lesions in the ventromedial hypothalamus of the mouse and a dramatic hyperphagia; since other salts of gold including thiocarbohydrates do not exert this effect, overeating occurs presumably because the glucose receptors within the ventromedial region that have taken up this toxic gold compound are subsequently destroyed (Mayer and Marshall, 1956).

On the other side of the fence, many experiments have somewhat impugned the idea of the hypothalamic glucose receptor. For instance, one's urge to eat frequently is not at all correlated with any systemic fluctuation in the concentration of glucose in the bloodstream (Janowitz and Ivy, 1949). Furthermore, the metabolism of cerebral glucose seems to be independent of the level of insulin (Stevenson, 1969). Finally, neither a severe insulin induced hypo glycemia produced in the ruminant (Baile and Mayer, 1968) nor the well-known hyperglycemia often observed in diabetic patients alters feeding behavior appreciably. Although a carbohydrate other than a 6-carbon sugar could be the factor that triggers the nutrient receptors in the brain-stem, it is interesting that the local elevation of glucose or dextrose in the hypothalamus of the monkey (Myers and Sharpe, 1968b; Sharpe and Myers, 1969) or rat (Epstein, 1960) fails to inhibit feeding behavior.

An animal in which the ventromedial hypothalamus is destroyed symmetrically usually exhibits the dramatic symptoms of hyperphagia and the concomitant syndrome of static obesity (Hetherington and Ranson, 1939; Brobeck et al., 1943). Even though the ventromedially lesioned preparation reacts to the palatability of a food substance by eating more of the food if it is appealing or less food if it is distasteful (Miller et al., 1950; Kennedy, 1953), the hyperphagic obese animal does not overeat after a certain level of body weight is attained (Kennedy, 1953). In other words, the animal with a ventromedial hypothalamic lesion achieves a level of static obesity around which it regulates its subsequent caloric intake with unique precision.

One explanation of this rests in the "lipostatic theory," which proposes that a humoral factor arising from the fat depots in the body triggers the feedback signals which provide the long-term regulation of energy balance once a certain weight level is finally reached. The elegant parabiotic experiments of Hervey (1959) support this notion. Again it should be emphasized that the postulated lipostatic receptors, whether they are of hypothalamic or extra-diencephalic origin, have not as yet been identified.

B. Neuroanatomical Basis of Feeding

A plethora of experiments followed the discovery by Anand and Brobeck (1951) of the severe aphagia and death from inanition produced by bilateral ablation of the lateral hypothalamus. The defect produced by such damage has been characterized as motivational, metabolic or due to motor failure (Morgane,

1961a and b; Baillie and Morrison, 1963). In a series of well-known studies, Teitelbaum and Epstein (1962) have characterized the stages by which a rat can recover from a devastating lesion of its lateral hypothalamus. If the animal is nursed and maintained until it accepts a palatable diet consisting of a nutritious liquid, recovery is almost always assured. Corresponding to these experiments are those in which electrical stimulation of a homologous portion of the lateral hypothalamus elicits spontaneous feeding, just as the stimulation of the ventromedial region tends to inhibit it (Delgado and Anand, 1953; Smith, 1956).

A vast amount of experimental information has tended to abrogate the concept of a hypothalamic center for either feeding or satiety (Grossman, 1968c; 1972). For example, the fiber system coursing out of the globus pallidus into the lateral hypothalamus is implicated in eating behavior, since its destruction evokes the same sort of aphagia as the lateral hypothalamic syndrome (Morgane, 1961). The chemical lesioning of the nigro-striatal system produces the same sort of lethal aphagia (Ungerstedt, 1971a). Similarly, circumscribed lesions of the midbrain tegmentum, red nucleus, amygdala, thalamic nuclei, septum pellucidum, hippocampus, cingulate gyrus and even frontal cortex have all variously enhanced or suppressed the intake of food of a variety of species (Stevenson, 1969; Hoebel, 1971). The diffuseness of the anatomical networks underlying the feeding response (Grossman, 1972) illustrates quite clearly that a sizeable number of nuclei and fiber pathways conventionally serve the functions of generalized activity, motor control, temperature regulation, emotionality, gastrointestinal motility, and the intricate facets of olfaction and the gustatory senses.

1. *Interaction with Other Functions*

Paralleling the anatomical intricacies of the hunger system is the complex functional interaction of food intake with other physiological and psychological processes (Grafe and Grünthal, 1929). As explained by Booth (1968c), the necessity of employing a double or even triple dissociation of the feeding response from other behaviors is apparent. To dissect out a specific chemical mechanism within an anatomical circuit involved in hunger would require first that each interaction be carefully deciphered and accounted for. These include drinking of water, a change in body temperature, learned temporal discriminations, motor movement or other generalized activity, painful gastric sensations or other condition. But why are these reactions not simply trivial?

If a chemical is applied to a given structure in the brain which in essence provokes a generalized excitatory state, the animal may simply eat chow from its food-well as a part of this excitation. Similarly, the response of gnawing could be misinterpreted as eating behavior if the animal happens to direct its teeth on a food pellet. Or, if the chemical agent blocks the heat production pathway in the brain-stem thereby causing hypothermia, the animal could feed secondarily because of this metabolic response to a thermogenic stimulus

(Spector *et al.*, 1968) rather than because of a direct activation of the feeding pathway.

2. *Technical Considerations*

A major technical difficulty always concerns the issue of defining just what does constitute a change in the feeding pattern of an animal. Let us consider that a control injection of saline into the hypothalamus causes the animal to eat 1 g of food, but that 1.5 g is consumed after a chemical is applied to the same site. Is that elevation in intake a significant one? Although statistical manipulations are easy to apply, they are difficult to interpret in respect to the internal condition of satiation. The time interval during which the animal eats spontaneously or fails to eat is another factor that is just as critical. Obviously, the palatability of the specific food offered to the animal will influence the magnitude of the food consumed, particularly should the chemical also modify the animal's sensory input.

The physical measurement of food intake is equally crucial in that the way that an animal such as a rodent consumes its food can influence the quantitation of the ingestive response. Pulverizing or gnawing a food pellet, spillage, and other variables associated with the act of eating always affect the validity of the intake measure. Such subtle aspects that contribute to the overall variance in the animal's intake require that any change in food intake be expressed in a gram value rather than as a percent change.

II. HYPOTHALAMIC HUNGER AND SATIETY MECHANISMS

The experimental evidence which is now coming to light suggests that not only glucose but other substances in the plasma may participate in the animal's behavioral response to hunger, to satiety or to both conditions. Although these chemical substances may be independent of those cerebral factors that are present endogenously in the brain-stem, they may also work in close conjunction with them. In addition, there may well be still other distinct chemosensitive mechanisms which act to establish the fundamental "set-point" that may determine the level of hunger, the regulation of body weight, lipid metabolism, glucose utilization and other essential processes. These "set-point" mechanisms are believed to be extant at birth and maintain the intrinsic level of energy exchange around which day to day regulation occurs (Veale and Myers, 1971).

A. Glucose Receptor Mechanisms

Although patterns of electrical activity in the ventromedial or lateral hypothalamus may simply constitute reflexive activity in these areas, there is strong evidence from EEG recordings (Anand *et al.*, 1961a and b), from the activity of single cells and other studies (Dunér, 1953) that specific glucoreceptors do exist in the hypothalamus. For instance, Forssberg and Larsson (1954) found that ^{32}P activity increased in the "feeding center" of the hungry rat when individual samples of ^{32}P-labelled tissue were analyzed. ^{14}C glucose activity possessed a similar trend showing that the physiological or metabolic activity of the hypothalamus may change during hunger produced by fasting the rat. Oomura *et al.* (1969) found that neurons in the lateral hypothalamus or ventromedial hypothalamus of the rat are reactive to glucose. As shown in Fig. 7-1, their discharge rates increase in response to a local excess in the concentration of the sugar. The firing rate of some lateral hypothalamic neurons is reduced and a few of these glucose-sensitive cells are equally responsive to Na^+. This would indicate that these neurons are also probably osmoreceptors as well. These findings correspond well with the micro-injection results of Peck and Novin (1971) discussed in Chapter 8.

Other evidence of the existence of glucose receptors has been taken from experiments in which 2-deoxy-D-glucose (2-DG) has been injected directly into the brain. This synthetic analogue of glucose acts to inhibit the local metabolism of glucose. When 2-DG is infused into the lateral hypothalamus of the rat, which would have the effect of reducing the regional store of glucose, the secretion of gastric acid increases substantially (Colin-Jones and Himsworth, 1970). One could imagine that the pangs of hunger that are correlated with an augmentation in gastric activity may be brought about by the local diminution of glucose within the lateral hypothalamus.

In support of the belief that the blockade of glucose metabolism by 2-DG could lead to feeding, presumably because of a lower glucose level in the lateral hypothalamus, is a preliminary report of Balagura (1971). When a high dose of 2-DG was administered in the lateral hypothalamus, a slight increase in food intake of less than 1 g above the control level occurred during a 30 minute test period. Similarly, crystals of 2-DG placed in the lateral hypothalamus of the rat on an *ad lib.* regimen evoked an average increase in food intake of 0.7 g (Balagura and Kanner, 1971). Surprisingly, when crystalline glucose itself is placed in the same areas, the rat increased its consumption of food by 0.4 g. A similar small increase in food intake was observed when the animal was deprived and the chemicals were deposited in the dorsomedial hypothalamus. These perplexing findings are nearly impossible to interpret since 2-DG is a biological antagonist of glucose, yet both substances appear to have the same local pharmacological effect on hypothalamic neurons in stimulating feeding. How the local application of 2-DG actually affects the cells of the hypothalamus is not clear. For instance, it could deplete glucose intracellularly, from extracellular fluid, or in the plasma within the local capillary supply. Overall, however, the findings thus far with 2-DG at least do not seem sufficiently strong to warrant a conclusion that the lateral hypothalamus or other parts of the hypothalamus contain glucose-receptive cells.

The ventromedial hypothalamus is also selectively sensitive to specific sugars in

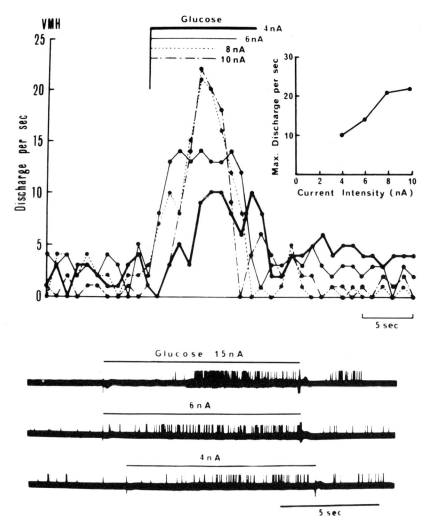

Fig. 7-1 Top, discharge rate of a typical VMH neuron before, during and after electro-osmotic application of various amounts of glucose through a micropipette. Inset, maximum discharge rate as a function of the amount of glucose applied. Bottom, the modulation of ongoing unit activity in another VMH cell by the administration of glucose. Strength of glucose application expressed in nA because only the current which was passed through the electrode could be measured in each experiment. The length of time the glucose stimulation lasted is indicated by the horizontal lines. Note the relatively long latency which indicates a glucose, rather than a current, effect. In this neuron, glucose was applied successively after 15, 6 and 4 nA. The shorter latencies in the latter two cases were probably due to accumulation of glucose in the vicinity of the cell. These cells were not affected by Na stimulation alone, which indicates that the effects are due to the glucose. (From Oomura *et al.*, 1969)

the glycogenic pathway. The EEG activity recorded directly from the ventro-medial hypothalamus increased following the local deposition of crystals of glucose-6-phosphate (GLU-6-P) in the ventromedial region of the rat, but declined when either glucose or fructose-6-phosphate (FRU-6-P) was applied at the same site (Gliddon, 1970). It is difficult to interpret these effects in terms of lateral hypothalamic-ventromedial hypothalamic control mechanisms for hunger and satiety until sufficient information is known about EEG activity of the lateral hypothalamus in response to these same sugars.

A direct test of the glucose receptor hypothesis has been made in both the rat and monkey. Epstein (1960) found that isotonic dextrose injected in very large volumes into the medial hypothalamus did not suppress or even interrupt the normal eating of the food-deprived rat. Similarly, Myers and Sharpe (1968b) reported that 5 or 15% dextrose infused into either the lateral or ventromedial hypothalamus of the rhesus monkey deprived of food for as long as 24 hours did not inhibit eating. Figure 7-2 illustrates the amount of food consumed by two monkeys after dextrose had been infused at the hypothalamic sites shown in the inset.

When glucose was micro-injected into feeding sites in the antero-lateral hypo-thalamus, so designated by prior injections of norepinephrine, the intakes of both food and water were attenuated in rats that had been primed to feed by bovine insulin given subcutaneously 20 minutes earlier (Booth, 1968b). To rule out the question of hypotonicity, isotonic glucose and saline controls were also run with no effect. However, because the animals curled up as if asleep following the intrahypothalamic injection of glucose and the water intake was equally reduced, Booth concluded that glucose does not exert a specific effect on the hypothalamic system for hunger. Thus, a glucose receptor hypothesis is not favored by these experiments. This corresponds with the view of Soulairac who showed that serum glucose concentrations and the degree of hunger fail to correlate (Soulairac, 1958).

With respect to the absence of a specific aphagic action of glucose on the hypothalamus, a noteworthy observation has been made by Panksepp and Nance (1972). In confirmation of the reports of others, glucose or glucose plus insulin injected in a large 2 μl volume into the rat's ventromedial hypothalamus had no effect on the immediate post-injection feeding behavior. However, the food intake over the day following the injection was somewhat reduced when the site of injection again was the VMH. Since a control infusion of urea or an injection of glucose in the lateral hypothalamus does not alter the ingestive pattern, the lag in this attenuation of eating might be related to a slow local metabolism of glucose in hypothalamic tissue. As suggested by Panksepp and Nance, a general malaise of unknown origin may also contribute to the change in the rat's feeding behavior.

In the mouse made diabetic with intravenous alloxan, the intraperitoneal injection of gold thioglucose (GTG) does not cause its typical effect of necrosis

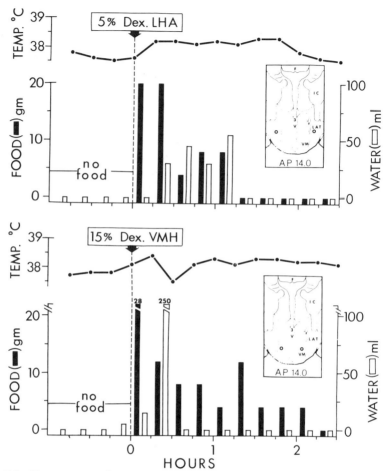

Fig. 7-2 Temperature, food and water intakes of two rhesus monkeys that were food deprived for 24 hours prior to bilateral 1 μl injections of dextrose in the hypothalamus. In one monkey, (Top) 5% dextrose (5% Dex) was given in the lateral hypothalamus (LHA) at zero hour. In the second monkey (Bottom) 15% dextrose (15% Dex) was micro-injected in the ventromedial hypothalamus (VMH). Insets portray diagrammatically the sites of each bilateral injection represented by each circle (o). Abscissa is time in hours. (From Myers and Sharpe, 1968b)

on ventromedial hypothalamic neurons (Debons et al., 1970). However, when insulin was micro-injected into the ventral hypothalamus, the usual GTG necrosis appeared. Since neuroanatomical and systemic controls verified the effect, these results suggest that the release of the pancreatic hormone may influence the hypothalamus directly in the restoration of the sensitivity to GTG of the satiety "center." In fact, the well-known hyperphagia noted in patients suffering from diabetis mellitus could well be mediated by the ventromedial hypothalamus as a result of insulin insufficiency.

B. Hypothalamic Factors for Hunger and Satiety

That an amino acid complex, conglomerate of lipids or other substances act in addition to glucose on the hypothalamus is certainly suspected by many workers in this field.

Evidence of a satiety factor has been obtained from studies of blood as well as neurophysiological investigations. After a fasted rat received a blood transfusion from another rat that had been satiated, the food intake of the first animal was diminished (Davis et al., 1967a). Although this unknown blood-borne factor can inhibit food intake, there is evidence at present that a factor is synthesized or present in the plasma of a food-deprived rat, which would in turn evoke feeding in a satiated animal after a similar blood transfusion. Thus, at the serum level, the condition of hunger seems to be correlated to a satiety factor. If the concentration of this factor in the blood falls below a certain critical level, this signals the absence of satiety, the net effect being feeding behavior.

The evidence that a potent chemical factor is released from the hypothalamus of a hungry animal was announced in 1967 by Myers at the New York Academy of Sciences. Either CSF drained from the third ventricle or perfusate collected by means of push-pull cannulae from the lateral hypothalamus of a hungry monkey caused spontaneous feeding in a fully satiated monkey when either of these two fluids was transfused to its lateral hypothalamus (Myers, 1969b). The latter effect is portrayed in Fig. 7-3. Even though the constituents of the perfusates were unknown, the results showed that an endogenous humoral substance can be collected upon its release from the cells of the fasted animal's hypothalamus. Furthermore, the activity of this substance is related to the level of deprivation of the donor animal.

The precise anatomical localization of the transfusion phenomenon and the characterization of the temporal aspects of the response have been described recently (Yaksh and Myers, 1972a). Documentation of two relatively stable humoral factors rather than one that underlies feeding has also been shown, again by the use of the push-pull transfusion procedure (Myers, 1967). Three basic types of experiments were performed. First, the donor monkey was deprived of food for 5 or 18 hours after which the hypothalamus was perfused and the collected effluent re-perfused at a homologous site in a recipient monkey. Second, the same procedure was repeated but both donor and recipient were satiated as an important control. Third, when individual monkeys were used, each of the animal's own hypothalamic perfusates was collected when it was fasted, and then re-perfused at the same site. This re-perfusion of the animal's own effluent was done some time later after the monkey had been fully fed.

In 10 out of 23 donor-recipient pairs of rhesus monkeys, the satiated recipient ate food generally in a magnitude depending on the hours of deprivation of the donor. The same result ensued in the single monkey when its own hypothalamic perfusate was re-perfused at the same site. The sites of release of this so-called

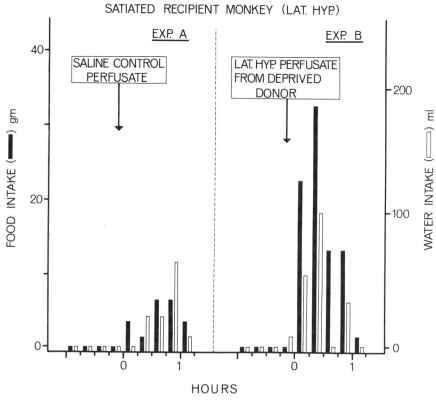

Fig. 7-3 Food and water intakes in grams of a fully satiated rhesus monkey after a 30 minute push-pull perfusion at 50 µl/minute of its lateral hypothalamus at the arrows. In *Experiment A*, the perfusate was physiological saline. In *Experiment B*, the perfusate was that which had been similarly perfused, immediately before the experiment began, through the lateral hypothalamus of another rhesus monkey donor that had been deprived of food for 18 hours. (Modified after Myers, 1969b)

hunger factor were identified by a commonality of characteristics: (1) their sensitivity to norepinephrine, which evoked feeding; (2) the morphological localization to the fiber system of the descending columns of the fornix; and (3) by the ability of the sites to release a norepinephrine-like substance when they were perfused after the monkey had been food-deprived overnight. Taken together, these findings support the concept that the concentration of a complex of factors including a noradrenergic-like substance is elevated in the hypothalamus during the hunger produced by withholding the animal's normal food ration. Subsequently, motivated feeding behavior, as reflected by the lever responses presented in Fig. 7-4, is caused by its presence in circumscribed loci in the hypothalamus of the monkey (Yaksh and Myers, 1972a).

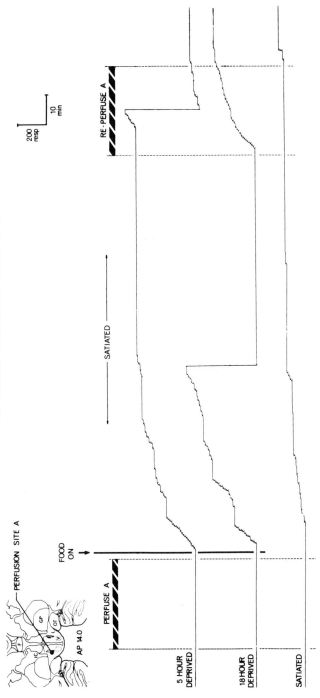

Fig. 7-4 Cumulative records of lever press responses for 1 g food pellets on an FR 10 schedule of reinforcement for three self-perfusion experiments shown at site A (inset) when animal was 5 hour deprived (top record), 18 hour deprived (middle record), or satiated (bottom record). At vertical dashed line food for deprived condition experiments was turned on and animal allowed to satiate, after which animal was again perfused (re-perfuse A) at site A with perfusate obtained earlier. Anatomical abbreviations are the same as Fig. 7-11. (From Yaksh and Myers, 1972b)

The first direct evidence of a hypothalamic satiety factor has also been described by Yaksh and Myers (1972a). In 13 pairs of monkeys, 9 recipients, which were deprived of food for up to 18 hours, ate substantially fewer banana pellets after the hypothalamus of each monkey was perfused with hypothalamic effluent collected from a donor that had been fully satiated. A typical inhibition of feeding is shown in Fig. 7-5. Two major differences were uncovered

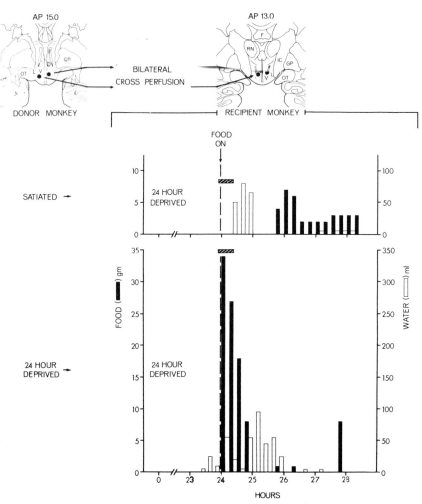

Fig. 7-5 Feeding (■) and drinking (□) responses of a 24 hour food-deprived recipient monkey following push-pull perfusion of perfusate at site shown at AP 13.0 (inset) obtained from site at AP 15.0 (inset) of donor animal which was satiated (top panel) or 24 hour food deprived (bottom panel). Abbreviations are the same a Fig. 7-11. (From Yaksh and Myers, 1972b)

between these and the foregoing experiments: (1) the perfusion sites, as exemplified in Fig. 7-5, in both donor and recipient monkeys were always close to midline in the plane of the ventromedial nucleus; and (2) in relation to evoked feeding, a sensitivity to norepinephrine injected at the perfusion sites was not correlated with the absence of feeding in the hungry recipient, the response being suppressed by perfusate collected from the hypothalamus of the satiated donor monkey. Since the suppression of food consumption often persisted for several hours after the hypothalamic transfusion had been completed (Fig. 7-5), the satiety factor is not only powerful pharmacologically but is also slow to be inactivated. The control perfusions between a hungry or normal donor and the fasted recipient rule out a nonspecific inhibitory effect. In addition, the behavior of the recipient monkey appeared to be normal in every other respect.

In a study somewhat related to the effects of a complex factor on the cells of the hypothalamus, Panksepp and Booth (1971) attempted to assess the direct effects of a collection of chemical substances other than glucose. A balanced amino acid solution containing 12 amino acids was micro-infused into the rat's hypothalamus. They found that this complex of essential amino acids reduced the rat's consumption of food by about 1 to 2 g, which was more than that caused by a solution of urea or NaCl injected similarly into the perifornical region. Thus, it is possible that a meal rich in protein could have some feedback influence on the hypothalamic region mediating feeding by way of amino acids circulating in blood.

A lipid soluble fatty acid such as prostaglandin may also be involved in the regulation of energy balance generally, or in the metabolism of fatty acids and glucose specifically. PGA_1, PGE_1, PGE_2 and other prostaglandins significantly reduce food intake when they are administered systemically (Scaramuzzi et al., 1971). Obviously, their effects on the fornical region remain to be determined.

C. Set-Point Mechanisms

As a result of the increase in body fat associated with the hyperphagia produced by ablation of the rat's ventromedial hypothalamus, Kennedy (1953) concluded that the animal's "lipostat" was disordered. Such a postulated lipostat would be an internal mechanism that in an unknown way sets and maintains the deposition of body fat at a relatively constant level. This view is contrasted somewhat with the idea of Miller et al. (1950) that a ventromedial lesion injures the regulatory system that somehow senses the condition of satiety. An outgrowth of Kennedy's lipostatic model is related to the typical aphagia and reduction in body weight observed following the ablation of a rat's lateral hypothalamus. For example, if a rat is starved to 80% of its body weight prior to the destruction of the lateral hypothalamus, it eats until it reaches a new but reduced level of body weight. In some cases the animal appears to be hyperphagic rather than aphagic after the lesion, but the overeating disappears as soon as the new point of under-weight is achieved and maintained (Powley and Keesey, 1970).

The cellular attributes in the hypothalamus that subserve such a set-point system for lipid metabolism and storage, weight maintenance or perhaps hunger itself are unknown. However, in connection with the ionic mechanism described in Chapter 6, which is believed to establish the set-point for body temperature, a similar type of mechanism may also provide the stability in local neuronal activity which would set the animal's intake of food. Evidence for the involvement of Na^+ and Ca^{2+} ions in this process has recently been presented.

1. Ion-Induced Feeding

In a freely-moving cat, spontaneous feeding was induced by the localized perfusion of a solution containing an excess of either Na^+ or Ca^{2+} ions (Myers and Veale, 1971b). The level of each cation was elevated within small, restricted regions of the hypothalamus by means of the push-pull cannula technique. As shown in Fig. 7-6, the eating response was entirely perfusion dependent. Although the latency to feed was longer following the perfusion of the Ca^{2+} solution, both of the cations in excess of their normal concentration in extracellular fluid evoked an intake of nearly 50 g of cat food. The sites of maximum sensitivity to sodium and calcium were the lateral hypothalamus and the ventromedial hypothalamus, respectively. Solutions of K^+ or Mg^{2+}, as well as an artificial CSF, had no effect on the cat's feeding behavior when perfused in the same way and at the same sites. If the same corollary is drawn with the maintenance of body temperature, these data could be taken to support the concept of an ionic set-point for weight regulation or perhaps hunger in the cat. The chief difference between a set-point for body temperature and one stabilizing body weight is the anatomical locus in the hypothalamus which is sensitive to the critical ratio of Na^+ to Ca^{2+} ions.

It is interesting that the injection of artificial CSF containing an excess in calcium ions into the cerebral ventricles of the rat also evokes spontaneous feeding (Myers et al., 1972). Of special significance is the fact that neither phentolamine nor propranolol, given earlier by the ventricular route, prevents this Ca^{2+}-induced feeding. These results provide evidence that an adrenergic compound is probably not the only substance in the complex anatomical circuit which mediates feeding in the rat. Moreover, probably another mechanism exists that is independent of the one responsible for hourly or even daily changes in the degree of appetite or satiety. In the human, obesity is often difficult to control primarily because of almost involuntary, compulsive eating. This behavior may be the end result of an aberration of the set-point which has been re-established at a higher, abnormal level. This internal set-point may be controlled by the ratio of Na^+ to Ca^{2+} ions in the hypothalamus, since a perturbation in the ratio, just as in the case of body temperature, alters the animal's response drastically.

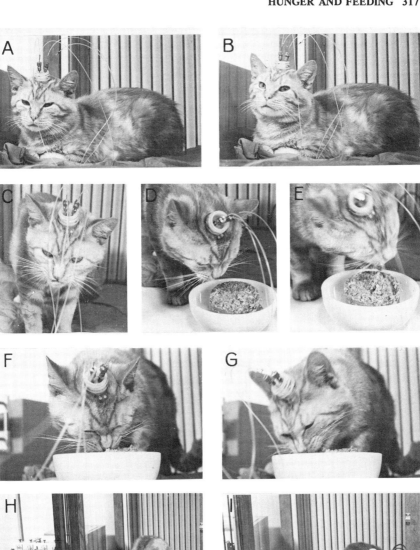

Fig. 7-6 Spontaneous feeding elicited by ionic stimulation in a satiated cat (A) following the start of a hypothalamic perfusion (B), with sodium 34.9 mM in excess of extracellular fluid. Within 3 minutes of the start of the perfusion, the animal arises (C), walks to the food dish (D) and begins eating voraciously (E). During the next 15 minutes (F, G, H), 50 g of Puss'n Boots cat food is consumed, after which the perfusion is stopped (I). The sites of the push-pull perfusion with sodium ions were located in the postero-lateral hypothalamus at coronal plane AP 8.0. (From Myers and Veale, 1971b)

III. ADRENERGIC RECEPTORS FOR FEEDING

The experimental beginning of the theory that an adrenergic mechanism in the hypothalamus constitutes a functional link in the control of feeding behavior was the observation that crystals of either epinephrine or norepinephrine placed in the perifornical region evoked eating in the satiated rat (Grossman, 1960). Since the catecholamine is heavily concentrated in this part of the brain, it was logical to assume a functional relationship between its presence and feeding behavior.

A more complete description of the phenomenon of adrenergic eating was given by Grossman (1962a), who also described the effects of adrenergic stimulation on drinking and feeding, respectively, in the 24 hour food or water deprived rat. Essentially, the same specificity of response was noted in that the fasted rat, in which carbachol was deposited in the hypothalamus, drank water rather than ate food. Similarly, the water-deprived rat, stimulated with crystals of norepinephrine at the same sites, ate food instead of consuming water. Both of these responses were abnormal in terms of the animal's physiological needs. The intrahypothalamic deposit of carbachol elicited lever pressing only for water, whereas a norepinephrine implant elicited lever responding for food only. Thus, the central motivational property of each of the substances was demonstrated independently. Satisfactory controls for local vasomotor effects, pH and osmotic tension were carried out. An overdose of carbachol evoked severe motor effects whereas a sedative action was produced by norepinephrine. The anatomical localization of the action of each amine on ingestion revealed that the fornical system and perhaps the medial forebrain bundle were involved. These same structures have been likewise implicated in an adrenergic feeding system in the primate (Yaksh and Myers, 1972b).

An incomplete but substantial blockade of normal eating or drinking in response to natural hunger and thirst occurs when adrenergic or cholinergic blocking agents are applied locally in the same areas in the rat where norepinephrine or carbachol evoked their respective ingestive response (Grossman, 1962b). Since the systemic administration of atropine blocks carbachol-induced drinking and ethoxybutamoxane antagonizes norepinephrine-induced feeding, the view was supported that independent cholinergic and adrenergic mechanisms function in the hypothalamus. Given in the hypothalamus, the precursors, dopamine or dimethylaminoethanol (DMAE), also evoke feeding or drinking, respectively; however, in each case the response was not as great. These differences are illustrated in Fig. 7-7. The issue of whether or not the action of the given agent is related to a neurohumoral event seemed to be clarified on the basis of the attributes of the blocking agents used and a variety of osmotic and vasomotor control experiments (Grossman, 1964c). Examples of the blockade experiments are shown in Fig. 7-8. An incomplete blockade of the ingestive effect produced by a chemical substance may be due to the

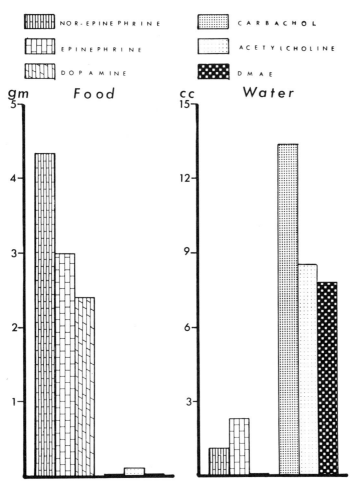

Fig. 7-7 Effects of adrenergic and cholinergic stimulation of the hypothalamus on food and water intake of sated animals during a 1 hour post-stimulation period. (From Grossman, S. P. 1964c. *Int. J. Neuropharmacol.* **3**:45–58. Pergamon Press, New York)

unilaterality of the drug implant. However, this phenomenon of partial antagonism also occurs when the blocking agent is injected into the cerebral ventricles, in which case both sides of the hypothalamus are bathed by an antagonist (Myers *et al.*, 1972).

A. Anatomical Aspects

In a careful anatomical study, Booth (1967) mapped the feeding areas in the diencephalon of the rat that were sensitive to norepinephrine injected in a

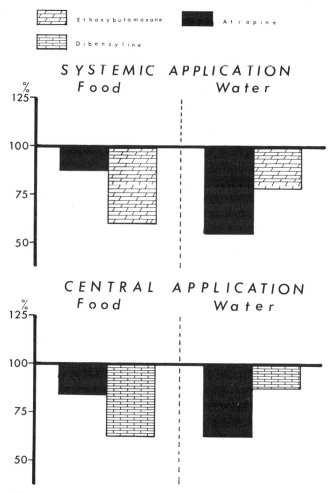

Fig. 7-8 Effects of systemically or centrally administered adrenergic (ethoxy-butamoxane or dibenzyline) and cholinergic (atropine) blocking agents on food and water intake of deprived animals. The results are expressed as a percentage of a base-line which represents the average of pre- and post-stimulation control tests. (From Grossman, 1964c)

single 6 μg dose. A feeding criterion was used of more than 1.2 g intake of wet mash above the base-line level, during the hour after the norepinephrine injection. The startling finding was that the sites at which the norepinephrine injection evoked feeding did not correspond to the classical morphological regions—the lateral or ventromedial parts of the hypothalamus which supposedly integrate the regulation of food intake in normal hunger. Further, the amine-sensitive loci did not extend beneath the internal capsule (Wagner and de Groot, 1963b). Instead, the great proportion of the anatomical scatter was far more rostral, and the region of reactivity encompassed the anterior hypothalamic area, medial forebrain bundle, and followed a course dorsally through the septal nuclei passing along the stria medullaris to the rostral thalamus. The anatomy of these sites is presented in Fig. 7-9. Thus, Booth (1967) concluded that the noradrenergic feeding pathway is an epithalamic one which projects between the limbic forebrain and limbic midbrain and lies parallel to the connections to the lateral hypothalamus. The use of wet mash without a dry food control may have influenced the interpretation of the distribution of these sites in that the water intake of these rats was nil.

A replication of Booth's study confirmed the evidence that the site of maximum sensitivity to norepinephrine in the rat is, in fact, the antero-lateral hypothalamus (Davis and Keesey, 1971) rather than the mid-portion of the lateral hypothalamus (Grossman, 1962a; Wagner and de Groot, 1963b). These sites are in fact anatomically distinct from those just lateral to the fornix, at which electrical stimulation evokes stimulus-bound feeding (Hoebel, 1971). Norepinephrine may also have a local action on the metabolic activity of cells of this rostral feeding circuit, since a hypoglycemia induced by insulin injected subcutaneously potentiates the norepinephrine feeding response (Davis and Keesey, 1971). The effect is similar to the enhancement of the noradrenergic feeding after food deprivation. Without a careful measurement of glucose levels, both in the serum and in hypothalamic tissue, this metabolic interpretation of the effect of norepinephrine remains speculative.

1. Sites in the Amygdala and Hypothalamus

In the rat deprived of food and water, which was trained on a VR-4 schedule to depress an individual lever, norepinephrine or epinephrine placed in the animal's ventral amygdala exerted differential effects. The responding on the food lever increased while the response for water decreased (Grossman, 1964a). Dibenzyline, carbachol, acetylcholine or GABA applied at the same site had the opposite effect in causing an enhancement of lever responding to obtain a water reward while the lever presses for food were depressed. Both atropine and hydroxylamine, a drug which ostensibly blocks the endogenous activity of GABA, reversed these effects and had an action similar to that of adrenergic stimulation of the food and water-deprived rat. Control experiments ruled out the possible side effects of the drugs on the amygdala. Since cholinergic or adrenergic stimulation of the amygdala of the satiated rat does not evoke spontaneous feeding or drinking, Grossman (1964a) proposed that descending impulses from the amygdala modulate the activity of hypothalamic ingestive centers. The amygdaloid influence on the hypothalamus may be inhibitory or excitatory or both. Although the large non-physiological concentrations of some of the substances used could yield effects that would be largely inhibitory, the reversal of the effects by pharmacological blocking agents administered systemically argues against an interpretation of nonspecificity. Corresponding to

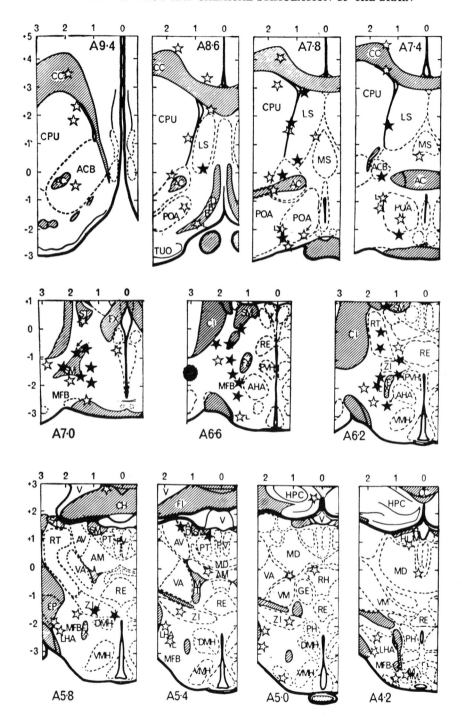

this is the fact that electrical stimulation of the amygdala does suppress feeding in the rat (White and Fisher, 1969). Presumably, the modulatory activity is brought about by activation of the ventromedial region via the stria terminalis. The sectioning of this pathway or ablating the ventromedial nucleus prevents such a stimulus-bound suppression in food intake.

In a further analysis of the motivational properties of norepinephrine-induced feeding, Coons and Quartermain (1970) found that the catecholamine injected into the lateral hypothalamus of the satiated rat evoked lever pressing for food on a continuous reinforcement or 30-second variable interval schedule. When the same animal was deprived of food for 24 hours, a similar injection depressed the rate of lever pressing for food when the partial reinforcement schedule was

---

Fig. 7-9 Injection sites at which norepinephrine elicited eating. Effective sites: solid stars; ineffective sites: open stars. Where two overlapping sites give the same behavior, only one is plotted. L, implant in a rat with a contralateral LHA lesion. Arrow above a site indicates that the placement was approached at an angle from the right-hand hemisphere. Projected on planes at intervals of 0.4 or 0.8 mm as in the atlas of de Groot (1963). Abbreviations are as follows: A, aqueductus cerebri (sylvius); AHA, area anterior hypothalami; LHA, area lateralis hypothalami; POA, area preoptic (medialis, lateralis); CE, capsula externa; CI, capsula interna; CLA, claustrum; AC, commissura anterior; CH, commissura hippocampi (commissura fornicis); CC, corpus callosum; PIR, cortex piriformis; MFB, fasciculus medialis telencephali (medial forebrain bundle); FI, fimbria hippocampi; FR, fissura rhinalis; M, foramen interventriculare (Monro); FX, fornix (corpus, columna); GP, globus pallidus; FD, gyrus dentatus (fascia dentata); DBB, gyrus diagonalis (diagonal band of broca); HPC, hippocampus (cornu ammonis); ACB, nucleus accumbens septi (area parolfactoria lateralis); ACE, nucleus amygdaloideus centralis; ACO, nucleus amygdaloideus corticalis; AME, nucleus amygdaloideus medialis; AD, nucleus anterodorsalis thalami; AM, nucleus anteromedialis thalami; AV, nucleus anteroventralis thalami; ARH, nucleus arcuatus hypothalami; CPU, nucleus caudatus/putamen; D, nucleus Darkschweitz; DMH, nucleus dorsomedialis hypothalami; EP, nucleus entopeduncularis; GE, nucleus gelatinosus thalami; HL, nucleus habenularis lateralis; HM, nucleus habenularis medialis; LS, nucleus lateralis septi; LT, nucleus lateralis thalami; MM, nucleus mammillaris medialis; MS, nucleus medialis septi; MD, nucleus mediodorsalis thalami; PT, nucleus parataenialis thalami; PVH, nucleus paraventricularis hypothalami; PV, nucleus paraventricularis thalami; PH, nucleus posterior hypothalami; PMV, nucleus premammillaris ventralis; RT, nucleus reticularis thalami; RE, nucleus reuniens thalami; RH, nucleus rhomboideus thalami; CL, nucleus subthalamicus (Luys); SO, nucleus supraopticus hypothalami; TS, nucleus triangularis septi; VE, nucleus ventralis thalami; VA, nucleus ventralis thalami pars anterior; VM, nucleus ventralis thalami pars medialis; VMH, nucleus ventromedialis hypothalami; PC, pedunculus cerebri; PM, pedunculus mammillaris; SM, stria medullaris thalami; ST, stria terminalis (Taenia semicircularis); MT, tractus mammillo-thalamicus (Vicq d'Azyr); OT, tractus opticus; TUO, tuberculum olfactorium; V, ventriculus cerebri; ZI, zona incerta. (From Booth, D. A. 1967. *Science.* **158**:515–517. Copyright 1967, by the American Association for the Advancement of Science)

introduced. Although the presence of norepinephrine in the lateral region may produce a partial motivational deficit similar to that observed in the rat with a lesion of the ventromedial nucleus, the sites of injection are probably crucial. That is, it would be important to determine whether norepinephrine would affect the motivated feeding when injected in the more sensitive sites found by Booth (1967) to be located in the anterior region, not the lateral.

To test the notion that norepinephrine evokes feeding by blocking the tonic inhibitory influence of the ventromedial hypothalamus on the lateral area, Herberg and Franklin (1972) made lesions in different parts of the ventromedial nucleus. After the posterior half of this nucleus was first destroyed, the rat subsequently became hyperphagic and obese. Thereafter, many of these rats did not feed after norepinephrine was injected at antero-lateral sites in the hypothalamus at which the amine earlier had evoked eating. Since norepinephrine was even found to have an anorexic effect on the hyperphagic rat, a simple hypothesis of disinhibition of the ventromedial region is probably not valid. Instead, Herberg and Franklin believe that norepinephrine acts to inhibit a pathway described by Chi (1970) which arises in the anterior hypothalamus and terminates in the posterior part of the ventromedial nucleus. Why norepinephrine evokes feeding along this pathway in the non-lesioned rat is not certain; nevertheless, as Booth (1967) had shown, the monoamine evokes feeding when acting at sites clearly separated from the region at which lesions disrupt feeding.

In respect to this finding, it is interesting further that the rat which is anorexic because of lesions placed in its lateral hypothalamus will begin to feed when norepinephrine is injected intraventricularly (Berger et al., 1971). This response has been observed in the intact rat (Myers and Yaksh, 1968). Conversely, phentolamine suppresses the feeding in a rat that has recovered from an ablation to its lateral hypothalamus. This could indicate that the proposed ascending adrenergic system (Fuxe, 1965), of which the medial forebrain is a part, may involve a lateral component.

2. Local Electrical Activity

Using the technique of an electrically evoked response from the tip of a combination recording electrode-cannula, Sutin et al. (1963) showed that catecholamines have opposite effects on the cells of the ventromedial hypothalamus of the cat. An injection or implant of crystals of norepinephrine or epinephrine enhances the local electrical responses within the ventromedial hypothalamus during stimulation of the septum. The same injection into the ventromedial region simultaneously depresses the evoked response following electrical stimulation of the amygdala. The injection of amphetamine into the ventromedial nucleus suppresses the response evoked from stimulation of either the septum or amygdala. No change in the ventromedially-evoked response was elicited by the local injection of 5 or 10% glucose or of 80 mU of insulin. These experiments would suggest that the action of an adrenergic substance within the hypothalamus may not simply be inhibitory.

In another important paper, Krebs and Bindra (1971) showed that norepinephrine has both excitatory and inhibitory effects when applied iontophoretically to units in the perifornical region of the rat. The anorexogenic agents, amphetamine and glucose often had effects on the firing pattern of the cells in this region that were identical to norepinephrine. Thus, the concept of a pure noradrenergic coding of hunger or satiety by a noradrenergic mechanism alone requires far more research at the unicellular as well as at the hypothalamic level.

B. Adrenergic Feeding in the Primate

The first reports of chemically elicited feeding in the primate described the effects of adrenergic compounds. In order of their potency, norepinephrine, epinephrine or dopamine injected into the lateral hypothalamus of the fully satiated rhesus monkey evoked voracious eating and prandial drinking (Myers and Sharpe, 1968b; Myers, 1969). ACh or carbachol injected in doses of 12 to 25 μg into the same region of the lateral hypothalamus prevented feeding and drinking in the hungry monkey that was fasted for up to 18 hours. This blockade of ingestive behavior persisted for nearly 2 hours and could be reversed by 12 μg atropine injected into the lateral hypothalamus. Smaller doses of ACh or carbachol did not inhibit feeding or drinking in the hungry animal, but ordinarily failed to evoke spontaneous drinking or feeding in the satiated monkey

Feeding can also be elicited in the satiated monkey by an injection of norepinephrine, epinephrine or dopamine at many other sites scattered throughout the hypothalamus and other parts of the diencephalon (Sharpe and Myers, 1969). Unlike the reports on the rat, water intake in the monkey is never suppressed by norepinephrine and, in fact, usually accompanies the ingestion of food pellets. The dose-dependent nature of norepinephrine-induced feeding and the drinking of water are shown in Fig. 7-10. Carbachol injected in doses as low as 1.5 μg at active adrenoceptive feeding sites failed to elicit ingestive responses in the satiated monkey and blocked feeding and drinking in the fasted animal. ACh and eserine also exerted this inhibitory effect which was reversible by atropine. At about 25% of the sites tested, 5-HT evoked drinking and a rather marginal feeding response, but only after a long latency.

The anatomical and functional independence of the actions of 5-HT and norepinephrine when micro-injected into the hypothalamus in identical doses has also been illustrated (Myers and Sharpe, 1968b). In the lateral hypothalamus of the monkey, 5-HT elicited mainly drinking of water whereas when it was injected into the anterior hypothalamus, the indolamine produced only hyperthermia or a transient fall followed by a rise in temperature. Similarly, norepinephrine infused in the lateral hypothalamus evoked only feeding and drinking with a short latency, but in the anterior hypothalamus produced only a hypothermic response.

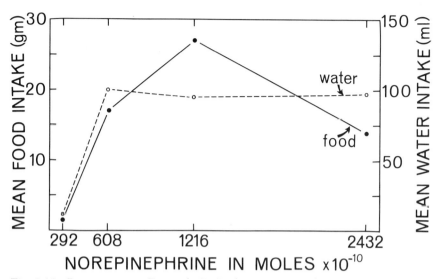

Fig. 7-10 Dose response. Eating (solid line) and drinking (dashed line) responses after four doses of norepinephrine were micro-injected into the diencephalon of the satiated monkey. (From Sharpe and Myers, 1969)

The powerful hyperphagic action of the catecholamines on the primate's hypothalamus occurs during an abnormal state. When the set-point temperature of a monkey was lowered by the perfusion of a solution of excess Ca^{2+} ions in the posterior hypothalamus, the monkey nevertheless ate biscuits after norepinephrine was injected into the rostral hypothalamus (Myers and Yaksh, 1972b). Thus, the hypothalamic response to adrenergic stimulation is not suppressed by excess Ca^{2+} or by the consequences associated with deep hypothermia.

Fig. 7-11. Anatomical mapping at nine coronal (AP) levels in the hypothalamus at which NE micro-injected in a dose of 5 to 12.5 μg base produces either a hypothermia of more than 0.4°C ($\blacktriangledown$) or feeding of more than 20 g with a latency of less than 15 minutes ($\bullet$) or both responses simultaneously ($\blacksquare$). Sites which are associated with no response are also indicated ($\circ$). Abbreviations are as follows: A, anterior hypothalamus; AC, anterior commissure; CA, caudate nucleus; CC, corpus callosum; D, dorsomedial nucleus of the hypothalamus; F, fornix; FF, fields of Forel/zona incerta; GP, globus pallidus; IC, internal capsule; L, lateral hypothalamus; MM, mammillary body; MT, mammillo-thalamic tract; NC, central nucleus of the thalamus; NP, paracentral nucleus of the thalamus; NR, reuniens nucleus of the thalamus; OC, optic chiasm; OT, optic tract; P, posterior hypothalamus; PN, paraventricular nucleus of the hypothalamus; PO, preoptic region; PP, cerebral peduncles; RN, reticular nucleus of the thalamus; S, septum; SN, substantia nigra; ST, subthalamic nucleus; V, ventromedial nucleus of the hypothalamus; VL, ventrolateral nucleus of the thalamus; VA, anterior ventral nucleus of the thalamus. (From Yaksh and Myers, 1972b)

1. *Anatomical Aspects*

An extensive anatomical mapping of sites within the primate's diencephalon has revealed several features of the feeding system. Multiple micro-injections of norepinephrine were made at a total of 179 sites in the hypothalamus of 36 monkeys (Yaksh and Myers, 1972b). At 16% of these sites, only feeding was elicited by norepinephrine. These loci were located mainly in the plane containing the columns of the fornix, ventromedial hypothalamus and lateral hypothalamus. At 11% of all of the loci located principally in the anterior hypothalamus, the injection of norepinephrine produced only a fall in temperature. Of special interest was the observation that at 5 injection sites, norepi-

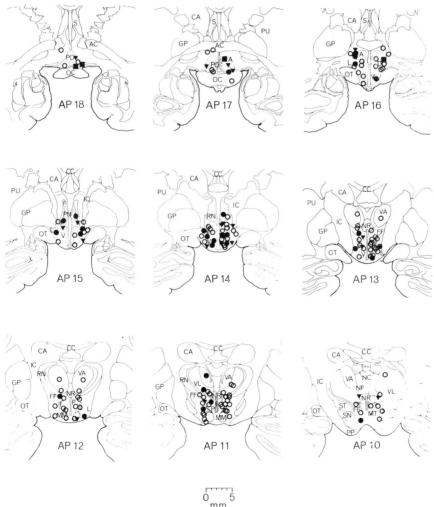

nephrine caused both eating and a drop in temperature simultaneously. These responses indicate a clear-cut overlapping and intermingling of the neuronal systems which are involved in both functions. In the main, however, the distinct functional separation of the norepinephrine sensitive sites observed more commonly reflects the individual nature of the separate anatomical pathways. Figure 7-11 illustrates the anatomical distinctiveness of the four classifications of norepinephrine-sensitive sites in the primate's diencephalon: (1) hypothermia; (2) feeding; (3) hypothermia and feeding; and (4) insensitive.

C. Pharmacological Specificity

An exceptionally extensive set of experiments completed by Booth (1968c) has helped to clarify some of the difficult questions raised by the phenomenon of norepinephrine-induced feeding behavior. A dose response relationship was first established in order to confirm the pharmacological findings of Miller *et al.* (1964). An examination of the volume relationship indicated that the optimal eating response was obtained with a 6 μg dose contained in 0.7 μl. Also, Booth showed that a slow infusion of the catecholamine solution did not produce feeding as reliably as a rapid injection. Phenoxybenzamine and phentolamine, both alpha adrenergic blocking agents, inhibited the norepinephrine-elicited feeding when either of the adrenolytic compounds was given earlier at the same site; however, propranolol, a beta receptor blocker, had no inhibitory effect on the eating evoked by norepinephrine. Desmethylimipramine (DMI), which retards the re-uptake of excess norepinephrine at the nerve terminals, also micro-injected just before norepinephrine, produced a time-dependent enhancement of norepinephrine feeding. A number of sympathomimetic amines such as phenylephrine, tyramine, octopamine, ephedrine or amphetamine injected intrahypothalamically did not possess any significant effect on food intake of the rat. Tyrosine, 5-HT and dopamine had a very weak and often delayed hyperphagic action, whereas histamine, normetanephrine and metanephrine were entirely without effect. Angiotensin produced no feeding but rather intense drinking of 6 to 19 ml of water within 30 minutes after 1.8 μg were micro-injected into the rat's hypothalamus. As a result of this thorough investigation, which is summarized graphically in Fig. 7-12, the specificity of

---

Fig. 7-12 Eating and drinking responses to intrahypothalamic injection of norepinephrine or other drugs. Hydrochlorides were used except where indicated by superior letters: a, bitartrate; b, oxalate. All solutions were 65 mM drug in 90 mM sodium chloride except as indicated by superior c, which was 2.5 mg of angiotensin amide per milliliter of 5% mannitol (Ciba). The four groups (A–D) contained 14, 10, 10 and 8 rats, with 8 common to all groups. Immediate responses (within 30 minutes from injection) are given to the left, late responses (30 to 60 and 60 to 90 minutes) to the right. Hatched bars, eating response; open bars, drinking response. Horizontal lines within bars give SEM for 0 to 30 minute and 30 to 90 minute periods. (From Booth, D. A. 1968c. *J. Pharmacol. Exptl. Ther.* **160**:336–348. The Williams and Wilkins Co., Baltimore)

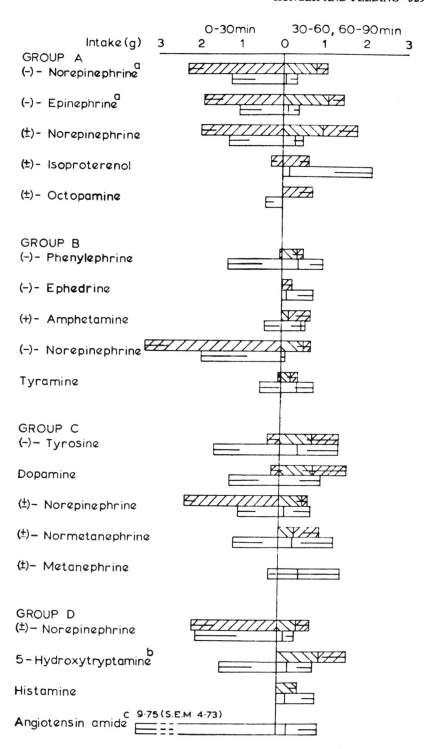

an alpha adrenergic mechanism in the diencephalic feeding circuit was dramatically illustrated.

Following up one of Booth's observations, Montgomery *et al.* (1969; 1971) also found that desmethylimipramine (DMI) caused an increase of about 1.5 g in food intake after DMI was micro-injected into the lateral hypothalamus of a rat deprived of food for 16 hours. When the animal was deprived of water or satiated on food, water or both, DMI did not facilitate the feeding response. Yet another clue is thus provided concerning the concept that the release of norepinephrine in the lateral hypothalamus occurs during natural hunger. By preventing its re-uptake, the feeding behavior is subsequently potentiated only when the rat is deprived of food.

In one of the most comprehensive studies utilizing the technique of chemical stimulation, Slangen and Miller (1969) demonstrated unequivocally, at least from a classical pharmacological standpoint, that the satiated rat eats following the intrahypothalamic injection of an adrenergic compound because of the stimulation of alpha-adrenergic receptors. Although substantial evidence does not really exist that drug receptors in the CNS correspond to those in autonomic ganglia (Chapter 1), this study does provide some extraordinary parallelisms between the activity of central and peripheral receptors. For example, when microinjected into the perifornical region, dopamine has the same hyperphagic effect as norepinephrine but is much less potent in terms of the magnitude of food

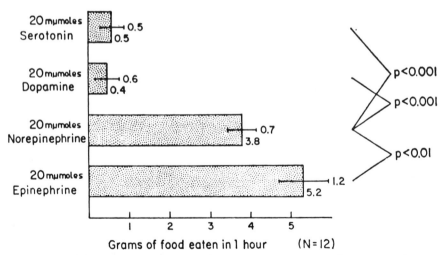

Fig. 7-13 Effects of intrahypothalamic administration of norepinephrine, dopamine, epinephrine, and serotonin on food intake by satiated rats during 1 hour. The numbers to the right of the bars give the group means and standard deviations (3 observations per drug per animal). All significant differences between the NE group mean and the other group means are indicated by their *p*-value. (From Slangen and Miller, 1969)

consumed and the latency to eat. These differences are probably due to the conversion of the precursor into the noradrenergic moiety. The relative potencies of epinephrine and the other monoamines are shown in Fig. 7-13. Isoproterenol, a beta agonist, fails to stimulate eating. Although the beta antagonist, propranolol, does not block norepinephrine-induced feeding, the alpha blocker, phentolamine, reduces norepinephrine feeding almost to nil. These sharp distinctions in antagonistic efficacy are shown in Fig. 7-14. Unfortunately, the effects of the two antagonists were not tested on epinephrine or dopamine-induced feeding which would seem to be essential since in the periphery, epinephrine possesses potent activity on beta receptors.

Confirming Booth's (1968c) earlier observation, Slangen and Miller (1969) also found that the inhibition of norepinephrine re-uptake into the presynaptic nerve terminals by desmethylimimipramine (DMI) potentiated norepinephrine feeding dramatically, again by keeping unbound norepinephrine in the synaptic region. The MAO inhibitor nialamide evoked eating when followed by tetrabenazine which prevents unbound, free norepinephrine from being incorporated into adrenergic granules. When the drug sequence was reversed and tetrabenazine was micro-injected before the MAO inhibitor, the rat did not eat. All in all, the totality of these pharmacological experiments biases the view rather convincingly that adrenergic receptors are involved in the feeding response following the administration of catecholamines in the rat's hypothalamus.

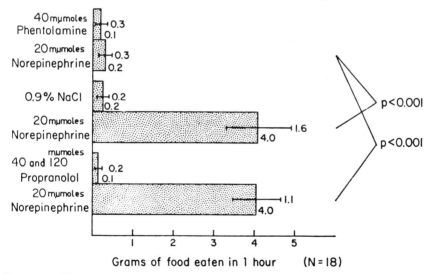

Fig. 7-14 Effects of intrahypothalamic administration of the α-blocking agent, phentolamine, and the β-blocking agent, propranolol, on food intake elicited by NE that was injected 1 hour later. The numbers to the right of the bars give the group means and standard deviations (3 to 4 observations per drug-combination per animal). All significant differences between group means are indicated by their p-value. (From Slangen and Miller, 1969)

1. *Receptor Agonists and Antagonists*

Dose-dependent eating has also been produced by chlorpromazine (CPZ) injected into the hypothalamus of the rat (Leibowitz and Miller, 1969). The magnitude of the response correlates well with the intensity of the feeding response produced by norepinephrine micro-injected into the same anatomical site. Although the duration of its action is much longer than that of norepinephrine, CPZ could mimic the effect of norepinephrine on hypothalamic neurons, or this phenothiazine could cause an increase in the regional release of the monoamine within the feeding circuit. If CPZ should block the hypothesized alpha receptors in the hypothalamus, such an action would be inconsistent with the pharmacological tests documented above.

Certain other compounds such as the adrenergic imidazolines are believed to possess powerful alpha receptor actions. When clonidine, a potent antihypertensive drug with alpha adrenergic properties is injected into the antero-lateral part of the hypothalamus of the satiated rat, the animal consumes food (Broekkamp and van Rossum, 1972). The magnitude of the eating response is about the same as that evoked by norepinephrine injected at the same locus. Another analogue, xylometazoline, had an even more potent effect on the rat's food intake when injected similarly. The specificity of alpha receptors in the clonidine-induced feeding was demonstrated when eating was blocked by a prior intrahypothalamic injection of phentolamine.

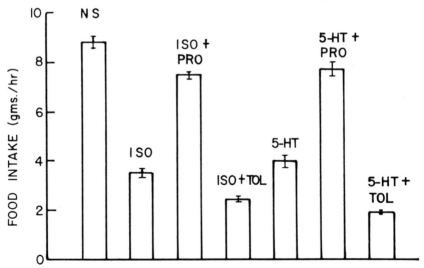

Fig. 7-15 Effect of isoproterenol, administered by the intrahypothalamic route, on food consumption in the food-deprived rat. NS, normal saline control; ISO, isoproterenol (37.0 μg); PRO, propranolol (44 μg); TOL, tolazoline (20 μg); 5-HT, serotonin (18 μg). Each group consisted of a minimum of ten animals. Analysis of p-values showed all data significant beyond $p < 0.01$. (From Goldman *et al.*, 1971)

Examining the antagonistic effects of drugs on feeding in the rat, Goldman *et al.* (1971) used alpha and beta blocking agents injected into the perifornical area of the hypothalamus in high doses and a large volume. The selective local antagonism of alpha receptors by either the beta receptor stimulation of isoproterenol or alpha receptor blockade of tolazoline reduced feeding in the rat that was fasted for 21 hours before the micro-injection. This hypophagic effect is portrayed in Fig. 7-15. Although beta and alpha receptors may indeed participate in a hypothalamic satiety mechanism, the specificity of the receptor mechanism is unclear from this study. That is, Goldman *et al.* found that 5-HT had an anorexic action as great as the beta agonist, isoproterenol. When 5-HT was injected together with tolazoline, the synergistic effect on the reduction of feeding was just as large as that produced by tolazoline mixed with isoproterenol.

In a series of brief reports Leibowitz (1970a and b) has extended the information about receptor specificity for ingestion. In an 18-hour food deprived rat, an intrahypothalamic injection of two beta receptor agonists, epinephrine and isoproterenol, suppressed feeding. This beta receptor reduction of feeding could be attenuated by a similar micro-injection of a beta antagonist, propranolol. As would be expected, the blockade of alpha receptors by an intrahypothalamic injection of phentolamine potentiated the reduced food intake in the hungry rat (Leibowitz, 1972). A composite picture of these results is presented in Fig. 7-16. Although the 1 μl injection would overlap both the ventromedial and lateral hypothalamic areas and an anatomical verification of the injection sites was not presented, Leibowitz concluded that alpha and beta receptors may function antagonistically in the hunger regulating mechanism. This does not correspond with the results of Grossman, Booth, Slangen and Miller who found that epinephrine evokes feeding.

Attempting to clarify this discrepancy, Leibowitz (1970b) reported that norepinephrine, epinephrine and phentolamine injected in a 1 μl volume at sites in the lateral hypothalamus, failed to affect the rat's feeding behavior. When these same compounds were injected into the ventromedial hypothalamus, they evoked eating, which was reduced by the alpha antagonists. When injected into the lateral hypothalamus, isoproterenol caused anorexia and the beta antagonist, propranolol, elicited feeding. If the raw data are examined closely (this chapter, section I, A), the change in gram intake usually reflects much less than a 20 to 40% shift in food consumption in either direction. For example, when infused into the ventromedial hypothalamus, propranolol reduced food intake from a control level of 9.3 to 8.4 g. Although this change was not considered to be significant, the increase from 6.0 to 7.1 g food intake produced by propranolol injected into the lateral hypothalamus was taken to be a significant enhancement. Although the perplexing question of pharmacological specificity of the receptors persists, it is interesting that the Duroc boar fasted for 24 hours reduces its food intake after isoproterenol is injected into the hypothalamus. Restoration of the pig's normal feeding response could be accomplished by a sim-

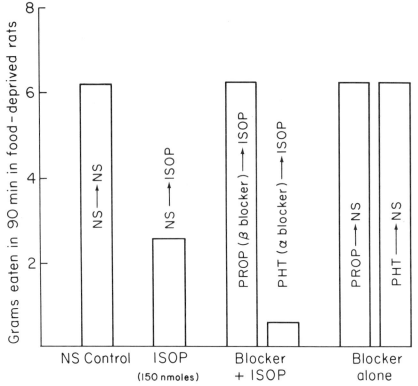

Fig. 7-16 Effect of perifornical hypothalamic injections of the relatively pure beta-adrenergic agonist, isoproterenol (ISOP), upon food intake in food-deprived rats, and the effects of the adrenergic blockers on this ISOP effect. The beta-adrenergic blocker is propranolol (PROP), the alpha-adrenergic blocker is phentolamine (PHT), and the control medium is normal saline (NS). All drugs were injected directly into the hypothalamus. The score is mean grams eaten during the first 90 minutes after injection. (From Leibowitz, 1972)

ilar injection of propranolol just prior to isoproterenol although the doses of each compound exceeded 300 μg (Jackson and Robinson, 1971).

Further research with antagonists and agonists that are injected in a limited volume, and careful histological analysis of the hypothalamic morphology will undoubtedly resolve the current discrepancies.

D. Destruction of Adrenergic Nerve Terminals

Using the procedure of histochemical fluorescence, Ungerstedt (1971b) has documented the fact that 6-OHDA is taken up by cells in the substantia nigra and caudate nucleus. This is followed by subsequent degeneration of dopamine- and norepinephrine-containing neurons in the nigro-striatal system. The initial depletion of the catecholamines is very rapid, taking place within 15 minutes. Then, intraneuronal auto-oxidation ensues which is characterized by the typical yellowish auto-fluorescence. A subsequent decrease in turnover of the mono-amines probably results in a marked interruption of the flow of nerve impulses in the aminergic pathways.

The functional relation of this observation to feeding was documented in an important paper by Ungerstedt (1971a). When norepinephrine and dopamine nerve terminals are destroyed as a result of local injections of 6-OHDA in the lateral hypothalamus and other areas of the rat brain, a marked adipsia and aphagia is produced. Unless the animal is fed by stomach tube, it becomes moribund. When 6-OHDA was injected in a region caudal to the substantia nigra (Fig. 7-17), which transected the ascending noradrenergic axons and thereby depleted the hypothalamus of most noradrenergic nerve terminals, the rat showed no signs of adipsia or aphagia. On the basis of the anatomical pathways depicted in Fig. 7-17, Ungerstedt concluded that the extent of

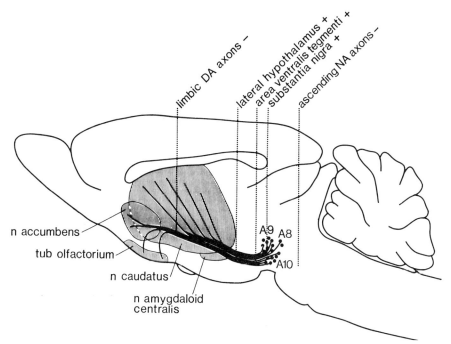

Fig. 7-17 Adipsia and aphagia after 6-OHDA lesions of the DA pathways. Sagittal outline of the nigro-striatal DA system and the meso-limbic DA system. A8–A10 are DA cell groups in the mesencephalon. A9 is the substantia nigra group. DA nerve terminals are found within the striped areas. Dotted lines indicate the sites of 6-OHDA injections. + signs indicate that adipsia and aphagia followed upon the 6-OHDA injection, while − signs indicate that the injection was ineffective. (From Ungerstedt, 1971)

dopamine denervation is the critical factor in the impairment of ingestive behavior. However, the degeneration of the nigro-striatal system is also linked with profound motor deficits. That is, akinesia, catalepsia and other severe motor symptoms become manifest after the 6-OHDA injections. Thus, the loss of the eating and drinking responses may be purely the net effect of a motor incapacity of the rat to move toward its food, open its mouth, bite, chew, lick, swallow and in essence, exact the sequence of coordinated muscular responses that every animal must perform to ingest a food substance.

Other investigators have also demonstrated the blockade of ingestive responses by 6-OHDA injected subcortically (Echavarria-Mage et al., 1972). Repeated bilateral injections of 6-OHDA in 4 μl volumes at 3 rostro-caudal sites in the lateral hypothalamus of the rat, which totalled as much as 24 μl caused a lethal aphagia and adipsia. Death occurred within 7 days in 14 out of 16 rats (Smith et al., 1972). The effects of 6-OHDA were believed to be on the lateral hypothalamus in spite of the fact that the volumes given exceed the entire dimension of the rat's hypothalamus if not most of the diencephalon. Nevertheless, the results were interpreted as supporting the idea that catecholaminergic neurons are required for drinking and eating.

When 0.5 μl volumes of 6-OHDA are injected into the rat's hypothalamus, the discrete anatomical regions that are affected by this chemotoxic substance can be ascertained (Myers and Martin, 1973). Although a fatal aphagia and adipsia may occur depending on the site at which 6-OHDA is micro-injected in the lateral or postero-lateral hypothalamus, or rostral mesencephalon, Myers and Martin found that the lethality of the effects can be totally reversed simply by offering the rat palatable food. Further, reduction of the animal's body weight prior to 6-OHDA injection can also ameliorate the effects of intrahypothalamic 6-OHDA. This would suggest that the catecholamine neurons may be involved also in the hypothesized calcium set-point mechanism for body weight.

Corresponding to the norepinephrine releasing effect of 6-OHDA, Evetts et al. (1972) found that small doses of 6-OHDA given in a large 1 to 5 μl volume evoked both feeding and drinking. When 6-OHDA was injected into the preoptic area, the effect lasted about 5 hours. These ingestive responses could be due to a known action of 6-OHDA in releasing norepinephrine from the preoptic area. The typical aphagia and adipsia that arise when 6-OHDA is injected into the lateral or postero-lateral hypothalamus or nigro-striatal system was not observed, and a preoptic injection of 6-OHDA or norepinephrine 4 to 5 days later in the same rats also evoked feeding. The equality in the blockade of the 6-OHDA induced eating by either an alpha or beta antagonist injected into the same site does not correspond to the typical attenuation of noradrenergic feeding by an alpha receptor antagonist only.

E. Palatability of Food and Other Factors

In 6 of 14 rats which ate after norepinephrine was micro-injected in the lateral hypothalamus, significantly more mash containing saccharin was consumed than when the rats were deprived of food altogether (Booth and Quartermain, 1965). The same sort of gustatory sensitivity is also observed with non-palatable food in relation to norepinephrine stimulation. Far less mash, adulterated with quinine, was consumed than by the same animal after it was fasted. Thus, the eating that is elicited by elevating the norepinephrine level in the rat's hypothalamus is qualitatively very different, in terms of taste factors at least, than either that of natural hunger following deprivation or that induced by electrical stimulation of the lateral hypothalamus.

Complementing this idea of Booth and Quartermain (1965) is the finding that although catecholaminergic stimulation of diencephalic sites in the rat evokes feeding, hoarding behavior is not affected (Blundell and Herberg, 1970). Ordinarily food deprivation or electrical current applied to the lateral hypothalamus both constitute excellent stimuli for the hoarding response. However, the animal does not hoard pellets even though the injection of norepinephrine into the antero-lateral hypothalamus causes the rat to eat. Thus, just as the sites in the rat's hypothalamus are different at which electrical stimulation and norepinephrine injections evoke feeding, the natural mechanisms seem to be equally divergent.

1. *Norepinephrine Drinking of "Food"*

Using Metrecal or sweetened condensed milk as the test substance, several investigators have found that either adrenergic stimulation or the blockade of alpha adrenergic receptors influences the intake of fluids. Most of these studies are considered in Chapter 8, "Thirst and Drinking."

The ingestion of Metrecal has been elicited by norepinephrine or epinephrine injected in a 5 μl volume purportedly into the lateral hypothalamus, ventromedial hypothalamus or globus pallidus (Wagner and de Groot, 1963b). Lidocaine or pentobarbital infused into the ventromedial hypothalamus has also elicited ingestion. A norepinephrine dose-response curve has also been obtained for the consumption of Metrecal which was diluted to the consistency of water (Miller *et al.*, 1964). In this instance, 0.8 to 37 μg of norepinephrine microinjected in a 1 μl volume into the lateral hypothalamus evoked the drinking of the nutrient. Since this fluid was selected over plain water, an interpretation was made that this response could be really designated as eating.

Contrary to these experiments are the reports of Margules (1969b; 1970a) who found that crystals of norepinephrine deposited in the medial forebrain bundle of the rat suppressed the drinking of milk, which was termed feeding. The test fluid was diluted condensed milk which may have been less like the Metrecal used by Miller *et al.* and more like water. Thus, the relative viscosity of the test fluid could easily explain this discrepancy. Somewhat surprisingly, phentolamine elicited the drinking of milk, presumably as a result of the local blockade of alpha receptors which enabled a selective domination of beta receptor activity. This phentolamine enhancement of drinking is illustrated in Fig. 7-18; however the phenomenon is difficult to reconcile with the fact that crystals of the beta

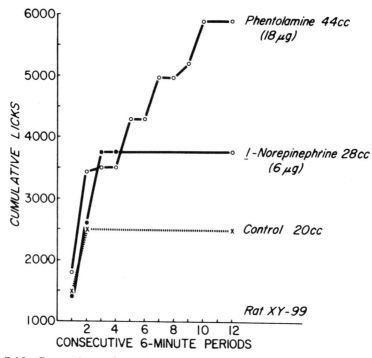

Fig. 7-18 Comparison of noradrenergic and phentolamine induced overeating at the same hypothalamic site. Total cubic centimeters of milk consumed is shown for each test. (From Margules, D. L. 1969b. *Life Sciences*. 8:693–704. Pergamon Press, New York)

blocker, propranolol, deposited similarly in the hypothalamus, exerted no effect on the drinking of milk. Clearly, more research is required in which a cafeteria approach would permit a rat to select its ordinary lab chow and water as well as other foods and fluids of varying texture, sapidity and nutritional value. In one such study, Montgomery and Armstrong (1973) found that adrenergic stimulation evoked a preference for wet food mash whereas carbachol elicited intake of water over other substances.

One possible resolution of the dilemma in the findings from different laboratories may rest simply in the time of day that norepinephrine is injected into the hypothalamus. According to Margules *et al.* (1972), crystals of norepinephrine applied to the lateral hypothalamus evoke drinking of undiluted condensed milk in an amount greater than the control level, when the rat is in the light. Under the condition of darkness, the amount of fluid drunk by the rat after an implant of norepinephrine at the same site is about the same as in the light but the volume was lower than the control values. The reason for the light-enhancing and dark-suppressing effects of norepinephrine on drinking is obscure. Undoubtedly, the circadian oscillation in the hypothalamic concentration and presumably the neuronal activity of the monoamine in distinct regions are intimately related to the response to the exogenous application of the catecholamine.

IV. CHOLINERGIC FEEDING

The explicit distinction of the hypothalamic coding of adrenergic feeding and cholinergic drinking was questioned almost as soon as the phenomena were described (Myers, 1964). Because of the inordinate complexity of the problem, as demonstrated by the reversals in a rat's ingestive response, cholinergic feeding or adrenergic drinking generally have not been examined extensively (Myers and Sharpe, 1968b). The variability of the response within the rat and the absence of this dual property of the two amines in any species other than the rat are serious issues.

The precise question of cholinergic-adrenergic coding of ingestive behavior was touched upon by Coury (1967) in extending the earlier work of others. In the great majority of structures contained within the Papez limbic pathways or the Nauta circuit, carbachol in crystalline form generally produces only drinking whereas crystals of norepinephrine only feeding. At a substantial number of sites in the hippocampus, anterior thalamus, cingulate gyrus and other structures, the crystalline carbachol elicited a drinking response. Except for the mammillary body, the hypothalamus was not explored. A mixed response of carbachol eating or norepinephrine drinking occurred at only 6% of the 184 sites stimulated with both substances, and norepinephrine-induced drinking occurred only once.

This sort of clear delineation has not always been found in similar studies with the rat or with other species as well (Myers and Sharpe, 1968b). For example, intrahypothalamic injections in a 0.5 μl volume of epinephrine or norepinephrine evoke drinking and other changes in behavior in the rat, whereas carbachol injected similarly elicits the following responses in order of their frequency: seizures, drinking, no response, feeding, ataxia or sleep (Myers and DeStefano, 1969). Although some sort of probabilistic pattern of responses to cholinergic stimulation seems to prevail (Robinson and Mishkin, 1968), feeding following cholinergic stimulation may depend on the experience of the animal, the site of hypothalamic stimulation as well as the order in which either carbachol or norepinephrine is injected into the hypothalamus. Table 7-1 summarizes the variety as well as frequency of responses observed following cholinergic (carbachol) or adrenergic (norepinephrine or epinephrine) stimulation of the hypothalamus and other regions of the rat's brain (Myers and DeStefano, 1969).

Intake of food significantly above the control level is also elicited by carbachol applied to the anterodorsal part of the hippocampus of the rat. This increase in eating occurs simultaneously with drinking and enhanced motor activity (Grant and Jarrard, 1968). More recently, Sciorelli et al. (1972) have found that crystals of carbachol deposited in the lateral hypothalamus of the rat evoked

TABLE 7-1 Overlap in food and water intakes in rats in the hour following micro-injections in a volume of 0.8 μl of carbachol, norepinephrine or Ringer solution. The sites of injections were the septum, nucleus reuniens or preoptic area. Since there were no differences in sensitivity to the drugs, the data from all sites were pooled. (From Myers and DeStefano, 1969)

Carbachol (N = 105)				Norepinephrine (N = 135)								Ringer (N = 78)	
0.7 μg		0.9 μg		2.0 μg		5.0 μg		10.0 μg					
Food	Water	Food	Water	Food	Water	Food	Water	Food	Water			Food	Water
1.8 g	9.3 ml	2.1 g	10.5 ml	1.4 g	3.3 ml	2.4 g	4.3 ml	2.7 g	2.3 ml			0.5 g	0.8 ml

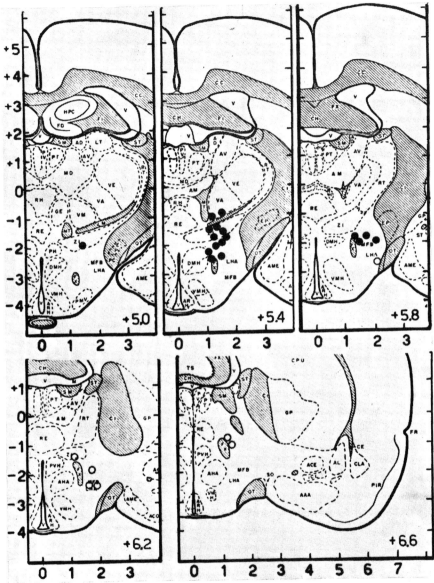

Fig. 7-19 ●, sites of rat diencephalon where stimulation by carbamylcholine and dibutyryl-adenosine-3′,5′-monophosphate elicited ingestive responses, and ○, sites of rat diencephalon where ingestive responses were elicited exclusively by carbamylcholine. Each point represents the localization of one cannula. For abbreviations, see Fig. 7-9. (From Sciorelli, G. *et al.*, 1972. *Brain Res.* 48:427–431. Fig. 3. Elsevier Publishing Co., Amsterdam, The Netherlands)

feeding in an amount twice that of the control. Figure 7-19 portrays the distribution of cholinoceptive sites in the diencephalon. The eating response was attenuated below the control level by hemicholinium and almost entirely blocked by atropine. In studies devoted primarily to the killing behavior in rats, Smith *et al.* (1970) made the striking observation that after 6 hours, food intake but not water intake had increased after crystals of carbachol had been deposited in the lateral hypothalamus. Although piloerection and salivation were also noted, no data on absolute grams of food consumed were presented.

A. Excitation and Blockade

A biphasic effect, drinking followed by feeding, is also produced by crystals of carbachol deposited at many sites in the limbic system of the rat (Wise, 1972). When water is withheld, those rats which did begin to feed did so with the same latency. They ate the same amount of food over the same 30 minute duration. These results reveal that cholinergic stimulation has a pharmacological effect of its own that is not the consequence of drinking or of the competing tendencies to eat or drink. Under food deprivation, the rat's feeding response to carbachol stimulation was inhibited for the first 10 minutes or so, which was not found by Myers and DeStefano (1969). Most interesting is the fact that with the experience of repeated applications of carbachol, the rat increased the amount of food consumed. Because of the variability of the anatomical site and the magnitude of effect, an averaging statistic applied to a group of rats in previous investigations could obviously obfuscate the hyperphagic action of cholinergic stimulation at certain sites.

When a solution of carbachol in a dose of 0.26 to 8.6 μg is micro-injected into the lateral hypothalamus or preoptic area of the rabbit, intense feeding occurs (Sommer *et al.*, 1967). After lower doses of carbachol from 0.06 to 1.0 μg are injected into the same structures, the rabbit drinks water. Although in the middle dose range eating and drinking were nearly equal, these ingestive responses, as shown in Fig. 7-20, are reciprocal to one another. The reaction of this species is really quite remarkable and reflects the divergence of responses produced by this cholinomimetic substance seen in the cat and monkey. Of direct bearing on this observation is the report of Kalyuzhnyi (1962) who found that crystals of carbachol inserted into the posterior hypothalamus of the rabbit improved the responding to obtain food, whereas norepinephrine reduced the feeding behavior.

From experiments with the rat in which physostigmine and amphetamine were given systemically, Stark *et al.* (1971) propose that there are both cholinergic and adrenergic controls over feeding in the central nervous system. For example, the anticholinesterase lowers the threshold for eating elicited by electrical stimulation of the lateral hypothalamus. On the other hand, the sympathomimetic agent raised the threshold for such eating. Whether or not a

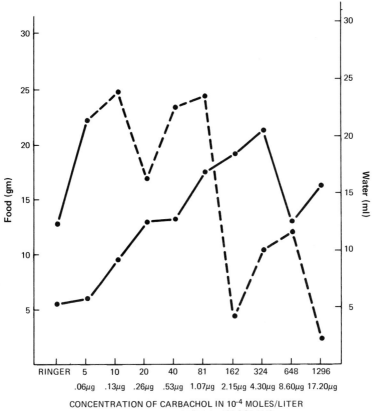

Fig. 7-20 Mean absolute food and water intake following injections of various concentrations of carbachol (.06 to 17.20 μg) and Ringer's solution. These data were obtained from eight animals. The solid line indicates food intake, and the dashed line indicates water intake. (From Sommer, S. R. *et al.*, 1967. *Science.* **156**:983–984. Copyright 1967, by the American Association for the Advancement of Science)

more generalized effect of these drugs on stimulating thresholds is responsible for these observations is not known, but in the rat, again more than one humoral factor seems to be involved in the feeding system.

The inhibition of feeding in the monkey by carbachol or ACh injected into the lateral or other areas of the hypothalamus may be due to a nonselective blockade of a cholinergic pathway for ingestive behavior in the primate. However, nicotine injected into the hypothalamus causes the monkey to drink water (Myers *et al.*, 1973). One possible explanation of this dilemma is that the proper receptor sites along the efferent pathway devoted to the feeding response have not been appropriately stimulated. In accord with the view of a cholinergic link in the feeding pathway (Myers and Sharpe, 1968b) are the results of stimulation of the hypothalamus or septum with atropine. When crystals of atropine were deposited in the ventromedial hypothalamus of the rat, lever responding for food declined (Grossman, 1966a). The consumption of food also fell when the cholinolytic agent was applied similarly to the septum of the rat (Kelsey and Grossman, 1969). In the cat, a dose-dependent suppression of feeding also has been reported when atropine was injected into the rostral hypothalamus (Nance *et al.*, 1971). These observations would not lead to the intransigent conclusion that when an acetylcholine system is blocked, the capacity to eat is abolished. But surely they accent the possibility that in at least three species an intact cholinergic pathway may be necessary for normal feeding behavior.

B. Cyclic AMP

The fact that cyclic AMP may function as a second messenger for norepine-phrine, acetylcholine or other neurohumoral substances has emphasized the importance of this nucleotide in the function of the brain (Gessa *et al.*, 1970). Already it has been implicated in the mechanism of the presynaptic release of transmitter substances.

In 1969, Breckenridge and Lisk discovered that an implant of crystals of cyclic AMP in the mammillary region of the rat caused a marked hyperphagia. The increase in food intake and subsequent gain in body weight continued for three days after the implantation.

Of special significance is the finding that cyclic AMP deposited in the lateral hypothalamus of the rat also evokes an immediate eating of food in an amount about double the control value (Sciorelli *et al.*, 1972). Although the intake of water also increases, the magnitude of food and water taken is not as great as that evoked by carbachol applied at the same site. The differences are il-lustrated in Fig. 7-21. When crystals of hemicholinium, which blocks entry into the neuron and thereby lowers ACh content, were applied to the hypo-thalamus one hour before cyclic AMP, both feeding and drinking were abolished. An implant of atropine had the same inhibitory action on the effects of cyclic AMP on ingestive behavior. These results support the contention that a cholinergic mechanism in the brain mediates the feeding response. Further, the action of cyclic AMP may be due mainly to the local release of ACh from synapses in the feeding pathway which, from the results of Breckenridge and Lisk (1969), may be caudal to the adrenergic system.

In a related study, Booth (1972) has recently found that cyclic AMP facilitated the learning of a preference or aversion for saccharin or salt flavored mash. The learned response depended on the site at which cyclic AMP was injected into the lateral hypothalamus or ventromedial hypothalamus as well as on the dose injected. Since cyclic AMP is involved metabolically in so many

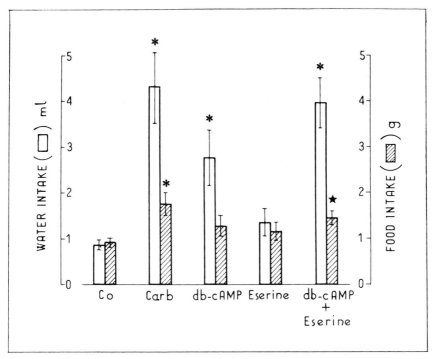

Fig. 7-21 Food and water intake of satiated rats during 1 hour (test period) immediately after cerebral stereotactical application of: Carb, carbamylcholine, db-cAMP, dibutyryl-adenosine-3′,5′-monophosphate; eserine alone or plus db-cAMP (eserine: db-cAMP = 1 : 2) into lateral hypothalamic area. Co, refers to food and water intake, during 1 hour (control period) prior to application of the substances. Means ± S.E. of 12 to 30 observations. *, $p < 0.001$; ★, $0.01 < p < 0.001$ (Student's t-test) as compared to control period. (From Sciorelli, G. et al., 1972. *Brain Res.* **48**:427–431. Fig. 1. Elsevier Publishing Co., Amsterdam, The Netherlands)

systems in the brain, biochemical processes other than those involving transmitter release may also occupy a focal if not inscrutable role in the control of feeding behavior.

V. INHIBITION OF FEEDING

Compounds including a putative transmitter substance may attenuate natural hunger by abolishing or reducing eating in a fasted animal. The mechanism by which such a blockade is achieved is not understood, although a reversible, transitory lesion is always one possibility. Another is that an actual inhibitory pathway may be excited by the chemical stimulus.

A. Drug and Hormonal Effects

Just as the presence of atropine at some sites in the brain of the rat can inhibit feeding, the central application of carbachol likewise may suppress ingestive behavior (Goddard, 1969). Originally, Grossman (1962a; 1964b) found that cholinergic stimulation of the hypothalamus, septum and other structures reduces food intake; similar results have been described for the cat (Milner et al., 1971) and other species such as the monkey (Myers, 1969b). Although its mechanism of action is unclear, in some instances carbachol may simulate a nerve blocker such as procaine. It may, in fact, be mimicking an effect that takes place at cholinergic inhibitory synapses which will be discussed further in some of the chapters to follow.

In a preliminary report, Singer and Montgomery (1968), using only one dose in an unknown volume, once again showed that norepinephrine could suppress drinking in the food-deprived or food-satiated rat when the catecholamine was injected into the amygdala. On the other hand, carbachol did not inhibit feeding when it was injected into the same amygdaloid locus of either the fasted or satiated rat. In a follow-up study, most of these results were confirmed (Singer and Kelly, 1972). In addition, carbachol was found also to reduce slightly (a) natural hunger that was induced by food deprivation for 6 or 17 hours, or (b) the feeding that follows an intrahypothalamic injection of norepinephrine. Phentolamine blocked only norepinephrine-induced feeding, not deprivation-induced feeding, but the single dose was 10 times less than that used by Leibowitz (1971). Here again we see the necessity of obtaining a dose-response curve in order to determine whether a blocking agent is acting as such or is simply a local toxicant.

In the rat fasted for 6 hours, amphetamine micro-injected into areas in which norepinephrine evokes feeding caused a dose-dependent suppression of food intake (Booth, 1967). The region of maximum sensitivity to amphetamine is also anterior to the classical lateral hypothalamic feeding area and corresponds to the noradrenergic sites mapped previously. Norepinephrine also reduced the overall food intake in the 22-hour deprived rat but not nearly to as great an extent as amphetamine. Thus, amphetamine could cause anorexia by releasing norepinephrine in such a large amount to be sufficient to block the normal neural activity of the feeding pathway.

Other drugs which have a slight anorexic effect when injected into the hypothalamus are 5-HT, yohimbine and methysergide (Singer et al., 1972). However, the decline in food intake is usually small and due possibly to a local generalized depression of the entire hypothalamus, since the 4 μl volumes that were injected would displace one entire side of the structure. In addition, the hypophagic effects are not nearly as marked as those seen when these agents are given systemically.

Whereas angiotensin has the property of evoking intense drinking when acting on the cells of the rostral hypothalamus (Chapter 8), the polypeptide at the same time seems to suppress feeding (McFarland and Rolls, 1972). When 1 to 2 μg of angiotensin are injected into the preoptic area of a rat that is pressing a lever to obtain food pellets, the rate of responding declines for about 30 minutes after the injection. The slope of the decrease in the response is portrayed in Fig. 7-22. Overall, angiotensin acts more quickly to evoke drinking than to suppress feeding, and its facilitating action on water intake is far more prolonged.

There is also a remarkable effect on the hypothalamus of gonadal hormones in

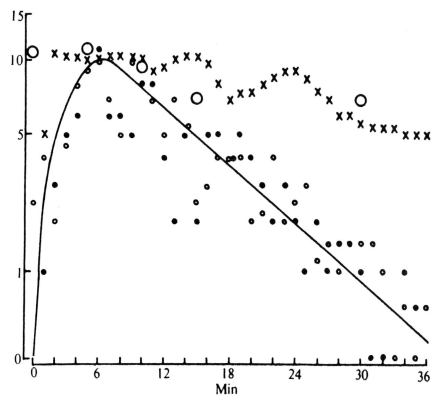

Fig. 7-22   Effect of 1 μg intracranial angiotensin on operant feeding and drinking. a, Depression of feeding in hungry rats following a single injection, showing data from two (open and closed small circles) of the rats tested (ordinate—control minus experimental score gives magnitude of depression in responses min^{-1}). b, Depression of feeding following multiple, computer controlled, injections. Solid line indicates the calculated impulse response. c, Stimulation of drinking in non-deprived rats following a single injection. Crosses give averaged results of the three rats tested (ordinate—responses min^{-1}). d, Amount consumed in drinking tests conducted at various intervals (abscissa) following a single injection (ordinate—ml water consumed).   Averaged results indicated by large circles. (From McFarland and Rolls, 1972)

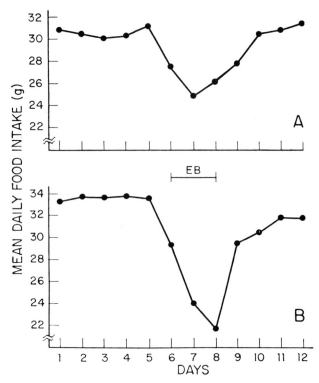

Fig. 7-23 Mean food intake before, during, and after stimulation of the ventromedial hypothalamus-arcuate region with estradiol benzoate. (Hormone was in the brain during days 6, 7, 8. Rats in A showed an average decrease of 10 to 20%; those in B a decrease > 20%.) (From Wade, G. N. and I. Zucker. 1970. *J. Comp. Physiol. Psychol.* **72**:328–336. Copyright 1970, by the American Psychological Association. Reprinted by permission)

terms of the regulation of energy balance. In the spayed female rat, estrogen not only alters the activity of the animal but also its food intake (Wade and Zucker, 1970). If an implant of estradiol is kept in place in the VMH for 3 days, the rat decreases its food intake, as illustrated in Fig. 7-23, by 10 to 20% during this interval. Estradiol deposited at other sites and an implant of other substances such as progesterone are generally without effect. Although the deposit of estradiol in the preoptic area does not alter ingestive behavior, Wade and Zucker found that estradiol increased locomotor activity; this verifies the finding of Colvin and Sawyer (1969). These results again suggest that there are two independent loci of chemoreceptive neurons in the hypothalamus that can mediate energy balance and the expenditure of energy.

B. Toxic and Reversible Chemical Lesions

In parallel with the observations on drugs that inhibit drinking (see Chapter 8), Bergmann *et al.* (1970a) have shown that glycosides or mercury salts implanted into the hypothalamus of the rat also cause a notable aphagia. Although the inhibition of feeding varies, it is ordinarily dose-dependent; the intensity is distinguishable by the drug used to produce the aphagia. After digitoxin or ouabain implants containing 8 to 16 μg or more of the salt are positioned in the hypothalamus, all of the rats die within 10 days. Other compounds, including ethacrynic acid, furosemide, chlormerodrin or mercuric acetate also cause a lethal aphagia but only after much higher doses are given. When the rat's water balance is maintained by a fixed volume of fluid injected systemically, the aphagia persists. This would indicate that these toxic agents may affect normal substrates involved in food and water intake in an independent fashion.

In a very clear experiment, Smith and Britt (1971) found that the implantation of gold thioglucose (GTG) directly into the ventromedial hypothalamus of a male and a female rat produced an increase in food intake of about 14 to 15 g per day over controls. As a technique to produce obesity, GTG evoked even greater feeding and gain in weight than electrolytic lesioning of the ventromedial hypothalamus. Gold-thiomalate and glucose implanted in control rats evoked only a slight elevation in food intake. In contrast to the pitfalls of high mortality and other problems associated with the systemic injection of GTG, the local application of GTG would seem to represent an erudite approach to the study of diencephalic glucose receptors as well as other functions including the release of humoral factors. Interestingly, Smith (1972) found that 2-deoxy-D-glucose could reverse the aphagia produced by GTG when both were deposited in the lateral hypothalamus of the rat. In the alloxan diabetic rat that does not gain weight, insulin placed together with GTG in the ventromedial hypothalamus resulted in a partial restoration of the normal course of growth.

1. *Procaine Blockade*

In spite of the massive lesions shown in the histology, an early study revealed that the repeated injections of procaine totaling as much as 20 μl over 2 hours elicited eating when the nerve blocker was injected into the ventromedial hypothalamus of the rat (Epstein, 1960). On the other hand, an injection of procaine into the lateral hypothalamus suppressed feeding in the fasted animal. Hypertonic NaCl injected into the ventromedial hypothalamus also reduced food intake. Dextrose did not interfere with normal eating when the sugar was infused bilaterally into the medial hypothalamus. More recently, Reynolds and Simpson (1969b) confirmed the hyperphagic action of procaine infused into the ventromedial region of the rat's hypothalamus.

By examining the anatomical correlates of the blockade of neural transmission in relation to food intake, Albert *et al.* (1970) found that eating was suppressed by the injection of a large volume and high concentration of procaine into several structures of the limbic system. In rats deprived only of food for 24 hours, it is significant that food intake was appreciably reduced when procaine was injected into the globus pallidus, the antero-lateral hypothalamus or directly into the lateral hypothalamus. The interval of nerve blockade, which did not cause any general motor or behavioral disturbance, lasted only 15 minutes. Just as important is the observation that feeding did not diminish after procaine was injected into the postero-lateral hypothalamus, preoptic area, amygdala or the caudate nucleus. Thus, the opinion that a divergent longitudinal circuit required for feeding passes through the globus pallidus and into the lateral and anterior hypothalamus is borne out (Morgane, 1961).

In fasted rats, procaine injected into a norepinephrine-sensitive area blocks the hyperglycemia observed when the trained animal is presented with a visual stimulus which had been previously associated with the opportunity to obtain food by lever pressing (Booth and Miller, 1969). Thus, the hypothalamic feeding system can influence the levels of blood glucose as evidenced by the local blockade of the glycemic response.

VI. CONCLUDING CONSIDERATIONS

Almost without exception, the rat has been used as the experimental test subject for investigating the chemical mechanisms in the brain-stem underlying eating behavior. This is in spite of the fact that the early observations on deficits in hunger or satiety were based on lesions and electrical stimulation of the hypothalamus of the cat or other large animal. In a way, the formulation of a model of hunger or feeding using an animal with such a diminutive diencephalon as the rat is unfortunate.

On an anatomical basis alone, the technical obstacles are nearly insurmountable in connection with almost every attempt to identify by chemical stimulation a functional group of neurons within a specific region. For example, the entire ventromedial nucleus is not as wide as the shaft of the cannula that delivers a chemical substrate. In this case, the lesion may supersede whatever effect the chemical may have. Of course, the same criticism may apply to the procedure of circumsection of fibers by rotational knife-cuts and other equally promising techniques that are so popular today. In essence, the validity of the investigation depends entirely upon the care that is taken to preserve the morphological elements that are at the heart of the ingestive function.

A. Experimental Aspects

A vast number of experiments have been completed in an attempt to isolate the chemically specific elements involved in feeding and hunger; but controversy and discrepancies still exist in large measure. There are three general sources of experimental inconsistency.

1. *The Food Substance*

The use of any foodstuff which is not the same as the ordinary dry laboratory biscuit introduces the ineluctable variable of palatability. Wetting the pellets to form a moist mash also alters the esculent nature of the food. By suddenly offering a delectable fluid such as Metrecal or milk to the animal in place of the dry lab biscuit, the test situation is confounded to such an awesome degree that it is impossible to factor out how much of the fluid is taken as a source of nutrient and how much as a sustentative of water balance. Whether or not the animal selects the fluid nutrient over water does not matter since this unknown proportion of food versus water cannot be resolved. At least a dry biscuit is not as ready a source of water.

2. Anatomical Precision

Histological identification of each site of stimulation is not routinely done; as a result, few anatomical maps have been constructed of loci that are reactive to an agonist or antagonist. What would seem to be mandatory is to establish the precise relationship of (a) the facilitation or reduction in eating by (b) a given chemical within (c) a specific locus in the diencepahlon. The reason for this is that in the hypothalamus alone there are at least five distinct anatomical components of the feeding system. Obviously, different results ought to be obtained when one chemical excites one pathway in contrast to another.

3. Technical Limitations

Considering the neuroanatomy of the feeding circuitry, it is unlikely that such issues as: (1) a zone of high density of a specific receptor site, (2) the chemosensitive area mediating satiety, or (3) the motor pathway required for eating can be resolved by the chemical procedures typically used today. For example, to inject a droplet of more than 0.2 to 0.5 μl into the diencephalon of the rat cannot elucidate an independent anatomical network of neurons that is already on a scale bordering on the subminiature. In the less commonly used but larger species such as the cat or monkey, 0.8 to 1.2 μl may even exceed the reasonable limits of an injection volume (Myers, 1971a). When necessary controls described in Chapter 2 are carried out for osmotic tension and pH, if a crystalline substance is applied or solution is injected, unwanted and cumbersome variables are ordinarily ruled out. The elaboration of a dose-response curve and the perspicuous usage of pharmacological antagonists and agonists are usually well worth the investigator's effort. In many instances they have yielded some fruits of clarification for a given feeding response.

But what can be concluded from an overall analysis of the experiments, taking into account species other than the rat?

B. Chemical Factors

Unlike the recent discoveries of the profound importance of peptides in the regulation of other vital functions including drinking (Chapter 8) and sleep (Chapter 9), an entanglement of loose ends surrounds the neurochemistry of the feeding system. The chemical nature remains to be unraveled of the potent hunger and satiety factors which are liberated within the diencephalon or into the corporeal circulation, or both. The most likely candidates which monitor the nutritional state of the animal are: (1) an amino acid complex of a unique sequence; (2) a lipid soluble fatty acid complex, or (3) a carbohydrate complex. In turn, these factors act on the chemosensitive elements or receptors located on cells that are in part delegated to activating or inhibiting the ingestion of a foodstuff.

One fact appears to be on a firm footing. A catecholaminergic mechanism in the brain-stem would seem to constitute a portion of the chemical link for feeding. From nearly every standpoint, norepinephrine is the most logical candidate as a modulator of the feeding mechanism. There are four reasons for this: (a) the hypothalamic action of adrenergic substances in eliciting spontaneous feeding in the rat and monkey; (b) the pharmacological antagonism by an alpha receptor blocker in the majority of experiments; (c) the evidence, albeit limited, that a catecholamine-like factor is released in the hypothalamus of a hungry animal; and (d) the general anatomical specificity, described in the next section, of the sensitivity to the monoamine. The randomness of the unit responses in the lateral hypothalamus to the iontophoretic application of amines (Krebs and Bindra, 1971) is mystifying in one sense but not in another (see Chapter 1, III. D.).

Obviously, more research must be completed before the role of dopamine in this system is known. Although the results of anatomical lesioning with 6-OHDA indicate that the precursor of norepinephrine may ultimately be involved, perhaps in the set-point for weight regulation (e.g., in the static phase of obesity), the central pharmacological evidence does not: dopamine is less potent and more sluggish in its action than norepinephrine. Another question is why norepinephrine fails to evoke feeding in the cat. Again, perhaps the right experiment has to be done and the appropriate locus searched out.

The apparent controversy about the specificity of adrenergic receptors in terms of which class signals satiety and which one signals hunger may be entirely artificial and based on a non-comparable means to an end. Surely, resolution will follow when individual researchers do their experiments at the same time of day or night, use a similar pabulum, control the dose and the volume of their injection and examine their anatomical material scrupulously. The caution should always be kept in mind that there are vitiating conceptual arguments against a humoral coding based on two or more types of CNS receptors. If a substance such as norepinephrine is released presynaptically onto the postsynaptic membrane, how could the monoamine recognize and select the receptor protein to which it should become attached—alpha, beta or other? No such discriminatory power is known to exist for norepinephrine in the central nervous system.

Not to be overlooked is the probable cholinergic link in the motor pathway which underpins the numerous components in the act of eating. Cholinergic synapses are thought to be located all along the efferent pathway for heat production, a vital portion of the totality of an animal's energy requirement, as well as along the closely related anatomical system for water balance (Chapter 8).

Curiously, feeding is switched off by angiotensin in the same way as an alpha antagonist given in the hypothalamus. In contrast, glucose applied to hypothalamic structures does not abolish feeding in spite of strong experimental support given to the idea of specialized glucose receptors. Yet both substances are blood-borne and are capable of being metabolized in cerebral tissue. The answer to these riddles awaits further research. The same is true for an ionic set-point mechanism based on the intrinsic ratio of extracellular sodium to calcium in the hypothalamus or other limbic structure (Myers and Veale, 1971). As appealing as such a set-point concept may be for weight regulation or the more elusory notion of hunger, the whole issue is still not settled concerning a set-point for weight around which the behavior of feeding is regulated and the ingestion of specific nutrients is monitored.

C. Morphological Factors

From the foregoing material, it is preposterous to label one anatomical region as a feeding center and another a satiety center. For example, the destruction of an animal's lateral hypothalamus after its body weight has been previously reduced by systemic fasting can be followed by a transient hyperphagia, not aphagia (Powley and Keesey, 1970). The oft-described recovery of eating behavior after the ablation of the lateral region certainly abjures the critical necessity of this part of the hypothalamus for feeding. The same probably holds true for the ventromedial nucleus (Rabin, 1972).

The anatomical bridgework between the ventromedial and lateral regions of the hypothalamus may be debated. The ventromedial hypothalamus could be part of the system that senses a shift in the plasma level of glucose or of different lipids, thus serving the function of so-called lipostatic and glucostatic monitoring. On the other hand, the lateral hypothalamic region most likely forms a portion of the pathway that carries the motor impulses such as chewing, biting and swallowing. The sensory aspects of taste and palatability also seem to have anatomical representation in the lateral hypothalamus.

Although the significance of the structures that comprise the rostral hypothalamus is not understood, the correlative nature of several functions including the centrally-induced release of thyroxin, the presence of osmoreceptors, and the origin of the heat production pathway is inescapable. As the cells in the anterior hypothalamus can be selectively stimulated by a catecholamine and perhaps other substances to evoke an ingestive response, the thermostatic element of feeding could indeed be integrated with the processes of thermal conservation and other metabolic activity.

Clearly, many anatomical systems for feeding, just as for thermoregulation and drinking, are organized in a somewhat redundant fashion. Destruction of one can lead to a functional, lifesaving take-over by another. Experiments using lesions or electrical stimulation have implicated such widely separated structures as the midbrain tegmentum, posterior hypothalamus, globus pallidus, reticular formation, nigro-striatal pathway, amygdala, septum, cerebral cortex and, of course, the lateral and ventromedial parts of the hypothalamus. An appraisal of these studies uncovers once more the rich integration of many structures in the limbic system that are delegated to the vital processes of energy metabolism, in the larger view, and the consumption of a meal, in the more narrow sense.

Although the anatomy of the chemical system underlying these processes has not yet been fully deciphered, several facts dovetail with other physiological information. Structures in close morphological contiguity with the fornical system are involved in the activation or cessation of ingestive behavior. In fact, the noradrenergic link with the limbic system in both the rat and monkey centers on the columns of the fornix. Two other important pathways, the medial forebrain bundle and the stria medullaris, also provide connections to the limbic system. Their part in the motivational aspect of eating behavior seems to be crucial but yet must be more fully explored.

VII. Master Summary Table
Chemicals that Exerted an Effect When Given at a Specific Site in the Brain

Chemical	Dose	Volume	Site	Species	State*	Response	Reference
Acetylcholine (ACh)	≈ 1 μg	crystal	Ventral amygdala	Rat	U	Reduced lever response for food	Grossman (1964a)
	25–50 μg	.5–1 μl	Lateral hypothalamus	Monkey	C	Dose-dependent blockade of feeding and drinking in fasted animal.	Myers (1969b)
ACh and Eserine	1.5–50 μg	1 μl	Hypothalamus	Monkey	C	Blockade of feeding and drinking at higher doses.	Sharpe and Myers (1969)
Amino acid complex	100 μg	1 μl	Hypothalamus	Rat	U	Suppressed feeding.	Panksepp and Booth (1971)
Amphetamine	37–74 μg	.2–5 μl	Ventromedial and lateral hypothalamus	Rat	U	Suppressed feeding.	Leibowitz (1970b)
	7.07–17.07 μg/kg	1 μl	Anterior hypothalamus	Rat	U	Anorexia.	Booth (1968a)
	10–50 μg	1 μl or crystal	Ventromedial hypothalamus (VMH)	Cat	A	Suppressed both septal and amygdala evoked responses in VMH.	Sutin et al. (1963)
Angiotensin II	1–2 μg	1 μl	Preoptic area	Rat	U	Suppressed feeding after food deprivation.	McFarland and Rolls (1972)
Atropine	≈ .5–5 μg	crystal	Ventromedial hypothalamus	Rat	U	Reduced lever responding to food or water.	Grossman (1966)
	12.5–50 μg	2 μl	Anterior preoptic area	Cat	U	Inhibition of feeding and drinking.	Nance et al. (1971)
	12 μg	.5–1 μl	Lateral hypothalamus	Monkey	C	Reversed cholinergic blockade of feeding and drinking.	Myers (1969b)
Ca^{2+}	5.21–20.04 μg/min	perfusion 50 μl/min	Ventromedial hypothalamus	Cat	U	Feeding in satiated animal.	Myers and Veale (1971b)

*U = unanesthetized and unrestrained; C = constrained, confined or curarized; A = anesthetized.

VII. Master Summary Table (Continued)

Chemical	Dose	Volume	Site	Species	State*	Response	Reference
Carbachol	≈ .5–1 µg	crystal	Ventral amygdala	Rat	U	Reduced lever response for food.	Grossman (1964a)
	≈ 1–3 µg	crystal	Antero-dorsal hippocampus, fornix, cingulum	Rat	U	Drinking, activity, feeding.	Grant and Jarrard (1968)
	≈ 5 µg	crystal	Lateral hypothalamus, nucleus reuniens, mammillary bodies, septum, hippocampus	Rat	U	Feeding.	Wise (1972)
	≈ .5–5 µg	crystal	Septum	Rat	U	Suppressed food intake.	Grossman (1964b)
	≈ 2–5 µg	crystal	Lateral hypothalamus	Rat	U	Increased food and water intake.	Sciorelli et al. (1972)
	.25 µg	1 µl	Amygdala	Rat	U	Inhibited eating and drinking.	Goddard (1969)
	.055 µg	?	Amygdala	Rat	U	Failed to block feeding in deprived or satiated rats.	Singer and Montgomery (1968)
	.33 µg	1 µl	Hypothalamus	Rat	U	Reduced NE or deprivation-induced eating.	Singer and Kelly (1972)
	.06–17.2 µg	?	Hypothalamus	Rabbit	U	Feeding at low doses.	Sommer et al. (1967)
	.1–1 µg	2 µl	Anterior hypothalamus, preoptic area and amygdala	Cat	U	Suppressed feeding and drinking.	Milner et al. (1971)
	.4–25 µg	1 µl	Hypothalamus	Monkey	C	Blockade of feeding and drinking at higher doses.	Sharpe and Myers (1969)
	1.2–25 µg	.5–1 µl	Lateral hypothalamus	Monkey	C	Dose-dependent blockade of feeding and drinking in fasted animal.	Myers (1969b)
Chlormerodrin	≈ 30–80 µg	crystal	Hypothalamus	Rat	U	Aphagia.	Bergmann et al. (1970a)

Substance	Dose	Volume/Form	Region	Species		Effect	Reference
Chlorpromazine (CPZ)	96–380 μg	1 μl	Perifornical region	Rat	U	Eating.	Leibowitz and Miller (1969)
Clonidine	1–53 μg	1 μl	Antero-lateral hypothalamus	Rat	U	Feeding.	Broekkamp and van Rossum (1972)
Cyclic AMP and Eserine	?	crystal	Lateral hypothalamus	Rat	U	Increased food and water intake.	Sciorelli et al. (1972)
Cyclic AMP	≃ 5–10 μg	crystal	Lateral hypothalamus	Rat	U	Increased food and water intake.	Sciorelli et al. (1972)
	≃ 250 μg	crystal	Mammillary region	Rat	U	Hyperphagia.	Breckenridge and Lisk (1969)
	1.8 μg	.9 μl	Lateral, ventro-medial hypothalamus	Rat	U	Feeding, associative preference for taste of food.	Booth (1972)
2-Deoxy-D-glucose (2-DG)	≃ 12 μg	crystal	Lateral hypothalamus	Rat	U	Increased feeding.	Balagura and Kanner (1971)
	25 μg	?	Lateral hypothalamus	Rat	U	Increased feeding.	Balagura (1971)
Desmethylimipramine (DMI)	.55 and 2.7 μg	1 μl	Lateral hypothalamus	Rat	U	Potentiated eating in fasted rats.	Montgomery et al. (1971)
	.73 and 2.7 μg	1 μl	Lateral hypothalamus	Rat	U	Enhanced feeding after fasting.	Montgomery et al. (1969)
	28 μg	7 μl	Antero-lateral hypothalamus	Rat	U	Suppression or enhancement of NE feeding.	Booth (1968c)
	106.6 μg	1 μl	Hypothalamus	Rat	U	Potentiated NE feeding.	Slangen and Miller (1969)
	107 μg	1–5 μl	Preoptic area	Rat	U	Blocked 6-OHDA feeding and drinking.	Evetts et al. (1972)
Dextrose	1400–1500 μg	28–30 μl	Medial hypothalamus	Rat	U	Does not inhibit feeding.	Epstein (1960)
Dibenzyline	≃ 1–5 μg	crystal	Perifornical region	Rat	U	Reduced eating after food deprivation.	Grossman (1962b)
Digitoxin	≃ 3–5 μg	crystal	Ventral amygdala	Rat	U	Reduced lever response for food.	Grossman (1964a)
	≃ 4–32 μg	crystal	Hypothalamus	Rat	U	Aphagia.	Bergmann et al. (1970a)
Dopamine (DA)	≃ 1–5 μg	crystal	Perifornical region	Rat	U	Feeding.	Grossman (1962b)

VII. Master Summary Table (*Continued*)

Chemical	Dose	Volume	Site	Species	State*	Response	Reference
Dopamine (DA)	3.8–19 µg	1 µl	Hypothalamus	Rat	U	Feeding in satiated rat.	Slangen and Miller (1969)
	25 µg	.5–1 µl	Lateral hypothalamus	Monkey	C	Feeding and drinking in satiated animal.	Myers (1969b)
	6–50 µg	1 µl	Hypothalamus	Monkey	C	Dose-dependent feeding.	Sharpe and Myers (1969)
Epinephrine (E)	≃ 1–5 µg	crystal	Lateral hypothalamus	Rat	U	Feeding.	Grossman (1960; 1962a)
	≃ 3–5 µg	crystal	Ventral amygdala	Rat	U	Lever response for food.	Grossman (1964b)
	3.7 µg	1 µl	Hypothalamus	Rat	U	Feeding in satiated rat.	Slangen and Miller (1969)
	5 µg	5 µl	Globus pallidus, ventro-medial and lateral hypothalamus	Rat	U	Drinking of Metrecal.	Wagner and de Groot (1963b)
	2.5–6 µg	.2–1 µl	Antero-lateral hypo-thalamus	Rat	U	Feeding.	Booth (1968c)
	7–13 µg	.2–.5 µl	Ventromedial hypo-thalamus	Rat	U	Feeding.	Leibowitz (1970b)
	33 µg	1 µl	Perifornical area of hypothalamus	Rat	U	Anorexia (β receptor).	Leibowitz (1970a)
	20–55 µg	1 µl or crystal	Ventromedial hypothalamus (VMH)	Cat	A	Enhanced septal-VMH evoked response and suppressed amygdaloid-VMH evoked response.	Sutin et al. (1963)
	12.5 µg	.5–1 µl	Lateral hypothalamus	Monkey	C	Feeding and drinking in satiated animal.	Myers (1969b)
	6–50 µg	1 µl	Hypothalamus	Monkey	C	Dose-dependent feeding.	Sharpe and Myers (1969)
Estradiol	?	crystal	Ventromedial hypothalamus	Rat	U	Depressed food intake.	Wade and Zucker (1970)

Substance	Dose	Form	Region	Animal	U/A	Effect	Reference
Ethacrynic acid	≈ 50–100 µg	crystal	Hypothalamus	Rat	U	Aphagia.	Bergmann et al. (1970a)
Furosemide	≈ 100 µg	crystal	Hypothalamus	Rat	U	Aphagia.	Bergmann et al. (1970a)
GABA	?	crystal	Ventral amygdala	Rat	U	Reduced lever response for food.	Grossmann (1964a)
Glucose	≈ 12 µg	crystal	Lateral hypothalamus	Rat	U	Increased feeding.	Balagura and Kanner (1971)
	50–90 µg	1 µl	Lateral hypothalamus	Rat	U	Blocked drinking, insulin-induced feeding, drowsiness.	Booth (1968b)
	200 µg	2 µl	Ventromedial hypothalamus	Rat	U	Suppressed long-term food intake.	Panksepp and Nance (1972)
	500 µg	50 µl	Hypothalamus	Cat	A	Decreased epinephrine and norepinephrine secretion from adrenal gland.	Dunér (1953)
Glucose-6-phosphate (GLU-6-P)	?	crystal	Ventromedial hypothalamus	Rat	A	Increased VMH electrical activity.	Gliddon (1970)
Glucose and Insulin	200 µg	2 µl	Ventromedial hypothalamus	Rat	U	Suppressed long-term food intake.	Panksepp and Nance (1972)
Gold thioglucose (GTG)	?	crystal	Ventromedial hypothalamus	Rat	U	Increased feeding, weight gain.	Smith and Britt (1971)
Gold thioglucose + 2-DG	≈ 10–25 µg	crystal	Lateral hypothalamus	Rat	U	Aphagia.	Smith (1972)
Gold thioglucose	≈ 10–25 µg	crystal	Lateral hypothalamus	Rat	U	No aphagia.	Smith (1972)
Gold thioglucose + Insulin	≈ 10–25 µg	crystal	Ventromedial hypothalamus	Rat	U	Hyperphagia after diabetic condition.	Smith (1972)
Hemicholinium	?	crystal	Lateral hypothalamus	Rat	U	Increased food and water intake.	Sciorelli et al. (1972)
6-Hydroxydopamine (6-OHDA)	.01–16 µg	1–5 µl	Preoptic area	Rat	U	Feeding and drinking.	Evetts et al. (1972)
	.2–16 µg	4 µl	Substantia nigra, caudate nucleus	Rat	A and U	Depletion of norepinephrine and dopamine in nerve terminals.	Ungerstedt (1971b)
	6–8 µg	3–4 µl	Lateral hypothalamus, central tegmentum, substantia nigra	Rat	U	Aphagia, catalepsia, akinesis.	Ungerstedt (1971a)

VII. Master Summary Table (Continued)

Chemical	Dose	Volume	Site	Species	State*	Response	Reference
6-Hydroxydopamine (6-OHDA)	4-32 µg	4 µl	Lateral hypothalamus.	Rat	U	Aphagia, adipsia.	Smith et al. (1972)
	20 µg	2 µl	Substantia nigra	Rat	U	Aphagia and adipsia; impaired shuttle box performance.	Echavarria-Mage et al. (1972)
Insulin	1-6 mU	2 µl	Hypothalamus	Mouse	A	Enhanced gold thioglucose necrosis in VMH.	Debons et al. (1970)
Isoproterenol	≈ 9 µg	crystal	Medial forebrain bundle	Rat	U	Suppressed drinking of quinine-milk.	Margules (1970b)
	5 µg	1 µl	Hypothalamus	Rat	U	No feeding.	Slangen and Miller (1969)
	37 µg	2 µl	Hypothalamus	Rat	U	Reduced feeding.	Goldman et al. (1971)
	20-40 µg	.2-.5 µl	Lateral hypothalamus	Rat	U	Anorexia.	Leibowitz (1970b)
	59.6 µg	1 µl	Perifornical area of hypothalamus	Rat	U	Anorexia (β receptor).	Leibowitz (1970a)
	333 µg	5 µl	Hypothalamus	Pig	U	Reduced feeding after deprivation.	Jackson and Robinson (1971)
LB-46	≈ 18 µg	crystal	Medial forebrain bundle	Rat	U	Increased drinking of quinine-milk.	Margules (1970b)
Lidocaine	20 µg	1 µl	Hypothalamus	Rat	U	Potentiated NE feeding.	Slangen and Miller (1969)
	50 µg	5 µl	Ventromedial hypothalamus	Rat	U	Drinking of Metrecal.	Wagner and de Groot (1963b)
Mercuric acetate	≈ 10-30 µg	crystal	Hypothalamus	Rat	U	Aphagia.	Bergmann et al. (1970a)
Methyl atropine	≈ 2-7 µg	crystal	Septum	Rat	U	Suppressed food and water intake.	Kelsey and Grossman (1969)
Methysergide	10 µg	4-4.5 µl	Lateral hypothalamus	Rat	U	Slight anorexia.	Singer et al. (1972)

Substance	Dose	Volume	Site	Species		Effect	Reference
Metrazol	500 μg	5 μl	Ventromedial hypothalamus	Rat	U	Reduced Metrecal drinking.	Wagner and de Groot (1963b)
Neostigmine	5 μg	5 μl	Ventromedial hypothalamus	Rat	U	Reduced Metrecal drinking.	Wagner and de Groot (1963b)
Nialamide	59.7 μg	1 μl	Hypothalamus	Rat	U	Feeding when tetrabenazine also given.	Slangen and Miller (1969)
Norepinephrine (NE)	≃ 1-3 μg	crystal	Limbic system, diencephalon	Rat	U	Feeding.	Coury (1967)
	≃ 1-5 μg	crystal	Lateral hypothalamus	Rat	U	Feeding.	Grossman (1960; 1962a)
	≃ 3-5 μg	crystal	Ventral amygdala	Rat	U	Lever response for food.	Grossman (1964a)
	≃ 25 μg	crystal	Lateral hypothalamus	Rat	U	Drinking of milk.	Margules et al. (1972)
	≃ 14-28 μg	crystal	Medial forebrain bundle	Rat	U	Suppressed milk drinking.	Margules (1970a)
	2.5-6 μg	.2-1 μl	Antero-lateral hypothalamus	Rat	U	Feeding.	Booth (1968c)
	5 μg	5 μl	Globus pallidus, lateral hypothalamus	Rat	U	Drinking of Metrecal.	Wagner and de Groot (1963b)
	5.5 μg	1-5 μl	Preoptic area	Rat	U	Blocked 6-OHDA feeding but enhanced drinking.	Evetts et al. (1972)
	6 μg	.67 μl	Hypothalamus	Rat	U	Feeding.	Booth (1967)
	6 μg	1 μl	Lateral hypothalamus	Rat	U	Greater eating of saccharin food than after deprivation.	Booth and Quartermain (1965)
	6.7 μg	1 μl	Perifornical area of hypothalamus	Rat	U	Feeding (α receptor).	Leibowitz (1970a)
	3-13 μg	.2-.5 μl	Ventromedial hypothalamus	Rat	U	Feeding.	Leibowitz (1970b)
	7.2-21.6 μg	.5-1 μl	Anterior hypothalamus	Rat	U	Feeding.	Davis and Keesey (1971)
	5-25 μg	.5 μl	Anterior hypothalamus	Rat	U	Food and water intake.	Avery (1971)

VII. Master Summary Table (Continued)

Chemical	Dose	Volume	Site	Species	State*	Response	Reference
Norepinephrine (NE)	8.7 μg	1 μl	Anterior hypothalamus	Rat	U	Anorexic effect after VMH lesion	Herberg and Franklin (1972)
	3.4–50.6 μg	1 μl	Hypothalamus	Rat	U	Feeding in satiated rat.	Slangen and Miller (1969)
	.8–64.8 μg	1 μl	Lateral hypothalamus	Rat	U	Drinking of Metrecal.	Miller et al. (1964)
	20 μg	1 μl	Lateral hypothalamus	Rat	U	Lever pressing for food only when satiated.	Coons and Quartermain (1970)
	20–55 μg	1 μl or crystal	Ventromedial hypothalamus	Cat	A	Enhanced septal-VMH evoked response and suppressed amygdaloid VMH evoked response.	Sutin et al. (1963)
	80 μg	2 μl	Nucleus centromedian of thalamus	Cat	U	Increased daily food intake.	Avery and Nance (1970a)
	40–160 μg	2 μl	Anterior hypothalamus, preoptic area, amygdala	Cat	U	Suppressed feeding and drinking.	Milner et al. (1971)
	10 μg	1 μl	Anterior hypothalamus	Monkey	C	Feeding during hypothermia.	Myers and Yaksh (1972)
	12.5 μg	.5–1 μl	Lateral hypothalamus	Monkey	C	Feeding and drinking.	Myers and Sharpe (1968b)
	5–12.5 μg	1–1.2 μl	Hypothalamus	Monkey	C	Feeding and drinking.	Yaksh and Myers (1972b)
	6–25 μg	.5–1 μl	Lateral hypothalamus	Monkey	C	Feeding and drinking in satiated animal.	Myers (1969b)
	6–50 μg	1 μl	Hypothalamus	Monkey	C	Dose-dependent feeding.	Sharpe and Myers (1969)
Novocaine (Procaine)	22.5 μg	1.1 μl	Lateral hypothalamus	Rat	U	Blocked hyperglycemia.	Booth and Miller (1969)
Ouabain	≃1–16 μg	crystal	Hypothalamus	Rat	U	Aphagia.	Bergmann et al. (1970a)

Drug	Dose	Volume	Site	Species	U	Effect	Reference
Oxymetazoline	1.5 µg	1 µl	Antero-lateral hypothalamus	Rat	U	Feeding.	Broekkamp and van Rossum (1972)
Pentobarbital	300 µg	5 µl	Ventromedial hypothalamus	Rat	U	Drinking of Metrecal.	Wagner and de Groot (1963b)
Phenoxybenzamine	4 µg	1 µl	Antero-lateral hypothalamus	Rat	U	Blocked NE feeding.	Booth (1968c)
Phentolamine	≈ 9–18 µg	crystal	Medial forebrain bundle	Rat	U	Drinking of milk.	Margules (1970a)
	3.5 µg	.7 µl	Antero-lateral hypothalamus	Rat	U	Blocked NE feeding.	Booth (1968c)
	4–8 µg	1–5 µl	Preoptic area	Rat	U	Blocked 6-OHDA feeding but enhanced drinking.	Evetts et al. (1972)
	12.7 µg	1 µl	Hypothalamus	Rat	U	Blocked NE feeding.	Slangen and Miller (1969)
	15 µg	1 µl	Antero-lateral hypothalamus	Rat	U	Feeding.	Broekkamp and van Rossum (1972)
	22 µg	1 µl	Perifornical area of hypothalamus	Rat	U	Potentiated β anorexia.	Leibowitz (1970a)
	10.33 µg	1 µl	Hypothalamus	Rat	U	Reduced only NE eating.	Singer and Kelly (1972)
	102 µg	4 µl	Ventromedial hypothalamus	Rat	U	Anorexia.	Leibowitz (1970b)
Potassium chloride (KCl)	2 µg	?	Occipital cortex	Rat	U	Drinking, eating, excitation.	Huston and Bureš (1970)
Procaine	10–150 µg	1–3 µl	Lateral hypothalamus	Rat	U	Suppressed feeding.	Epstein (1960)
	10–150 µg	1–3 µl	Ventromedial hypothalamus	Rat	U	Feeding.	Epstein (1960)
	100 µg	2 µl	Globus pallidus, anterior and lateral hypothalamus	Rat	U	Reduced food consumption in deprived rat.	Albert et al. (1970)
	50–750 µg	1–15 µl	Ventromedial hypothalamus	Rat	U	Slight eating.	Reynolds and Simpson (1969b)

VII. Master Summary Table (Continued)

Chemical	Dose	Volume	Site	Species	State*	Response	Reference
Propranolol	11.8-35 µg	1 µl	Hypothalamus	Rat	U	Failed to block NE feeding.	Slangen and Miller (1969)
	41 µg	1 µl	Perifornical area of hypothalamus	Rat	U	Reversed β anorexia.	Leibowitz (1970a)
	103 µg	.2-.5 µl	Lateral hypothalamus	Rat	U	Increased feeding.	Leibowitz (1970b)
	368 µg	10 µl	Hypothalamus	Pig	U	Restored feeding after iso-proteronol blockade.	Jackson and Robinson (1971)
Ribonuclease	300 µg	5 µl	Dorsal hippocampus	Rabbit	U	Blocked conditioned reflex to obtain food.	Tushmalova and Melkova (1970)
Serotonin (5-HT)	4 µg	4-4.5 µl	Lateral hypothalamus	Rat	U	Slight anorexia.	Singer et al. (1972)
	18 µg	2 µl	Hypothalamus	Rat	U	Reduced feeding.	Goldman et al. (1971)
	12.5 µg	.5-1 µl	Lateral hypothalamus	Monkey	C	Feeding and drinking.	Myers and Sharpe (1968a)
	6-25 µg	1 µl	Hypothalamus	Monkey	C	Drinking followed by eating.	Sharpe and Myers (1969)
Sodium Chloride (NaCl)	15.63-40.10 µg/min	perfusion 50 µl/min	Lateral hypothalamus	Cat	U	Feeding in satiated animal.	Myers and Veale (1971b)
	50-200 µg	1-4 µl	Ventromedial hypothalamus	Rat	U	Suppressed feeding.	Epstein (1960)
	50-200 µg	1-4 µl	Lateral hypothalamus	Rat	U	Feeding.	Epstein (1960)
Sotalol (MJ-1999)	4-8 µg	1-5 µl	Preoptic area	Rat	U	Blocked 6-OHDA feeding and drinking.	Evetts et al. (1972)
Tolazoline	20 µg	2 µl	Hypothalamus	Rat	U	Reduced feeding.	Goldman et al. (1971)
Yohimbine	1.8-18 µg	4-4.5 µl	Lateral hypothalamus	Rat	U	Slight anorexia.	Singer et al. (1972)

8 Thirst and Drinking

I. INTRODUCTION

There are a great many well recognized facts about the maintenance of body water and the regulation of salt balance. They are derived in large measure from the salient contributions made over the last half of the century by renal and electrolyte physiologists (see Wolf, 1958; Wayner, 1964). As exemplified in the outstanding, recent reviews of Andersson (1971a and b), Hoebel (1971), Share and Claybaugh (1972), and Fitzsimons (1972), an enormous number of investigations have been conducted in four major spheres: (1) peripheral osmotic detectors; (2) central thirst receptors; (3) the homeostatic role played by the kidneys; and (4) the behavioral determinants of drinking behavior.

As we have witnessed in the central systems underlying other vegetative functions, the exceptional balance between the peripheral and central mechanism for controlling body water is also finely tuned. That there are receptors in the mouth, stomach and other parts of the periphery as well as in the brain itself that monitor the conditions which bring about thirst or the craving for water or that signal the state of adequate hydration is now well documented. But as one would imagine, the central neural control mechanism which processes the input that belies a critical imbalance in body water, one way or the other, is the subject of intensive research, specific controversy and generalized debate. How this information is translated by a humoral or transmitter event in the brain-stem into the most common of motor acts—drinking a fluid—is exceedingly complex.

A. Development of Thirst

Water is continually lost from the body through the different processes of evaporation and excretion. To sustain normal bodily function, an adequate level of water must be maintained in both the extracellular fluid as well as intracellular fluid compartments. Andersson (1971b) has presented a simplified explanation of three of the main controlling factors which provide the stimuli for drinking.   Figure 8-1 portrays diagrammatically the conditions of hydration, dehydration and water balance, and the following principles explain the relationships between these conditions.

Na^+ is present primarily in the extracellular fluid compartment, i.e., outside the cell, every cell, regardless of its location in the body. Although water can pass readily across the cell membrane, in and out of the intracellular compartment, Na^+ is ordinarily prevented from entering the cell to any degree by an essential inborn feature of the cell membrane—its relative impermeability to this cation.

When an excess amount of Na^+ is taken into the system, which thereby raises

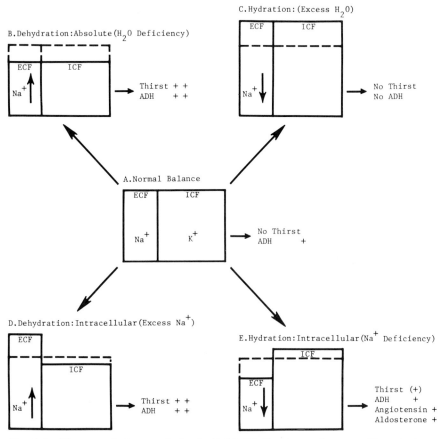

Fig. 8-1 Diagram of changes in body fluid distribution and composition during negative and positive water and salt balances. To the right of the diagrams are indicated compensatory factors aimed to restore normal balance. ECF. Extracellular fluid compartment; ICF. Intracellular fluid compartment; ADH. Antidiuretic hormone. (Modified after Andersson 1971b)

the concentration of Na^+ in the extracellular fluid, water diffuses out of the cell so as to restore the crucial osmotic balance extracellularly. But this intracellular depletion of water causes an *intracellular dehydration* (often called "cellular" or "relative") and a subsequent osmotic disturbance (Fig. 8-1D).

When there is insufficient Na^+ in the system, water then passes from outside the cell membrane into the cell causing a state of *extracellular dehydration* (i.e., intracellular hydration). But under this condition, the volume of the blood is reduced (*hypovolemia*) causing a volumetric disturbance (Fig. 8-1E).

When a water deficit is incurred, the state of *absolute dehydration* ensues. The net result is a reduction of water stores in both intracellular and extracellular compartments. Nevertheless, the proportion of water between both of the compartments is not disturbed (Fig. 8-1B). Consequently, an *increase in the relative* concentration of Na^+ occurs in the extracellular water in the absence of any change in the absolute level of Na^+.

B. Compensatory Responses

A shift in the osmotic tension of the blood during either absolute dehydration (Fig. 8-1B) or intracellular dehydration (Fig. 8-1D) results in a net increase in the relative, but not absolute, concentration of extracellular Na^+ and a net decrease in the actual amount of intracellular water. Such a shift results in thirst, the release of antidiuretic hormone (ADH) and the drinking of water.

The re-instatement of the normal balance in body water is accomplished by a number of remarkable responses including the simple act of seeking water (Blass, 1968). For example, both kinds of dehydration evoke the liberation of ADH from the posterior lobe (neurohypophysis) of the pituitary gland. ADH then acts within the renal tubules of the kidney to facilitate reabsorption of water into the blood. Thus, the excretion of water is prevented by the hypophyseal secretion of ADH during all three types of water deficit. This hormone acts by (a) diluting the relative concentration of an excess in Na^+ ions following intracellular dehydration and (b) diminishing the production and output of urine during hypovolemia and during absolute dehydration. Ever since Linazasoro and his colleagues demonstrated that nephrectomy inhibits drinking which can be re-instated by a systemic injection of kidney extract (Linazasoro *et al.*, 1954; Jiménez-Díaz *et al.*, 1959), the pivotal role of the kidney directed toward the restoration of water balance has been recognized.

A second factor that is as important as ADH in the mechanism for maintaining water balance is angiotensin II. When the blood supply to the kidney declines during hypovolemia, let us say, the kidney reacts swiftly by liberating renin. This hormone then acts on a liver globulin to form angiotensin which is then converted into angiotensin II. A primary functional property of this polypeptide circulating in the plasma is to constrict the blood vessels. By this action, angiotensin can thereby maintain normal blood pressure as well as deviations that are incurred in the face of a reduced blood volume, i.e., the hypovolemia of extracellular dehydration. Second, angiotensin mediates the release of aldosterone from the adrenal glands. This vital hormone causes the kidney to reabsorb sodium in order to minimize the further loss of sodium during the condition of extracellular dehydration. Again as indicated in Fig. 8-2, the reabsorption helps to maintain the volume of blood and enhance the blood pressure response. Third, angiotensin can evoke the release of ADH from the pituitary. Finally, as we shall see in the next section, angiotensin II causes water-seeking behavior.

In summary of Figs. 8-1 and 8-2, two kinds of regulation are generally acknowledged: (1) osmotic and (2) volumetric. The osmotic factors regulating body water center on the act of drinking and the simultaneous actions of ADH. As a result of some elegant research, it is now clear that specialized cells in the brain act as osmoreceptors or osmodetectors (Vincent et al., 1972). These cells are located in the rostral hypothalamus and alter their firing pattern perhaps because of a slight shrinkage in their size in response to an intravascular or local salt challenge.

During extracellular dehydration when Na$^+$ is low and extracellular water is reduced, drinking nevertheless does occur. In this case, a volume receptor in the

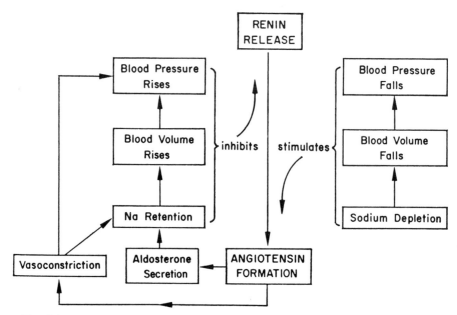

Fig. 8-2 A schematic portrayal of some speculations on the possible homeostatic role of the renin-angiotensin system. (From Douglas, W. W. 1970. *In: The Pharmacological Basis of Therapeutics*, Fourth Edition. L. S. Goodman and A. Gilman (eds.), pp. 663–676. Copyright 1970, The Macmillan Co., New York)

kidney causes the mobilization of angiotensin which presumably acts at certain sites in the nervous system (Fitzsimons, 1971a). Thus, specialized cells in a restricted part of the brain can respond either to an osmotic or a volumetric disturbance.

C. Central Pathways

In a series of classical papers, Ranson and his colleagues have shown that hypothalamic lesions positioned so as to cut through the pathways to the neurohypophysis prevent ADH release (Fisher *et al.*, 1938). A subsequent polyuria, marked polydipsia and a shift in urine composition develop rapidly, and the animal displays the symptoms of diabetes insipidus. These important observations led Verney (Verney, 1947; Jewell and Verney, 1957) to undertake the now renowned experiments in which hypertonic saline was infused into the blood supply of the supraoptic nucleus. Since such an infusion provoked an increased release of ADH, the concept of "osmoreceptor" gradually evolved. Later, other investigators discovered that solutions of different osmotic equivalents affect the discharge pattern of single neurons in this region (Joynt, 1964; Brooks *et al.*, 1970).

In addition to the rostral hypothalamus, the lateral, ventromedial and posterior parts of the hypothalamus have also been implicated in the drinking mechanism. Moreover, the lesioning or stimulation of other structures in the limbic system including the amygdala, septum, hippocampus or corpus striatum may severely alter drinking behavior or even ADH activity (Fitzsimons, 1972). Furthermore, because of the incompatible observations related to the absence of an effect of intraventricular sucrose or urea, Andersson (1971b) has proposed that the ionic composition of the cerebrospinal fluid rather than osmotic tension may exert an influence over ADH release as well as upon the sensation of thirst.

D. Practical Issues

What constitutes drinking behavior as opposed to feeding is still a question open to debate. However, in this chapter we shall consider drinking to be the ingestion of any fluid in a known volume. For instance, if a rat ingests a given quantity of a watered-down solution of sucrose, condensed milk, ethanol or other liquid, this behavior is not designated as eating even though calories may be simultaneously taken. In spite of a high caloric value of a solution of ethanol or the nutritious constituents of a fluid such as Metrecal, the magnitude of water consumed would preclude any sort of generalization that denotes eating. In fact, in experiments in which drinking is called feeding, the compelling controls usually are not done. Offering the animal the choice of solid pelletized food, water, a nutrient solution, a palatable non-nutrient solution, and perhaps an aversive substance would help to distinguish the factors responsible for the ingestion of a substance after a chemical is applied to brain tissue. These factors include: water balance, a caloric deficit, gnawing, nonspecific motor activity, preference for a sweetened compound, or a specific hunger such as that for sodium.

In regard to adequate controls, the application of NaCl as crystals or in an 0.9% solution to the hypothalamus or other structure is undoubtedly an insufficient procedure. In view of the presence of osmosensitive cells, an artificial CSF or other balanced physiological solution should be employed.

Other technical ramifications which may make an experimental finding difficult to interpret are: (1) the size of the lesion produced by the cannula and injection, since even a partial ablation of the lateral, rostral or other hypothalamic area interferes with normal water drinking; (2) the level to which an animal is deprived of water, food, or both substances; (3) the time of day of the experiment in that circadian rhythm may influence water balance; (4) the general experimental set-up including the kind of drinking tube or watering spout; and (5) the interaction of effects produced by a change in temperature, general activity, the symptoms of seizure or food intake itself.

A most pertinent consideration is how one defines the suppression or enhancement of drinking behavior by a centrally given drug or chemical. If the volume taken is 50% of the control value, is that a significant drinking response? That is, does a decline in drinking from 20 to 10 ml have the same meaning as a reduction from 2 to 1 ml? In essence, the way that the measures are expressed and evaluated becomes crucial when considering the chemical nature of the drinking circuit.

II. THIRST RECEPTORS IN THE HYPOTHALAMUS

The osmotic pressure of arterial blood coursing from the internal carotid artery to the supraoptic nucleus is considered to be a principal trigger for the release of ADH. Osmoreceptors located in or about the supraoptic nucleus activate the pathway of the neurosecretory cells which terminate in the posterior pituitary, where ADH is liberated into the rich network of capillaries. Vincent and Hayward (1970) have presented convincing evidence of two types of osmosensitive neurons in the hypothalamus of the monkey. They are (a) specifically responsive to an intra-arterial infusion of hypertonic saline, or (b) nonspecifically responsive to the saline infusion or to other arousing sensory stimuli.

A. Osmoreceptors: Evidence from Stimulation

In the first of a series of classical papers to test Verney's (1947) hypothesis of osmoreceptor signals for thirst, Andersson (1952) showed that a hypertonic solution of NaCl injected into the anterior hypothalamus of the goat evoked intense drinking of up to 2.5 liters of water. Even though the 100 μl volume of the injection was so large that the NaCl spilled over into the ventricle, an injection into other parts of the hypothalamus was not as effective in eliciting the intake of water. Thus, the first direct evidence was presented that cells in the rostral hypothalamus react to an increased osmotic pressure and in so doing, evoke the behavioral response of drinking.

In a further test, Andersson (1953) demonstrated that at points close to the fornix and paraventricular nucleus, the polydipsic effect of hypertonic NaCl was most intense. When control injections were made into the ventricle of the goat, the effect was less pronounced. Moreover, no drinking occurred after the intra-hypothalamic injection of normal or hypotonic saline. The short latency of the response for fluid would rule out both a "dry mouth" interpretation to account for the effect as well as the possibility that polydipsia was secondary to an initial polyuria. This latter sequence is noted always in diabetes insipidus which develops after the infundibular stalk is sectioned (Richter, 1935).

When a much smaller volume in the range of 3 to 10 μl of hypertonic saline is micro-injected into the hypothalamus of the goat, the onset of drinking varies between 30 to 60 seconds (Andersson and McCann, 1955). Imbibition of water continues for about 5 minutes and from 2 to 8 liters are consumed. The region most sensitive to the NaCl lies between the goat's mammillo-thalamic tract and the columns of the fornix. Although electrical stimulation of the same locus caused a similar polydipsia, the drinking is characterized by being more stimulus bound in nature. Figure 8-3 illustrates the appearance of a typical goat after electrical stimulation or NaCl is applied to its hypothalamus.

In an extensive anatomical investigation, Peck and Novin (1971) mapped those diencephalic sites in the rabbit that are sensitive to hypertonic solutions of NaCl, sucrose and urea. In only one anatomical zone, the rabbit's lateral preoptic area, illustrated in Fig. 8-4, did the NaCl or sucrose injection evoke the intense drinking of water. At some sites in the dorsal and lateral hypothalamus, NaCl also produced feeding, gnawing, scratching or other behavior. Hypertonic urea used as a control failed to cause any consistent intake of water. This negative result would be expected, since urea diffuses readily into cells whereas saline and sucrose are, respectively, excluded actively and passively from the intracellular space. In tests of fluid preference the osmotic stimulation of the preoptic area by NaCl or sucrose causes the rabbit to select water over a weak saline solution, even though the rabbit ordinarily chooses a salty solution. Of special significance is the finding that hypertonic NaCl injections into the lateral or dorsal hypothalamus elicited drinking of the normally preferred saline solution. These results show unequivocally that in the rabbit a circumscribed osmosensitive region of the hypothalamus, as portrayed in Fig. 8-4, is specifically sensitive to cellular dehydration.

Additional supportive evidence was obtained in another species by Blass and Epstein (1971) who found that hypertonic NaCl or sucrose causes the rat to drink water when either solution is injected into the lateral preoptic area. The potency and specificity of the polydipsic response is shown in Fig. 8-5. It is interesting that distilled water injected into the same region reduces the ingestion

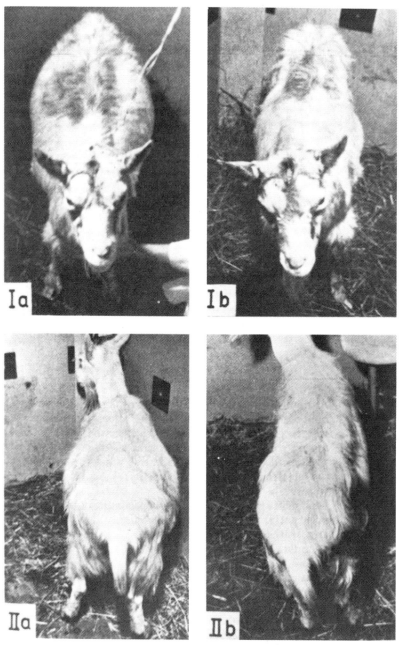

Fig. 8-3 The appearance of two goats (experiment I and II) after overhydration induced by electrical stimulation (Ia and IIa) and their appearance 15 hours later when most of the water had been excreted (Ib and IIb). (From Andersson and McCann, 1955)

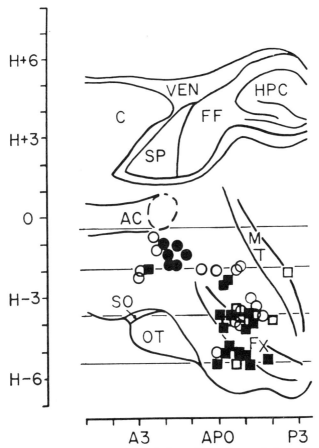

Fig. 8-4 Schematic sagittal section of the rabbit diencephalon taken through the plane joining the fornix and mammillo-thalamic tracts to indicate the distribution of sensitive loci. The horizontal lines indicate the level of the sections. Abbreviations: AC. anterior commissure; C. caudate nucleus; FF. fimbria of fornix; FX. fornix; HPC. hippocampus; VEN. lateral ventricle; MT. mammillo-thalamic area; SO. nucleus supraopticus; OT, optic tract; SP. septum. Symbols: drinking induced by cellular dehydration [●]; drinking induced by saline [○]; eating induced by saline [■]; gnawing, scratching, or licking induced by saline [□]. (From Peck, J. W. and D. Novin. 1971. *J. Comp. Physiol. Psychol.* 74:134–147. Copyright 1971, by the American Psychological Association. Reprinted by permission)

of water elicited by an intraperitoneal injection of saline but not by renin. This inhibition is illustrated in Fig. 8-6. Thus, when cellular dehydration occurs naturally, a rather restricted zone of osmotic sensitivity in the rostral hypothalamus determines the consequent drinking response. That the tonicity of the injection site is an extremely critical factor is absolutely clear in that only 180 mM of NaCl cause drinking.

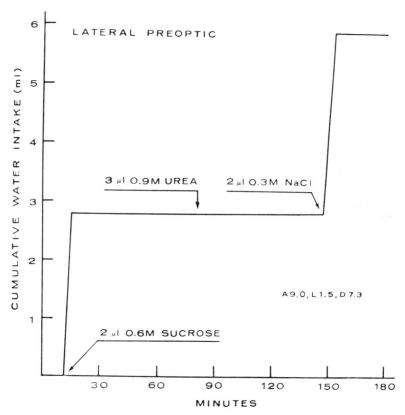

Fig. 8-5 Specificity of drinking to hypertonic solutions injected into the LPO. Hypertonic saline and sucrose elicited drinking. Hyperosmolal urea did not. (From Blass, E. M. and A. N. Epstein. 1971. *J. Comp. Physiol. Psychol.* 76:378–394. Copyright 1971, by the American Psychological Association. Reprinted by permission)

B. ADH Release Mechanism

In an extraordinary early experiment, Pickford (1947) demonstrated the anatomical specificity of ACh on a selected region in the hypothalamus of the dog. After 2 to 40 μg of ACh were injected into the supraoptic nucleus, the flow of urine during water diuresis was substantially inhibited. This reduction in output was prolonged by the addition of eserine to the injection solution, which corresponds perfectly with the expected facilitating effect of the anticholinesterase. These pharmacological results led Pickford to the hypothesis that ACh is released at the level of the supraoptic nucleus, which in turn induces the secretion of ADH from the posterior lobe of the pituitary into the bloodstream. To pinpoint the morphological specificity of this dramatic effect, ACh was injected

DRINKING INDUCED by 2 ml, 2M NaCl IP

O 2 µl 0.15M NaCl ic   ● 2 µl Distilled HOH ic

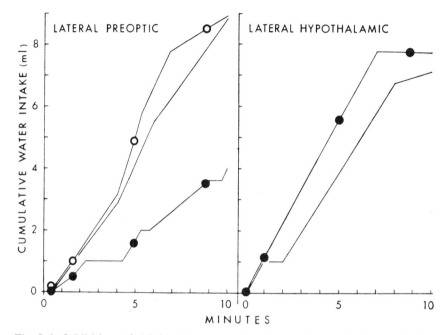

Fig. 8-6 Inhibition of drinking to systemic cellular dehydration by 2 µl injections of distilled water into the LPO. Intracranial injections of isotonic saline into the LPO did not inhibit drinking, nor did injections of distilled water into the lateral hypothalamic area (right panel). (From Blass, E. M. and A. N. Epstein. 1971. *J. Comp. Physiol. Psychol.* 76:378–394. Copyright 1971, by the American Psychological Association. Reprinted by permission)

into the lateral hypothalamus or mammillary bodies; the urine flow did not change. Thus, the first direct evidence was presented of a central cholinergic mechanism underlying the excretion of body water.

As a further test of the idea that ACh could be a transmitter involved in ADH release in the supraoptic nucleus, additional experiments with the powerful anticholinesterase, diisopropylfluorophosphate (DFP), were carried out in Pickford's laboratory. DFP combines irreversibly with cholinesterase, and when it was injected into the supraoptic nucleus of the dog, it stopped urine flow immediately (Duke *et al.*, 1950). Then a profound polyuria followed that lasted for 4 to 19 days. The normal urine flow in response to the injection of ACh in the supraoptic nucleus returned only after approximately 3 to 4 months. This remarkable sequence of events could be explained on the basis of two successive stages: (1) a mutually elevated level of ACh caused by DFP, which is followed by (2) a paralyzing action on the cells of the supraoptic nucleus of an abnormally high concentration of ACh which persists. Although the longevity in the recovery of a normal pattern of urinary excretion is notable, this is in accord with the well-known toxicity of DFP.

C. Angiotensin II Receptors

Angiotensin II has a direct excitatory effect on single neurons of the supraoptic nucleus of the cat. The polypeptide increases their firing rate almost instantaneously when applied iontophoretically (Nicoll and Barker, 1971). Since the response of cortical and other individual neurons not involved in cardiovascular and volume regulation is unaffected, the specificity of this local augmentation in activity is probable. Thus, angiotensin, if it passes into this part of the CNS from the systemic circulation, may also release ADH from the neurosecretory cells of the supraoptic nucleus through its effect on ACh.

In 1968, the first report appeared of the polydipsic effect of angiotensin on the central nervous system. Booth (1968c) found that 1.8 µg of angiotensin injected into the antero-lateral hypothalamus of the rat elicited a spontaneous intake of water that averaged 9.8 ml. This initial discovery was not only fortuitous but at the same time valid. That is, a control for the local vascular effects of angiotensin was intrinsically provided by other control injections that were done by Booth to rule out the possible vasoactive action of adrenergic substances which produced eating (Chapter 7).

Although the doses given were not cited, Hendler and Blake (1969) localized the polydipsic action of angiotensin II to the anterior hypothalamus of the rat. An implant of crystals of the peptide did not produce drinking when deposited in the ventromedial or posterior hypothalamus. Also, an implant of aldosterone had no effect whatsoever on water intake. A significant rise in blood pressure also occurred when the angiotensin compound was applied to sites in the rostral hypothalamus. It is interesting that the amount of water consumed by 24-hour deprived rats was attenuated when the norepinephrine was implanted in the anterior and ventromedial sites or when carbachol was applied in the postero-lateral hypothalamus.

When a rat is in a normal state of water balance, angiotensin II evokes a dose-dependent drinking of water. This response occurs if the peptide is injected as shown in Fig. 8-7, into the septum, anterior hypothalamus, the most sensitive preoptic area, and also the lateral and ventromedial hypothalamus (Epstein et al., 1970). Doses of either 0.5 or 1 µg seemed to be maximal (Fig. 8-7); the drinking response was repeatable and described as motivated. Although carbachol and renin also elicited drinking when injected at the same hypothalamic loci, the significant point was that the volume ingested was not nearly as great. Further, when vasopressin, epinephrine, norepinephrine, aldosterone and brady-

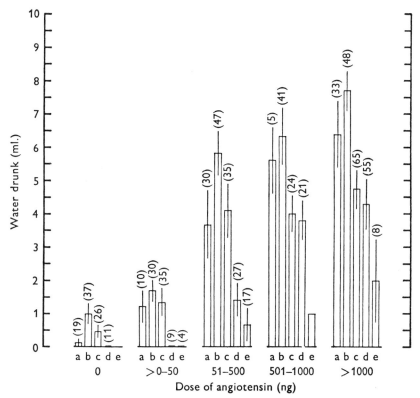

Fig. 8-7 The relationship between the mean amounts of water drunk and the intracranial dose of angiotensin. Results for all animals have been grouped together according to the range of doses used and the anatomical locus of the cannula tip. Note the decrease in sensitivity as the locus of injection is moved from (a) the septal region, (b) the preoptic region and (c) the anterior hypothalamic area, where sensitivity is highest, to (d) the lateral hypothalamic area and (e) the ventromedial hypothalamic region where sensitivity is lower. The vertical lines on the bars represent 1 SE of the mean on either side of the mean. The numbers in parentheses are the number of observations. (From Epstein *et al.*, 1970)

kinin were injected at homologous sites, there was no significant change in water intake. As a result of these convincing observations, Epstein *et al.* concluded that angiotensin II is the natural hormone mediating water balance and drinking behavior. When the stimulus from the kidney activates the production of angiotensin in a concentration high enough to exert a direct action on the chemoreceptive region in the hypothalamus, the animal seeks out water and drinks. The intensely motivating property of the peptide has been shown by Rolls *et al.* (1972) in that a rat will depress a lever to obtain water at the same rate as an animal deprived of fluid for 24 hours.

Fitzsimons (1971b) then found that renin-induced drinking in the rat is characterized by a much longer latency and duration than angiotensin II. These striking differences are graphically demonstrated in Fig. 8-8. However, angiotensin I and the synthetic tetradecapeptide, renin substrate, were as effective as angiotensin II in evoking the drinking of water as were two other angiotensin II octapeptides. In the doses injected, the hexapeptide and pentapeptide forms had little or no dipsogenic activity, nor did bradykinin, vasopressin, oxytocin, cyclic AMP or saline. These results on renin and angiotensin I suggest that a converting enzyme is present in the angiotensin II sensitive zone of the rat's hypothalamus, which could give rise to angiotensin II locally. Alternatively, these compounds may mimic angiotensin II or have a pharmacological action of their own that may involve the release of another humoral factor or transmitter.

The efficacy of angiotensin in inducing a rat to drink water continues even after a 60 minute interval when water is withheld (Rolls and Jones, 1972). When the rat's access to its water tube was not delayed, the animal stopped drinking in about 8 minutes after the angiotensin was injected into the rostral hypothalamus. As one would expect, the satiation to the intragastric fluid load rather than the local inactivation of angiotensin is responsible for the cessation

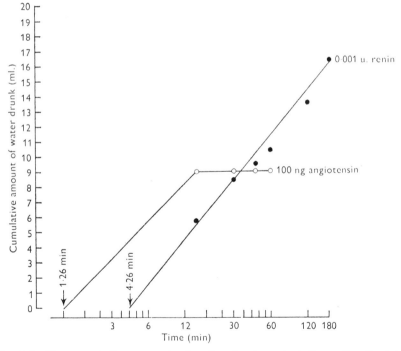

Fig. 8-8 The cumulative amount of water drunk against time after the intracranial injection of 0.001 Goldblatt u. renin (●) or 100 ng angiotensin II (○). Each curve is the mean obtained from ten rats. The onset of drinking is indicated by the arrow and the mean latency is given. (From Fitzsimons, 1971b)

of drinking. A similar result is obtained when isotonic sodium chloride is offered
as the test fluid instead of water. Slightly more of the saline solution is consumed probably because the rat prefers its taste or because of some unknown
post-ingestional factor. Using a test solution of 1.5% sodium chloride, Covian *et
al.* (1972) found that water was selected preferentially over the saline in response
to an injection of angiotensin into the septum.

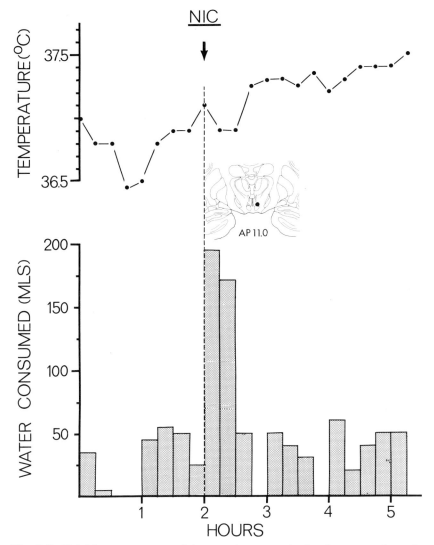

Fig. 8-9 Drinking responses and temperature record of a rhesus monkey after
5 μg nicotine were injected at coronal plane AP 11.0 in a volume of 1 μl at a site
within the fasciculus princeps dorsal to the mammillary body (inset). (From
Myers *et al.*, 1973)

1. Angiotensin-Nicotine Drinking

The rhesus monkey is an animal which does not drink reliably in response to the chemical stimulation of its brain without eating food (Myers, 1969b). However, Myers *et al.* (1973) found that nicotine produced a mammoth intake of up to 365 ml of water within 30 minutes after a micro-injection at 18 of 153 sites in the hypothalamus and mesencephalon. One such bout of hyperdipsia is presented in Fig. 8-9. An anatomical analysis of the injection sites revealed that most of the nicotine-sensitive loci were clustered within and around the mammillary complex. Surprisingly, angiotensin II exerted an identical dipsogenic effect when it was micro-injected at the homologous sites, portrayed in Fig. 8-10, in the caudal hypothalamus. This region is in direct contrast to the area of maximum sensitivity in the rat, which is reportedly the rostral hypothalamus. Because of the large volumes injected into the rat's brain by Epstein *et al.* (1970), somewhat more caudal sites may actually have been stimulated. In view of the morphological concordance of nicotine and angiotensin-active sites (Fig. 8-10), Myers *et al.* hypothesized that the renal polypeptide activates the release of ACh from cholinergic synapses of efferent neurons along a drinking pathway. This transmitter would act at nicotinic receptor sites in the primate's brain, since carbachol stimulation can block a monkey's drinking response which is reversed by the injection of the muscarinic antagonist, atropine, at the same hypothalamic site (Myers, 1969b).

2. Antagonism of Angiotensin Drinking

An exceptionally pertinent observation was made by Giardina and Fisher (1971). Methyl atropine failed to block the angiotensin- or isoproterenol-induced water intake of the rat when the cholinolytic was implanted in the septum 10 minutes before either of the other two dipsogenic compounds. Therefore, the drinking produced by angiotensin or the beta-adrenergic agonist could act by a mechanism that is independent of a muscarinic-type cholinergic thirst circuit, as described in the next section. More important is the fact that the isoproterenol given peripherally in a dose one-fourth of the intrahypothalamic dose used by Leibowitz (1971) caused an intake of water in a volume much greater than that when

---

Fig. 8-10 Morphological mapping within six coronal planes of the sites in the diencephalon and mesencephalon of the rhesus monkey at which 1 μg angiotensin in a 1 μl volume elicited intense drinking of water (●) or no change in water intake (o). Anatomical structures are abbreviated as follows: a. cerebral aqueduct; d. dorsomedial nucleus; ff. fields of Forel; f. fornix; gp. globus pallidus; ic. internal capsule; l. lateral hypothalamus; m. mammillary body; mp. mammillary fasciculus princeps; mt. mammillo-thalamic tract; n. nucleus ruber; np. nucleus paracentralis; nr. nucleus reuniens; nv. ventrolateral nucleus of the thalamus; ot. optic tract; p. posterior hypothalamus; pp. cerebral peduncles; pv. paraventricular nucleus; r. reticular nucleus; s. nucleus subthalamicus; sn. substantia nigra; 3V. third ventricle; va. anteroventral nucleus of the thalamus; vm. ventromedial nucleus. (From Myers *et al.*, 1973)

Angiotensin → Drinking

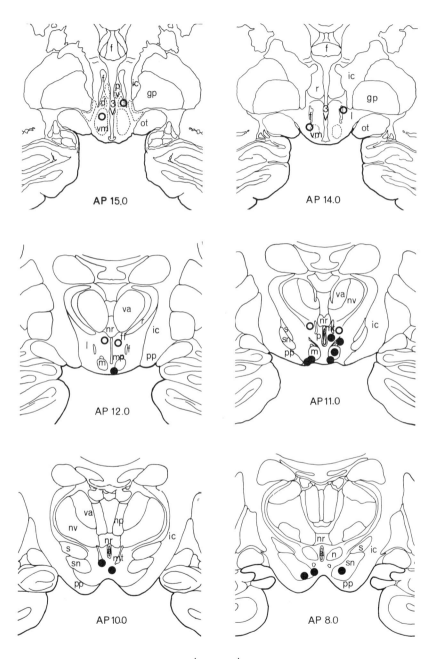

the β agonist is given centrally. This confirms the idea of Lehr *et al.* (1967) and the hypothesis of Houpt and Epstein (1971) that the drinking elicited by a beta-adrenergic agonist is a result of a peripheral effect. Isoproterenol drinking is blocked by nephrectomy, which further suggests that the mechanism is the activation of the renin-angiotensin pathway, and the subsequent excitation of the anterior-preoptic area by angiotensin. A dose-response relationship would be required to substantiate this notion.

Another important correlation of angiotensin-sensitive sites with cholinoceptive loci revealed that the hydrated rat ingested water after either substance was injected into 80% of the hypothalamic sites tested (White *et al.*, 1972). The overall volumes consumed were similar in response to both compounds but did not necessarily correlate with the selective sensitivity of an individual site. While two cholinolytic agents, atropine or scopolamine, failed to reduce angiotensin-induced drinking, they did exert their characteristic inhibiting action on carbachol drinking. The alpha-adrenergic blocker, phentolamine, also did not prevent the drinking of water following the angiotensin micro-injection. The intake of a hypertonic saline solution offered to the rat when angiotensin was micro-injected was avoided in much the same way as the aversion to the saline that follows carbachol stimulation (Stricker and Miller, 1968).

When a systemic dose of atropine (10 mg/kg) was given which will block the polydipsia induced by an intrahypothalamic injection of carbachol, the drinking elicited by a solution of angiotensin or NaCl injected into the lateral preoptic area of the rat was only partially attenuated by the cholinergic antagonist (Blass and Chapman, 1971). When atropine was injected directly into the rat's preoptic area, the resultant drinking caused by systemic renin was only mildly attenuated. Following an intraperitoneal injection of sodium chloride, the central injection of atropine also failed to inhibit drinking caused by this form of systemic cellular dehydration. Thus, if a blockade by the neuromuscular antagonist can be accepted as an end-point, muscarinic receptors and/or a muscarinic-type cholinergic pathway is probably not the exclusive mediator of the thirst which arises from an imbalance in body fluid economy. Apparently, other neurohumoral factors in the hypothalamus and other structures must participate in the drinking response. In this regard, Covian *et al.* (1972) failed to note a blockade of angiotensin induced drinking following intra-septal injections of atropine, propranolol, phentolamine or methysergide.

An intricate relationship between the volumetric control ostensibly mediated by angiotensin and osmometric regulation involving NaCl may eventually be established anatomically. Andersson and his colleagues have hypothesized that angiotensin could act by way of the third cerebral ventricle to facilitate the transependymal transport of sodium ions to those cells in the hypothalamus which release ADH (Andersson and Westbye, 1970) or other cells that influence blood pressure (Andersson *et al.*, 1971). When angiotensin II is mixed with a solution of isotonic glucose or urea and then infused into the ventricle of a goat, the drinking response is much less then when the angiotensin is infused together with NaCl (Andersson et al., 1970). Finally, Daniels-Severs et al. (1971) believe that angiotensin and salt balance are directly related and, in fact, the polypeptide could impinge upon the appropriate cells in the brain so that a local condition of hyperosmolality would be detected. In this connection, very small doses of angiotensin given intraventricularly in the rat evoke drinking along with elevated plasma corticosterone levels (Daniels-Severs et al., 1971).

III. CHOLINERGIC THIRST SYSTEM

Ever since the original report of Grossman in 1960 that crystals of either ACh or carbachol placed in the hypothalamus of the rat evoked spontaneous drinking (Grossman, 1960), this observation has been one of the most widely witnessed in this field—literally thousands of times in laboratories scattered throughout the world from North Ryde to Utrecht. Unfortunately, all of these experiments have been done only with the rat and a generalization of the phenomenon to other species has not materialized (Myers and Sharpe, 1968b). The reasons for this disturbing note on the one hand, but the compelling assortment of facts in support of the role of ACh in thirst on the other (Levitt, 1971) will be discussed at the conclusion of this chapter.

In the first study of the central effect of a putative transmitter on ingestive behavior, Grossman (1960) showed that crystals of carbachol or ACh elicited drinking when deposited in a dose probably far less than that described. Of the original conclusions set forth, two were erroneous: (1) that adrenergic stimulation did not evoke drinking as a main effect, which was refuted later (Myers, 1964b; Margules, 1970a and b; Leibowitz, 1971); and (2) the density of cells sensitive to the cholinomimetic was highly concentrated in the lateral hypothalamus. In spite of this, the preliminary evidence constituted an important breakthrough in this field which was followed by a spate of research.

In the 24-hour water-deprived rat, drinking was potentiated by carbachol applied to the perifornical region of the hypothalamus (Grossman, 1962a). A rat reportedly would also depress a lever only to obtain water following carbachol application. Thus, a motivated component of chemical stimulation was demonstrated for the first time. Later that year, the pharmacological specificity of the excessive intake of water in response to cholinergic stimulation was shown when Grossman (1962b) applied crystals of atropine just before carbachol at the same site. The amount of water that the rat drank was suppressed substantially.

Following closely on the heels of these early studies was another in which the one, two or three tap method (Chapter 2) was introduced for tamping crystals of a drug into the brain of a rat (Stein and Seifter, 1962). In addition to confirming Grossman's report, synthetic muscarine was found to produce as "good" a drinking response as carbachol. Since nicotine had only a weak effect, muscarinic synapses in the hypothalamus were implicated in the rat's drinking of water. Additional strength to this supposition was provided by the equal blockade by crystals of atropine of the drinking elicited by either muscarine or carbachol.

With this set of findings, the notion of an ACh mediated mechanism in the brain for drinking evolved, and the cholinergic receptor sites were believed to be muscarinic, at least for the rat.

A. Anatomy of the Thirst Circuit

In a classical paper, Fisher and Coury (1962) soon repudiated the idea of a specific anatomical locus underlying drinking. They reported that cholinergic stimulation of widespread sites in the hippocampus, septum, thalamus and hypothalamus evoked the polydipsic response, with the most sensitive area lying in the dentate fasciculus of the hippocampus. The conclusion was thus drawn that a cholinergic pathway corresponding to the Papez anatomical "circuit" mediates the sensation of thirst and the behavior of drinking. Parenthetically, five instances of feeding also occurred after crystals of carbachol were implanted (Chapter 7), but the anatomical areas of stimulation were not specified. In 1964, these findings were presented in terms of the anatomical pathways diagrammed in Fig. 8-11 (Fisher and Coury, 1964). Later, Coury (1967) showed that at most sites throughout the limbic system, excluding the hypothalamus, which follow the pathways of the Papez system, carbachol elicited only drinking. In contrast to feeding, these results seem to reflect a far wider anatomical diffuseness underlying the drinking behavior of the laboratory rat.

A dose-dependent drinking response can be obtained whether carbachol is injected in an 0.9% NaCl solution or as crystals in a mixture of dextrose at any of a large number of sites. These include the lateral, anterior or posterior parts of the hypothalamus, the preoptic area, anterior thalamus, hippocampus, fornix or corpus callosum (Levitt et al., 1970). The volume and threshold are similar in each instance. However, the average latency to drink after the injection of a carbachol solution, independent of site, was 3.5 minutes but 6.5 minutes after the crystals of the drug were deposited. The distance of the carbachol placement to the ventricle was not a factor. Instead, the sites again appeared to be part of a larger and diffuse trajectory of interconnected neurons that spans the entire limbic system.

A further examination of the anatomical characteristics of the rat's central thirst circuit revealed that after the implantation of crystalline carbachol into the antero-dorsal but not postero-ventral portions of the hippocampus, the rat drank water (Grant and Jarrard, 1968). The general level of activity also increased following cholinergic stimulation of this antero-dorsal region. Water intake but not activity level was enhanced when carbachol was placed also in the fornix or cingulum. A part of these results was replicated by Mountford (1969) who not only placed carbachol in the hippocampal formation but also in the adjacent lateral ventricle. Water intake was significantly above the control levels following stimulation of the hippocampus. In confirming the earlier results of Myers and Cicero (1968) and Khavari *et al.* (1968), Mountford found that the rat did not increase its fluid consumption significantly when the cholinomimetic was deposited directly in the ventricle. As Grant and Jarrard (1968) observed, carbachol also caused some eating as well.

The anatomy of the thirst circuit has also been investigated by the use of a cholinolytic compound. If atropine is implanted at a site in the limbic system of the rat at which carbachol previously had produced drinking, then the anticholinergic agent inhibits the intake of water elicited by carbachol implanted at another active site at which carbachol always evoked drinking (Levitt and Fisher, 1966). Thus, each of the anatomical components of the proposed thirst circuit seems to be functionally related to acetylcholine.

In extending the work of Fisher's group, Singer and Montgomery (1969) showed that the amygdala is closely integrated with the lateral hypothalamus. Atropine injected in the fornix of the rat blocks the drinking produced by carbachol injected into the amygdala. Similarly, carbachol injected in both of

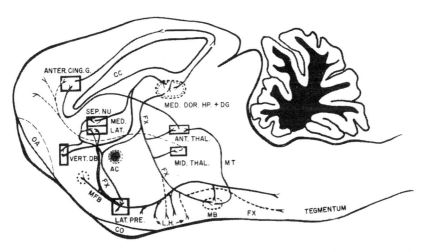

Fig. 8-11 A schematic representation of brain structures and pathways which are involved in the cholinergic stimulation-drinking response relationship. AC. anterior commissure; CC. corpus callosum; CO. optic chiasma; FX. fornix; LH. lateral hypothalamus; MB. mammillary bodies; MFB. medial forebrain bundle; MT. mammillo-thalamic tract; OA. olfactory area; ANTER. CING. G. anterior cingulate gyrus; ANT. THAL. anterior thalamus; LAT. PRE. lateral preoptic region; MED. DORS. HP and DG. medial dorsal hippocampus and area of dentate gyrus; MID. THAL. mesial thalamic nuclei; SEP. NU. medial and lateral septal nuclei; VERT. DB. diagonal band of Broca; >—< two way connections between regions so marked. (From Fisher and Coury, 1964)

SIMPLIFIED FISHER-COURY CIRCUIT

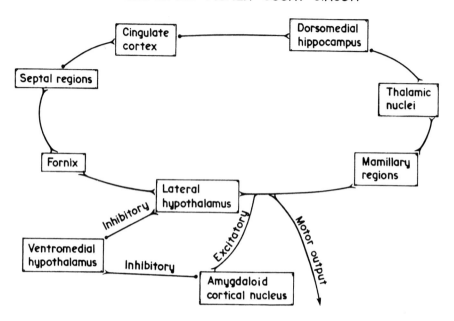

MODULATORY CIRCUIT

Fig. 8-12 Diagrammatic representation of functional relationships between Fisher-Coury (lateral hypothalamus-septal area) circuit, amygdaloid circuit and ventromedial hypothalamic circuit. The Fisher-Coury circuit is the initiating circuit underlying drinking behavior, and is inhibited by activity in the ventromedial hypothalamic circuit during satiety. Activation of the Fisher-Coury circuit activates the amygdaloid circuit, which in turn inhibits the ventromedial hypothalamic circuit, thus releasing the Fisher-Coury circuit from ventromedial inhibition, and thereby augmenting its activity. (From Singer, G. and R. B. Montgomery. 1970. *Life Sciences.* 9:91–97. Pergamon Press, New York)

these structures simultaneously caused the rat to drink more than that observed when the cholinomimetic was injected into the lateral hypothalamus alone. Although the modulatory influence of the amygdala may be indirect, it would seem to be an essential component of the drinking circuit as witnessed by the effect of the anticholinergic in nullifying the cholinergic action on the hypothalamus. Similarly, the spontaneous drinking seen after carbachol is injected into the septum (Singer and Montgomery, 1970) is either enhanced by carbachol or blocked by atropine when these cholinomimetic or anticholinergic substances were injected simultaneously into the amygdala. This relationship is similar to the amygdaloid-hypothalamic interaction. Figure 8-12 presents a simplified version of the Fisher-Coury circuit (Fig. 8-11) depicting the possible connections between each of the limbic structures involved in the modulatory part of the central thirst system.

1. *Sensitivity of Sites*

The diagonal band of Broca (tractus diagonalis) of the rat is particularly sensitive to the application of carbachol, atropine or methyl atropine (Terpstra and Slangen, 1972a). In terms of the blockade of carbachol-induced drinking, as little as 0.15 μg of atropine injected in this structure before 1.3 μg of the cholinomimetic reduced the intake of water by 90%. This dose of atropine is about 3 to 10 times lower than that used in earlier studies in which the cholinergic antagonist blocked drinking when applied at other sites in the limbic system.

In a related study, drinking was elicited by injecting carbachol in a dose of 1 μg or less into the subfornical organ (Routtenberg and Simpson, 1971), a structure that has had only a recent history in the drinking literature. Carbachol injected through a 24 gauge cannula placed into the third ventricle at a site close to the subfornical organ also evoked the spontaneous intake of water. However, the dose required to produce an equal effect was significantly greater and the latency much longer than when applied to the subfornical tissue. Therefore, a ventricular hypothesis is again not upheld (Chapter 2) to explain carbachol's action in which the drug leaves the tissue, enters the ventricle where it is diluted, and returns to tissue to elicit an effect.

Perhaps the site in the brain most sensitive to carbachol is indeed the subfornical organ. Simpson and Routtenberg (1972) have gone to great pains with a 34 gauge injector needle and a sensible 0.5 μl volume to obtain a dose-response curve for water intake following the injection of carbachol in this structure. As little as 0.05 μg of the cholinomimetic elicited drinking with a latency that was much shorter than a similar injection into the lateral hypothalamus given in a significantly larger volume. A composite comparison of the potency of carbachol at different sites is shown in Fig. 8-13. The possibility that the subfornical organ is part of the monitoring system for sodium ions or molecules of angiotensin is raised since a lesion of this structure produces a partial adipsia. Unfortunately, this reduction in water intake lasts for only one day. However, the morphological position, the capillary network and the neurosecretory cells contained in the subfornical organ taken together would suggest that this structure may be an important link in the cholinergic thirst circuit.

Crystals of acetylcholine, eserine, or a combination of both reportedly placed in the third ventricle evoke drinking, which does not occur when the substances are deposited in the lateral ventricle (Chiaraviglio and Taleisnik, 1969). However, the histological reconstructions revealed that nearly all of the designated placements that were reactive to the cholinergic substances were located in the medial septal nucleus, fornix or preoptic area. In any event, the cannula assembly was 0.6 mm in diameter which is much wider than the third ventricle of the rat. Hence, the needle obviously encroached upon the tissue of the medial preoptic or anterior hypothalamic area, regions that are highly sensitive to the application of a cholinergic substance in terms of dipsogenic activity (Fisher and Coury, 1962).

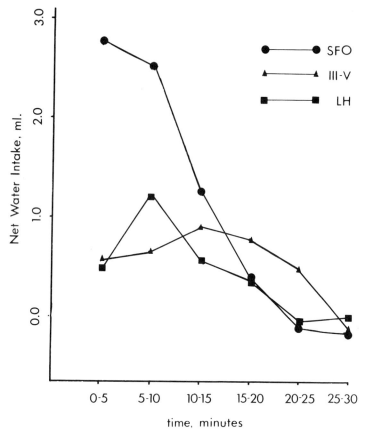

Fig. 8-13 Net water intake as a function of successive 5-minute periods for animals with all dosage levels of carbachol applied to subfornical organ (SFO), interventricular foramen (III-V), or lateral hypothalamus (LH). Point on ordinate for all groups is mean water intake for 5 minute intervals during baseline (unstimulated) periods. (From Simpson, J. B. and A. Routtenberg. 1972. *Brain Res.* **45**:135–152. Fig. 4. Elsevier Publishing Co., Amsterdam, The Netherlands)

2. *Lesions of the Circuit*

In the rat in which a lesion is placed in the lateral hypothalamus, carbachol fails to elicit the typical drinking pattern when the drug is injected into highly sensitive sites within the anterior or posterior hypothalamus (Wolf and Miller, 1964). Carbachol did, however, produce drinking if lesions were positioned more rostrally or posteriorly. After the usual 1 to 3 week period of recovery following lateral lesions at which time the volume of water consumed returns to 70% or 80% of the normal daily intake, carbachol nevertheless failed to elicit drinking when injected at the same sites even after 6 weeks. Thus, the lateral hypothalamic area is perhaps more crucially involved than any other in the cholinergic circuit. Clearly, a pathway alternative to the cholinergic one must be utilized in the drinking system so that normal fluid balance is maintained after the rat recovers from the destruction of its lateral hypothalamus.

A very interesting observation by Parks *et al.* (1971) showed that the polydipsic response to crystals of carbachol implanted in the lateral septal nucleus was totally abolished for at least 30 days after the lateral hypothalamus had been lesioned bilaterally. Surprisingly, when the situation was reversed and the septal nuclei were ablated, intense drinking occurred when carbachol was deposited in the lateral hypothalamus. These differences in drinking are presented in Fig. 8-14. As mentioned previously, the septum may facilitate the impulses for thirst along the principal pathway to the hypothalamus in a way similar to that of the ventral amygdala (Grossman, 1964b). It would seem that the hypothalamus receives the primary motorial confluence of all anatomical systems involved in the intake of water and for that matter ingestive behavior in general.

A unilateral lesion of the hypothalamic site at which carbachol ordinarily elicits drinking will also abolish the typical drinking response after carbachol crystals are deposited in the lateral septum or anterior thalamus of the rat (Stein and Levitt, 1971). Again, a lesion of either the septal or the thalamic structure fails to prevent drinking produced by carbachol placed at other points in the limbic system. When atropine is deposited directly in a lesioned site, the rat's drinking was effectively abolished. Thus, the muscarinic blocking agent selec-

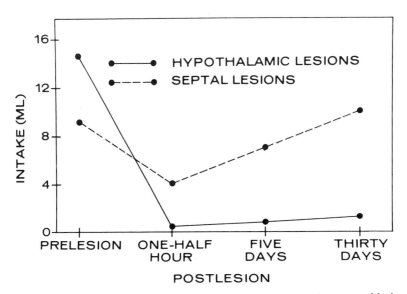

Fig. 8-14 Average water intake for animals with hypothalamic or septal lesions. (From Parks *et al.*, 1971)

tively attaches to cholinergic receptors within a local region and does not act simply by causing a temporary, functional lesion.

B. Pharmacology of the Thirst Circuit

When carbachol is implanted in the septum of a fasted or satiated rat, the drinking of water increases. At the same time, carbachol may suppress the food intake even in the animal that has been deprived of food (Grossman, 1964b). Although implants of epinephrine or norepinephrine in the amygdala attenuate the lever pressing for water in the water-deprived rat, carbachol, ACh or Dibenzyline, an alpha receptor blocker, enhances the lever responding for water when the drugs are deposited at the same site (Grossman, 1964a). GABA also possesses a cholinomimetic action on drinking when inserted into the amygdala, which was blocked by prior implants of hydroxylamine, a GABA antagonist. Montgomery and Singer (1969b) failed to replicate this finding in that their rats did not drink after GABA was injected in the ventral amygdala. Solutions of GABA were injected at sites in the amygdala homologous to those of Grossman and in a volume of 0.5 to 1 μl in five different concentrations. Since hydroxylamine prevents the degradation of GABA and should potentiate any local effect of GABA, crystals of GABA apparently do not act as a neurohumoral excitant but probably block an inhibitory influence on drinking that might emanate from the amygdala.

After Levitt (1969) had tamped carbachol into the rat's septum, anterior thalamus or anterior midbrain in order to establish reliable drinking, the actions of 13 substances were tested. Only atropine and scopalamine were found to block cholinergic drinking reliably when deposited either at the site of carbachol stimulation or at one of the other sites in the thirst circuit. Generally, there was a greater blockade when the drug was placed at a different site. Compounds in addition to the muscarinic blockers which reduced cholinergic-induced drinking by more than 30% when implanted at distant sites were acetylcholinesterase, hemicholinium, phenoxybenzamine, pentobarbital, procaine, strychnine and picrotoxin. The absence of dose-response data, however, precludes any speculation about the pharmacological specificity of the inhibition of drinking by these substances.

Atropine has also been shown to interfere with the motivated component of thirst (Grossman, 1966a). When crystals of this muscarinic blocker were deposited in the ventromedial hypothalamus of the rat, the animal ceased to lever press to secure droplets of water. Placed in the septum, atropine also suppresses drinking when the measure of water intake is taken at 1- or 24-hour intervals (Kelsey and Grossman, 1969). A typical blockade of drinking by atropine placed in the highly sensitive diagonal band of Broca (Terpstra and Slangen, 1972a) is illustrated in Fig. 8-15.

The assertion that ACh or carbachol induced drinking, even though blocked by atropine, represents an actual functional response rather than a nonphysio-

% inhibition

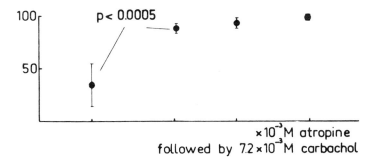

× 10^{-3} M atropine
followed by 7.2 × 10^{-3} M carbachol

water intake in ml

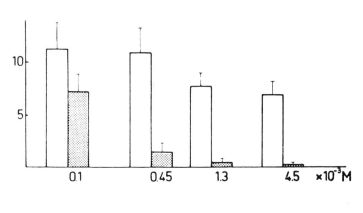

☐ carbachol preceded by mock injection

▨ carbachol preceded by atropine

Fig. 8-15 The effect of different doses of atropine on the water intake elicited by carbachol stimulation. The results are expressed as the mean ± SE of the values obtained. In the upper part of the figure the inhibiting effect is expressed as the percentage of inhibition, putting the water intake elicited by 7.2 nmol of carbachol at 100%. In the bottom of the figure the effect is expressed as the amount of milliliters of water drunk after carbachol stimulation only and after atropine and carbachol stimulation. (From Terpstra and Slangen, 1972a)

logical effect has been strengthened by the experiments of Miller and Chien (1968). Eserine, an anticholinesterase which prevents the degradation of ACh and thereby elevates the endogenous store of this presumed central transmitter, evokes drinking when the drug is injected into the preoptic area of the water satiated rat. It enhances an even greater intake in the rat deprived of food and water for 5 hours. The resultant inference that cholinergic synapses exist in the preoptic area was supported by the anatomical findings of Levitt and Boley (1970). They demonstrated that eserine produces drinking in the rat at virtually all carbachol-sensitive sites in every limbic structure that was tested. Atropine injected at a contralateral site also blocked the eserine-induced imbibition of water with the same latency of 4 minutes.

A replication of many earlier observations by Antunes-Rodrigues and Covain (1971) again demonstrated that the drinking induced by carbachol injected into the septum of the rat is blocked by the prior administration of atropine at the same site. In addition, tap water was preferred over isotonic saline when the choice was offered.

In a study in which a 1 μl injection was made in the fiber system instead of in a nucleus, carbachol but not eserine caused the rat to drink (Levitt and O'Hearn, 1972). These surprising results indicate that the cholinomimetic may act on axons in the central nervous system to depolarize the membrane of the neurons in the thirst system. The fact that atropine injected into the fornix also blocked drinking following a carbachol injection in the septum suggests that the fiber bundle is equally sensitive to the presence of the anticholinergic drug. Of course, there may be axonal spreading to cholinoceptive sites at the synapse, which would render this supposition invalid. Obviously, a study using a radiotracer is called for.

C. Relation to Natural Thirst

The hypothesis that the phenomenon of cholinergic drinking is an analogue to natural thirst has been the subject of some controversy. A rational case for this concept was presented by Khavari and Russell (1966) who found that a rat which was deprived of fluid or a water-sated rat stimulated by a carbachol implant in the lateral hypothalamus ran a T-maze in an identical manner for water reinforcement. The behavioral test, therefore, shows that cholinergic stimulation and a water deficit have the same net effect on the animal.

Although the level of deprivation is known to affect the magnitude of the drinking response induced by a carbachol implant, Russell et al. (1968) concluded that a water deficit entailed by 3 hours of deprivation constituted an optimal interval. After a 24-hour period, the percent increase in the rat's water intake was insignificant. Even though the actual volumes of water were not denoted, the results fit the innovative model of Russell et al. in which the drinking activity of the rat is dependent entirely upon the channel capacity of the system for water balance.

Along these same lines, the ingestion of water by a rat that has been deprived of fluid for 23 hours is not altered by an implant of either atropine or scopalamine in the septum or anterior thalamus (Levitt, 1968). However, if food is made available to the animal at the same time in the test cage, then the rat drinks about 10% less water. This reduction can probably account for the extra space occupied intragastrically by the food that was eaten, another factor that would surely influence channel capacity.

As explained above, atropine deposited at one site can block the drinking induced by carbachol placed at another site in the rat's limbic thirst "circuit." However, the implantation of atropine at any of three structures, the septum, anterior thalamus or lateral hypothalamus, of a rat deprived of water for 23 hours does not reduce the volume of water usually consumed as a result of such deprivation (Levitt and Fisher, 1967). This important finding shows that drinking due to a water deficit is not neuropharmacologically identical to carbachol-stimulated drinking. Although somewhat at odds with an earlier report (Grossman, 1962b) in which atropine did depress the water intake of a fluid-deprived rat, the animal in this latter study had sustained a unilateral lesion which in itself could intensify the local antagonistic response to a cholinergic blocking agent.

Further evidence has been presented on the question of whether a natural thirst mechanism is related to a cholinergically-induced ingestion of water. Lumping together the information on carbachol implants at all sites in the septum, thalamus and hypothalamus of the rat, Krikstone and Levitt (1970) found that carbachol enhanced drinking of water remarkably after a deprivation interval. This facilitation is represented for three levels of deprivation in Fig. 8-16. Atropine had virtually no inhibitory action on the rat's water intake regardless of the number of hours that the rat was deprived of fluid. For example, after water was withheld for 23 hours, the control rats drank an average of 19 ml, whereas those rats in which atropine was deposited bilaterally drank 17 ml of water. Phenoxybenzamine did not affect the drinking response. Thus, the polydipsic responses to cholinergic stimulation and to a water deficit are ostensibly mediated by a different central pathway or mechanism.

Additional support for this conclusion of Krikstone and Levitt (1970) was provided by Spencer and Holloway (1972) who again demonstrated the potentiation of deprivation-induced drinking in the rat by carbachol implanted at several sites in the limbic system. When the animal was deprived of water, the same sort of enhancement of water intake arose except after 2 days of water deprivation when the animal's intragastric capacity was reached in terms of a load of fluid of about 25 ml. Eserine, however, failed to potentiate the deprivation-induced intake of water, which would again support the notion that

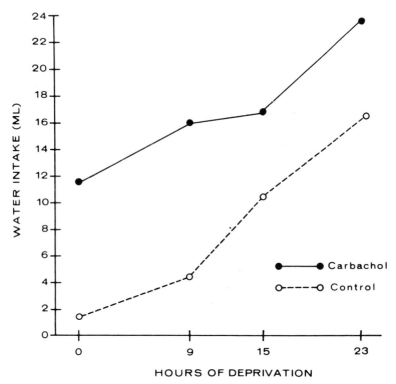

Fig. 8-16 Interaction of cholinergic stimulation with level of water deprivation. (From Krikstone, B. J. and R. A. Levitt. 1970. *J. Comp. Physiol. Psychol.* 71:334–340. Copyright 1970, by the American Psychological Association. Reprinted by permission)

a component of natural thirst is not necessarily mediated by a cholinergic pathway.

1. *Osmotic Activation and Cholinergic Thirst*

The drinking that is aroused by an intraperitoneal injection of hypertonic saline is attenuated by as much as 52% by methyl atropine, a more potent antimuscarinic than the sulfate salt, when it is injected into either of two of the most sensitive areas of the rat's thirst circuit, the medial septum or nucleus reuniens (Block and Fisher, 1970). In the thirsty animal, a similar implant of atropine reduces water intake by 65% after 6 hours of fluid deprivation, but only by 35% in the 23-hour deprived rat. These observations suggest than an osmotic disturbance brought about by a fluid debt or by an excess in extracellular sodium, either of which leads to drinking of water, is only partly mediated by a cholinergic system. Again we have the difficult question raised by a partial blockade which may be due to: (1) an alternative anatomical pathway; (2) a dose effect; or

(3) an alternative neurohumoral substrate that serves the central control of thirst and drinking behavior.

Asking the question in another way, does a cholinergic mechanism facilitate osmotic thirst? After 3.0 ml of 15% NaCl were given subcutaneously in the rat, an implant of carbachol at any of several loci in the limbic system did, in fact, increase even further the volume of water consumed (Levitt and Buerger, 1970). Atropine given at the same cholinoceptive sites reduced only partially the salt arousal drinking as well as that evoked by an implant of carbachol and systemic hypertonic saline given simultaneously. Thus, the synergism of cholinergic stimulation with an osmotic challenge corresponds precisely to that of water deprivation (Krikstone and Levitt, 1970). The local anticholinergic effect of atropine in partially attenuating both types of drinking is likewise almost identical. Figure 8-17 shows the magnitude and similarity of the atropine antagonism.

In confirming these effects, Terpstra and Slangen (1972b) also showed that the ingestion of water, induced by an interval of fluid deprivation or by a systemic injection of hypertonic saline, was blocked only about 20% by either atropine or

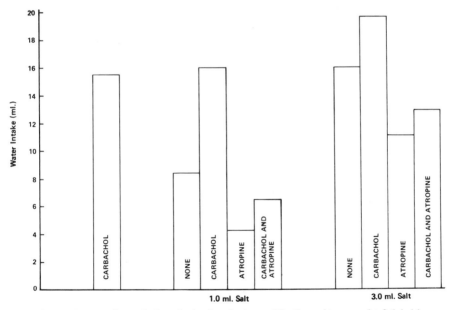

Fig. 8-17 Interaction of chemical stimulation with the salt arousal of drinking. The first bar shows mean water intake following brain stimulation with carbachol in positive drinking sites with no peripheral salt injection. The next two groups of bars show mean water intake following a 1.0 or 3.0 ml injection of hypertonic salt alone, no chemical stimulation, "None" in the figure, or in combination with each of the three brain stimulation conditions. (From Levitt and Buerger, 1970)

methyl atropine injected into the diagonal band of Broca (tractus diagonalis) of the rat. Even at this exceptionally sensitive cholinoceptive site in the drinking circuit, intact cholinergic synapses do not seem to be crucial for the consumption of water evoked by an aberration in water stores or a state of hypertonicity.

Norepinephrine has been claimed to be a more potent blocker than atropine of natural, deprivation-induced thirst or the osmotic thirst evoked by a salt solution administered systemically (Singer and Kelly, 1972). The cholinolytic injected into the hypothalamus of the rat failed altogether to alter salt arousal drinking. But again, the question of dose equivalence when testing the efficacy of two drugs, norepinephrine and atropine, must first be ascertained by a careful dose-response analysis. Statistics notwithstanding, a valid comparison of the results from different laboratories of a partial blocking effect would require some similarity in experimental technique, a situation which one rarely finds.

2. Temporal Decay of Drinking

By delaying the access to water of a rat in which carbachol had been injected into the lateral preoptic area, curves of decreasing water intake, presented in Fig. 8-18, were obtained for four different intervals of delay (Quartermain and Miller, 1966). If the rat was allowed water immediately after stimulation, about 7 times more water was taken than if an hour elapsed before water was made available (Fig. 8-18). When the animal was placed on a VI 1 minute schedule of reinforcement, the ordinary duration of drinking of 20 minutes ordinarily seen when water was continuously available was distributed evenly over nearly an hour. Thus, internal feedback from receptors in the system is just as responsible for the termination of cholinergically-induced drinking as the temporal dissipation of the drug in brain tissue.

Although the volume of water consumed was not cited, Feider (1967) found that a rat would persist in licking a water tube even if as much as a two-hour delay was interposed between the time that carbachol was deposited in the hypothalamus and the water tube was presented to the rat. This lack of decay of the licking or drinking effect of carbachol was believed to support the idea that feedback signals of water satiation are required to terminate the drinking evoked by cholinomimetic stimulation of the hypothalamus.

Pooling data from stimulation sites in the septum and thalamus, Levitt (1970) showed that atropine still blocked carbachol drinking to some degree after it was implanted in one cholinoceptive drinking site 1, 2, 6 or 24 hours before carbachol was applied to a contralateral site. As expected, the inhibitory efficacy of the anticholinergic substance declined over time.

Although both eserine and diisopropylfluorophosphate (DFP), injected into the lateral preoptic area of the rat, elicit drinking of water of essentially the same magnitude, the availability of water to the rat differentiated the actions of these two cholinesterase inhibitors (Winson and Miller, 1970). Eserine still elicited a significant intake of over 3 ml of water after a 20 minute delay in the

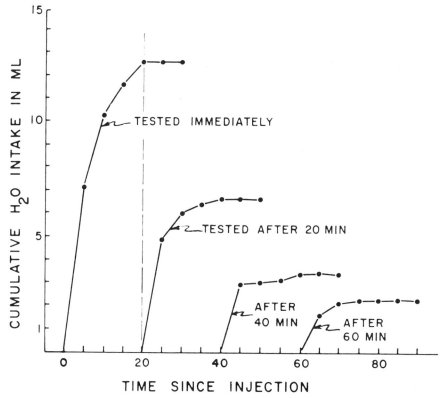

Fig. 8-18   Mean cumulative water intake plotted at 5-minute intervals for four delay conditions.   (From Quartermain, D. and N. E. Miller. 1966. *J. Comp. Physiol. Psychol.* 62:350–353.   Copyright 1966, by the American Psychological Association.   Reprinted by permission)

presentation of the water spout.   On the other hand, DFP evoked drinking even after a 90 minute delay.   The longer-lasting potency of DFP is probably related to its partial irreversibility and the prolonged anti-enzymatic action which the compound exerts on cholinesterase metabolism.   However, since the effect on water intake lasts no longer than 3 to 4 hours, an isoenzyme of cholinesterase may be re-synthesized at the local region of micro-injection.

D.   Palatability of Fluid

A rat offered a choice between water and a 25% solution of sucrose prefers to drink the sweet fluid over water after carbachol is implanted in the medial septal area (Gandelman *et al.*, 1968).   When the fluids were presented separately, the carbachol-injected animal drank between 8 to 10 ml of either fluid.   Since the rat preferred water over the sucrose after deprivation, it would appear that cholinergic drinking differs qualitatively from a deprivation-induced imbibition of fluid. In fact, the acetylcholine synapse may be equally as involved in the sensory component of fluid ingestion as in the control of water balance.

Carbachol-induced drinking is also directly related to the palatability of a solution of NaCl which was determined earlier (Stricker and Miller, 1968). Thus, carbachol drinking may not simply be reflexive but may contain a motivational element. Interestingly, Stricker and Miller showed that neither serum electrolytes nor osmolarity were significantly altered in the rat analyzed 10 minutes after an injection of carbachol into the anterior hypothalamus. Although this would be expected since no water was ingested by the animal before it was sacrificed, the possibility is ruled out that cholinergic stimulation of the hypothalamus on its own could influence directly the osmotic tension of the blood.

A rat deprived of fluid for 23 hours drinks a solution of ethanol in the preferred range to the point of ataxia when 4, 8 and 12% solutions are offered simultaneously (Cicero and Myers, 1969). However, when carbachol is injected into one of four cholinoceptive sites in the limbic system thirst circuit, which evokes spontaneous drinking of up to 20 ml of water, each solution of ethanol is rejected. Even the lowest concentration of 4%, which is well within the preferred range, was refused by the rat after a carbachol injection. Therefore, the noxious gustatory or olfactory qualities of alcohol could have been accentuated by cholinergic stimulation. In any case, water deprivation and carbachol injections do not evoke the same sort of drinking response for this intoxicating fluid.

When a rat is (a) exposed to quinine-adulterated water, (b) forced to drink on an intermittent schedule, or (c) must depress a lever to obtain a water reward, substantially less drinking occurs after carbachol is deposited in the preoptic area than after the animal is deprived of water for 23 hours (Franklin and Quartermain, 1970). Although deprivation and carbachol stimulation produce comparable drinking when water is freely available, the concomitant introduction of a motivational component in obtaining fluid leads to a reduction in the volume taken. Probably, water deprivation affects all of the central systems underlying thirst, whereas the activating properties of carbachol at a single anatomical locus is not nearly as pervading or powerful a stimulus.

E. Relationship to Other Functions

Although the drinking response following cholinergic stimulation of the hypothalamus has been described by many workers (e.g., Davis et al., 1967b), other processes are often affected at the same time. For example, accompanying the drinking of water evoked by carbachol implanted into the rat's lateral hypothalamus are increases in activity as well as a reduction in sleeping and resting. These responses are in contrast to those of sham controls of norepinephrine-implanted rats (Blanchard and Blanchard, 1966). These indices, rated by an independent observer for only 20 minutes after the injection, did not include measurements of EEG activity.

Applied to the medial septum of the rat, carbachol also causes a sharp increase in activity in an open chamber. There is a negative correlation between the animals that exhibit the most activity and those that drink the largest volume of water (Greene, 1968). Therefore, the change in the general responsiveness of the rat cannot be attributed to an altered thirst drive.

Crystals of carbachol deposited in the septum, preoptic area and an unidentified area bordering the ventral thalamus and red nucleus also cause a simultaneous intake of water as well as a fall in the core temperature of the rat (Hulst and deWied, 1967). It is often difficult to say whether one effect causes the other or whether they are independent events. In several cases, the rat drank when the temperature was rising but in 18 of 22 experiments, the fall in temperature generally paralleled the ingestion of water; in 8 of 13 experiments, a rise in temperature usually was not accompanied by drinking. The sites of stimulation were very close at which the cholinomimetic exerted one effect or another. In the same species, Avery (1971) showed that drinking was also accompanied by a rise in body temperature when carbachol was micro-injected in solution into the anterior hypothalamus. The interacting effects of drinking water to overcome an elevated body temperature are at once apparent but at the same time difficult to segregate. Similarly, the site of action of carbachol drinking is closely allied to the locus in the lateral hypothalamus at which crystals of the cholinomimetic elicit species-specific killing behavior in the rat (Bandler, 1969; 1970) (Chapter 11).

Repeating the experiments of Fisher and Coury (1962; 1964), Hulst (1972) verified the fact that the rat drinks water after crystals of carbachol are deposited within 17 different structures in the limbic system related to the Papez (1937) emotion-motivation circuit. In addition, Hulst again showed that hypothermia or hyperthermia could develop simultaneously after the cholinomimetic was implanted. However, if water was withheld, the drop in temperature often ensued anyway. This means that a carbachol-induced hypothermia may not simply be due to an intragastric load of cold water but rather is independent of a cholinergic pathway for thirst. The cholinergic pathway for heat production, which may be blocked by crystals of carbachol, seems to be anatomically overlapping and probably intertwined (Chapter 6).

Cortical spreading depression produced by 25% KCl solution applied to the surface of the rat's cortex prevents the ingestion of water motivated either by central cholinergic stimulation or by the natural thirst of water deprivation (Levitt and Krikstone, 1968). After crystals of carbachol are deposited in the septum, the normal polydipsia is totally abolished after the application of bilateral spreading depression. The unilateral infiltration of the KCl solution had no effect. This inhibition of drinking lasts over an hour and can probably be attributed to a generalized abolition of cortical and subcortical pathways subserving all behavior and has nothing to do with the specific mechanism involving thirst.

In the satiated rat, drinking and, in some cases, feeding follow a more localized wave of cortical spreading depression induced by a solution of KCl infused into the occipital lobe 1 mm below the surface of the cortex (Huston and Bureš, 1970). This behavior could be elicited up to 10 to 15 times in one session. Excitatory behavior, including wall climbing, consistently preceded the ingestive responses, so the effect of KCl on this part of the brain may be on a generalized release of motivational systems. That is, a functional rebound of the subcortical structures to the cortical depression may occur.

Cholinergically-induced drinking does, however, survive nephrectomy or uretic ligation; therefore, it seems to be independent of the renin-angiotensin system. After the surgical intervention of kidney function, the rat drinks approximately the same amount of water in response to crystals of carbachol deposited in the medial septal nucleus as the sham-operated controls (Antelman et al., 1972). This would not be entirely unexpected, since the cholinergic synapses that mediate drinking are likely to be on the efferent as well as afferent side of the neuronal link.

Following the discovery of Breckenridge and Lisk (1969) on the effect of cAMP on feeding, Rindi et al. (1972) also found that drinking could be evoked in the rat by the dibutyryl derivative of cyclic AMP. This response was obtained only when crystals of cyclic AMP were deposited in the rat's lateral hypothalamic area, which confirms the observation of Fitzsimons (1971) that cyclic AMP had no effect on drinking when deposited in the rostral hypothalamus. However, the volume consumed was by no means as large as that following a similar implantation of carbachol. Apparently, cAMP could act on the complex, but as yet incompletely understood, mechanism of storage and release of ACh within the hypothalamic pathway mediating drinking.

In the absence of water, carbachol injected into the lateral hypothalamus of the rat suppresses its food intake when only the rat's lab chow is available (Beideman and Goldstein, 1970). After food had been offered and refused in the test chamber during five successive tests of the effect of carbachol, water was immediately selected over food on the sixth test when the choice between food and water was presented to the rat. Although this kind of specificity is not always seen (see Chapter 7), the switching behavior from drinking to eating and back again that has been reported when homologous sites in the lateral hypothalamus of the rat are stimulated electrically (Valenstein et al., 1970) may not be facilitated by a chemical substance injected at the same locus. Hence, the specificity of a chemical agent in terms of a local action on neurons is contrasted to that of electrical stimulation.

IV. ADRENERGIC MECHANISMS OF DRINKING

In the first study which departed totally from the concept of separate cholinergic thirst-adrenergic hunger systems, Myers (1964b) reported that 5 μg of epinephrine injected in an 0.5 μl volume into the perifornical region of the rat evoked an intake of up to 8 ml of fluid. In each test, water and 5 and 10% ethanol were offered. In this free choice situation, the two most aversive fluids were avoided if water was available, indicating again that palatability affects the chemically elicited drinking (Cicero and Myers, 1969). When the water tube was withdrawn, 5% ethanol was nevertheless consumed and if only 10% ethanol was available, then a small volume of this solution was taken. In repeated preference tests after intrahypothalamic injections of epinephrine, the rats drank water only and refused the more noxious ethanol.

The patterns of drinking presented in Fig. 8-19 for a representative rat indicate that the gustatory features of alcohol as well as its pharmacological effect were learned with each successive adrenergic-induced drinking experience. These observations of epinephrine-induced drinking in the rat opened up a Pandora's box of consternation, mainly because cholinergic synapses were at that time thought to be solely responsible for the chemical mediation of fluid consumption (Wayner, 1964). Although the fact that epinephrine stimulates beta-adrenergic receptors was not elaborated upon by Myers (1964b), participation of alpha-adrenergic receptors in the central thirst circuit is also a possibility.

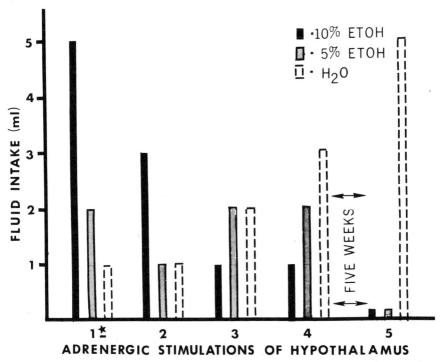

Fig. 8-19 Patterns of fluid intake in a three choice test as a result of successive adrenergic stimulation of the ventromedial hypothalamus. Starred stimulation indicates ataxia and anesthesia following drinking. (From Myers, 1963)

402 HANDBOOK OF DRUG AND CHEMICAL STIMULATION OF THE BRAIN

Although the anterior hypothalamic preoptic area mediates cholinergic drinking and adrenergic eating, crystals of norepinephrine deposited in the preoptic area of the rat deprived of food for 24 hours evoke drinking of water. Carbachol placed at the same locus reduces the drinking if the animal is water-deprived for 24 hours (Hutchinson and Renfrew, 1967). Norepinephrine-induced drinking may be related to the postulated heat loss mechanism which has been anatomically localized in precisely the same region of the rat's hypothalamus (Chapter 6). If this were the sole explanation, however, the reduction of drinking following carbachol stimulation during the water-deprived state would be difficult to interpret. However, this inhibitory effect could be linked to a cholinergic heat production mechanism in the rat (Myers and Yaksh, 1968) which is undoubtedly influenced by an imbalance in body water.

Crystals of the beta agonist, isoproterenol, implanted in the lateral hypothalamus of the rat were found not to elicit drinking (Lehr et al., 1967), although the intrahypothalamic doses were perhaps too low to have the systemic effect of a beta agonist on drinking proposed by Houpt and Epstein (1971). Lehr et al. demonstrated the polydipsic action of isoproterenol after its systemic administration and the antidipsic effect of propranolol, a beta receptor blocker, given similarly. A direct reciprocal action of beta and alpha receptor activity within a CNS mechanism was therefore first hypothesized, although perhaps prematurely, for the regulation of body water.

Even though norepinephrine, not epinephrine, is contained in high concentration in the hypothalamus and exerts an effect on alpha receptors primarily, the adrenergic drinking of water or other fluids induced by epinephrine injected into the hypothalamus of the rat (Myers, 1964b) could be attributable to an action on beta receptors. Isoproterenol injected into the lateral hypothalamus enhances drinking in the fully sated or water-deprived rat (Leibowitz, 1971). The hyperdipsia was attenuated by a similar micro-injection of propranolol or by norepinephrine, the latter effect being the same as that reported by Grossman (1962a). Phentolamine and carbachol, also injected into the lateral hypothalamus, evoked drinking in satiated or deprived rats, the latter effect differing from that reported by Hutchinson and Renfrew (1967). Although these findings may support some of the earlier observations, the intrahypothalamic dose of isoproterenol given by Leibowitz exceeds by several times the systemic threshold dose for spontaneous drinking in the water replete rat.

In a further experiment, Montgomery et al. (1971) found that in addition to the effect on feeding, desmethylimipramine (DMI) also injected in the lateral hypothalamus causes drinking in the fully satiated rat. Because this tricyclic antidepressant prevents the re-uptake of norepinephrine presynaptically, the endogenous levels of the catecholamine would be thereby elevated. Although the average volume consumed of 4 ml is slightly less than that reported by Myers (1964b), an adrenergic component of water balance is again implicated. Perhaps endogenous norepinephrine could mimic epinephrine's local action on the cells of the hypothalamus in producing drinking.

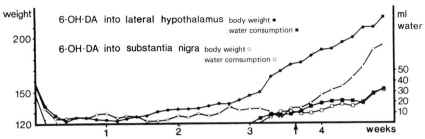

Fig. 8-20 Water consumption and body weight after bilateral degeneration of the nigro-striatal DA system induced by 6-OHDA injection at two different sites. Two representative animals. The arrow indicates when tube-feeding is discontinued. (From Ungerstedt, 1971a)

A. Destruction of Catecholaminergic Neurons

As described in Chapter 7, the localized destruction of noradrenergic and dopaminergic nerve terminals by a micro-injection of 6-OHDA into the diencephalon causes a marked adipsia and aphagia which is ordinarily fatal (Ungerstedt, 1971a). This powerful effect on ingestive behavior occurs when the 6-OHDA is given in the substantia nigra or at sites scattered along the longitudinal axis of the lateral hypothalamus (Smith *et al.*, 1972). The long-term detrimental effect on water intake of 6-OHDA after its injection into either the lateral hypothalamus or substantia nigra is shown in Fig. 8-20.

Although these findings are again suggestive of the involvement of the catecholamine fiber pathways in water regulation, an interpretation of these lesions presently requires extensive research. For example, a generalized 6-OHDA impairment of afferent impulses to the sensory elements related to tasting and selecting a fluid may arise. Equally possible is a subsequent dysfunction of the efferent pathways over which the impulses travel for the appropriate motor movements essential for lapping up and swallowing a liquid.

Directly related to these ideas is the observation that the certain death of a rat in which 6-OHDA is injected intrahypothalamically is avoidable (Myers and Martin, 1973). The lethal refusal of water and food can be reversed in most instances simply by offering the rat a palatable diet (Chapter 7). Prandial drinking of water in volumes sufficient to maintain the animal in water equilibrium occurs at once. Thus, the sensation of the taste of the substance or other oral factor may again play a pivotal role in the centrally evoked or inhibited drinking response.

B. Drinking of Palatable Liquids and Nutrients

In a sort of shot-gun study, a total of 17 drugs seemingly taken off the shelf were injected in high concentration and a large 5 μl volume into the hypothalamus of the rat (Wagner and de Groot, 1963b). The drinking of a Metrecal solution, which was called eating, occurred following the injection of a number of these chemicals (see Master Summary Table). Undoubtedly, the effects correspond to those of an intraventricular injection because of the volume given (Myers, 1966). Yet some of the compounds purportedly exerted different effects if injected into the ventromedial as opposed to the lateral hypothalamus. In the fasted rat, for example, lidocaine injected into the ventromedial nucleus evoked drinking but suppressed it when injected into the lateral hypothalamus or globus pallidus.

In another study in which the consumption of a palatable and nutritious fluid was termed feeding, Miller *et al.* (1964) injected 1 µl of norepinephrine to establish a dose-response curve for the drinking of a highly palatable Metrecal solution. Drinking of water after a similar injection of a carbachol solution was also accompanied by the ingestion of between 1 to 2 g of dry rat chow at the higher doses. Although between 1 and 2 ml of water were also drunk when the effective doses of norepinephrine elicited Metrecal drinking, the preference for the highly palatable Metrecal, shown in Fig. 8-21, illustrates that a discrimination based on gustatory or olfactory cues is made during the drinking induced by an adrenergic substance injected into the hypothalamus of the rat. The important difference in the response of ingesting pellets or fluid following adrenergic stimulation may be based solely on the experience of the animal or on the overall palatability of the food or liquid which is offered (Myers, 1964b).

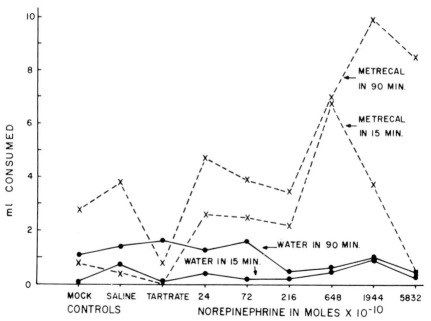

Fig. 8-21 Effect of different doses of norepinephrine in lateral hypothalamus on consumption of liquid food and water. (From Miller *et al.*, 1964)

1. *Adrenergic Satiety Mechanism*

Citing salient peripheral evidence and selected central studies, Margules (1969b) made a very strong case for a startling new concept—a noradrenergic satiety mechanism in the hypothalamus. Using as the reinforcer a very palatable and preferred substance, dilute condensed milk, Margules found that phentolamine, an alpha blocker, enhanced the drinking of milk; in contrast, the ingestion of milk was suppressed by norepinephrine. The compounds were both applied as crystals to the medial forebrain bundle of the rat. Although the results are in conflict with all previous observations of feeding induced by norepinephrine, they do correspond with the inhibitory action of the catecholamines on drinking reported as a hypothalamic effect (Grossman, 1962a). Generally, a high dose of the crystals was used, since low doses did not cause licking a spout for milk. A high dose of phentolamine, by the same token, could act initially to cause a local release of norepinephrine which may evoke an ingestive response (Leibowitz, 1971).

An extension of these findings revealed that the rat drank milk in response to the local application of phentolamine only when the injector cannula was placed bilaterally and symmetrically in the rat's medial forebrain bundle (Margules, 1970a). When the milk was mixed with quinine, the rats consumed less of the solution in response to the phentolamine. Norepinephrine also suppressed the intake of the quinine-adulterated milk, but enhanced the intake of sweet milk in that from 18 to 28 cc were consumed. This result is illustrated in Fig. 8-22. Propranolol, a beta receptor blocker, not only failed to enhance or suppress the intake of milk but also did not affect the licking rate for this fluid. This does not correspond with the effect that propranolol has on water intake (Leibowitz, 1971). A case could be made for a central noradrenergic satiety mechanism based on several incidental observations including the evoked release of norepinephrine by amphetamine, a potent appetite suppressant (Carr and Moore, 1969). The argument that lab chow is unpalatable would not support the norepinephrine satiety theory, since norepinephrine has been found by many investigators to evoke an intake of 3 to 5 g of dry pellets in a very short interval.

The beta-agonist, isoproterenol, reduces the rat's intake of quinine adulterated milk when crystals of the drug are implanted bilaterally in the MFB. A conditioned suppression with repeated administration was believed to occur (Margules, 1970b). The beta receptor blocking agent, *dl*-4-(2 hydroxy-3-isopropylaminopropoxy)-indole (LB-46), elevated the licking rate but not the intake of a bitter milk solution. Margules concluded that beta-adrenergic receptors in the perifornical area may participate in taste aversions, both unconditioned and conditioned. Unfortunately, no dose response was obtained and, of course, other catecholamines that were not tested may have been responsible for the effects. The crucial test of a beta receptor phenomenon in addition to dose and the relationship to other antagonists is whether an endogenous substrate evokes the same response when applied at the same site.

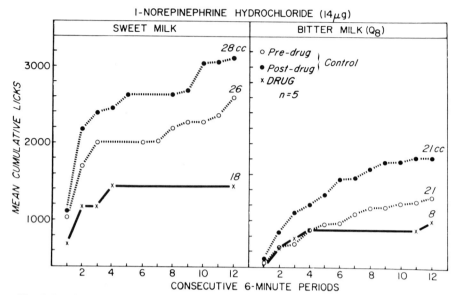

Fig. 8-22 Effect of direct bilateral application of 14 µg of *l*-norepinephrine on licking responses and total intake of sweet and bitter milk. (From Margules, D. L. 1970a. *J. Comp. Physiol. Psychol.* 73:1–12. Copyright 1970, by the American Psychological Association. Reprinted by permission)

V. CENTRAL BLOCKADE OF DRINKING

Carbachol or ACh injected into the hypothalamus of the conscious monkey blocks, rather than elicits, drinking even after the monkey has been water-deprived (Myers, 1969b). Atropine injected into the same hypothalamic area reverses this blockade in the thirsty monkey. This would indicate that the cholinomimetic inhibition of drinking in the monkey is through muscarinic receptors. As cited earlier (Section C), angiotensin and nicotine implanted at certain caudal sites evoke intense drinking of over a third of a liter of fluid (Myers *et al.*, 1973), indicating that the muscarinic blockade by carbachol probably overrides the nicotinic receptors. In another study, Sharpe and Myers (1969) extended this observation to include an ACh-eserine mixture which when infused into the lateral hypothalamus again prevented ingestive behavior. Injected into the rabbit's hypothalamus, carbachol in low doses evokes only feeding but at higher doses, some drinking is produced (Sommer *et al.*, 1967). Thus, the complexity of the system could be resolved in terms of the number as well as category of fiber systems that are excited in the diencephalic areas mediating thirst.

In the cat, a single high dose of carbachol injected into the ventromedial thalamus also reduces the intake of water and bar pressing for milk (Avery and Nance, 1970); however, a nonspecific motor deficit caused by the tetanizing properties of the drug in high doses cannot be excluded. Either carbachol in low doses or norepinephrine injected into the hypothalamus in a very high dose causes in most instances a suppression of water intake and of eating of dry cat food (Milner *et al.*, 1971). Unfortunately, both measures of ingestive behavior were lumped together. Although in a few experiments both carbachol and norepinephrine shift the percent of intake upwards, a high dose of the catecholamine may simply depress neuronal activity in a nonspecific manner. Further, a dose-dependent reduction in feeding and drinking is also produced in the cat by an injection of atropine into the anterior, preoptic area, with a somewhat greater effect on the water intake (Nance *et al.*, 1971). In this species, atropine may actually cause a temporary chemical lesion rather than alter the synaptic activity of a specific chemical pathway for ingestive behavior.

Glucose injected in the rat's lateral hypothalamus also blocks drinking, reduces feeding and induces drowsiness (Booth, 1968b). Although tonicity controls were run, the local presence of the sugar may have caused simple inactivation rather than a direct effect on thirst receptors.

A. Adipsia of Toxic Drugs

Chlorothiazide is a potent diuretic drug when given systemically. When implanted into the hypothalamus of a normal rat or one made thirsty by hypertonic saline given subcutaneously, the drug inhibits water intake (Gutman and Chaimovitz, 1966). The antidipsic action of the drug may have as one of its sites of effect the hypothalamic neurons underlying thirst.

Ouabain implanted bilaterally in a large number of areas including the medial forebrain bundle and the ventromedial and lateral hypothalamus of the rat also causes adipsia and even suppresses the normal drinking response to hypertonic saline given subcutaneously (Bergmann *et al.*, 1967). This adipsia persisted for several days and often led to fatal dehydration. The localization of this effect suggests that the glycoside is acting directly on osmoreceptors, perhaps to block active Na^+ transport. However, the simultaneous inhibition of food intake to less than one-half of the normal level or more for a five-day period would suggest a more generalized toxic effect to all the cells mediating ingestive behavior.

The behavioral action of a drug implanted into the hypothalamus does not necessarily follow its diuretic activity since the cardiac glycosides, ouabain and digitoxin, are the most potent in terms of their blockade of water intake. Although a long-lasting adipsia or an inhibition of salt-arousal drinking is produced in the rat by a variety of heterogeneous chemicals (Bergmann *et al.*, 1968a), their principal structural commonality is the aromatic sulphonamide group which if not present, as in the case of diazoxide, renders the compound devoid of antidipsic activity.

In spite of the fact that the implants were distributed over a 2 mm area of the rat's hypothalamus, digitoxin, ethacrynic acid and furosemide prevented drinking even after saline was given subcutaneoualy (Bergmann *et al.*, 1968b). Large doses caused convulsions and death. Control animals in which 100 μg of talc were implanted similarly regained their normal consumption of water after 2 to 3 days. Also, control implants in the thalamus or hippocampus did not affect drinking. Although these drugs have various diuretic or antidiuretic potencies, their common antidipsic action could be related to their ability to inhibit the active transport of sodium. If effective locally, the normal function of osmoreceptor neurons in the hypothalamus may be disrupted. Toxicity is still a major question, however, in any interpretation.

The bilateral deposition of crystals of mercury derivatives at sites scattered throughout the hypothalamus of the rat also causes adipsia, aphagia and ultimately death. These reactions were correlated generally with the estimated doses (Bergmann *et al.*, 1968c). The failure of a salt challenge to induce drinking as well as the delayed onset of the symptoms, which often did not reach their full scope until after 2 to 3 days, were particularly notable. An implant of one of the mercurials into the thalamus had either no effect or a reduced effect if the dose was much higher. Both the mercury derivatives and ethacrynic acid, which prevent normal or salt arousal drinking, also suppressed the drinking evoked by hypovolemia that is produced by a subcutaneous injection of polyethylene glycol (Bergmann *et al.*, 1968d). Although the mechanisms underlying hypovolemic and hypertonic thirst may be different in terms of their actions on aldosterone and ADH secretion, both classes of toxic drugs block the hypothalamic pathways which underlie the drinking that arises from a perturbation in plasma osmolality.

The same drugs which have a potent antidipsic action when implanted in the hypothalamus of the rat also exert a direct effect on kidney function (Gutman *et al.*, 1971a). Such compounds as furosemide, hydrochlorothiazide, ethacrynic acid and phenformin produce a large increase in the volume of urine excreted over a 4-day interval. At the same time, osmolality is decreased. Although no anatomical evidence was provided and dose responses were not obtained, it is possible that these powerful anti-dipsogens have an effect on the osmoreceptors in the rostral hypothalamus that trigger ADH release.

In a follow-up experiment, Gutman *et al.* (1971b) found that ouabain causes a marked increase in sodium excretion in the urine when crystals of the drugs are deposited in the lateral hypothalamus, but only a slight effect when placed in the medial hypothalamus. This ouabain-induced natriuresis disappears completely after the rats are adrenalectomized. The results support the idea that a neurogenic control over sodium balance is mediated by the adrenal glands. A possible mechanism could be the reduction in mineralocorticoid production, which is thought to be brought about by a shift in the angiotensin or potassium levels in the plasma.

In order to sort out the reasons why the cardiac glycoside, ouabain, causes diuresis when given systemically, as well as when implanted in the hypothalamus, Gutman *et al.* (1970) repeated their experiments. Again, ouabain crystals deposited in the lateral hypothalamus of the rat depressed water intake, caused a relative increase in urine production, but lowered the osmolality of the urine. Adrenalectomy did not alter these responses to a hypothalamic implant of ouabain. After a rat was deprived of water and food for an unspecified interval, ouabain inserted in the lateral area still evoked a hypotonic polyuria, but had no effect when implanted in the ventromedial area. These results suggest that a peripheral diuretic often used therapeutically in the human patient in the control of hypertension can exert a direct effect on the central release of antidiuretic hormone (ADH) with no apparent involvement of the adrenal gland. A partial impairment or blockade of the osmoreceptors in the supraoptic nucleus could account for the presumed decline in ADH output. However, osmoreceptors have not been identified anatomically in the parts of the hypothalamus at which Gutman *et al.* found ouabain to possess its effective renal action.

VI. CONCLUDING CONSIDERATIONS

The rapid strides taken recently in the study of the central mechanisms responsible for water balance have brought to light facts of unusual significance. When compared to most other topics considered in this book, an understanding does seem closer at hand of the neurochemical processes underlying thirst and the resultant drinking behavior. Outstanding contributions from laboratories throughout the world form the basis of this optimistic view.

Unquestionably, the micro-injection experiments have provided some very powerful evidence which correlates with data on single neurons, for the existence of specialized thirst receptors that are anatomically localized in the diencephalon. A locus sensitive to hypertonicity in the region contiguous to the supraoptic nucleus (Blass and Epstein, 1971; Peck and Novin, 1971) would seem to monitor a condition of extracellular dehydration due either to an absolute dehydration from a lack of water or to an excess in the relative concentration of sodium in the parenchyma. The suggestion of Andersson (1971a) that the ependymal wall or sites close to it possess osmoreceptors also cannot be excluded, because part of the 2 μl volume used to identify the region of maximal reactivity to an osmotic challenge in the rat could have spilled over into the animal's cerebral ventricle.

Equally as impressive is the evidence of a volumetric sensor system that is mediated through the action of angiotensin II on neurons in the hypothalamus. At present the precise region containing receptors for this polypeptide has not been localized with absolute certainty by a micro-injection experiment. The target region which is the primary anatomical candidate is the supraoptic nucleus itself, at least in the rat. The special sensitivity to angiotensin of single neurons in and around this structure (Nicoll and Barker, 1971) almost constitutes the molecular proof in support of the behavioral response of drinking.

The exact relationship between the water seeking behavior evoked by the injection of angiotensin into the hypothalamus and a hyperosmotic challenge within the same anatomical area is still unclear. Presumably there is a close tie if not functional overlap between each of these two types of central stimuli to drink. Yet to be settled are two important matters: (1) the entry of the chemical trigger into the brain, and (2) the physiological level of plasma angiotensin. Of course, it is well known that sodium can alter the firing pattern of a single hypothalamic neuron when acting from the blood supplied in the microvasculature. Whether angiotensin also passes into the same hypothalamic region of receptivity in a physiologically effective amount has not been demonstrated. It would seem, nonetheless, that different chemical substances possess the capacity to evoke drinking perhaps by utilizing the same neuronal route. Although individual mechanisms may have evolved within that pathway, the net result on homeo-stasis is the same—achievement of water balance.

A. Cholinergic Pathway

From the time of the pioneering work of Pickford and her colleagues on the role of acetylcholine in the release of ADH, the role of this neurotransmitter in thirst has been studied intensively in the experimental animal. Even the human patient experiences the sensation of dryness of the mouth when an anticholinergic drug is injected into the globus pallidus (Nashold, 1959).

An evaluation of the research described in Section III of this chapter documents the importance of cholinoceptive neurons in the morphological components of the thirst system. A consistent drinking response is evoked by a cholinomimetic at sites scattered throughout the limbic lobe. Because of this intimate relationship, one would surmise that an osmotic or volumetric signal to the primary receptor sites for thirst in the supraoptic nucleus, or associated structures connected by fiber pathways to this nucleus, is transmitted to the limbic system by way of a distinct cholinergic pathway.

The purpose of such widespread representation of a thirst signal is not immediately apparent. Presumably, an intensely motivated urge to drink in the face of a water deficit occasioned by a factor such as heat or exercise is sufficient reason enough. In fact, one could envisage that if the resources of the entire body are dominated by the urge to reinstate water balance, many parts of the limbic system would be recruited to direct the behavior of the animal to the fluid. In terms of survival, such motivated activity has a very decided temporal urgency.

One detail that is not trivial requires explanation. Why does atropine fail to block entirely the imbibition of water following an osmotic perturbation, hypo-volemia or an elevated level of angiotensin II? By the same token, how does this antagonist of muscarinic receptors inhibit drinking caused by a cholinomimetic applied in any of the structures in the limbic system circuitry for thirst?

First, atropine is almost always used as the receptor antagonist because of the early implication of the muscarinic receptor. The recent discovery of nicotinic-like receptor sensitivity in the hypothalamus of the monkey and at sites homologous to those reactive to angiotensin demonstrates that drugs that occupy nicotinic and other classes of receptors must be tested and evaluated.

Second, carbachol is ordinarily used as the test chemical instead of ACh or a mixture of ACh and an anticholinesterase. As described in most pharmacology texts, the drug acts as a chelon, or as a cholinergic blocking agent and exerts many other potent effects. As enumerated in Chapter 10, carbachol is a powerful convulsant and, in fact, a seizure focus is easily produced by its local application to neural tissue. Therefore, its exclusive usage is unwise. An injection or application in a single dose is strategically incorrect because the local concentration of carbachol will determine its action on the neuron, glial structure or contiguous circulation.

Third, intracellular dehydration may affect neurons other than those within a primary hypothalamic zone of osmoreceptors and volume receptors. A water deficit may secondarily be detected, albeit less intensively, by all of the receptive elements in the limbic system. Thus, when a cholinolytic is applied at one site in this neuronal network, the remainder of the system compensates for this unitary blockade, so that the animal nevertheless consumes water. The built-in redundancy in the limbic circuitry would seem to have great utility if purely for the element of survival.

Obviously, all regions of the limbic system are not devoted specifically to the ingestion of fluid. An experiment with a blocking agent may necessarily elucidate only a small fraction of the relationship of the region to another vital function served by an acetylcholine (carbachol) sensitive locus. A lack of body water is inexorably bound up with thermoregulatory control, the animal's subsequent emotional state, the type of feeding, the dynamics of each excretory process, the composition of the interstitial fluid, blood pressure and other functions of varying relative significance.

B. Receptor Sensitivity

Angiotensin, acetylcholine, sodium chloride, epinephrine, cyclic AMP and other compounds applied to distinct regions of the brain evoke drinking. The reasons why they do so are related just as much to the neuroanatomy of the system as the probability that each endogenous chemical substance may hinge upon the activity of another. The very fact that morphological differences exist between species insofar as angiotensin-sensitive sites, or that cholinergic drinking is a peculiar phenomenon of the laboratory rat, emphasizes the critical need for comparative anatomical investigation. Morphological maps in at least two species must be constructed in order to delineate the specific receptor properties of each region implicated in the drinking response.

From information gathered already on the rat alone, we know that there is indeed a regional difference in terms of the maximum reactivity to a chemical. In this species the most sensitive anatomical region to an injection of a given chemical is as follows: cyclic AMP in the perifornical area; carbachol in the subfornical organ or diagonal band of Broca; and a hypertonic salt solution in the anterolateral hypothalamus.

Clearly, the sensitivity of a very select constellation of neurons to each of these compounds must be carefully compared along a dose-continuum. Which substance is more potent in regard to the latency to drink a fluid and the volume of that fluid ingested? What site is most sensitive to each substance? Since one substance could work through the release of another, or alternatively modify the threshold of neuronal excitation by changing the membrane sensitivity to another compound, such a dose or site analysis would help to distinguish a primary from a secondary trigger (Chapter 13).

Although the drinking in response to the injection of a catecholamine into hypothalamic tissue could constitute a peripheral response, it is interesting that angiotensin drinking can be attenuated by the application of a catecholamine blocking agent to the same site. However, even though haloperidol, a dopaminergic antagonist, is most effective (Fitzsimons, 1972), it must be remembered that this drug abolishes locomotor activity (Costall et al., 1972a and b) which could account for the cessation of drinking just as easily.

Finally, the drinking response to epinephrine or norepinephrine could well be related to some aspect of energy metabolism. For example, the neurons along the thermoregulatory pathway that signal a condition of overheating (Chapter 6) are thought to utilize a catecholamine. If all afferent systems are called into play to initiate a compensatory heat loss, then a part of the catecholamine activation would consist of an immediate intake of water either for cooling of the body or to rectify the loss of water due to perspiration or tachypnea. In examining the mechanism of water intake, a temperature measure as well as the usual monitoring of food intake would help to define ultimately which receptors in a given region mediate a pure response to an adrenergic, cholinergic or peptidergic stimulus.

VII. Master Summary Table
Chemicals that Exerted an Effect when Given at a Specific Site in the Brain

Chemical	Dose	Volume	Site	Species	State*	Response	Reference
Acetylcholine (ACh)	?	crystal	Hypothalamus	Rat	U	Drinking.	Davis et al. (1967b)
	≃1 µg	crystal	Ventral amygdala	Rat	U	Lever response for water.	Grossman (1964a)
	≃1–5 µg	crystal	Lateral hypothalamus	Rat	U	Drinking.	Grossman (1960; 1962a)
	≃2.5–3 µg	crystal	Septum, fornix, preoptic area	Rat	U	Drinking.	Chiaraviglio and Taleisnik (1969)
	2–40 µg	4 µl	Supraoptic nucleus	Dog	A	Inhibited rate of urine flow, diuresis.	Pickford (1947)
	25–50 µg	.5–1 µl	Lateral hypothalamus	Monkey	C	Dose-dependent blockade of feeding and drinking in fasted animal.	Myers (1969b)
ACh and Eserine	≃2.5–3 µg	crystal	Septum, fornix, preoptic area	Rat	U	Drinking.	Chiaraviglio and Taleisnik (1969)
	7 µg + 1–2 µg	4 µl	Supraoptic nucleus	Dog	A	Inhibited rate of urine flow, diuresis.	Pickford (1947)
	1.5–50 µg	1 µl	Hypothalamus	Monkey	C	Blockade of feeding and drinking at higher doses.	Sharpe and Myers (1969)
Angiotensin II	?	crystal	Anterior hypothalamus	Rat	U	Drinking, rise in blood pressure.	Hendler and Blake (1969)
	≃15–20 µg	crystal	Septum	Rat	U	Drinking.	Giardina and Fisher (1971)
	1 µg	1 µl	Septum, anterior thalamus, lateral hypothalamus.	Rat	U	Water drinking, aversion to hypertonic saline.	White et al. (1972)
	1 µg	1 µl	Rostral hypothalamus	Rat	U	Drinking.	Fitzsimons (1971b)

*U = unanesthetized and unrestrained; C = constrained, confined or curarized; A = anesthetized.

VII. Master Summary Table (Continued)

Chemical	Dose	Volume	Site	Species	State*	Response	Reference
Angiotensin II	1 μg	1 μl	Septum	Rat	U	Water preference over saline.	Covian et al. (1972)
	10 ng	1 μl	Preoptic area	Rat	U	Drinking after water was withheld for 60 minutes.	Rolls and Jones (1972)
	10–50 ng	1 μl	Preoptic area	Rat	U	Lever pressing to obtain water.	Rolls et al. (1972)
	1 μg	1 μl	Preoptic area	Rat	U	Drinking.	Blass and Epstein (1971)
	1–2 μg	1 μl	Preoptic area	Rat	U	Evoked drinking after food depression.	McFarland and Rolls (1972)
	1.5 μg	1 μl	Preoptic area	Rat	U	Drinking reduced by peripheral atropine.	Blass and Chapman (1971)
	1.8 μg	.7 μl	Antero-lateral hypothalamus	Rat	U	Drinking.	Booth (1968c)
	.005–4 μg	1–2 μl	Rostral hypo-thalamus, septum	Rat	U	Drinking.	Epstein et al. (1970)
	.5–1 μg	1 μl	Hypothalamus	Monkey	C	Water drinking.	Myers et al. (1973)
Atropine	?	crystal	Septum, anterior thalamus	Rat	U	Reduced salt arousal drinking.	Levitt and Buerger (1970)
	?	crystal	Septum, thalamus, hypothalamus	Rat	U	Slight reduction of deprivation drinking.	Krikstone and Levitt (1970)
	?	crystal	Ventral amygdala	Rat	U	Reduced lever response for water.	Grossman (1964a)
	≃.5–5 μg	crystal	Septum	Rat	U	Reduced drinking.	Grossman (1964b)
	≃.5–5 μg	crystal	Ventromedial hypothalamus	Rat	U	Reduced lever responding to food and water.	Grossman (1966a)
	≃1–3 μg	crystal	Septum, anterior thalamus	Rat	U	Reduced thirst in presence of food.	Levitt (1968)

≈1–3 µg	crystal	Septum, cingulate gyrus, fornix, thalamus, midbrain	Rat	U	Blockade of carbachol drinking.	Levitt and Fisher (1966)
≈1–3 µg	crystal	Septum, nucleus reuniens	Rat	U	Partially blocked salt arousal and deprivation drinking.	Block and Fisher (1970)
≈1–5 µg	crystal	Perifornical region	Rat	U	Reduced drinking after water deprivation.	Grossman (1962b)
≈2–3 µg	crystal	Contralateral thalamus	Rat	U	Blocked drinking.	Levitt (1970)
≈2–3 µg	crystal	Septum, anterior thalamus, mesencephalon	Rat	U	Blocked cholinergic drinking.	Levitt (1969)
≈2–3 µg	crystal	Septum, anterior thalamus, lateral hypothalamus	Rat	U	Blocked carbachol drinking but not deprivation drinking.	Levitt and Fisher (1967)
≈2–7 µg	crystal	Septum	Rat	U	Suppressed food and water intake.	Kelsey and Grossman (1969)
≈2.5–3 µg	crystal	Septum, lateral hypothalamus, anterior thalamus	Rat	U	Blocked drinking.	Stein and Levitt (1971)
≈15–20 µg	crystal	Septum	Rat	U	Blockade of carbachol but not angiotensin or isoproterenol drinking.	Giardina and Fisher (1971)
.069–1.25 µg	1 µl	Amygdala	Rat	U	Blocked LH carbachol drinking.	Singer and Montgomery (1969)
.48–90 µg	1 µl	Tractus diagonalis	Rat	U	Inhibited carbachol drinking.	Terpstra and Slangen (1972b)
.069–1.25 µg	1 µl	Lateral hypothalamus	Rat	U	No effect on amygdaloid carbachol drinking.	Singer and Montgomery (1969)
.069 µg	1 µl	Septum	Rat	U	Did not affect drinking.	Singer and Montgomery (1970)

VII. Master Summary Table (*Continued*)

Chemical	Dose	Volume	Site	Species	State*	Response	Reference
Atropine	.21 μg	1 μl	Amygdala	Rat	U	Blocked septal carbachol drinking.	Singer and Montgomery (1970)
	1.25 μg	1 μl	Hypothalamus	Rat	U	Blocked carbachol but not salt or natural thirst.	Singer and Kelly (1972)
	.03–1.5 μg	1 μl	Diagonal band of Broca	Rat	U	Blockade of drinking.	Terpstra and Slangen (1972a)
	2 μg	1 μl	Septum, anterior thalamus, hypothalamus	Rat	U	Blockade of eserine drinking.	Levitt and Boley (1970)
	2.5 μg	1 μl	Fornix, hippo-campal commissure, corpus callosum	Rat	U	Blocked cholinergic drinking.	Levitt and O'Hearn (1972)
	2.5 μg	1 μl	Septum, anterior thalamus, lateral hypothalamus	Rat	U	Failed to block angiotensin drinking.	White et al. (1972)
	.1–16 μg	2 μl	Preoptic area	Rat	U	Partially reduced renin drinking, but not salt arousal drinking.	Blass and Chapman (1971)
	150 μg	2 μl	Septum	Rat	U	Blocked carbachol drinking but only attenuated deprivation drinking.	Antunes-Rodrigues and Covian (1971)
	12.5–50 μg	2 μl	Anterior, preoptic area	Cat	U	Inhibited feeding and drinking.	Nance et al. (1971)
	12 μg	.5–1 μl	Lateral hypothalamus	Monkey	C	Reversed cholinergic block-ade of feeding and drinking.	Myers (1969b)
Carbachol	?	crystal	Anterior hypothala-mus and ventrome-dial hypothalamus	Rat	U	Drinking.	Hendler and Blake (1969)

Dose	Form	Site	Species		Effect	Reference
?	crystal	Lateral hypothalamus	Rat	U	Drinking at some sites.	Lehr et al. (1967)
?	crystal	Anterior hypothalamus, preoptic area	Rat	U	Reduced drinking in water deprived animal.	Hutchinson and Renfrew (1967)
?	crystal	Lateral hypothalamus	Rat	U	Drinking; activity, reduction in sleep.	Blanchard and Blanchard (1966)
?	crystal	Medial septal nucleus	Rat	U	Drinking after nephrectomy.	Antelman et al. (1972)
?	crystal	Medial septum	Rat	U	Increased open field activity; drinking.	Greene (1968)
$\approx .01–2.5\ \mu g$	crystal	Lateral hypothalamus, anterior thalamus, fornix	Rat	U	Drinking.	Levitt et al. (1970)
$\approx .5–1\ \mu g$	crystal	Ventral amygdala	Rat	U	Lever response for water.	Grossman (1964a)
$\approx .5–5\ \mu g$	crystal	Septum	Rat	U	Drinking.	Grossman (1964b)
$\approx 1\ \mu g$	crystal	Hippocampus	Rat	U	Drinking.	Mountford (1969)
$\approx 1–3\ \mu g$	crystal	Limbic system	Rat	U	Drinking.	Fisher and Coury (1962)
$\approx 1–3\ \mu g$	crystal	Septum, cingulate gyrus, fornix, thalamus, midbrain	Rat	U	Drinking.	Levitt and Fisher (1966)
$\approx 1–3\ \mu g$	crystal	Limbic system, diencephalon	Rat	U	Drinking.	Coury (1967)
$\approx 1–3\ \mu g$	crystal	Antero-dorsal hippocampus, fornix, cingulum	Rat	U	Drinking, activity and feeding.	Grant and Jarrard (1968)
$\approx 1–3\ \mu g$	crystal	Lateral septum	Rat	U	Drinking blocked by bilateral spreading depression.	Levitt and Krikstone (1968)
$\approx 1–5\ \mu g$	crystal	Lateral hypothalamus	Rat	U	Drinking.	Grossman (1960; 1962a)
$\approx 2–3\ \mu g$	crystal	Septum, thalamus, hypothalamus	Rat	U	Enhanced deprivation drinking.	Krikstone and Levitt (1970)
$\approx 2–3\ \mu g$	crystal	Septum, anterior thalamus	Rat	U	Enhanced salt arousal drinking.	Levitt and Buerger (1970)

VII. Master Summary Table (*Continued*)

Chemical	Dose	Volume	Site	Species	State*	Response	Reference
Carbachol	$\simeq$ 2–3 μg	crystal	Septum, thalamus	Rat	U	Drinking.	Levitt (1970)
	$\simeq$ 2–3 μg	crystal	Septum, anterior thalamus, lateral hypothalamus	Rat	U	Drinking.	Levitt and Fisher (1967)
	$\simeq$ 2–3 μg	crystal	Lateral hypothalamus	Rat	U	Drinking 5 days after septal lesion.	Parks *et al.* (1971)
	$\simeq$ 2–3 μg	crystal	Septum	Rat	U	Drinking abolished by LH lesions.	Parks *et al.* (1971)
	$\simeq$ 2–5 μg	crystal	Lateral hypothalamus	Rat	U	Increased food and water intake.	Sciorelli *et al.* (1972)
	$\simeq$ 2.5–3 μg	crystal	Septum, lateral hypothalamus, anterior thalamus	Rat	U	Drinking that was abolished by LH but not septal or thalamic lesions.	Stein and Levitt (1971)
	$\simeq$ 3–5 μg	crystal	Lateral hypothalamus	Rat	U	Motivated drinking.	Khavari and Russell (1966)
	$\simeq$ 5 μg	crystal	Septum, preoptic area, red nucleus, anterior hypothalamus	Rat	U	Drinking.	Hulst and deWied (1967)
	$\simeq$ 5 μg	crystal	Limbic system (17 structures)	Rat	U	Drinking, hypothermia, hyperthermia.	Hulst (1972)
	$\simeq$ 5–10 μg	crystal	Septum	Rat	U	Drinking sucrose in preference to water.	Gandelman *et al.* (1968)
	$\simeq$ 5–10 μg	crystal	Septum	Rat	U	Drinking.	Giardina and Fisher (1971)
	$\simeq$ 10–20 μg	crystal	Perifornical region	Rat	U	Drinking.	Stein and Seifter (1962)
	.44 μg	1 μl	Lateral preoptic area	Rat	U	Less motivated drinking than under deprivation.	Franklin and Quartermain (1970)

Dose	Volume	Site	Species	U	Effect	Reference
.018–.33 μg	1 μl	Lateral hypothalamus	Rat	U	Drinking.	Singer and Montgomery (1969)
1.32 μg	1 μl	Tractus diagonalis	Rat	U	Drinking.	Terpstra and Slangen (1972b)
.009–.44 μg	.5 μl	Amygdala	Rat	U	Drinking in deprived rats.	Russell et al. (1968)
.018–.33 μg	1 μl	Amygdala	Rat	U	Facilitated LH carbachol drinking.	Singer and Montgomery (1969)
.027–.33 μg	.5–1 μl	Amygdala	Rat	U	Drinking.	Montgomery and Singer (1969b)
.055 μg	1 μl	Amygdala	Rat	U	Enhanced septal carbachol drinking.	Singer and Montgomery (1970)
.25 μg	1 μl	Amygdala	Rat	U	Inhibited eating and drinking.	Goddard (1969)
.018 μg	1 μl	Septum	Rat	U	Drinking.	Singer and Montgomery (1970)
.01–2.5 μg	1 μl	Septum, preoptic area	Rat	U	Drinking.	Levitt et al. (1970)
.06–2 μg	2 μl	Septum	Rat	U	Preference for water over saline.	Antunes-Rodrigues and Covian (1971)
.35–.96 μg	.8–2.2 μl	Anterior hypothalamus	Rat	U	Enhanced or suppressed drinking of palatable NaCl solution.	Stricker and Miller (1968)
.44–1.32 μg	1 μl	Anterior, lateral, posterior hypothalamus	Rat	U	Drinking abolished after LH lesions.	Wolf and Miller (1964)
.44 μg	1 μl	Preoptic area	Rat	U	Drinking dependent on interval after drug.	Quartermain and Miller (1966)
.046–.44 μg	1 μl	Lateral hypothalamus, preoptic area, septum	Rat	U	Drinking after deprivation.	Spencer and Holloway (1972)

VII. Master Summary Table (*Continued*)

Chemical	Dose	Volume	Site	Species	State*	Response	Reference
Carbachol	.5 µg	.4 µl	Lateral hypothalamus	Rat	U	Drinking in sated or deprived animal.	Leibowitz (1971)
	.8 µg	1 µl	Lateral hypothalamus	Rat	U	Drinking.	Beideman and Goldstein (1970)
	.01–1 µg	.5 µl	Subfornical organ	Rat	U	Drinking.	Routtenberg and Simpson (1971)
	.01–2.6 µg	1 µl	Diagonal band of Broca	Rat	U	Dose-dependent drinking of water.	Terpstra and Slangen (1972a)
	.05–1 µg	.5 µl	Subfornical organ	Rat	U	Drinking.	Simpson and Routtenberg (1972)
	.5–12.5 µg	1 µl	Lateral hypothalamus, ventromedial hypothalamus	Rat	U	Dose-dependent drinking of water.	Miller *et al.* (1964)
	.7–.9 µg	.8 µl	Septum, nucleus reuniens, rostral hypothalamus	Rat	U	Drinking of water but not ethanol.	Cicero and Myers (1969)
	1–4 µg	1 µl	Rostral hypothalamus, septum	Rat	U	Drinking.	Epstein *et al.* (1970)
	2 µg	1 µl	Septum, anterior thalamus, hypothalamus	Rat	U	Drinking.	Levitt and Boley (1970)
	2.5 µg	1 µl	Fornix, hippocampal commissure, corpus callosum	Rat	U	Drinking.	Levitt and O'Hearn (1972)
	2.5 µg	1 µl	Septum, anterior thalamus, lateral hypothalamus	Rat	U	Water drinking, aversion to hypertonic saline.	White *et al.* (1972)
	3–8 µg	.5 µl	Anterior hypothalamus	Rat	U	Water intake.	Avery (1971)

Substance	Dose	Volume	Site	Animal		Effect	Reference
	5 μg	?	Hypothalamus	Rat	U	Licking water tube after water was delayed.	Feider (1967)
	.06–17.2 μg	?	Hypothalamus	Rabbit	U	Drinking at high doses.	Sommer et al. (1967)
	.1–1 μg	2 μl	Anterior hypothalamic preoptic area, amygdala	Cat	U	Suppressed feeding and drinking.	Milner et al. (1971)
	.5–4 μg	1–4 μl	Thalamus, caudate nucleus, other limbic structures	Cat	U	Inhibited bar-pressing for milk.	Hull et al. (1967)
	16 μg	2 μl	Nucleus centromedian of thalamus	Cat	U	Reduced water intake.	Avery and Nance (1970)
	.4–25 μg	1 μl	Hypothalamus	Monkey	C	Blockade of feeding and drinking at higher doses.	Sharpe and Myers (1969)
	1.2–25 μg	.5–1 μl	Lateral hypothalamus	Monkey	C	Dose-dependent blockade of feeding and drinking in fasted animal.	Myers (1969b)
Chlormerodrin	≈ 20–60 μg	crystal	Hypothalamus	Rat	U	Adipsia, aphagia, death.	Bergmann et al. (1968c)
Chlorpropamide	≈ 100–200 μg	crystal	Hypothalamus	Rat	U	Adipsia.	Bergmann et al. (1968a)
Chlorothiazide	?	crystal	Hypothalamus	Rat	U	Inhibited water intake.	Gutman and Chaimovitz (1966)
	≈ 100–200 μg	crystal	Hypothalamus	Rat	U	Adipsia.	Bergmann et al. 1968a)
Cyclic AMP	≈ 5–10 μg	crystal	Lateral hypothalamus	Rat	U	Increased food and water intake.	Sciorelli et al. (1972)
	≈ 5–10 μg	crystal	Lateral hypothalamus	Rat	U	Drinking.	Rindi et al. (1972)
Cyclic AMP and eserine	?	crystal	Lateral hypothalamus	Rat	U	Increased food and water intake.	Sciorelli et al. (1972)
Desmethyl-imipramine	.55–2.7 μg	1 μl	Lateral hypothalamus	Rat	U	Drinking in satiated rats.	Montgomery et al. (1971)
	107 μg	1–5 μl	Preoptic area	Rat	U	Blocked 6-OHDA feeding and drinking.	Evetts (1972)

VII. Master Summary Table (Continued)

Chemical	Dose	Volume	Site	Species	State*	Response	Reference
Diamox	≈100-200 µg	crystal	Hypothalamus	Rat	U	Adipsia.	Bergmann et al. (1968a)
Dibenzyline	≈3-5 µg	crystal	Ventral amygdala	Rat	U	Lever response for water.	Grossman (1964a)
Digitoxin	≈.5-4 µg	crystal	Hypothalamus	Rat	U	Adipsia following saline load.	Bergmann et al. (1968d)
Diisopropylfluoro-phosphate (DFP)	.1-50 µg	1 µl	Preoptic area	Rat	U	Drinking after long delay.	Winson and Miller (1970)
	120 µg	20 µl	Supraoptic nucleus	Dog	A	Inhibition of urine flow.	Duke et al. (1950)
Dimethylamino-ethanol (DMAE)	≈1-5 µg	crystal	Perifornical region	Rat	U	Drinking.	Grossman (1962b)
Dopamine (DA)	25 µg	.5-1 µl	Lateral hypothalamus	Monkey	C	Feeding and drinking in satiated animal.	Myers (1969b)
Epinephrine	≈3-5 µg	crystal	Ventral amygdala	Rat	U	Reduced lever response for water.	Grossman (1964a)
	5 µg	.5 µl	Perifornical region, hippocampus	Rat	U	Drinking water and ethanol.	Myers (1964b)
	5 µg	5 µl	Globus pallidus, ventromedial and lateral hypothalamus	Rat	U	Drinking of Metrecal.	Wagner and de Groot (1963b)
	12.5 µg	.5-1 µl	Lateral hypothalamus	Monkey	C	Feeding and drinking in satiated animal.	Myers (1969b)
Eserine	≈2.5-3 µg	crystal	Septum, fornix, preoptic area	Rat	U	Drinking.	Chiaraviglio and Taleisnik (1969)
	12 µg	1 µl	Preoptic area	Rat	U	Drinking.	Miller and Chien (1968)
	18.8 µg	1 µl	Lateral hypothala-mus, preoptic area, septum	Rat	U	Drinking only when non-deprived.	Spencer and Holloway (1972)

Substance	Dose	Route	Site	Species		Effect	Reference
	12 µg	1 µl	Preoptic area	Rat	U	Drinking after delay.	Winson and Miller (1970)
	20 µg	1 µl	Fornix, hippocampal commissure, corpus callosum	Rat	U	No drinking.	Levitt and O'Hearn (1972)
	20 µg	1 µl	Septum, anterior thalamus, hypothalamus	Rat	U	Drinking.	Levitt and Boley (1970)
Ethacrynic acid	≈30 µg	crystal	Hypothalamus	Rat	U	Increased urine output, reduced osmolality.	Gutman et al. (1971a)
	≈40 µg	crystal	Hypothalamus	Rat	U	Adipsia after hypovolemia.	Bergmann et al. (1968b)
	≈4–25 µg	crystal	Hypothalamus	Rat	U	Adipsia following saline load.	Bergmann (1968d)
Fructose-6-phosphate (FRU-6-P)	?	crystal	Ventromedial hypothalamus	Rat	A	Inhibited VMH electrical activity.	Gliddon (1970)
Furosemide	≈80 µg	crystal	Hypothalamus	Rat	U	Increased urine output, reduced osmolality.	Gutman et al. (1971a)
γ-aminobutyric acid (GABA)	≈40–160 µg	crystal	Hypothalamus	Rat	U	Adipsia following saline load.	Bergmann (1968d)
	?	crystal	Ventral amygdala	Rat	U	Lever response for water.	Grossman (1964a)
	.0051–.74 µg	.5–1 µl	Amygdala	Rat	U	No drinking.	Montgomery and Singer (1969b)
Glucose	50–90 µg	1 µl	Lateral hypothalamus	Rat	U	Blocked drinking.	Booth (1968b)
Hemicholinium	?	crystal	Lateral hypothalamus	Rat	U	Increased food and water intake.	Sciorelli et al. (1972)
Homosulphanilamide	≈100–200 µg	crystal	Hypothalamus	Rat	U	Adipsia.	Bergmann et al. (1968a)
Hydrochlorothiazide	≈100 µg	crystal	Hypothalamus	Rat	U	Increased urine output, reduced osmolality.	Gutman et al. (1971a)
	≈100–200 µg	crystal	Hypothalamus	Rat	U	Adipsia.	Bergmann et al. (1968a)

VII.   Master Summary Table (Continued)

Chemical	Dose	Volume	Site	Species	State*	Response	Reference
6-Hydroxydopamine (6-OHDA)	.01–16 µg	1–5 µl	Preoptic area	Rat	U	Feeding and drinking.	Evetts (1972)
	4–32 µg	4 µl	Lateral hypothalamus	Rat	U	Aphagia.	Smith et al. (1972)
	6–8 µg	3–4 µl	Lateral hypothalamus, central tegmentum, substantia nigra	Rat	U	Adipsia, catalepsia, akinesis.	Ungerstedt (1971a)
dl-4-(2-Hydroxy-3-isopropylamino-propoxy)-indole (LB-46)	≈18 µg	crystal	Medial forebrain bundle	Rat	U	Increased drinking of quinine-milk.	Margules (1970b)
Hydroxylamine	≈1–2 µg	crystal	Ventral amygdala	Rat	U	Reduced lever response for water.	Grossman (1964a)
Isoproterenol	?	crystal	Lateral hypothalamus	Rat	U	No consistent effect on drinking.	Lehr et al. (1967)
	≈9 µg	crystal	Medial forebrain bundle	Rat	U	Suppressed drinking of quinine-milk.	Margules (1970c)
	≈15–20 µg	crystal	Septum	Rat	U	Drinking.	Giardina and Fisher (1971)
	40 µg	.4 µl	Lateral hypothalamus	Rat	U	Drinking in sated or deprived animal.	Leibowitz (1971)
Lidocaine	50 µg	5 µl	Ventromedial hypothalamus	Rat	U	Drinking of Metrecal.	Wagner and de Groot (1963b)
Mercuric acetate	≈10 µg	crystal	Hypothalamus	Rat	U	Increased urine output, reduced osmolality.	Gutman et al. (1971a)
	≈5–15 µg	crystal	Hypothalamus	Rat	U	Adipsia, aphagia, death.	Bergmann et al. (1968c)
	≈20 µg	crystal	Hypothalamus	Rat	U	Adipsia after hypovolemia.	Bergmann et al. (1968b)
Metrazol	500 µg	5 µl	Ventromedial hypothalamus	Rat	U	Reduced Metrecal drinking.	Wagner and de Groot (1963)

Substance	Dose	Form	Region	Animal		Effect	Reference
Muscarine	≈10–20 µg	crystal	Perifornical region	Rat	U	Drinking.	Stein and Seifter (1962)
Neostigmine	5 µg	5 µl	Ventromedial hypothalamus	Rat	U	Reduced Metrecal drinking.	Wagner and de Groot (1963)
Nicotine	≈10–20 µg	crystal	Perifornical region	Rat	U	Drinking (weak effect).	Stein and Seifter (1962)
Norepinephrine (NE)	2–10 µg	1 µl	Hypothalamus	Monkey	C	Water drinking.	Myers et al. (1973)
	?	crystal	Anterior hypothalamus, preoptic area	Rat	U	Drinking in food deprived animal.	Hutchinson and Renfrew (1967)
	?	crystal	Anterior hypothalamus, ventromedial hypothalamus	Rat	U	Reduced drinking.	Hendler and Blake (1969)
	≈3–5 µg	crystal	Ventral amygdala	Rat	U	Reduced lever response for water.	Grossman (1964a)
	≈4–28 µg	crystal	Medial forebrain bundle	Rat	U	Suppressed milk drinking.	Margules (1969b; 1970a)
	≈25 µg	crystal	Lateral hypothalamus	Rat	U	Drinking of milk.	Margules (1972)
	5 µg	5 µl	Globus pallidus, lateral hypothalamus	Rat	U	Drinking of Metrecal.	Wagner and de Groot (1963b)
	21.59 µg	?	Amygdala	Rat	U	Suppressed drinking in food deprived or satiated rats.	Singer and Montgomery (1968)
	5.5 µg	1–5 µl	Preoptic area	Rat	U	Blocked 6-OHDA feeding but enhanced drinking.	Evetts (1972)
	20 µg	.4 µl	Lateral hypothalamus	Rat	U	Reduced drinking in water deprived animal.	Leibowitz (1971)
	.8-64.8 µg	1 µl	Lateral hypothalamus and ventromedial hypothalamus	Rat	U	Drinking of Metrecal.	Miller et al. (1964)
	1.3–10 µg	1 µl	Hypothalamus	Rat	U	Blocked thirst.	Singer and Kelly (1972)
	5–25 µg	.5 µl	Anterior hypothalamus	Rat	U	Food and water intake.	Avery (1971)

VII. Master Summary Table (Continued)

Chemical	Dose	Volume	Site	Species	State	Response	Reference
Norepinephrine	40–160 μg	2 μl	Anterior hypothalamus, preoptic area, amygdala	Cat	U	Suppressed feeding and drinking.	Milner et al. (1971)
	5–12.5 μg	1–1.2 μl	Hypothalamus	Monkey	C	Feeding and drinking.	Yaksh and Myers (1972b)
	6–25 μg	.5–1 μl	Lateral hypothalamus	Monkey	C	Feeding and drinking in satiated animal.	Myers (1969b)
	12.5 μg	.5–1 μl	Lateral hypothalamus	Monkey	C	Feeding and drinking.	Myers and Sharpe (1968a)
Ouabain	≈1 μg	crystal	Hypothalamus	Rat	U	Increased urine output, reduced osmolality.	Gutman et al. (1971a)
	≈1–2 μg	crystal	Hypothalamus	Rat	U	Adipsia after saline loading.	Bergmann et al. (1967)
	≈4 μg	crystal	Lateral hypothalamus	Rat	U	Natriuresis. Reduced water intake and urine osmolality; increased urine output.	Gutman et al. (1970; 1971b)
Pentobarbital	300 μg	5 μl	Ventromedial hypothalamus	Rat	U	Drinking of Metrecal.	Wagner and de Groot (1963b)
Phenformin	≈30 μg	crystal	Hypothalamus	Rat	U	Increased urine output. reduced osmolality.	Gutman et al. (1971a)
Phentolamine	≈9–18 μg	crystal	Medial forebrain bundle	Rat	U	Milk drinking.	Margules (1969b; 1970a)
	4–8 μg	1–5 μl	Preoptic area	Rat	U	Blocked 6-OHDA feeding but enhanced drinking.	Evetts (1972)
	13 μg	1 μl	Septum, anterior thalamus, lateral hypothalamus	Rat	U	Failed to block angiotensin drinking.	White et al. (1972)
	102 μg	4 μl	Lateral hypothalamus	Rat	U	Drinking in sated or deprived animal.	Leibowitz (1971)

Substance	Dose	Volume	Brain site	Species	C/U	Effect	Reference
Potassium chloride (KCl)	2 µg	?	Occipital cortex	Rat	U	Drinking, eating, excitation.	Huston and Bureš (1970)
Propranolol	≈18 µg	crystal	Medial forebrain bundle	Rat	U	No effect.	Margules (1970a)
	84 µg	.4 µl	Lateral hypothalamus	Rat	U	Reduced drinking in deprived animal.	Leibowitz (1971)
Renin	1 mU	1 µl	Rostral hypothalamus	Rat	U	Drinking.	Fitzsimons (1971b)
	5-15 mU	1 µl	Rostral hypothalamus, septum	Rat	U	Drinking.	Epstein et al. (1970)
Scopolamine	≈1-3 µg	crystal	Septum, anterior thalamus	Rat	U	Reduced thirst in presence of food.	Levitt (1968)
	≈2-3 µg	crystal	Septum, anterior thalamus, mesencephalon	Rat	U	Blocked cholinergic drinking.	Levitt (1969)
	2.5 µg	1 µl	Septum, anterior thalamus, lateral hypothalamus	Rat	U	Failed to block angiotensin drinking.	White et al. (1972)
Serotonin (5-HT)	12.5 µg	.5-1 µl	Lateral hypothalamus	Monkey	C	Feeding and drinking.	Myers and Sharpe (1968a)
	6-25 µg	1 µl	Hypothalamus	Monkey	C	Drinking followed by eating.	Sharpe and Myers (1969)
Sodium chloride (NaCl)	?	crystal	Anterior hypothalamus	Rat	U	Reduced drinking after deprivation.	Hendler and Blake (1969)
	5.25-35.06 µg	.5-2 µl	Preoptic area	Rat	U	Drinking.	Blass and Epstein (1971)
	28.05 µg	2 µl	Preoptic area	Rat	U	Drinking reduced by peripheral atropine.	Blass and Chapman (1971)
	62.5 µg	2 µl/min	Preoptic area	Rabbit	U	Drinking of water.	Peck and Novin (1971)

428 HANDBOOK OF DRUG AND CHEMICAL STIMULATION OF THE BRAIN

VII. Master Summary Table (Continued)

Chemical	Dose	Volume	Site	Species	State	Response	Reference
NaCl	62.5 μg	2 μl/min	Lateral and dorsal hypothalamus	Rabbit	U	Drinking or eating.	Peck and Novin (1971)
	1.5–2 mg	100 μl	Anterior hypothalamus	Goat	U	Polydipsia, diuresis.	Andersson (1952)
	1.5–2.5 mg	100–150 μl	Medial hypothalamus	Goat	U	Drinking, diuresis.	Andersson (1953)
	60–200 μg	3–10 μl	Hypothalamus	Goat	U	Polydipsia.	Andersson and McCann (1955)
Sotalol hydro-chloride (MS-1999)	4–8 μg	1–5 μl	Preoptic area	Rat	U	Blocked 6-OHDA feeding and drinking.	Evetts (1972)
Sucrose	410.76 μg	2 μl	Preoptic area	Rat	U	Drinking.	Blass and Epstein (1971)
	787.3 μg	2 μl/min	Preoptic area	Rabbit	U	Drinking.	Peck and Novin (1971)
Sulphadiazine	≃ 100–200 μg	crystal	Hypothalamus	Rat	U	Adipsia.	Bergmann et al. (1968a)
Tetradecapeptide renin	1 μg	1 μl	Rostral hypothalamus	Rat	U	Drinking.	Fitzsimons (1971b)
Tolbutamide	≃ 100–200 μg	crystal	Hypothalamus	Rat	U	Adipsia.	Bergmann et al. (1968a)
Water	—	2 μl	Preoptic area	Rat	U	Attenuated salt arousal drinking.	Blass and Epstein (1971)

9
Sleep and Arousal

I. INTRODUCTION

The phenomenon of sleep is not only fascinating in its own right but is one of the most puzzling of all of our vital functions. From all scientific quarters come the speculations about the very purpose of sleep. How we enter into somnolence, which serum factor, if any, promotes the state of sleep, and the possible hypnogenic mechanisms within the brain have been the subject of vast enquiry. Literally dozens of reviews, books, symposia and collaborative monographs have appeared on every aspect of sleep and waking over the last two decades alone. Epitomizing these and appearing in a single volume are the insightful and comprehensive treatises of Jouvet (1972) and Moruzzi (1972).

The lack of agreement on detail and the general controversy surrounding even the definition of sleep and the various states of arousal underscore the redoubtable complexity of the phenomenon itself (Morgane, 1972). Certainly, all organ systems in the body benefit in one way or another by the cyclicity in sleep and arousal. Generally, it is conceded that sleep is a restorative process that enables the brain and other bodily structures to recover from what Sherrington called "wear and tear." The consequences of the recovery processes are a reinstatement of physiochemical balance or homeostasis of the cerebral structures essential to survival. In most mammals the recuperative process is a relatively slow one, for fully one-third of one's entire life is occupied in this remarkable state.

On appearance, the behavioral symptoms of sleep can be described in terms of a postural change, the closure of the eyelids, an increased depth but decreased rate of respiration, and generalized immobility. However, sleep is a complex sequence of events which cannot be attributed to a static circumstance—an absence in cerebral activity. In fact, dynamic changes occur in the electrical activity of the cortex and subcortical structures.

Even though somewhat imprecise and a physiological oversimplification, the continuum of sleep is nonetheless divided heuristically into the following three electroencephalographic categories: (1) wakefulness which is characterized by a desynchronized EEG pattern consisting primarily of low voltage waves of high frequency; (2) deep or slow-wave sleep (SWS), during which time the pattern of the EEG is synchronized and dominated by rhythmic high voltage waves that occur less frequently; and (3) paradoxical sleep (PS) which is typified by bursts of fast-wave EEG activity, rapid eye movements (REM) and perhaps dreaming. To discuss or interpret experiments on sleep, a common ground based upon these EEG parameters is now considered to be an incontrovertible requisite (Morgane, 1972).

A. Anatomical Significance of the Brain-Stem

Classical experiments utilizing the techniques of transection, local ablation or electrical stimulation have uncovered the anatomical regions in the brain-stem concerned with arousal. Specifically, the reticular formation of the lower brain-stem is the major anatomical substrate implicated in the normal sleep-wakefulness pattern.

After the cerebrum is neurologically isolated by a complete mesencephalic transection (*cerveau isolé*), the acute preparation remains in a comatose state from which arousal is never possible (Bremer, 1935). However, the important demonstration by Villablanca (1962) that a sleep-waking cycle is eventually observed in the animal's cortical EEG means that the intrinsic rhythmicity in sleep-wakefulness may be quite independent of lower brain-stem control. After a decortication, the chronically sustained animal shows some features of normal sleep-waking cyclicity and even almost typical EEG patterns recorded from subcortical leads. Of course, as Moruzzi (1972) has rightly emphasized, lesions placed in the reticular formation, raphé nuclei, cerebellum, thalamus, hypothalamus and other subcortical structures can cause effects ranging from a subtle imbalance between paradoxical and slow-wave sleep to a total abolition of waking behavior.

In spite of the inertia of the sleep response, characterized by the long latency following electrical stimulation of the midline structures in the thalamus, Hess's (e.g., 1954, 1957) discovery has stood as a great landmark in sleep physiology. Arousal from sleep or EEG desynchronization can be triggered by a stimulating current applied to the reticular formation (Moruzzi and Magoun, 1949), whereas basal forebrain stimulation evokes synchronization of the EEG and behavioral sleep (Sterman and Clemente, 1962).

Figure 9-1 shows schematically the reticular core system (Morgane and Stern, 1972). It is comprised of ascending and descending pathways that link this system to diencephalic and other subcortical structures as well as to the neocortex. Within this reticular core are presumably the neurochemical substrates which provide the checks and balances for maintaining the levels of activation and wakefulness as well as sleep.

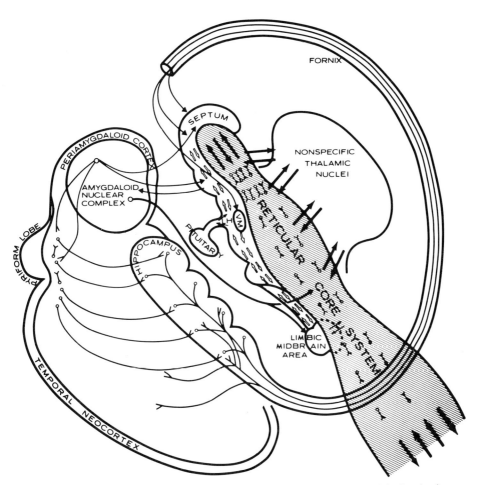

Fig. 9-1   Drawing showing the well-developed relations between limbic forebrain areas and the reticular core of the brain-stem. In reality, a study of the patterns of neural assembly indicates that the entire limbic forebrain area, nonspecific thalamic nuclei, and hypothalamus represent the forebrain and diencephalic extensions of the reticular formation.   The limbic midbrain area actually is a component of the reticular core system based on its neural architecture and patterns of neuronal assembly. However, for descriptive purposes this paramedian region of the mesencephalon is often delimited as limbic midbrain area, specifically comprising the ventral tegmental area of Tsai, the nucleus centralis superior of Bechterew, and the ventral and dorsal (deep) tegmental nuclei of Gudden, this latter nucleus buried in the central half of the central gray surrounding the cerebral aqueduct. (From Morgane and Stern, 1972)

B. Neurohumoral Correlates

Alternate accumulation and dissipation of humoral constituents in a morphologically circumscribed region of the brain would seem to account for the reciprocal activation and deactivation of the arousal system. This could explain the residual antagonism of sleep-wakefulness states that is restored in the well-nursed cat recovering from a mesencephalic transection.

An issue of major dimensions in this field today is the nature of the postulated hypnogenic circuit. Is such an anatomical circuit mediated by one humoral factor or more? How do parts of the system function in congruence with one another? On the basis of a number of studies involving certain lesions and drugs, Jouvet (1967) has proposed that the ratio of serotonin to norepinephrine within the brain-stem maintains each of several different states of sleep. The balance in the release of these monoamines presumably operates in much the same way as is hypothesized to occur in the anterior hypothalamus in the control of body temperature (Chapter 6).

When cerebral serotonin is depleted by the drug p-chlorophenylalanine (pCPA), slow-wave sleep is reduced and symptoms of insomnia develop. Similarly, when the raphé nuclei which contain large stores of serotonin are lesioned, the animal's state of wakefulness again predominates. Here, the implicit action of serotonin is apparent.

The nucleus coeruleus contains a dense conglomeration of noradrenergic nerve terminals. When this mesencephalic nucleus is lesioned, several attributes of paradoxical sleep disappear. Further, drugs that interfere with the synthesis of norepinephrine such as disulfiram or α-methyl-p-tyrosine (αMpT) suppress paradoxical sleep (Jouvet, 1972). An overall interpretation then of the monoamine theory of sleep suggests that the neuronal release of serotonin within the midbrain could evoke deep sleep, whereas the synaptic liberation of norepinephrine would trigger the paradoxical state. These two coordinated aminergic actions thus would provide the necessary balance between the two major states of sleep, both of which are necessary for physical as well as mental stability. That the serotonin mechanism in the raphé complex may somehow prime the catecholamine component in the locus coeruleus in order to activate fast-wave sleep also is an intriguing possibility (Jouvet, 1969).

The serotonergic, noradrenergic and dopaminergic systems discussed in reference to sleep and arousal are summarized in Fig. 9-2. The anatomical pathways and the group of nuclei have been derived elegantly from a number of important mapping studies utilizing histochemical fluorescence (e.g., Fuxe et al., 1968).

1. Other Sleep Substances

At the turn of this century Piéron and his French colleagues discovered that CSF collected from a sleep-deprived dog and injected subsequently into the cisterna

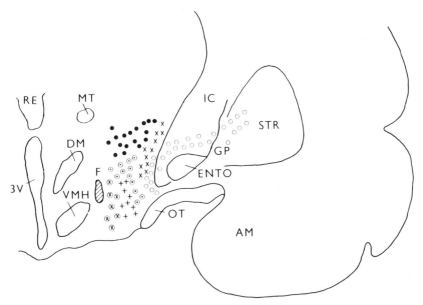

Fig. 9-2   Schematic drawing of the cat brain in frontal section through the middle of the hypothalamus at the level of the ventromedial nucleus. The entire region lateral to the column of the fornix, extending to the internal capsule, comprises the lateral hypothalamic area, which is the bed nucleus of the medial forebrain bundle. Note the parcellation of this bundle based on chemical coding (chemospecificity determined by histofluorescence mapping) and that the serotonergic, noradrenergic, and dopamine systems occupy particular positions within the bundle. This topographic separation allows each chemically coded circuit to be manipulated independently.   Cholinergic systems also in this bundle are not shown.   •, Dorsal noradrenergic system; ⊙, ventral noradrenergic system; ⊗, medial serotonergic system; +, lateral serotonergic system; ○, nigro-striatal dopamine system; x, mesolimbic dopamine system; RE, reuniens nucleus of thalamus; 3V, third ventricle; MT, mammillo-thalamic tract; DM, dorsomedial hypothalamic nucleus; VMH, ventromedial hypothalamic nucleus; F, fornix; OT, optic tract; ENTO, entopeduncular nucleus; GP, globus pallidus; STR, neostriatum (putamen and caudate nuclei); IC, internal capsule; AM, amygdala. (From Morgane and Stern, 1972)

magna of a normal dog caused the recipient animal to sleep for several hours (Legendre and Piéron, 1910; 1912). Variations on this astounding observation have met with mixed success, probably because of the inordinate number of physiological and other variables (Pappenheimer *et al.*, 1967; Ringle and Herndon, 1969). As will be discussed later, Monnier and his co-workers have recently been able to identify a plasma-dialyzable factor that induces sleep in a normal rabbit (Monnier and Hösli, 1965).

Acetylcholine has also been implicated in brain-stem arousal mechanisms as a result of a number of pharmacological experiments employing cholinergic agonists and antagonists (Jouvet, 1972). An ascending cholinergic pathway has been traced by Shute and Lewis (1967) which dovetails anatomically with this notion. To confound the situation, Hernández-Peón and his colleagues have postulated, on the basis of chemical stimulation experiments, a cholinergic sleep circuit. This arises as a descending pathway in the medial forebrain bundle. When a cholinomimetric substance is applied to certain spots in the cat's forebrain, deep sleep as measured behaviorally and electrographically is reportedly produced. However, the possible role of the release of endogenous ACh in triggering the sleep responses is far from clear. Arousal, rage and autonomic effects are evoked by cholinergic stimulation, even simultaneously in the same experiment.

How can we contend with the fact that many naturally occurring substances may induce behavioral or EEG manifestations of sleep when they are injected into the brain? Does each of these play a part in the humoral mechanism of sleep? Is it possible that a difference in laboratory technique, inadequacy in human observation, or a failure to exercise adequate controls contributes to the differences in the results contained in individual research reports?

Because of the sensitivity of the sleep phenomenon and the preparation itself, a dose-response analysis is probably of paramount importance in this field. For example, with the injection into the mesencephalon of a single dose of a drug, it is impossible to determine whether the compound (a) blocks an arousal or excitatory pathway because of a local overdose which swamps receptor sites, or (b) mimics the natural release in a reciprocal inhibitory pathway of a natural neurohumoral factor. In either case, the same net effect would ensue – sleep.

Obviously, numerous controls are required. As Pappenheimer et al. (1967) have warned, an animal such as the laboratory cat may sleep much of the time away, literally taking cat naps. In our laboratory, we have often observed particularly in the afternoon that if a cat is moved about and has its electrode leads connected to a recording instrument, or is given some sort of an intracerebral injection, the cat will often search out a corner, curl up and go to sleep. Had we just infused a drug after all this manipulation, it would have been easy to misinterpret the animal's response as a direct action of the chemical on the infused structure. Finally, two compounds assumed to have the same physiological action probably cannot be used interchangeably since acetylcholine may produce sleep whereas carbachol evokes intense rage when both substances are applied to one area (Yamaguchi et al., 1964).

II. MONOAMINES AND SLEEP

Although scant, some direct anatomical evidence of the participation of the monoamines in the control of sleep, its activation or suppression, has been recently documented. In spite of the fact that many of the micro-injection experiments do correspond with those studies involving more peripheral methods, a thorough-going analysis of the localization of a chemical's action has yet to be accomplished.

A. Serotonin and EEG Synchronization

After serotonin is injected via the bloodstream or into the cerebral ventricle of the cat, the ocular and EEG signs of synchronized EEG sleep are quickly seen. Presumably, serotonin acts on receptor sites in the area postrema which can apparently be penetrated by the indoleamine through the systemic route (Koella and Czicman, 1966). The specificity of the synchronization was supported by the finding that the local application of methysergide on the area postrema by means of a cotton pellet soaked in this serotonin antagonist reversed the EEG hypersynchrony.

An important investigation by Bronzino et al. (1972b) revealed that in the anesthetized cat the application of serotonin to the region of the area postrema, again by a cotton pledget soaked in a solution of the indoleamine increases the synchronization of the EEG. The duration of serotonin's effect on the EEG pattern lasts only about 40 minutes even though the sponge was left on the exposed tissue. Probably the serotonin receptors become saturated. The hypersynchrony that is characterized by an increase in low frequency waves at the same time that the fast-wave components decline occurs in all cats in which serotonin is applied only within the area postrema. This result would give further support to the idea that this amine plays a key role in the sleep-organizing or controlling process. Since the effect of serotonin is so highly localized, it is likely that the area postrema could be an important anatomical link in the hypnogenic circuit subserving slow-wave sleep. In this region, the permeability of the blood brain barrier is proportionately greater than in most other areas.

Even though technical details were not presented, Morgane and Stern (1972) have recently summarized the effect of serotonin injected into midbrain raphé nuclei of the cat. Ordinarily, serotonin does not affect the animal's sleep profile. However, after pCPA is given systemically in order to deplete central serotonin stores, the interval of slow-wave sleep increases at the expense of waking, but with no change in paradoxical or REM sleep. Since pCPA on its own causes insomnia, the local elevation of serotonin in the raphé complex probably serves to replace the depleted fraction of the indoleamine and to restore the normal balance in humoral factors.

When a large volume of 5-HTP or DOPA, the respective precursors of serotonin and norepinephrine, is injected into different parts of the bulbo-pontine region of the rabbit, the resultant pattern of EEG activity is different. Distinguishing the structures injected according to a functional rather than anatomical basis, Ledebur and Tissot (1966) were able to show that 5-HTP given more posteriorly evokes the typical features of EEG sleep. Infused more anteriorly, 5-HTP causes bursts of desynchronization and ocular movements characteristic of REM sleep.

No matter where it is injected in the pontine-bulbar area, DOPA exerts the same effect as when given intravenously: neocortical desynchronization, lack of awareness and reduction in muscle tone. Probably this result occurs because of the huge dose and volume that may have duplicated a systemic injection.

Crystals of melatonin implanted into the preoptic area or nucleus centralis medialis of the cat's thalamus produce an increase in high voltage slow waves in an EEG record taken from the hippocampus or other subcortical structure (Marczynski et al., 1964). These changes are illustrated in Fig. 9-3. However, the latency of 15 to 30 minutes was unusually long and the duration of EEG sleep was 2 to 3 hours. Even though serotonin also produces sleep when injected at similar sites, Marczynski et al. postulated that melatonin may play a role in sleep-wakefulness. In view of the latency of the effect, an alternative interpretation is that this pineal factor probably mimics serotonin in acting on trypt-aminoceptive structures.

B. Catecholamines and Level of Arousal

Ordinarily, an injection of a catecholamine into the hypothalamus of the cat causes a condition of somnolence. However, when a rat is treated with α-methyl-p-tyrosine (αMpT), a drug which depletes brain-stem catecholamines, it responds somewhat differently to a micro-injection of a small dose of norepinephrine into the preoptic area or mesencephalic reticular formation (Torda, 1968). In the αMpT-treated rat that is asleep, norepinephrine temporarily arouses the animal. The duration of both paradoxical and deep sleep is shortened, thereby extending the period of wakefulness. Although the catecholamine-depleting action of αMpT is not as selective as originally thought, the capacity of norepinephrine to reverse its soporific effect could reflect the participation of the endogenous amine in the brain-stem mechanism of wakefulness and general arousal.

Catecholamines infused into the brain of a bird generally suppress activity, induce sleep, lower blood pressure, diminish oxygen consumption and evoke hypothermia (Marley and Stephenson, 1970). Although α-methyl-norepine-phrine and isoprenaline possess identical actions when infused into the chick's brain, their potencies vary, with isoprenaline about half as active as α-methyl-norepinephrine. A prior infusion of phenoxybenzamine prevents all of the effects of the three catecholamines, whereas propranolol attenuates only the bird's hypothermia. The qualitative differences in these effects would suggest that in the chicken's hypothalamus, the actions of these amines are mediated largely through alpha receptors.

In examining the question of arousal and sleep following an intrahypothalamic injection of a catecholamine in the bird, Marley and Nistico (1972) found that an intraventricular dose at least 5 to 20 times larger than a hypothalamic dose was required to produce an equivalent response. Figure 9-4 illustrates the change in the chicken's electrocortical activity from a low amplitude, high frequency

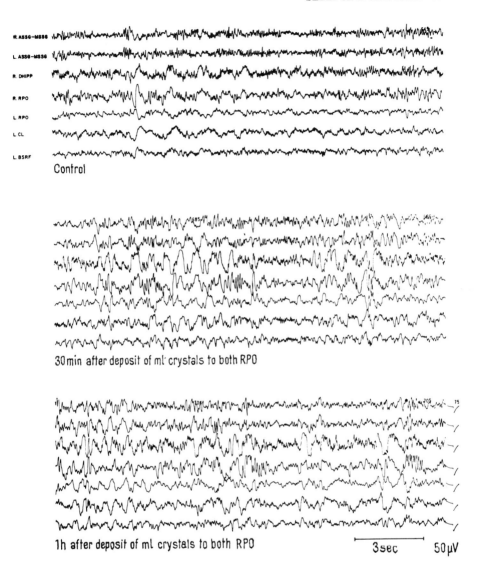

Fig. 9-3 Representative EEG record from an unanesthetized cat: before, and 30 and 60 minutes after the administration 15 μg per cannula of melatonin to the left and right preoptic region. Note the high amplitude waves in the right dorsal hippocampus (R. DHIPP), right and left preoptic region (R. RPO, L. RPO) and left nucleus centralis lateralis (L. CL). The remaining abbreviations: ASSG, anterior suprasylvian gyrus, MSSG, medial syprasylvian gyrus, BSRF brain-stem reticular formation. (From Marczynski *et al.*, 1964)

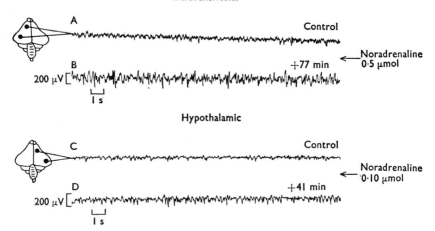

Fig. 9-4 Electrocortical activity from two adult fowls. A, C, Control alert electrocortical potentials. B, Large amplitude (100–400 μV), 5–8 Hz sleep electrocortical potentials 77 minutes after intraventricular noradrenaline. D, Smaller amplitude (60–140 μV), 6–8 Hz typical sleep potentials 41 minutes after intrahypothalamic infusion of noradrenaline. (From Marley and Nistico, 1972)

pattern to high voltage slow activity after the two doses of norepinephrine were given. After the inhibition of monoamine oxidase by systemic mebanazine, the action of the catecholamines on sleep was enhanced. Dopamine which has only very little effect on the bird produced deep sleep which lasted for 3 hours. Cyclic AMP and adenosine infused into the hypothalamus after systemic aminophylline administration also evoked behavioral and electrocortical sleep. However, dibutyryl cyclic AMP infused similarly suddenly aroused the animal; the chicken became alert, vocalized, moved about and the EEG showed spiking activity. These opposite and dramatic responses are difficult to understand in terms of the possible role of cyclic AMP as a second messenger for neurohormones such as the catecholamines.

Slow-wave sleep is also evoked when cyclic AMP is infused in a large dose into the fastigial nucleus of the cerebellum (Gessa *et al.*, 1970). Since the doses used to produce sleep were out of any physiological range and the latency of effect was 10 to 30 minutes, a biochemical change secondary to a direct action of the nucleotide is probably responsible for the response.

III. ACETYLCHOLINE: SLEEP OR ACTIVATION?

Given by the systemic route, acetylcholine, anticholinesterases, nicotine and other cholinergic agonists induce cortical EEG activation and behavioral arousal. Even though the action of atropine and other antagonists is still uncertain, the release of acetylcholine in the brain-stem and cortical structures has been implicated historically in sleep-wakefulness mechanisms (Dikshit, 1935) and in the general level of an animal's state of arousal (see Jouvet, 1972).

A. Cholinergic Sleep Circuit

Before the untimely death of the illustrious Mexican physiologist, Hernández-Peón, he and his collaborators published what has come to be regarded as a classical series of papers in sleep research. In 1962, Hernández-Peón first reported that crystalline ACh applied in the posterior hypothalamus of a cat resulted in a sleep often so deep that a strong nociceptive stimulus failed to disturb the animal. Although no details were given, norepinephrine placed at some of the same loci produced alertness and motor hyperactivity.

Two other brief reports described sites in the cat's hypothalamus and mesencephalon at which ACh evoked excitation or sleep (Hernández-Peón et al., 1962; Hernández-Peón and Chávez-Ibarra, 1963). In some animals, an initial alertness for a brief interval preceded the more prolonged period of drowsiness and the relaxed state. Nevertheless, Hernández-Peón and his co-workers proposed that sharply segregated zones, drawn in Fig. 9-5, articulated the pathways extending from the forebrain as follows: (1) a sleep circuit traversing the medial forebrain bundle to the dorsal tegmentum; (2) an alerting pathway extending from the septum to the lateral mesencephalic reticular formation; and (3) a rage pathway projecting from the septum through the dorsal hypothalamus and into the periaqueductal gray matter. At that time the possibility was, of course, not considered that the local concentration of ACh deposited in an unknown dose was so high that a tetanizing blockade of synaptic transmission had occurred which would deactivate the neurons serving arousal.

In a more complete account, Hernández-Peón et al. (1963) showed that along a limbic pathway, extending from the preoptic region to the pons, crystals of ACh or carbachol, again in an unspecified dose, evoked sleep within 20 seconds to 4 minutes. Spindles and high voltage slow waves characterized the lighter phases of sleep. The EEG records obtained from the muscles of the cat's neck were also diminished in amplitude. The high amplitude, oscillating eye movements of REM sleep also occurred during the phase of deep sleep. The anatomical analysis showed that sleep was induced by cholinergic stimulation of the septum, MFB, fibers of the fornix and other related structures and nuclei. At similar sites, tranquilization, alertness, autonomic changes and rage could also be produced. Taken together, these two conflicting sets of results are difficult to interpret, mainly because coronal or sagittal maps were not constructed to determine what percent of the sites were sleep sites, what percent were rage sites, and whether some sort of anatomical specificity for either response existed. At many sites, norepinephrine evoked responses similar to those of ACh, which is again perplexing.

Evidence of a possible regional cholinergic blockade due to a high local con-

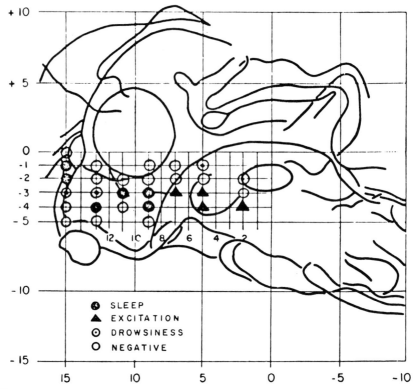

Fig. 9-5 Map summarizing the points in which acetylcholine produced either drowsiness, sleep, alertness or no effect. Stereotaxic coordinates are in millimeters. (From Hernández-Peón, R. and G. Chávez-Ibarra. 1963. *EEG Clin. Neurophysiol.* 24:188–198. Elsevier Publishing Co., Amsterdam, The Netherlands)

centration of carbachol or ACh was also presented by Hernández-Peón (1965), who described experiments in which the depth of sleep was so great that "the cat could not be aroused by nociceptive stimuli." This state would virtually correspond to one of anesthesia or stupor that is observed on injection of a cholinomimetic substance into the cerebral ventricle of the cat (Feldberg, 1963) or into the ventricle of the human patient (Henderson and Wilson, 1936). Interestingly, the severity of the effect of the cholinergic drug could be vitiated by crystals of atropine if applied previously to the same locus. The sites at which ACh evoked sleep in addition to those mentioned earlier include the cingulate gyrus, pyriform cortex, pre-pyriform cortex, the basal forebrain, medial thalamic nuclei, caudate nucleus, globus pallidus, claustrum, putamen, pons and the lower portion of the cervical spinal cord. Figure 9-6 shows typical EEG records of sleep produced by ACh deposited in the pyriform cortex. Although

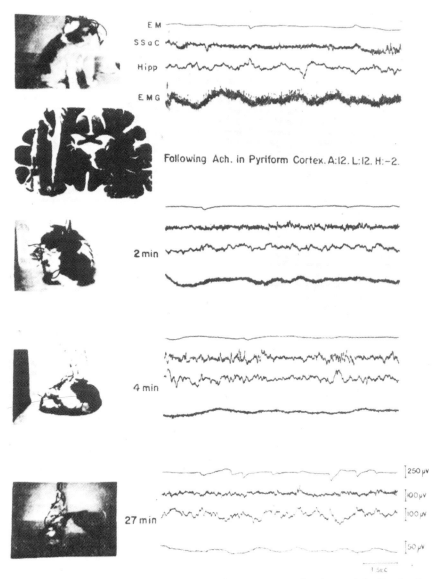

EM

SSaC

Hipp

EMG

Following Ach. in Pyriform Cortex. A:12. L:12. H:-2.

2 min

4 min

27 min

250 μv

100 μv

100 μv

50 μv

1 sec

Fig. 9-6 Sleep produced by application of minute crystals of acetylcholine in the pyriform cortex at the point marked by the arrow. EM, eye movements; SSaC, suprasylvian anterior cortex; Hipp, hippocampus; EMG, electromyogram of the neck muscles. (From Hernández-Peón, R. 1965. *Progress in Brain Research.* **18**:96–115. Fig. 3. Elsevier Publishing Co., Amsterdam, The Netherlands)

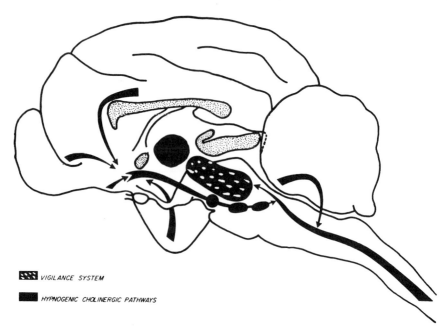

VIGILANCE SYSTEM

HYPNOGENIC CHOLINERGIC PATHWAYS

Fig. 9-7 Diagram illustrating the anatomical substrate of the sleep system disclosed by localized cholinergic stimulation. The system is composed of two components: a descending component with corticofugal projections from the pyriform cortex, the orbital surface of the frontal lobe and the anterior part of the gyrus cinguli which converge upon the limbic midbrain circuit extending down to the ponto-mesencephalic tegmentum. A midline thalamic area is shown. The descending component joins at the pontine level with an ascending component originating in the spinal cord. (From Hernández-Peón, R. 1965. *Progress in Brain Research.* 18:96–115. Fig. 10. Elsevier Publishing Co., Amsterdam, The Netherlands)

the exceptional diffuseness of the sleep system raises the suspicion that the effect of acetylcholine crystals applied to the structure are relatively nonspecific, Fig. 9-7 presents a speculative view of how the cholinergic vigilance-hypnogenic systems may be anatomically separated.

In a pharmacological extension of this work, Velluti and Hernández-Peón (1963) found that atropine applied at posterior sites in the sleep circuit blocks the sleep evoked by ACh or eserine deposited in the preoptic area. The anatomical relationship is illustrated schematically in Fig. 9-8. The cholinergic blocking agent also prevents sleep when applied at the same preoptic site just before ACh. Since eserine induces sleep in the same way as ACh, and because atropine blocks the effect of both ACh and eserine, Velluti and Hernández-Peón concluded that the natural release of ACh is in all likelihood the mechanism for the transmission of signals for sleep.

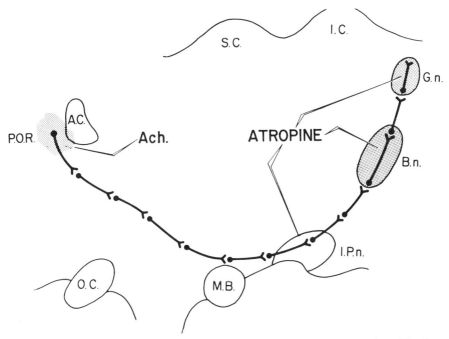

Fig. 9-8 This diagram illustrates the blocking effect of atropine placed in the interpeduncular nucleus (I.P.n.), or in Bechterew's (B.n.) or Gudden's (G.n.) nuclei upon sleep otherwise induced by acetylcholine applied in the medial upper pre-optic region. (From Velluti and Hernández-Peón, 1963)

Related to this supposition is the crucial nature of the dose of the chemical given in a structure of the central nervous system. In determining the resultant sleep pattern, this fact has been demonstrated lucidly by Kostowski (1971). When 5 μg of ACh is injected into the pons of the cat, the neocortical EEG becomes synchronized. On the other hand, 15 μg of ACh at the same site desynchronizes the EEG. Eserine produces the same synchronizing response as a lower dose of ACh, whereas the effect of nicotine or atropine injected into the pons is similar to the higher dose — EEG desynchronization. Although the pontine raphé area is exceedingly complex, these pharmacological findings indicate that the EEG synchronizing mechanism could depend on the stimulation of muscarinic receptors; conversely, cortical desynchronization is related to the activation of nicotinic receptor sites within the same morphological area.

Cholinergic stimulation of still more posterior sites within the pontine reticular formation of the cat with a muscarinic agent or carbachol evokes paradoxical sleep including rapid movement of the eyeballs, synchronized hippocampal activity, and atonia (George et al., 1964). These effects are prevented or reversed by an injection of atropine at the same site. Of great importance is the finding that serotonin, norepinephrine, epinephrine, dopamine or nicotine failed to cause any changes whatsoever when any of the drugs were injected at the same site in doses of up to 10 μg. Although this finding is not in agreement with that of Cordeau *et al.* (1963) or others, the postulate pertaining to a cholinergic mechanism underlying the hypnogenic pathway is again upheld.

B. Cholinergic Arousal System

In 1961, Myers found that in the freely moving cat, epinephrine applied at sites throughout the hypothalamus including the preoptic area caused weakness, stupor, drowsiness and what appeared behaviorally to be deep sleep (Myers, 1964a). Cholinergic stimulation with either carbachol or ACh in solution or in crystalline form at homologous sites only aroused the cat and elicited emotional excitation. With a higher dose the animal became enraged. As described more fully in Chapter 11, ACh or a cholinomimetic drug injected in sites in the limbic system corresponding to those described by Hernández-Peón ordinarily tended to arouse an animal and heighten its emotional behavior rather than to induce sleep.

An attempt was made by Macphail and Miller (1968) to reconcile the two conflicting reports of Hernández-Peón *et al.* (1963) and Myers (1964a) to determine whether cholinergic stimulation of identical spots in the hypothalamus did produce sleep or an affective defense reaction. Repeating the previous experiments, they stimulated sites homologous to those that were thought to comprise the cholinergic hypnogenic sleep circuit. The results of Myers were confirmed in that: (a) sleep was never observed; (b) autonomic arousal and behavior responses of the defense reaction were elicited; and (c) these latter effects were not localized to particular areas of the hypothalamus. Macphail and Miller offered several explanations for the discrepancies. One is the possibility of differences between crystals and solution, but this was rejected on the basis of Myers's use of both. Another possibility is that Hernández-Peón may have failed to exercise adequate controls, since cats may fall asleep spontaneously in a quiet environment. Interestingly, Vahing *et al.* (1971) have confirmed that affective reactions are evoked by ACh injections into the cat's hypothalamus; however, behavioral inhibition and possibly sleep were also observed by these Russian workers when ACh was given in the lateral hypothalamus.

Additional results contradicting the idea of a cholinergic sleep system were reported by Peñaloza-Rojas and Zeidenweber (1965). Although the olfactory bulb of the cat was the site of stimulation, a local injection of a low dose of epinephrine evoked EEG synchronization and a postural response indicative of sleep. In contrast, ACh injected similarly produced the opposite effect. As shown in Fig. 9-9, electrocortical and behavioral arousal occurred with the EEG showing mostly alpha and beta rhythms. This investigation failed to confirm any hypnogenic effect of ACh in the cat.

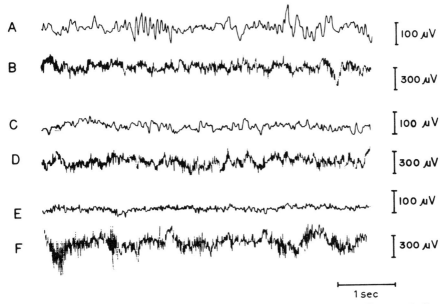

Fig. 9-9 Effect of the application of acetylcholine within the olfactory bulb upon the EBOG (lower tracings) and EEG (upper tracings). A and B: before injection during somnolence. C and D: 1 minute after injection simultaneously with sleep-like posture. E and F: 5 minutes after injection, during alertness induced by auditory stimulation. (From Peñaloza-Rojas, J. H. and J. Zeidenweber. 1965. *EEG Clin. Neurophysiol.* **19**:88–90. Elsevier Publishing Co., Amsterdam, The Netherlands)

Rather perplexing results were reported by Yamaguchi *et al.* (1964). The sleep evoked by crystals of ACh deposited in the preoptic area purportedly lasted for 30 to 60 minutes, the same duration as that produced by serotonin deposited similarly. Since the hydrolysis of ACh is so rapid without the enzymatic protection of eserine or another anticholinesterase, ACh should probably have had little or no effect. An implant of carbachol produced the more typical effect of rage and a defense reaction. Although given in approximately one-sixth the dose, it was not understood at that time why carbachol should have such a different effect than ACh. Norepinephrine produced sleep when deposited in the thalamus, but had some autonomic effects when placed in the preoptic area. An interpretation of these results is difficult since information on the localization of sites or controls was not given.

When 10 μg crystals of carbachol were placed close to the aqueduct in the mesencephalon of the cat, an intense emotional arousal occurred first; then an episode of REM sleep followed that is illustrated in Fig. 9-10 (Baxter, 1969). The paradoxical sleep was so deep that the cat could not be awakened even by a strong peripheral stimulus. It is possible that the initial excitatory effect of

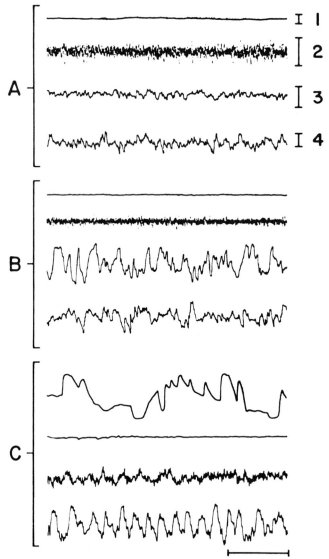

Fig. 9-10   Recordings obtained during typical relaxed wakefulness (A); slow-wave sleep (B); and carbachol-induced REM sleep (C). Numbers to the right in (A) show order and calibration voltages (200 μV) for all three conditions: (1) eye movements; (2) neck muscle potentials; (3) cortical activity; and (4) hippocampal activity.   Note the marked eye movements, loss of muscle activity, cortical activation, and high amplitude hippocampal theta rhythm in (C). Normal REM sleep records were similar to that shown in (C) except that maximal hippocampal theta was approximately one-half the amplitude shown here. Time: 1 second. (From Baxter, 1969)

cholinergic stimulation was followed by depression because of the slow degradation of carbachol or the prolonged tetanizing effect of such a high dose.

In an interesting experiment, Langlois and Poussart (1969) demonstrated that cortical EEG waves similar in appearance to sleep spindles were evoked by ACh injected into the caudate nucleus of the cat. Further, the spindling was blocked by 5 μg of atropine injected earlier. However, they correctly interpreted the electrocortical activity and concluded that it was not related to sleep. The cat which had been curarized moved its eyes, and followed the experimenter about the room with its eyes, indicating that the animal was fully awake. In addition, their pattern of occurrence was not the same as actual sleep spindles.

Corresponding to the excitatory effects of carbachol injected into the hypothalamus of the pigeon (Macphail, 1969) are the results of Marley and Seller (1972) who found that muscarine infused into the diencephalon or myelencephalon of the chick produces arousal. The bird became alert and electrocortical activity paralleled the increase in motor movements. These effects are shown in Fig. 9-11. Scopolamine, the powerful anti-muscarinic compound, antagonized the action of local muscarine but only if infused before the cholinomimetic. The cholinoceptive pathway for arousal which seems to exist in the brain-stem of a nonmammalian species seems to share a similar muscarine receptor mechanism as the mammal.

A so-called chemitrode to micro-inject, to stimulate electrically or record simultaneously the electrical activity of a site was used to investigate the EEG effects of altering the local adrenergic activity (Trzebski, 1960). Epinephrine, norepinephrine or an inhibitor of monoamine oxidase given repeatedly in a large 10 μl volume in the cat's hypothalamus or mesencephalon caused an increase in local electrical activity characterized by rapid but high voltage synchronization. The report is difficult to interpret because of the long latency of the response and lack of anatomical localization.

Courville et al. (1962) were among the first to speculate that adrenergic and cholinergic systems function antagonistically in the brain-stem reticular formation. In the "encephale isole" cat immobilized by Flaxedil, the amplitude of cortical potentials evoked by electrical stimulation of the optic chiasm varied according to the substance that was injected into the pons. Epinephrine in a large volume caused an increase in the amplitude of the potentials which began within 1 to 2 minutes and lasted 2 to 4 minutes. Conversely, ACh generally caused a decrease in the amplitude which was somewhat longer lasting than the effect of epinephrine. Procaine injected similarly mimicked epinephrine when given in the pons, but mimicked ACh when infused in the mesencephalon.

After giving an intra-arterial injection of norepinephrine or epinephrine directly into the cerebral circulation of the cat, without recirculation, Mantegazzini et al. (1959) observed that an arousal or desynchronization of the EEG did not occur. This is opposite to that seen when the catecholamines are injected into the general circulation. Thus, these monoamines could not possibly be the

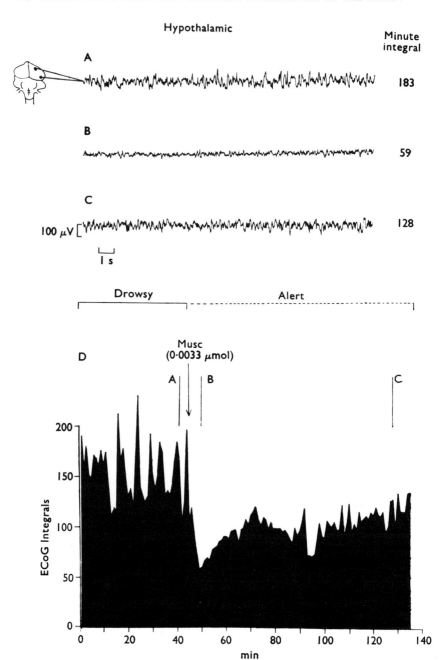

Fig. 9-11 Records of electrocortical activity (A–C) and histogram of integrated electrocortical activity (D) in an unanesthetized, unrestrained 13-day chick. Intervals corresponding to A, B and C are indicated in the histogram and integrals

chemical mediators for the ascending reticular activating or arousal systems, a conclusion contrary to what Bonvallet, Dell, Bradley and many of the other workers believed in the 1950s on the basis of systemic injections.

Yet, a few years later Cordeau et al. (1963) disputed the findings of Mantegazzini. When given in a large 20 μl volume, 20 μg of epinephrine aroused a sleeping cat and desynchronized the EEG when injected into the mesencephalic or pontine reticular formation. ACh injected in the same dose and volume had an opposite effect in producing behavioral sleep and in causing EEG synchronization. In some cats, salivation and retching occurred during an injection and "a few seconds later, he sank quickly to the floor of the cage . . . and remained motionless thereafter!" (Cordeau et al., 1963). Because of obvious mechanical and other problems associated with the method of injection into these lower brain-stem structures and the probability that the effects were partly systemic, these early findings are difficult to evaluate.

IV. IONIC BALANCE AND SLEEP

In an extraordinary account of the results of an early experiment, Demole (1927) found that all physiological systems typically depressed during anesthetic-like sleep could be similarly affected by calcium. When a solution of calcium chloride was injected in the region dorsal to the optic chiasm (Fig 9-12) or infundibulum of the rabbit or cat, sleep-like symptoms appeared which were dependent largely on the concentration of the calcium "*Eingespritzung*." The deep sleep and atonia are illustrated in Fig. 9-13. When calcium was infused in the thalamus or when potassium chloride was injected in a corresponding area, a pattern of sleep did not appear. Instead, potassium evoked hypertonia, tremor, stupor and increases in respiratory and heart rates. Except for the limitations imposed by the large volumes used, Demole's anatomical mapping revealed that the region of maximal sensitivity to the cations is localized within the inferior diencephalon, i.e., the hypothalamus.

Repeating Demole's experiment, Marinesco et al. (1929) found some differences in the latency and duration of sleep which depended on the site of injection and the concentration of the calcium chloride solution. Calcium in the thalamus of the cat seemed to cause pain probably because of the mechanical lesion attendant to the large volume given. This, of course, would prevent subsequent sleep. Intense agitation and excitement followed a similar injection

---

for the corresponding minute of electrocortical activity are given on the right of the trace. A, Control drowsy electrocortical activity. B, Electrocortical arousal accompanied by reduction in electrocortical integrals after micro-infusion of muscarine into the hypothalamus; electrocortical arousal extended to both hemispheres. C, Return of drowsy activity in the electrocorticogram. (From Marley and Seller, 1972)

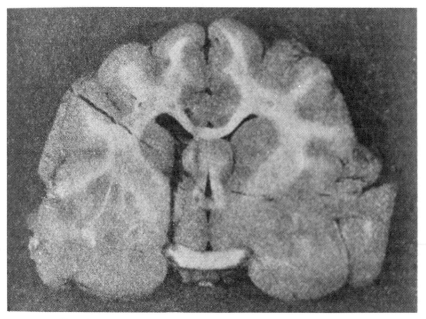

Fig. 9-12 The frontal section of a cat brain. The sleep-inducing injection of CaCl$_2$ is localized in the region of the nucleus supra-chiasmaticus in gray matter at a position dorsal and lateral to the optic chiasm. (From Demole, 1927)

of potassium which was then followed some 3 to 4 hours later by sleep. In both instances, the quantity of the injection was probably damaging. In addition, part of the volume injected certainly passed into the third ventricle.

In contrast to the anatomical loci at which an injection of an amine or carbachol has been reported to evoke sleep are those mapped by Veale and Myers (1971) following the localized perfusion of calcium. Using the push-pull technique to maintain an aberrant ionic concentration for 30 to 40 minutes, they found that behavioral sleep, as illustrated in Fig. 9-14, was evoked by 10.4 mM excess calcium in the perfusate. This was accompanied by high voltage EEG activity, recorded from the occipital as well as the frontal cortex. The sites sensitive to calcium were nearly all within the posterior hypothalamus and mammillary region, as shown in Fig. 9-15.

Figure 9-16 illustrates a typical EEG recording obtained from a cat in which 10.4 mM excess calcium was perfused simultaneously at two bilateral sites in the caudal hypothalamus. The EEG records were sampled at five 1-hour intervals prior to the beginning of the perfusion and at 5-minute intervals throughout the course of the 40-minute perfusion. When the animal was awake prior to the effect of excess calcium, the electrical activity was characterized by low voltage desynchronized waves. Characteristic sleep-like waves distinguished by higher

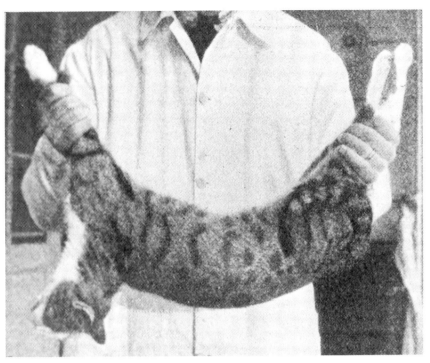

Fig. 9-13 Appearance of deep sleep and hypotonia in a cat after the injection of 2 mg of CaCl$_2$ in nucleus supra-chiasmaticus shown in Fig. 9-12. (From Demole, 1927)

voltage, and in some instances, by synchronization, occurred during the calcium perfusion. When the animal was aroused by a sudden noise such as a clap of the hands or by touching a hindfoot, the typical desynchronization of the cortical electrical activity resulted, as shown in Fig. 9-16.

The description is noteworthy of the behavioral effects of calcium: ". . . During the calcium-induced sleep, signs of drowsiness became apparent within 5 to 15 minutes following the start of perfusion. These included a decline in the cat's activity, the respiratory rate, body temperature and muscle tonus as well as dilatation of the ear vessels and constriction of the pupils. After the animal lay down and closed its eyes, it respired deeply at a rate of about 16 per minute; the cat, however, could be aroused easily by a sudden noise or by handling. When forced to move, it showed no signs of motor impairment or loss of muscle coordination, and if left undisturbed for a few minutes, the animal would go to sleep immediately. Figure 9-14 shows the typical appearance of a cat in which calcium in a concentration of 10.4 mM in

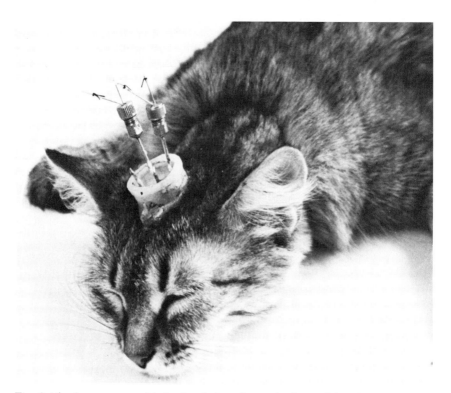

Fig. 9-14 Appearance of behavioral sleep in a cat when calcium in a concentration of 10.4 mM in excess of normal Krebs solution was perfused within the posterior hypothalamus. (From Veale and Myers, 1971)

Fig. 9-15 Anatomical mapping at eight coronal (AP) planes of sites within the hypothalamus of the cat at which calcium ions were perfused by means of push-pull cannulae. Sites are shown at which Ca 2.4 or 10.4 mM above the concentration in extracellular fluid produced sleep (●) during or following a 30 minute perfusion, or did not alter the level of arousal (○). The scales are in millimeters ah, anterior hypothalamic area; ca, anterior commissure; cho, optic chiasm; cin, internal capsule; cm, central medial nucleus of the thalamus; cs, subthalamic nucleus; db, diagonal band of Broca; en, endopeduncular nucleus; f, fornix; fmb, medial forebrain bundle; ff, fields of Forel; lh, lateral hypothalamic area; mm, medial mammillary body; mt, mammillo-thalamic tract; nac, nucleus accumbens; nbo, supraoptic nucleus; niv, interventricular nucleus of the thalamus; npr, prothalamic nucleus; ph, posterior hypothalamic area; pp, cerebral peduncle; re, nucleus reuniens; rpo, preoptic tract; tro, optic tract; vmh, ventromedial nucleus; zi, zona incerta; 3v, third ventricle. (From Veale and Myers, 1971)

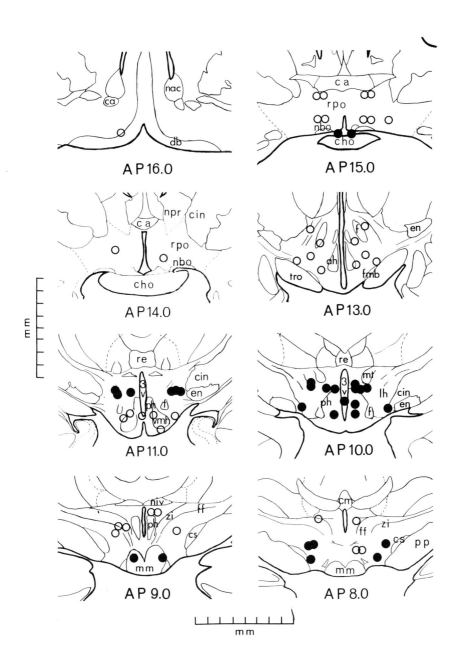

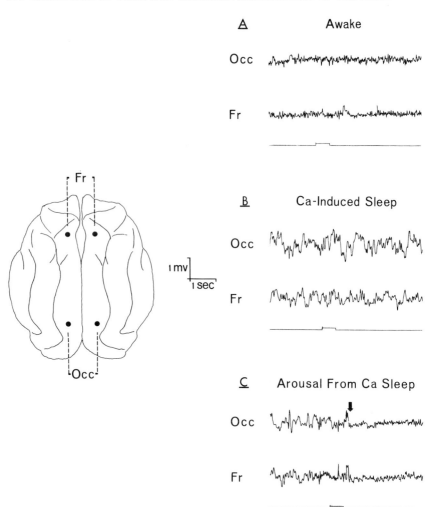

Fig. 9-16 Representative EEG records obtained from cortical electrodes implanted in a cat. The records were taken (A) prior to perfusion of calcium when the cat was awake; (B) during calcium-induced sleep; and (C) when the cat was suddenly aroused from the sleep-like state and typical desynchronization resulted in the EEG pattern. Occ, occipital; Fr, frontal. The time base is shown for each set of tracings with the time mark indicating an interval of 0.6 second. (From Veale and Myers, 1971)

excess of the normal Krebs solution was perfused in the posterior hypothalamus. In this case, the cat did not even respond to the repeated use of flashbulbs for photographic purposes, during what is best described as a deep sleep."

The effect on the mesencephalic reticular formation of substances designated as neural excitants such as potassium, sodium citrate (a Ca^{2+} chelating agent) and Coramine (a barbiturate antagonist) were compared with neural depressants that included calcium, procaine and pentobarbital (Nakajima, 1964). Injected bilaterally into the midbrain of the rat, the excitants caused alertness, fear, immobilization and withdrawal behavior. On the other hand, the depressants evoked some hyperactivity after the injection of a low dose but, in general, a loss of muscle tone, collapse and coma following a higher dose. Lever pressing for food pellets was suppressed by a high concentration of either calcium or potassium. From this result, the level of arousal is perhaps not related to the drive to obtain food but rather to the functional activity of the reticular formation. A curvilinear relationship between arousal and behavioral performance is established in that behavior becomes less efficient as either end of the continuum of arousal is approached. That is, any sort of hyperactivity interferes with the performance of a given task in exactly the same way as sedation.

V. DRUGS AND AROUSAL

A diencephalic injection, if given in a sufficient volume, can induce somnolence not because of the chemical introduced into tissue but rather because of a lesion. A case report of one monkey described just such a neurological deficit including a drooping posture, depressed activity and a comatose condition (Karasszon, 1968) after 500 μl of polio virus were injected on each side of the thalamus of a rhesus monkey. The neuropathological symptoms could be traced to a necrotizing hemorrhagic lesion in the diencephalon.

Similarly, certain drugs may alter the arousal pattern by virtue of their local anesthetic action (Sahlgren, 1934) or their irritative property. For example, cobalt introduced in the mesencephalic reticular formation profoundly alters the sleep-wakefulness rhythm of a cat for over three months (Mancia and Lucioni, 1966). Although the periods of synchronized or desynchronized sleep were shortened drastically, the cat was behaviorally alert and attentive but was somewhat fearful. The irritative focus would correspond to the morphological area involved in persistent arousal.

A. Local Anesthesia

When a film of silicone rubber cement is deposited over the lumen of the tip of a cannula, a chemical in a gaseous state will diffuse through this artificial membrane. Using this so-called chemode, Folkman et al. (1968) found that three commonly used anesthetics have an action on the midbrain reticular formation of the cat. Light sleep, EEG spindles and analgesia were produced by teflurane and methoxyflurane gas diffusing into mesencephalic sites. Cyclopropane was far less potent when delivered by this route, whereas nitrous oxide, which is known to diffuse through such a silicone rubber membrane had no effect on the cats which remained alert.

The anatomical specificity of the action of these anesthetics is, however, somewhat suspect. For example, Wilkinson *et al.* (1971) have shown that teflurane gas diffusing through a membrane-tipped cannula into the cat's thalamus or hypothalamus produces postural repose, typical slowing of the EEG activity and sleep spindles. They did find, however, that cats exposed to focal suppression by teflurane in unspecified frontal white matter showed no behavioral or electrographic signs of drowsiness or sleep.

Following the lead of Sahlgren (1934), other workers have shown that after a bilateral injection of sodium pentobarbital into the amygdala, hippocampus, thalamus, hypothalamus or the head of the caudate nucleus of the cat, only the caudate was sensitive to this barbiturate anesthetic (Leighton and Jenkins, 1970). Following its micro-injection, pentobarbital evoked behavioral sedation and a deactivation of the EEG, as shown in Fig. 9-17. The EEG recording from the frontal cortex was characterized by an increase in voltage within about 6 minutes after the injection. Thus, the caudate nucleus would also seem to participate in the synchronizing mechanism of cortical electrical activity.

Slow-wave, high amplitude EEG wave activity may also increase following the application of chlorpromazine derivatives to the mesencephalic reticular formation of the rat (Grossman, 1968a). However, the amplitude of local electrical

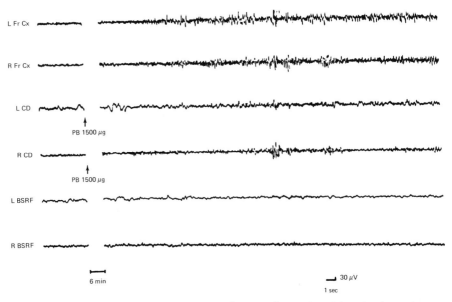

Fig. 9-17   Six minutes after pentobarbital (1500 μg) was placed into both caudate nuclei (heads). (From Leighton and Jenkins, 1970)

activity is only slightly modified by infusion of meprobamate in large doses and volumes into the amygdala of the conscious monkey (Delgado *et al.*, 1971a). Although the ataractic agent has an effect on the electrical activity of structures in the limbic system, its direct effect on nerve cells in the non-metabolized form is minimal.

The electrical activity of the cortex is aroused more intensely and for a longer duration when the caudal medulla is blocked by a local injection of Novocaine (Bonvallet and Bloch, 1961). Even though this preliminary report did not include the concentration or volume of Novocaine given, the data suggest that a very posterior inhibitory mechanism is brought into action when the reticular activating system of a cat is aroused. Hippocampal theta rhythm can be observed after the crystalline application or injection of carboline into the dorsal part of this structure in the cat (Trabka, 1967); however, there were no behavioral manifestations of sleep that accompanied the slowing of the EEG waves.

B. Endogenous Substances and Sleep

ACTH injected in a large volume into the hypothalamus, caudate nucleus or other subcortical structure evokes a peculiar syndrome in the cat termed yawning and stretching (Gessa *et al.*, 1967). The latency of the action of the trophic hormone was only 12 to 20 minutes, an interval which perhaps represents the time required for ACTH to reach the receptors in the median eminence. Although the meaning of the cat's stretching of its limbs and yawning is unclear, these responses could be mediated by overlapping neurons that are involved in controlling sexual activity, arousal, wakefulness or related behavior.

After a rabbit is stressed by immobilization, the incidence of paradoxical sleep is markedly reduced for 6 to 8 hours (Kawakami *et al.*, 1965). An implant of crystalline cortisone in the hypothalamus prevents this reduction in the episodes of paradoxical sleep. These results could reflect some sort of extrinsic influence of ACTH in generating a diurnal rhythm for paradoxical sleep. Interestingly, estradiol injected in minute volumes into the hypothalamus of the cat has the capacity to synchronize the EEG pattern recorded from the cortex (Morelli, 1968), and estradiol applied similarly to the hypothalamus or other areas of the rabbit brain may also influence slow-wave and paradoxical sleep (Faure, 1968). The precise relationships of the neuroendocrine factors, however, remain to be determined.

The typical orienting reaction of a conscious cat to a "psst" or other sensory stimulus is attenuated by crystals of GABA applied in an enormous dose of 700 to 800 μg in the hippocampus (Rogozea *et al.*, 1969). Spontaneous synchronization of hippocampal neurons likewise disappeared within 2 to 6 minutes after GABA was deposited, and signs of hippocampal theta rhythm were likewise absent. Evoked potentials from the hippocampus following repetitive auditory stimulation were similarly suppressed by GABA. In spite of the dose, this amino acid may be involved in the local processing of sensory input in the temporal lobe.

GABA injected in a large volume into the hippocampal-amygdaloid region of the rhesus monkey reduces spontaneous EEG activity and may induce sleep as measured behaviorally and determined electrographically by the incidence of high voltage, slow waves (Delgado *et al.*, 1971b). Glutamate given similarly in the same area causes a transitory increase in low voltage, fast EEG activity which progressed in several monkeys to a generalized motor convulsion. In spite of the dramatic shift in the monkey's EEG patterns, usually no significant change in lever pressing for food, grooming or walking was observed. That GABA and glutamate may somehow function in a balanced way to sustain the normal neuronal function in this part of the limbic system could be implied from these results.

Enzymes such as phospholipase A or C or pronase reduce EEG amplitude and the cortical evoked potentials when they are injected in low doses into the lateral geniculate body of the cat (Hafemann *et al.* 1970). However, hyaluronidase injected in a dose of 300 μg seemed to possess a toxic effect on the EEG. This enzyme caused a progressive increase in EEG amplitude until seizure activity occurred. Even though the mechanism involved in these responses remains obscure, polysaccharide material present extracellularly is perhaps essential to the maintenance of the electrical stability of the neuronal membrane.

VI. CONCLUDING CONSIDERATIONS

Sleep induced by stimulating a structure in the brain with a chemical is subject to the same sort of questions of interpretation as that produced by electrical stimulation. Does the chemical trigger the synchronization of cortical and subcortical electrical activity as registered by the EEG? Is it just as likely that a drug inhibits the ascending pathways for arousal rather than activates the anatomical system for sleep? What is the relationship between chemically evoked somnolence and the natural, diurnal sleep that has the distinguishing feature of periodicity?

The issue of natural versus artificially-induced sleep plagues all researchers in this field. There is increasing awareness, for example, that the behavioral sleep following forced sleep deprivation has unusual EEG characteristics. In fact, the hypersomnia displayed by a cat that has just been sitting vigilantly for many hours upon a brick set in the middle of a tub of water is characterized by EEG patterns quite apart from those recorded while the animal takes a morning nap in a warm, quiet and darkened room after a large meal. Dement (1972) has gone so far as to conclude that it may be impossible for a sleep deprivation study to give clear answers about the purpose of this major behavioral state.

Quantification of each of the many facets of sleep is yet another horrendous problem that we face in evaluating the material in this chapter. Unlike recordings of body temperature in °C or of ingestive behavior in terms of grams of food or milliliters of water consumed, the typical measures of sleep are not sharply defined. Recently, the sleep researcher has taken great strides to quantitate accurately the electrographic alterations in the sleeping or waking brain. Fourier and other modern mathematical techniques have been coupled with careful computer analyses of the changes in cortical potentials generated during the various stages of arousal. Nevertheless, clear-cut sleep profiles of these stages, as well as the distinctions between the behavioral appearances of sleep are intricate and often deceptive. Even the one species which is conventionally used for sleep research has not escaped from sharp criticism. Pappenheimer *et al.* (1967) are of the opinion that the laboratory cat may be "ill-suited" for the biological assay of sleep-promoting factors, since it may naturally sleep away much of a 24-hour period.

A. Hypnogenic Factors

Ever since the work of Pieron in the early 1900s, the existence of a blood-borne sleep factor has been suspected. Recently, Monnier and his co-workers have carried out an intriguing set of investigations utilizing the technique of linking together the circulatory systems of two rabbits. After the thalamus of one rabbit is stimulated with electric current, the second rabbit goes to sleep after a given latency (e.g., Monnier and Hösli, 1965). Thus, a pharmacologically potent sleep factor whose release is electrically evoked in the first animal is carried via the systemic circulation to the other rabbit.

Following these original crossed circulation experiments, Monnier and his collaborators have obtained important new evidence that a hypnogenic factor is present in the brain of the sleeping animal (Monnier and Hatt, 1971; Monnier and Schoenenberger, 1972). A sleep hemodialysate has been isolated from the cerebral blood supply which when injected into the cerebral ventricle of an awake and unrestrained rabbit causes a significant increase in the duration of delta sleep. The somnolent potency of the sleep dialysate isolated earlier does change when subjected to freezing, thawing, storage, an alteration in pH, lyophilization or heating. The efficacy in the sleep activity of the dialysate is lost in varying degrees when it is tested later by the intraventricular route in an awake animal. Thus, the response of the recipient rabbit depends directly upon the physical-chemical conditions to which the factor is exposed. From their analysis, Monnier *et al.* believe that the hypnogenic activity of the dialysate is not due to a protein but rather to an organic compound of low molecular weight, probably a peptide. In this connection, it is interesting that Pappenheimer *et al.* also believe that the factor present in the CSF of the sleep-deprived goat, which reduces the activity or level of arousal on injection of the CSF into the ventricle of a cat or rat, is also a substance of low molecular weight.

Using the cerebral cross-perfusion technique of Myers (1967b), Drucker-Colín *et al.* (1970) discovered that the effluent collected by means of a push-pull perfusion of the mesencephalic reticular formation of a sleep-deprived cat also exerts a physiological effect. This perfusate evokes fast-wave sleep when delivered to the same morphological region of an awake recipient cat. The potential importance of this demonstration is undeniable in that a factor is clearly released from neuronal tissue which is either independent of or similar to the hypnogenic factor present in the bloodstream. Moreover, the approach to the problem in terms of evoked release is unquestionably a promising one which if continued using an appropriate control ought to dovetail with the results of chemical stimulation experiments.

It would not be surprising if one or more of the states of sleep is indeed triggered by a peptide (Monnier and Schoenenberger, 1972). We know already that at least three peptidergic releasing factors present in the hypothalamus are essential for gonadal function and reproductive behavior. Another blood-borne peptide, angiotensin II, has been implicated in thirst and the mechanism for water balance. Thus, if another of this family of chemical compounds is ultimately isolated in mammalian tissue as a humoral link in the mechanism underlying sleep, the cross-functional coincidence would be more than monumental. Above all, it would point to the likelihood that other peptides, as yet unidentified, could be involved in the monitoring and control of other vegetative or primitive functions including feeding and emotional behavior.

B. Biogenic Amines

To make a definitive statement about the function of the endogenous brainstem amines during sleep requires information based on a sound experimental footing. At the present time, there is simply not enough direct evidence. Up until now, the role of the amines has been ascertained primarily on the basis of two lines of attack: (1) the action of peripherally administered drugs such as reserpine, pCPA or αMpT, and (2) the effect of discrete lesions of midbrain raphé and other nuclei that contain monoamines. Although the results of chemical stimulation with serotonin and the catecholamines are exiguous, they are consistent in several instances with the drug and lesion studies (Morgane and Stern, 1972; Jouvet, 1972). Nevertheless, prodigious research is required along many fronts using well-controlled stimulation procedures. In addition, studies of the local release, turnover and uptake of amines are equally essential with respect to their dynamic activity during the various stages of arousal.

Parenthetically, an assay of the biochemical content of the whole brain of an animal or even its entire mesencephalon in this context would seem to be fruitless. Within the mesencephalon alone, the locus coeruleus and at least one raphé nucleus presumably play entirely different roles in the synchronizing process of sleep. The duration of REM sleep, the balance between paradoxical and slow-wave sleep and the circadian periodicity of sleep may well be paced by these different anatomical structures.

Given the limited number of facts, it is still very likely that a cholinergic mechanism in the lower brain-stem mediates the arousal of the cortex by way of a thalamic relay. For example, a cholinergic substance injected into the thalamus of the cat may evoke cortical synchronization and spindles (Endröczi *et al.*, 1963b). Conversely, cholinergic stimulation of the lower brain-stem at the level of the reticular formation desynchronizes the neocortical EEG. The cholinergic activity in the brain-stem could correspond to the nonspecific and diffuse activating system.

In Jouvet's (1972) theory, ACh is involved in the maintenance of EEG and behavioral arousal on the one hand and the "executive mechanism" controlling paradoxical sleep on the other. In this scheme, serotonin neurons initiate slow-wave sleep by means of the release of the indoleamine. Neurons releasing catecholamines activate the fast cortical activity thereby heralding paradoxical sleep. However, none of these fascinating speculations accommodate conceptually a cholinergic triggering of slow-wave sleep. Thus, the initial hypotheses of Hernández-Peón made many years ago are still left unresolved.

VII. Master Summary Table
Chemicals that Exerted an Effect when Given at a Specific Site in the Brain

Chemical	Dose	Volume	Site	Species	State*	Response	Reference
Acetylcholine (ACh)	?	crystal	Preoptic area, interpeduncular nucleus, tegmentum	Cat	U	Sleep.	Velluti and Hernández-Peón (1963)
	?	crystal	Limbic structures, hypothalamus and mesencephalon, pons	Cat	U	Sleep, alertness.	Hernández-Peón et al. (1963)
	?	crystal	Hypothalamus, mesencephalon	Cat	U	Hyperactivity, alertness, sleep.	Hernández-Peón and Chávez-Ibarra (1963)
	≃30 µg	crystal	Preoptic area	Cat	U	EEG and behavioral sleep.	Yamaguchi et al. (1964)
	2–4 µg	10 µl	Olfactory bulb	Cat	U	EEG arousal.	Peñaloza-Rojas and Zeiden-weber (1965)
	2–5 µg	5–10 µl	Thalamus	Cat	A	Cortical EEG spindles.	Endröczi et al. (1963b)
	2–5 µg	5–10 µl	Reticular formation	Cat	A	Cortical and hippocampal desynchronization.	Endröczi et al. (1963b)
	5 µg	4–5 µl	Pons	Cat	A U	EEG synchronization.	Kostowski (1971)
	15 µg	4–5 µl	Pons	Cat	A U	Neurocortical EEG desynchronization.	Kostowski (1971)
	20 µg	.2 µl	Caudate nucleus	Cat	A	Sleep-like EEG "spindles."	Langlois and Poussart (1969)
	20 µg	10 µl	Pontine reticular formation	Cat	C	Decreased amplitude of cortical potentials.	Courville et al. (1962)
	20 µg	20 µl	Reticular formation	Cat	U	Sleep, EEG synchronization.	Cordeau et al. (1963)

*U = unanesthetized and unrestrained; C = constrained, confined or curarized; A = anesthetized.

Substance	Dose	Volume	Site	Species		Effect	Reference
Adrenocorticotrophic hormone (ACTH)	20 µg	5 µl	Hypothalamus, caudate nucleus, basal ganglia	Cat	U	Yawning, stretching.	Gessa et al. (1967)
Adenosine	26.7–107 µg	1–2 µl	Hypothalamus	Chicken	U	Sleep after aminophylline.	Marley and Nistico (1972)
Atropine	?	crystal	Preoptic area, interpeduncular nucleus, tegmentum	Cat	U	Alertness or blockade cholinergic sleep.	Velluti and Hernández-Péon (1963)
	1 µg	1–2 µl	Pons (reticular nucleus)	Cat	U	Prevented syndrome of paradoxical sleep.	George et al. (1964)
	10 µg	4–5 µl	Pons	Cat	A U	Neurocortical EEG desynchronization.	Kostowski (1971)
Calcium (Ca^{2+})	6–25 µg	2 µl	Mesencephalon, reticular formation, superior colliculi	Rat	U	Behavioral sedation, coma, suppression.	Nakajima (1964)
	5.21–20.84 µg/min	perfusion 50 µl/min	Postero-lateral hypothalamus	Cat	U	Behavioral and EEG sleep, catatonia.	Veale and Myers (1971)
	50–500 µg	12.5–25 µl	Infundibular region	Cat Cat Rabbit	A U U	Sleep.	Clöetta and Fischer (1930)
	500–2000 µg	100 µl	Hypothalamus	Cat	U	Reversible behavioral sleep, respiration decline.	Marinesco et al. (1929)
	250 µg–2000 µg	25–50 µl	Hypothalamus	Rabbit Cat	U U	Anesthetic-like sleep.	Demole (1927)
Carbachol	?	crystal	Lateral hypothalamus	Rat	U	Drinking, activity, reduction in sleep.	Blanchard and Blanchard (1966)
	?	crystal	Limbic structures, hypothalamus and mesencephalon pons	Cat	U	Sleep, alertness.	Hernández-Péon et al. (1963)
	≃10 µg	crystal	Mesencephalon	Cat	U	REM sleep.	Baxter (1969)
	.14–3.9 µg	1 µl	Hypothalamus	Cat	U	Failed to obtain sleep.	Macphail and Miller (1968)

VII. Master Summary Table (*Continued*)

Chemical	Dose	Volume	Site	Species	State*	Response	Reference
Carbachol	.2-5 µg	1-2 µl	Pons (reticular nucleus)	Cat	U	Atonia, tremor, EEG desynchronization, paradoxical sleep.	George et al. (1964)
	2-5 µg	5-10 µl	Thalamus	Cat	A	Cortical EEG spindles.	Endröczi et al. (1963b)
Carboline	≈15-30 µg	crystal	Hippocampus	Cat	A	Theta rhythm.	Trabka (1967)
	50-150 µg	10-20 µl	Hippocampus	Cat	A	Theta rhythm.	Trabka (1967)
Chlorpromazine derivatives	5 µg	crystal or 1 µl	Mesencephalic reticular formation	Rat	U	Increased EEG high voltage, slow waves.	Grossman (1968a)
Cobalt	≈10 mg	crystal	Mesencephalic reticular formation	Cat	U	Reduced sleep periods, persistent arousal.	Mancia and Lucioni (1966)
Coramine	500 µg	2 µl	Mesencephalon, reticular formation, superior colliculi	Rat	U	Alertness, fear, convulsions.	Nakajima (1964)
Cortisone	≈200 µg	crystal	Supraoptic region, ventromedial nucleus, median eminence	Rabbit	U	Prevents stress-induced blockade of paradoxical sleep.	Kawakami et al. (1965)
Cyclic AMP	34.7-208 µg	1.2 µl	Hypothalamus	Chicken	U	Sleep after aminophylline.	Marley and Nistico (1972)
Dibutyryl cyclic AMP	49.1-196 µg	1-2 µl	Hypothalamus	Chicken	U	Hyperactivity.	Marley and Nistico (1972)
	200-500 µg	5-10 µl	Cerebellum	Rat Cat	U	Sedation, slow-wave sleep.	Gessa et al. (1970)
Cyclopropane	?	?	Mesencephalic reticular formation	Cat	U	Somnolence.	Folkman et al. (1968)
Dopamine (DOPA)	19-190 µg	1-2 µl	Hypothalamus	Chicken	U	Sleep after MAO inhibition.	Marley and Nistico (1972)
	38-114 µg	1-2 µl	Striatum	Chicken	U	Arousal and involuntary movements.	Marley and Nistico (1972)

Compound	Dose	Volume	Site	Species	Code	Effect	Reference
Epinephrine	1000 µg	10 µl	Pons, medulla	Rabbit	C	EEG desynchronization of neocortex.	Ledebur and Tissot (1966)
	1–50 µg	1 µl (or crystal)	Hypothalamus (all areas)	Cat	U	Motor impairment, sleep, stupor.	Myers (1964a)
	2–4 µg	10 µl	Olfactory bulb	Cat	U	EEG patterns of sleep.	Peñaloza-Rojas and Zeiden-weber (1965)
	10 µg	10 µl	Posterior hypothalamus, mesencephalic reticular formation	Cat	A	Increased amplitude and frequency of MRF potentials.	Trzebski (1960)
	20 µg	10 µl	Pontine reticular formation	Cat	C	Increased amplitude of cortical potentials.	Courville et al. (1962)
	20 µg	20 µl	Reticular formation	Cat	U	Arousal from sleep and EEG desynchronization.	Cordeau et al. (1963)
Eserine	?	crystal	Preoptic area, interpeduncular nucleus, tegmentum	Cat	U	Sleep.	Velluti and Hernández-Peón (1963)
	10 µg	4–5 µl	Pons	Cat	A U	EEG synchronization.	Kostowski (1971)
Estradiol	2–5 µg	.4–1 µl	Medial hypothalamus	Cat	A	Synchronized the cortical EEG.	Morelli (1968)
γ-Aminobutyric acid (GABA)	≈700–800 µg	crystal	Hippocampus	Cat	U	Suppressed evoked synchronization.	Rogozea et al. (1969)
	2.06–30.9 mg	20–300 µl	Hippocampus, amygdala	Monkey	C	Reduced spontaneous EEG activity, sleep.	Delgado et al. (1971b)
Harmine	10–100 µg	10 µl	Posterior hypothalamus, mesencephalic reticular formation	Cat	A	Increased amplitude and frequency of MRF potentials.	Trzebski (1960)
Hyaluronidase	300 µg	1.5 µl	Lateral geniculate	Cat	C	Enhanced spontaneous EEG activity.	Hafemann et al. (1970)
5-Hydroxytryptophan (5-HTP)	1000 µg	10 µl	Pons, medulla	Rabbit	C	EEG sleep or REM-like activity.	Ledebur and Tissot (1966)

VII. Master Summary Table (Continued)

Chemical	Dose	Volume	Site	Species	State*	Response	Reference
Iproniazid	100–1000 μg	10 μl	Posterior hypothalamus, mesencephalic reticular formation	Cat	A	Increased amplitude and frequency of MRF potentials.	Trzebski (1960)
Isoprenaline	13.92–27.85 μg	.5 μl	Hypothalamus	Chicken	U	Behavioral and EEG sleep.	Marley and Stephenson (1970)
Melatonin	≃15–30 μg	crystal	Preoptic area, central medial nucleus of thalamus	Cat	U	EEG and behavioral sleep.	Marczynski et al. (1964)
Meprobamate	600 μg	100 μl	Amygdala	Monkey	C	Decreased amplitude in focal electrical activity.	Delgado et al. (1971a)
Methoxyflurane	?	?	Mesencephalic reticular formation	Cat	U	Sleep and hypalgesia.	Folkman et al. (1968)
α-Methyl-norepinephrine	5.50 μg	.5 μl	Hypothalamus	Chicken	U	Behavioral and EEG sleep.	Marley and Stephenson (1970)
Methysergide (UML)	1.5 μg	?	Area postrema	Cat	A	Blocked 5-HT synchrony of EEG sleep.	Koella and Czicman (1966)
Muscarine	.99 μg	1 μl	Myelencephalon, diencephalon	Chicken	U	Behavioral arousal, EEG alerting.	Marley and Seller (1972)
Nembutal	120 μg	2 μl	Mesencephalon, reticular formation, superior colliculi	Rat	U	Behavioral sedation, coma, suppression.	Nakajima (1964)
Nicotine	5 μg	4–5 μl	Pons	Cat	A, U	Neurocortical EEG desynchronization.	Kostowski (1971)
Norepinephrine (NE)	4.23–63.37 μg	.5 μl	Hypothalamus	Chicken	U	Behavioral and EEG sleep.	Marley and Stephenson (1970)

	Dose	Volume	Location	Species	U/C/A	Effect	Reference
	?	crystal	Lateral hypothalamus	Rat	U	Resting and sleeping.	Blanchard and Blanchard (1966)
	.002–.007 µg	1 µl	Preoptic area, mesencephalic reticular formation	Rat	U	Reduced deep and paradoxical sleep after systemic αMpT.	Torda (1968)
	?	crystal	Limbic structures, hypothalamus, mesencephalon, pons	Cat	U	Arousal and rage.	Hernández-Peón et al. (1963)
	?	crystal	Hypothalamus, mesencephalon	Cat	U	Excitation.	Hernández-Peón and Chávez-Ibarra (1963)
	≃20–30 µg	crystal	Thalamus	Cat	U	Sleep.	Yamaguchi et al. (1964)
	10 µg	10 µl	Posterior hypothalamus, mesencephalic reticular formation	Cat	A	Increased amplitude and frequency of MRF potentials.	Trzebski (1960)
Oxotremorine	.2–10 µg	1–2 µl	Pons (reticular nuclei)	Cat	U	Atonia, tremor, EEG desynchronization, paradoxical sleep.	George et al. (1964)
Pentobarbital	1000–3000 µg	2–6 µl	Caudate nucleus	Cat	U	Sedation, EEG deactivation.	Leighton and Jenkins (1970)
Phenobarbital	2000 µg	10 µl	Infundibular region	Rabbit	U	Sleep reaction.	Sahlgren (1934)
Phenoxybenzamine	68 µg	2 µl	Hypothalamus	Chicken	U	Sleep.	Marley and Stephenson (1970)
Phospholipase A	.71 µg	1 µl	Lateral geniculate	Cat	C	Reduced EEG amplitude.	Hafemann et al. (1970)
Phospholipase C	.71 µg	1 µl	Lateral geniculate	Cat	C	Reduced evoked potentials.	Hafemann et al. (1970)
Poliomyelitis virus	?	500 µl	Thalamus	Monkey	U	Somnolence	Karasszon (1968)

VII. Master Summary Table (Continued)

Chemical	Dose	Volume	Site	Species	State*	Response	Reference
Potassium (K$^+$)	6–22 µg	2 µl	Mesencephalon, reticular formation, superior colliculi	Rat	U	Alertness, fear, convulsions.	Nakajima (1964)
	2000–3500 µg	100 µl	Hypothalamus	Cat	U	Excitation; delayed sleep.	Marinesco et al. (1929)
Procaine	100 µg	2 µl	Mesencephalon, reticular formation, superior colliculi	Rat	U	Behavioral sedation, coma, suppression.	Nakajima (1964)
	?	?	Pontine reticular formation	Cat	C	Increased amplitude of cortical potentials.	Courville et al. (1962)
	?	?	Caudal medulla	Cat	A	Antagonism of reticular excitation.	Bonvallet and Bloch (1961)
	40 µg	1–2 µl	Pons (reticular nuclei)	Cat	U	Prevented syndrome of paradoxical sleep.	George et al. (1964)
Pronase	10 µg	1 µl	Lateral geniculate	Cat	C	Reduced evoked potentials	Hafemann et al. (1970)
Scopolamine	43.8 µg	1 µl	Myelencephalon, diencephalon	Chicken	U	Blocked muscarinic arousal.	Marley and Seller (1972)
Serotonin (5-HT)	?	?	Mesencephalon	Cat	U	Increased slow-wave sleep (after pCPA).	Morgane and Stern (1972)
	≃20 µg	crystal	Preoptic area	Cat	U	EEG and behavioral sleep.	Yamaguchi et al. (1964)
Sodium citrate	3 µg	2 µl	Mesencephalon, reticular formation, superior colliculi	Rat	U	Alertness, fear, convulsions.	Nakajima (1964)
Teflurane	?	?	Mesencephalic reticular formation	Cat	U	Light sleep, EEG spindles.	Folkman et al. (1968)
	?	?	Thalamus, hypothalamus	Cat	U	Behavioral sleep, EEG spindles.	Wilkinson et al. (1971)

10 Sensory and Motor Systems

I. INTRODUCTION

The independent pathways which carry sensory information and motor commands throughout the central nervous system have been teased out in great detail in the last 30 years. The spinal cord, the thalamus and other major structures of great synaptic density have been examined studiously by electrophysiologists whose purpose is to establish the functional connections of these systems.

The rationale of chemically exciting a structure in the brain has been quite different. One principal question has centered on the issue of whether major sensory pathways are mediated by one class of transmitter or several. Another major objective has been to ascertain the biochemical nature of certain pathological conditions including epilepsy and Parkinsonism. Do these disease states of central origin arise as a result of a local humoral imbalance within a given cortical or subcortical structure?

A. Sensory Pathways

The various ascending spinal pathways synapse at several junctions along the afferent system. Although the release of ACh from the cerebral cortex (e.g., Mitchell, 1963) and from subcortical structures (e.g., Phillis *et al.*, 1968; Myers and Beleslin, 1970) has been demonstrated, a major question is how a transmitter could participate in the passage of a sensory signal across respective subcortical synapses to its ultimate destination. For instance, within the important relay network of the thalamus, are synapses coded by a specific humoral substance according to a particular sensory modality? In addition to the much needed micro-injection studies for mapping these systems chemically, this problem is another that would be amenable to the technique of perfusion of an isolated area of the thalamus for collecting the substances released locally during sensory bombardment.

Another issue of major import is the chemical nature of the postulated engram underlying the perception of pain. By what humoral mechanism is a nociceptive stimulus processed in cerebral structures so that the individual seeks to withdraw, avoid or otherwise escape a noxious stimulus or painful condition? By what chemical mediator is a nociceptive message transmitted? Fulminating pain perceived after a peripheral or internal injury is also not well understood with regard to the anatomical locus of the sensation (e.g., Sternbach, 1968). When particularly protracted, ill-defined secondary changes occur in the central nervous system that are linked with emotional and autonomic syndromes (Selye, 1956).

Some research has been undertaken to determine the central site of action of an opiate or other drug (see review of Herz and Teschemacher, 1971). Although these compounds possess an analgesic effect and can ameliorate or abolish the sensation of pain, the precise mechanism by which they affect a select element of cortical or subcortical tissue is largely unknown.

B. Motor Functions

To identify a transmitter factor which carries an efferent impulse along a multi-synaptic pathway is the goal of many research workers. But the main thrust in this field has been directed towards the understanding of the chemical basis for the remarkable disturbances often seen in normal function.

That a local chemical aberration within a specific structure could give rise to a particular muscular dysfunction has been recognized for many years. For example, the particularly high concentration of cholinesterase in the hippocampus (Burgen and Chipman, 1951) might provide a clue for the role of acetylcholine in affective disorders, in certain aspects of acquired motor behavior, or in epileptic discharges. In consideration of the fact that the corpus striatum contains much of the total content of dopamine in the brain and that a lesion to this structure can impair one's normal motor response in one of several ways, it is easy to surmise that a malfunction in dopamine release or the metabolism of this amine would have the same overall effect (Hornykiewicz, 1966). Thus, the well-known Parkinsonian disorders such as paralysis agitans or postencephalitic Parkinsonism may evolve following a local, permanent pathological change in the metabolism or other neuronal activity of a humoral substance. As we shall see in this chapter, the abnormal physiological and behavioral manifestations of such an alteration of a substrate make this supposition a very attractive one.

A totally different question dealt with in these studies is the central site of action of neuroleptics and other drugs. When given systemically, these compounds affect drastically ordinary muscular activity and can produce defects in coordination, catalepsy and other serious signs. Over and above the question of the central site and mechanism of action, investigations of convulsant agents have been devoted also to the etiology of the various forms of epilepsy. Attempts to simulate the neuropathology of temporal lobe epilepsy by the application of a chemical agent acting locally have met with considerable success. In fact, the neurohumoral basis for some facets of the disease is beginning to be placed on a sound footing. From chemical stimulation studies, one could deduce that a long-term regional change in neurohumoral function is at the heart of the malady of intermittent attacks of EEG seizure and muscular convulsion.

II. MODIFICATION OF SENSORY INPUT

A shift in pain threshold is widely used as an end-point for examining the central chemical mechanism sustaining somatosensory input. Up until the present time, very little research has been undertaken in which visual, auditory, olfactory or gustatory modalities have been modified specifically by the local application of a drug to brain tissue.

Blockade of the visual system of the cat at the level of the thalamus has been accomplished in an elegant experiment by Hafemann et al. (1969). Using only 0.5 μl of tetrodotoxin injected into the lateral geniculate body, they showed that the puffer fish poison blocked the typical evoked potentials both in the geniculate and visual cortex when light was flashed into the cat's eyes. Such a unilateral blockade is shown in Fig. 10-1. Although the effect is reversible, a high dose of tetrodotoxin causes nystagmus, focal spiking of the EEG and a strong tendency for the cat to turn toward the side of the micro-injection.

A similar interference with cortical evoked potentials can also be produced by GABA or GABOB (γ-amino-β-hydroxybutyric acid) applied directly to the sensory or motor cortex (Matsumoto et al., 1971). When the ventro-basal complex of the cat's thalamus is stimulated electrically, the usual spike potentials are inhibited in a concentration-dependent manner by a solution of either amino acid.

A. Reaction to Pain

Noteworthy contributions have been made independently by two groups of German workers who have investigated the function of acetylcholine in subcortical structures involved in nociceptive reactions. At a symposium held in 1967, Herz and Metyš (1968) first reported that two cholinomimetics, oxotremorine and carbachol, injected into the septum of the rat elevate the animal's pain threshold. When the tail was shocked, vocalizations and the typical motor defense reaction were considerably reduced. In this structure, cholinergic synapses could thus mediate the depression of sensory reactivity.

When injected into a variety of different subcortical or brain-stem structures, a cholinomimetic has the capacity to alter the threshold for a nociceptive or painful stimulus rather remarkably. Using electrical current applied to the root of the rat's tail or to the tooth pulp of the rabbit, Metyš et al. (1969a) found

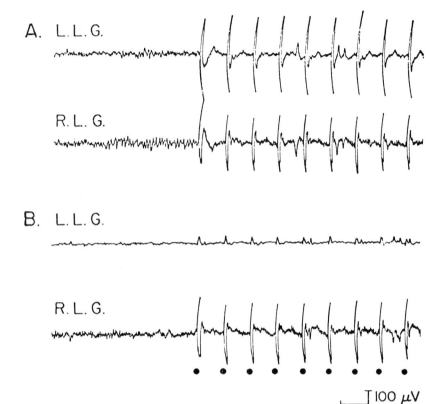

Fig. 10-1   Effect of tetrodotoxin (TTX) on photic evoked potentials. A, Control.   B, Forty minutes after introduction of 0.005 μg TTX into LLG. The dots indicate flashes. (From Hafemann, D. R. *et al.*, 1969. *Brain Res.* **12**:363–373. Fig. 2. Elsevier Publishing Co., Amsterdam, The Netherlands)

that several regions of the brain examined were differentially sensitive to the local concentration of a given cholinomimetic. Injected into the septum or mesencephalon, 0.3 μg of carbachol induced a pronounced elevation in the threshold for nociceptive stimulation. As shown in Fig. 10-2, 20 times this dose had to be injected into the caudate nucleus or hippocampus to produce an equivalent reduction of the pain response. Oxotremorine was somewhat less effective than carbachol, and arecoline was even less potent. In view of these differences in pharmacological sensitivity of the afferent pathway which is in stark contrast to the motor responses elicited following cholinergic stimulation of the caudate nucleus or hippocampus, it would seem that a cholinergic sensory system does mediate pain sensibility in the mesencephalon and thalamus as well as in the septum.

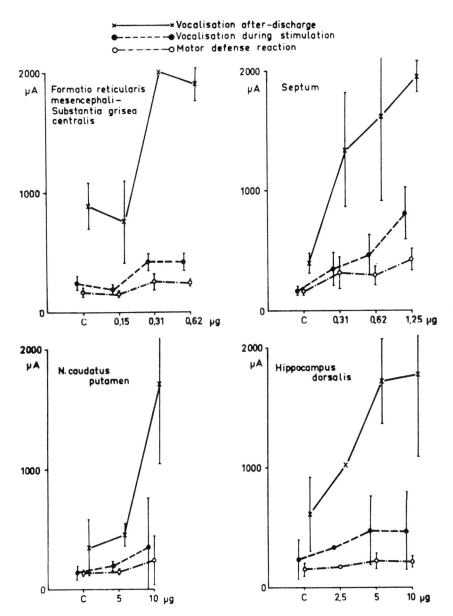

×————×Vocalisation after-discharge
●- - - - -●Vocalisation during stimulation
○—·—·—·○Motor defense reaction

Formatio reticularis mesencephali–Substantia grisea centralis

Septum

N. caudatus putamen

Hippocampus dorsalis

Fig. 10-2 Anti-nociceptive action of carbachol following intracerebral micro-injection into various brain areas in rats. Mean threshold values within 20 minutes after the injection with confidence limits ($P = 0.05$) in μA. Groups of 4 to 7 animals for each structure. C, saline injection. (From Metyš, J. *et al.*, 1969. *Int. J. Neuropharmacol.* 8:413–425. Pergamon Press, New York)

Either arecoline or oxotremorine injected into the medulla of the decerebrate or intact rat blocked the "tail-flick" reaction which is a well-defined reflexive response to a nociceptive stimulus (Andreas and Oelssner, 1969). This inhibition of a spinal pain reflex could be due to an activation by these cholinomimetics of a muscarine-like receptor of the Renshaw cell, which would thereby block the respective spinal motor neuron. The fact that atropine given peripherally antagonized the effect of the two drugs gives further support to this idea. However, because of the large volume given, the injection was almost equivalent to an intraventricular injection.

An extension of this previous study was done by Andreas and Staib (1971) to localize further the effect of the cholinomimetic. In spite of the large 10 μl volume infused, they contend that the reticular formation is apparently the region most sensitive to the local action of oxotremorine. Thus, a spinal inhibitory mechanism for a nociceptive sensation could be mediated in the rat through a suprasegmental system that articulates with the reticular formation. Curiously, Grossman (1968b) reports quite an opposite effect of cholinergic stimulation of the rat's mesencephalic reticular formation. The effect of a sensory stimulus is enhanced to such an extent by carbachol deposited in the midbrain that a startle response is evoked simply by a gentle tactile stimulus. The anatomical evidence described above by Metyš and his colleagues also does not support the observation of Andreas and Staib (1971), since the thalamus was most sensitive to cholinergic stimulation (Metyš et al., 1969a). Interestingly, Guerrero-Figueroa et al. (1966a) have shown that ACh applied to the caudate nucleus or septum can either excite or suppress sensory evoked potentials.

Once again, the dose, the volume and other technical matters could easily account for these discrepancies. Clearly, the demonstration of a pharmacological antagonism of the central receptors in the pain pathway and evidence of the extent of diffusion of the injected chemical would help to resolve these issues.

B. Central Action of Morphine and Procaine

For the relief of intractable pain in the human, Mandl (1951) found that the intracerebral infiltration of procaine or phenol was highly effective. When either was infused into the frontal lobe about 8 to 9 cm below the surface of the cortex, the unbearable agony usually associated with terminal carcinoma abated. Mandl's terse clinical description of the success of this procedure is most notable indeed:

> ". . . . Case 3.—Male, 47 years of age. Exploratory thoracotomy. Infiltration on July 5, 1950. Died September 25, 1950. The first infiltration made the patient free of pains for 50 days, the second one until his death. Result: excellent."

When a rabbit is exposed to a powerful heat lamp whose rays are focused on the nose or thigh, morphine acts centrally to inhibit the withdrawal from this painful stimulus (Tsou and Jang, 1964). An injection of a low dose of morphine in the periventricular or periaqueductal gray matter produces the greatest analgesic effect. For the most part, an injection into various sites in the thalamus and mesencephalon is without effect. Thus, it would appear that a principal site of action of morphine in raising the pain threshold is the network of neurons in the central gray in a region that is very close to the third ventricle. The antagonistic actions of nalorphine are also pinpointed to this locus.

In a preliminary report, Metyš et al. (1969b) found that morphine was as effective as a cholinomimetic substance in raising the threshold for various nociceptive reactions in the rat. The two regions of greatest sensitivity to either of the drugs were the hypothalamus and mesencephalon.

When applied to the medial portion of the hypothalamus, subthalamus or mesencephalon of the rabbit, morphine attenuated the nociceptive licking response to electrical stimulation of tooth pulp (Herz et al., 1970a). Figure 10-3 illustrates the anatomical region of maximum sensitivity to morphine. Although bilateral and unilateral injections did not seem to differ in overall effect, an injection into the lateral hypothalamus seemed to cause an increase in vigilance, whereas the rabbit became hyperexcitable, vocalized and tried to escape following the injection of morphine into the periaqueductal gray matter. A dose of 20 to 40 μg was much higher than that required to produce the same effect via the ventricular route. This suggests that the micro-injection was acting indirectly on another more distant structure such as one forming the aqueduct. Thus, the dose given in the periaqueductal gray may have been too high and caused excitation.

According to Lotti et al. (1965), the analgesic effect of morphine on the rat, as assessed by the absence of withdrawal of the tail upon pinching, could not be localized to any part of the hypothalamus. Instead, 50 μg of morphine in a volume of 1 μl elicited analgesia when it was injected at nearly all sites. Using a hot plate upon which the rat was placed, Foster et al. (1967) found that the reaction time to the hot plate stimulus increased significantly after 25 μg of morphine were injected in the rostral hypothalamus; however, the localization of the injected sites was admittedly imprecise. The smaller dose used, however, could account for the fact that morphine did not have such an anatomically widespread action.

III. GROSS MOTOR FUNCTION

A large number of motor symptoms have been observed following the chemical stimulation of various segments of the neuraxis. These range from a mild change in locomotor activity to a grand mal convulsion. Abnormal EEG manifestations including focal discharges are often correlated with a disturbance in motor activity.

As early as 1937 the Canadian physiologist, Miller (1937), showed that blotting paper soaked in eserine and applied to the surface of the cat's motor cortex

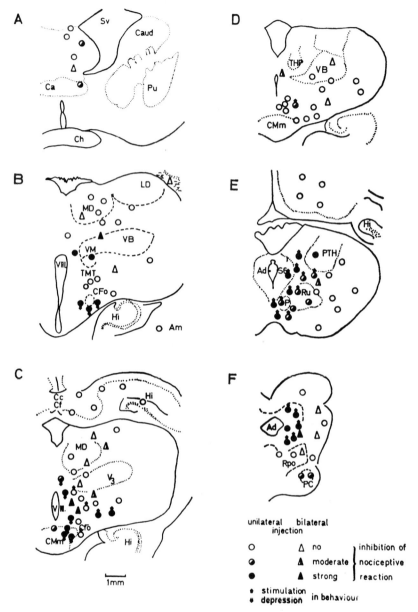

Fig. 10-3 Diagram to show effectiveness of morphine when applied by micro-injection into various brain structures. The graphs A through F refer to planes between septum and midbrain according to the atlas of Gerhard (1968). Moderate effect: an increase in stimulation threshold of 200 to 500%; strong effect: an increase of > 500%. In most experiments, 40 μg morphine were applied unilaterally, or 2 X 20 μg bilaterally. (From Herz, A. *et al.*, 1970. *Neuropharmacology*. 9:539–551. Pergamon Press, New York)

caused an intense activity in the contralateral limbs. Within a few seconds the fore or hind leg developed a tremor which was followed by rigidity and a powerful clonus. This chemical elevation in ACh activity also sensitized the cortex to punctate electrical stimulation as well. Similarly, when Miller (1943) positioned filter paper saturated in an ACh solution on the XII nerve nuclei located on the floor of the cat's fourth ventricle, he observed movements of the tongue, elevation of the palate and dilatation of the mouth. That the hypoglossal nucleus has a cholinergic innervation for deglutition was thus proposed over 30 years ago.

A. Locomotor Activity

Circling to the same side or opposite to that of unilateral stimulation is produced in the rabbit or cat by cholinergic substances applied to the caudate nucleus and other subcortical structures (Nashold and Gills, 1960). The extent and direction of these walking movements are dependent on the site at which the crystals are applied. Vertical and rotational movements of the head can also be elicited from cholinergic stimulation of a large number of sites. The contralateral circling produced by carbachol applied to the caudate of the rabbit was verified by Stevens et al. (1961) in later observations of the cat. They also observed that the limbs contralateral to the side of the cholinergic stimulation were also left weak. Contralateral circling movements have also been described by Myers (1964a) following cholinergic stimulation of the lateral and posterior parts of the hypothalamus of the cat.

Some chemically unspecific motor effects are caused in the cat by several crystalline substances tamped into brain-stem structures in 200 μg amounts (Nashold et al., 1965). Carbachol, eserine, strychnine or reserpine implanted in the red nucleus or in the substantia nigra usually evoked ipsiversive head turning, circling, some ataxia and, in several instances, an abnormal righting reflex. In contrast to the effect of electrical stimulation of these structures, none of the chemicals produced tremor or other Parkinsonian signs.

1. Caudate Nucleus

Besides the involvement of the caudate nucleus in gross locomotor activity, this structure may play a part in finer motor control. For example, the application in a toxic dose of carbachol, alumina cream or penicillin to the head of the caudate evokes a vertical nystagmus in the cat (Szekely and Spiegel, 1963). Significantly, however, the deposition of these substances in the lateral or third ventricle elicits identical symptoms; thus, their oculogyric action could be on any one of several diencephalic or mesencephalic sites.

When the anticholinesterase diisopropylfluorophosphate (DFP) is injected in a relatively high dose in the caudate nucleus of the rabbit, the animal begins to circle in a direction contralateral to the side of the injection (White, 1956; White and Himwich, 1957). In the anatomical controls, DFP injected at other sites exerts no motor effect, except when injected in the medulla and ventromedial thalamus. Metrazol and mecholyl also evoke contralateral turning when given in very high milligram doses. This was the first evidence since Miller's early work that a chemical mechanism is involved in motor control which can be modified if cholinesterase is depleted in a subcortical region.

In contrast to the result of a lesion of the caudate nucleus after which the animal rotates ipsiversively, localized spreading depression produced by KCl micro-infused into the caudate nucleus of the rat or rabbit causes contralateral circling movements (Weiss and Fifková, 1963). These responses are similar to those produced by electrical stimulation of this structure. This paradoxical response may be due to continual functional impairment of a sufficient number of cells which maintain the rotational movement or to a blockade of just those cells which exert an inhibitory influence on extrapyramidal activity.

Excitatory, autonomic and motor effects were produced by N-methyl-aspartic acid (NMA) injected in a high dose and in a large volume into the caudate nucleus of the cat (Baker, 1972). The rapid latency of onset and the failure of the cholinergic antagonist, scopolamine, to block this activity would indicate that NMA is acting directly on a subcortical system by action on receptors other than cholinergic ones. In fact, this amino acid could mimic an electrical current in terms of its capacity to depolarize neurons.

The general activity of an animal may also depend upon a cholinergic inhibitory mechanism in the septal-hippocampal system. Crystalline atropine applied to sites in the dorsal or ventral hippocampus or the septum causes a rat to increase its locomotor activity (Leaton and Rech, 1972). That the anticholinergic action of atropine presumably blocks the system that inhibits motor movement has also been supported by other experiments with mice. When injected into the hippocampus of a mouse of the DBA strain, scopolamine enhances exploratory behavior which is characterized by rearing, wall-leaning or the sniffing of objects (van Abeelen et al., 1972). On the other hand, neostigmine diminishes all three varieties of exploratory activity and induces a freezing response. A dose-response analysis of this inhibition is presented in Fig 10-4. In another strain, the C57BL/6 mouse, a similar injection of scopolamine reduces exploration. As a result, the cholinergic mechanism in the hippocampus implicated in overall general activity may be genetically as well as chemically determined.

2. Corpus Striatum and Catecholamines

In addition to the localized destruction of adrenergic nerve terminals, 6-hydroxy-dopamine (6-OHDA) injected into the substantia nigra of the rat produces ipsiversive turning and generalized motor asymmetry (Ungerstedt, 1968). These symptoms are consistent with those seen after conventional electrolytic lesions. The bodily rotation of the 6-OHDA lesioned rat is also elicited by handling and enhanced further by intraperitoneal amphetamine. This behavioral response is illustrated in Fig. 10-5 for three doses of amphetamine (Ungerstedt and Arbuthnott, 1970). Perhaps the degree to which dopamine receptors within the

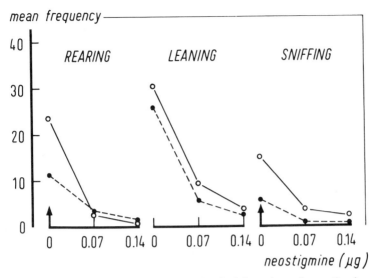

Fig. 10-4 The effect of intrahippocampal administration of neostigmine upon the frequencies per 15 minutes of three exploratory acts in inbred mouse strains DBA/2 (closed circles) and C57BL/6 (open circles). The DBA/2 groups comprise 13 (saline), 12 (0.07 μg), and 14 (0.14 μg) animals; the C57BL/6 groups comprise 13, 14, and 14 animals, respectively. Their median scores closely approach the mean values presented. Significant strain differences ($p < 0.05$) are indicated by arrows on the abscissae. All drug groups differ significantly ($p < 0.02$) from their saline controls. (From van Abeelen et al., 1972)

intact nigro-striatal system are stimulated by amphetamine determines the intensity of the abnormal motor responses.

Pretreatment of a rat with the MAO inhibitor, nialamide, enhances contralateral turning and asymmetric posture with adducted limbs, evoked by an injection of dopamine into the corpus striatum. Norepinephrine and apomorphine have the same effect, presumably as the result of their stimulation of dopaminergic receptors (Ungerstedt et al., 1969). Conversely, chlorpromazine causes ipsilateral turning possibly because it blocks the dopamine receptor sites. It is difficult to know why dopamine without MAO inhibition did not produce this effect even if a high dose in excess of that capable of being degraded by available MAO was micro-injected. Nevertheless, these data are not in conflict with the supposition that both cholinergic and dopaminergic systems may play an integral part in extrapyramidal motor function.

Metatyramine protects the stores of dopamine in the corpus striatum of the rat from depletion by systemic reserpine (Andén et al., 1970). When 15 mg of metatyramine in a volume of 300 μl were infused over a 5-hour period, the content of dopamine was much higher at the end of this interval than in the control contralateral striatum. During this period, the rat rotated toward the side oppo-

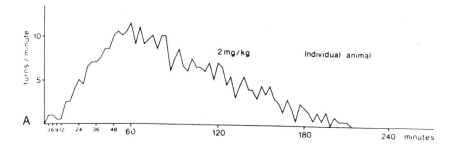

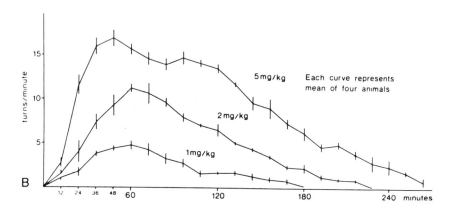

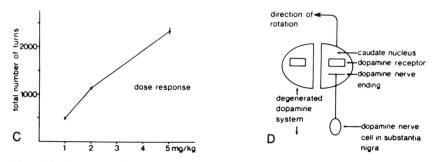

Fig. 10-5 Rotational behavior after amphetamine. A, Rotation curve showing a single animal that received amphetamine, 2 mg/kg. The drug was given at time zero. The small peak during the first 9 minutes was due to the activation caused by handling and injection. The mean rotational speed in turns per minute towards the left lesioned side is plotted for each 3-minute period. B, Rotational behavior after 1, 2 and 5 mg/kg amphetamine. Each curve represents the mean rotational speed for four animals. The average rotational speed and the standard error of the mean are plotted for each 12-minute period. The curves differ clearly

site to the infusion possibly as a consequence of the elevated stores of dopamine in the neostriatum.

Profound sensorimotor incapacitation evolves in the cat after the dopaminergic system of its substantia nigra is lesioned chemically. A direct injection of 6-OHDA in a large volume into the tegmental structure of the cat causes contralateral or ipsilateral circling until the cat collapses. Other symptoms are an ataxic gait, some flexor rigidity, limb hyperextension and the loss of the ability to step or jump downward. Although Parkinsonian tremor does not occur, these findings signify the vital importance of an intact nigro-striatal or nigro-thalamic projection for normal sensorimotor function (Frigyesi *et al.*, 1971).

After 59 or 65 μg of dopamine or norepinephrine, respectively, are injected into the hypothalamus or corpus striatum of the rat, the animal becomes restless, runs carelessly, grooms and licks itself (Benkert and Köhler, 1972). Because of the inordinately high doses and the large 3 μl volume which would be taken up easily by the locally rich blood supply, the hyperactivity could be due to the well-known energizing action of the catecholamines acting by the systemic route.

B. Stereotypy Behavior

So-called stereotypy behavior of the rat includes continuous sniffing, licking, biting and perhaps compulsive gnawing. This sort of activity interrupted with cataleptic pauses appears after a mixture of dopamine and scopolamine or scopolamine alone is injected into the corpus striatum (Fog *et al.*, 1967). Thus, the stereotyped behavior produced by amphetamine given by the systemic route may be mediated by acetylcholine, dopamine or both biogenic amines in this region of the brain.

1. *Cholinergic and Dopaminergic Activation*

A systemic injection of apomorphine or dopamine (DOPA) causes compulsive gnawing behavior in the rodent, presumably by a mechanism situated in the extrapyramidal system. Crystals of both apomorphine and DOPA implanted into the dorsal caudate nucleus and globus pallidus, but not in more lateral or ventral areas, evoke an identical gnawing response in the rat (Ernst and Smelik, 1966). Certainly, sites mediating this motor reaction, shown in Fig. 10-6, are apparently in the corpus striatum. Cholinergic stimulation of the presumed dopaminergic

---

in their rise, peak value and duration. C, Total number of turns plotted against dose of amphetamine. Each point represents four animals. The vertical lines represent standard error of the mean. D, Schematic representation of the experimental situation. The left nigro-striatal dopamine system is degenerated by an intracerebral injection of 6-OHDA. Activation of the remaining dopamine system will cause the animal to rotate towards the left lesioned side. (From Ungerstedt, U. and G. W. Arbuthnott. 1970. *Brain Res.* 24:485–493. Fig. 2. Elsevier Publishing Co., Amsterdam, The Netherlands)

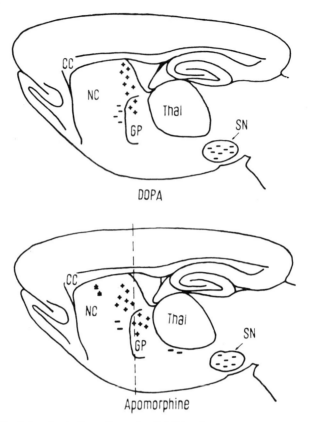

Fig. 10-6 (Top) Implantation sites of L-DOPA, shown in sagittal section of rat brain.   + = gnawing behavior; − = ineffective. (Bottom) Implantation sites of apomorphine, shown in sagittal section. (From Ernst and Smelik, 1966)

fiber system in the nigro-striatal pathway causes the rat to gnaw the wire mesh of its cage floor compulsively (Smelik and Ernst, 1966). Although this response was not quantified, it was evoked by eserine crystals after a very long latency of 30 minutes. It lasted 1 to 2 hours and was thought by Smelik and Ernst to be due to the local release of dopamine. A build-up of acetylcholine is an equally tenable explanation.

Crystals of acetylcholine placed in tegmental structures have been reported to evoke bizarre stereotyped changes in the posture of the rat, which were characterized mainly by standing (Davis et al., 1967b). These standing responses are elicited by cholinergic activation of loci in the dorsomedial rather than ventro-lateral aspect of the midbrain reticular system.

Either hydroxyamphetamine or dopamine injected into the corpus striatum evokes stereotyped behavior in a rat previously made cataleptic by systemic reserpine (Fog and Pakkenberg, 1971). That norepinephrine is not involved in the "compulsivity" was shown when this catecholamine injected in the same region did not induce the repetitive responses. Thus, the finding that hydroxy-amphetamine mimics the action of dopamine suggests that its action is mediated by way of a dopaminergic neuronal mechanism within the caudate-putamen complex. A locus of action other than the striatum is suspect, however, since the autoradiographic counts actually showed that the 5 μl volume passed up the shaft of the cannula. The highest density of grains appeared superficially in the homolateral cortex. In the 24-hour reserpinized rat, Fuxe and Ungerstedt (1970) found that apomorphine injected into the neostriatum in a low dose evokes stereotyped walking, but intense biting with a higher dose. The receptors in the corpus striatum were probably supersensitive since apomorphine injected alone had little effect.

The rat's stereotypy behavior induced by an injection of amphetamine into the caudate-putamen complex or globus pallidus is exaggerated significantly by pretreatment with atropine given intraperitoneally (Costall *et al.*, 1972). Corresponding to this, the cholinomimetic, arecoline injected into the globus pallidus reduces the amphetamine stereotypy within 30 seconds. Haloperidol, a dopamine antagonist, injected also into the pallidum, has an even greater inhibitory action on the stereotypy. Thus, further evidence is offered for a dopaminergic-cholinergic interaction within both the neostriatal and pallidal systems.

The antagonism of the cholinergic component of the dopaminergic-cholinergic system in the basal ganglia potentiates rather dramatically stereotyped behavior in the rat. The injection of several cholinolytics including atropine, orphenadrine or phenglutarimide into the globus pallidus or corpus striatum enhances gnawing, biting, licking and other compulsive behaviors (Costall and Naylor, 1972a). These results support the general view that a reciprocal balance in the release of dopamine and acetylcholine in these subcortical structures determines the magnitude of amphetamine stereotypy. Nonetheless, it should be emphasized that the destruction by electrolytic lesions of the noradrenergic nerve terminals in the lateral amygdaloid nucleus reduces stereotyped behavior induced by apomorphine (Costall and Naylor, 1972b). Therefore, an exclusive dopaminergic system mediating all of the components of stereotypy behavior can probably be ruled out.

In the cat, dopamine, L-dopa or *d*-amphetamine also induces stereotypy behavior when the amines are injected in a large 10 μl volume into the caudate nucleus (Cools and van Rossum, 1970); these effects do not appear until after a period of 10 minutes has elapsed. One might expect the delay to be due perhaps to some sort of metabolic conversion; however, norepinephrine injected into the same area of the caudate nucleus does not evoke stereotyped behavior in the cat, a finding opposite to that of the rat (Ungerstedt *et al.*, 1969). A further analysis of the limb movements produced by an intra-caudate injection of L-dopa or dopamine reveals that the activity can be classified into classical athetoid or choreiform hyperkinesis (Cools, 1972). These movements are characterized by rhythmic alternating hyperextension and flexion of muscle groups in the animal's limb and paw. Interestingly, the cat tries to lick and clean the affected limb.

2. *5-HT or Copper Metabolism*

Serotonin also causes compulsive gnawing behavior, after a latency of 1 to 2 hours, when injected into the corpus striatum of a rat pretreated with a MAO inhibitor. An implant in the striatum of 5-HTP, apomorphine or eserine had no effect (Hadžović and Ernst, 1969). When either 5-HT or 5-HTP was implanted in the substantia nigra, with or without MAO-I pretreatment, tremor but no gnawing appeared 15 to 100 minutes later and lasted for 30 to 150 minutes. The reason for the long latency is not clear; however, diffusion, overdose, or some regional uniqueness of 5-HTP decarboxylase in the substantia nigra may account for these findings. Again, tremor could have really been the shivering related to a hyperthermic action of 5-HT in the rat after an initial fall in temperature occurred.

In an extension of this earlier work, Hadžović (1971) found that 5-HT and 5-HTP implanted in the lateral hypothalamus of the rat evoke some signs of heat production as well as other unrelated responses, in all probability because of the enormous overlap of systems which were affected by the large doses of the indoleamine. After a latency of 5 to 20 minutes, 5-HT or 5-HTP evoked tremor, piloerection, stereotypic movements of the head and forelimbs, and occasionally salivation. Compulsive gnawing was also produced by 5-HT. Thus, it would appear that there are multiple sites of action of amines in evoking stereotyped motor movements. Clearly other measures such as body temperature and water intake should be recorded, and thorough pharmacological controls are required. In line with this, the results of the peripheral administration of L-dopa and 5-HTP, after central stores of monoamines are depleted, indicate that the central effect of dopamine on the extrapyramidal system is mediated by the release of an endogenous substance other than serotonin (Ernst, 1972).

Beads of copper salt deposited in the caudate nucleus of the cat evoke a burst of obstinate treading of the animal's feet in an attempt to move pointlessly against a wall (Butcher and Fox, 1968). After the copper was implanted, intermittent periods of lethargy and motionlessness occurred for several hours. Since other salts used as controls did not have these severe effects on the cat's behavior, abnormal copper metabolism within the neostriatum may contribute to certain of the neuropathologic conditions of the extrapyramidal system.

3. *Catalepsy*

What is probably a chemical lesion rather than chemical stimulation is produced by a local injection of alumina cream. When this substance was infused in a 200 μl volume in the caudate nucleus of the cat, catatonia, ataxia, the loss of ingestive responses and other severe motor dysfunctions arose (Spiegel and

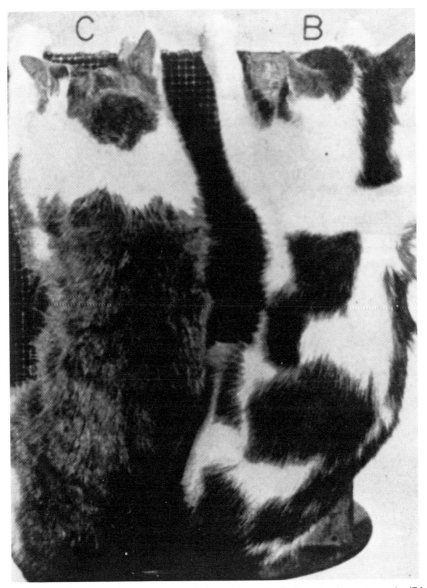

Fig. 10-7 Cat in striatal catatonia (C) and one in bulbocapnine catatonia (B) in hanging position, supporting themselves with forepaws on the top of the cage. (From Spiegel, E. A. and E. G. Szekely. 1961. *Arch. Neurol.* 4:55–65. Copyright 1961, the American Medical Association)

Szekely, 1961). Active catalepsy, illustrated in Fig. 10-7, in which the animal's paws or body remain suspended for some time in an abnormal position, was clearly evident. Even after extirpation of both the frontal pole and the homolateral motor cortex, the syndrome still developed. However, since large lesions of the amygdala prevented the syndrome, the striatal-fugal fiber system which mediates catatonia may have an important link with the amygdaloid nuclei. The inability of a cat with chemically induced striatal catatonia to pounce upon a mouse is portrayed in Fig. 10-8.

After a bilateral micro-injection of a phenothiazine or thioxanthene into the corpus striatum of the rat, the stereotyped behavior of compulsive sniffing, licking and biting induced earlier by 10 mg/kg amphetamine is totally abolished (Fog *et al.*, 1968). Instead, however, catalepsy develops which lasts for 15 to 30 minutes. Certain other drugs such as amobarbitone injected intrastriatally do not diminish the amphetamine stereotypy (Fog *et al.*, 1969). A number of quaternary derivatives injected into the corpus striatum of the rat do act to block the stereotypy produced by a subcutaneous injection of *d*-amphetamine (Fog *et al.*, 1971). These include haloperidol, beneperidol, floropipamide and oxypertine. Following their intrastriatal injection, the stereotyped responses are suddenly converted into catalepsy which is interrupted by bouts of hyperactive

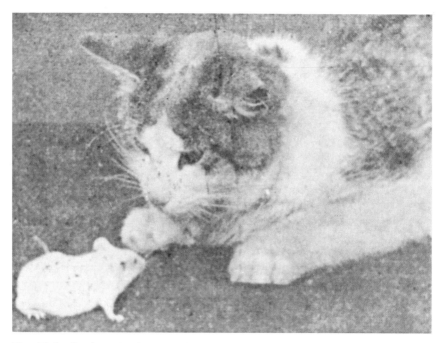

Fig. 10-8 Cat in striatal catatonia staring at a mouse. (From Spiegel, E. A. and E. G. Szekely. 1961. *Arch. Neurol.* 4:55–65. Copyright 1961, the American Medical Association)

locomotor activity. Again, the antagonism of the amphetamine stereotypy may be brought about through a dopaminergic mechanism (Randrup and Munkvad, 1970).

A catatonia-like state also may occur in the cat following the localized push-pull perfusion of a solution containing excess calcium ions within the posterior hypothalamus (Veale and Myers, 1971). Figure 10-9 illustrates the posture of such a cat with its left fore-paw remaining in place after being placed over its back. The effects of calcium can best be portrayed by the following description:

"Catatonia-like responses were also observed after perfusion with excess calcium ions within several isolated regions of the hypothalamus. Figure 10-9 illustrates the position of a cat in which the posterior portion of the lateral hypothalamus at AP 10.0 was perfused with a calcium solution 10.4 mM in excess of the normal extracellular fluid. The signs of deep sleep accompanied by catatonia appeared within 15 minutes of the start of perfusion. When one of the animal's limbs was placed in an unnatural position, as shown in Fig. 10-9, the cat often remained motionless for as long as 2 minutes. In this case,

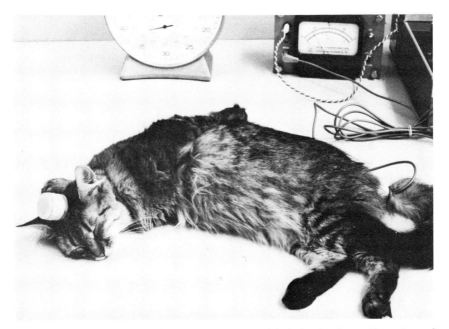

Fig. 10-9 Catatonic-like state in association with behavioral manifestation of sleep following the perfusion of calcium ions 10.4 mM in excess of normal Krebs solution within the posterior hypothalamus. The animal remained motionless even if its limb was placed in an unnatural position as shown. (From Veale and Myers, 1971)

the pupils were constricted and the nictitating membrane covered more than half of the surface of each eye. Nevertheless, the cat retained its normal blink reflexes and would withdraw its leg to deep pressure or a nociceptive stimulus. In other tests of catatonia, the cat would remain for several minutes with its paws placed on an elevated block, and when forced to change its position, the cat moved in a slow but coordinated manner. With the higher concentration of calcium, when signs of catatonia were observed, the effects of the calcium lasted for as long as 5 hours, after which the normal behavioral characteristics returned fully."

IV. TREMOR

Ordinarily, gross limb movement is easily differentiated from smaller muscle fasciculations. Frequently, the latter merges into the former. As in the case of intense shivering, more and more muscle groups are mobilized and a transition occurs from fine movement to a total motion of the extremities. Thus, some distinction between shivering and tremor may be made on the basis of magnitude of limb movement. Obviously, an electromyographic recording helps to answer some of the questions pertaining to the quantitation of the repetitive and rhythmic movement of a muscle complex.

In dealing with the issue that we have seen in the previous section of the central interaction between chemically evoked heat production and myotonic activity, a reasonable solution is always to record core temperature itself, vasomotor responses and even O_2 consumption. These measures would sort out, by the process of elimination, the primary local action of a compound at a given site. When differential latencies are recorded for each physiological response, the measure takes on even greater significance. For example, if vasoconstriction precedes an increase in muscular fasciculations at the same time that the temperature rises, the pathway mediating a thermogenic response rather than a tremorogenic system may be activated. On the other hand, if there is no essential physiological change until after a sequence of rhythmic motor movement begins, then it is more safe to conclude that a tremor mechanism has been selectively stimulated.

A. Tremorogenic Substances

In addition to a family of unique drugs that have the capacity to evoke tremor, the part played by two endogenous humoral substances, acetylcholine and dopamine, has been examined extensively.

In a preliminary report, Spiegel et al. (1965) found that the injection of 1 mg of L-dopa in a 20 μl volume into the caudate nucleus of the cat reinstates spontaneous limb movements after they had been previously blocked by 200 μg of carbachol injected similarly. When a more permanent bradykinesia was induced in the rat by an injection of tungstic acid into its caudate nucleus, L-dopa also counteracted the lack of motor activity (Spiegel *et al.*, 1968). The injection of L-dopa at the same site in the caudate nucleus increased the movement of the rat and its running speed in response to an auditory or nociceptive stimulus.

An initial attempt to localize the tremorogenic effect of oxotremorine was made by George *et al.* (1966) who injected this compound at sites in the mesencephalon and rostral hypothalamus of the cat. Injected at pontine-mesencephalic sites, oxotremorine produced tremor as reflected in the electromyographic records presented in Fig. 10-10. These changes were simultaneously accompanied by EEG desynchronization, atonia and sleep. Arousal and emotional changes occurred when the drug was injected into the hypothalamus. Thus, it would appear that several physiological systems, including perhaps one of the efferent pathways for shivering and the maintenance of body temperature, were activated simultaneously. Unfortunately, temperature was not recorded.

Both tremorine and oxotremorine evoke tremor when either is injected in a large 3 μl volume in the globus pallidus, caudate nucleus, substantia nigra or red nucleus of the rat. Although there is some difference in the magnitude of tremor, the substantia nigra and red nucleus are more sensitive to a single dose of oxotremorine (Cox and Potkonjak, 1969).

INTRACEREBRAL OXOTREMORINE (2 μg)

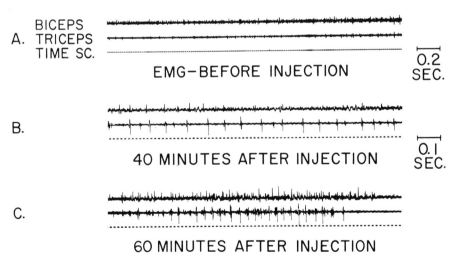

Fig. 10-10 EMG records showing onset of tremor and change in tremor frequency following intrapontine injection of oxotremorine. Time marker: 60 c/s. (From George, R. *et al.*, 1966. *Int. J. Neuropharmacol.* **5**:27–34. Pergamon Press, New York)

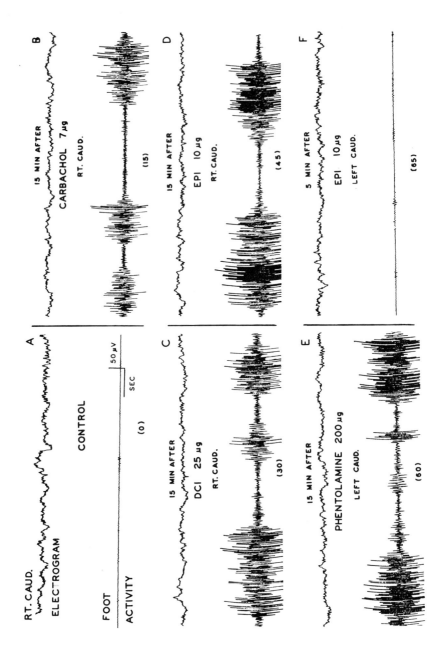

A substantial contribution to our understanding of the central mechanism governing tremor has been made by Connor, Baker, Rossi, Lalley and their associates.   When Connor *et al.* (1966b) injected carbachol into the caudate nucleus of the cat, a persistent hind limb tremor arose.   Then a rise in temperature occurred and focal EEG changes evolved from spike activity into a full-blown seizure pattern.   Metrazol and procaine did not produce these effects, nor did a similar injection of carbachol into other sites in the brain including the hippocampus, reticular formation, hypothalamus or third ventricle.   Procaine temporarily abolished the tremor when injected also into the same region of the caudate, which indicates that the action of the cholinomimetic could be a localized one in spite of the volume of the infusion.   Of all of the cholinomimetics tested in the cat, their order of tremorogenic potency judged on the basis of dose is carbachol > bethanechol > methacholine > acetylcholine (Connor *et al.*, 1966a).   When injected into the caudate nucleus, antagonists of muscarinic but not nicotinic receptors block the carbachol-induced tremor at the very height of its activity.   From this finding, the central mechanism for tremor seems to be mediated by a muscarinic type of synapse in the complex neural network that connects structures of the basal ganglia to those in the brain-stem and spinal cord.

Since the caudate nucleus has such high concentrations of dopamine and norepinephrine, the effects of several catecholamines have also been examined in the cat by Connor *et al.* (1967).   Injected into the caudate nucleus after carbachol had been applied there to induce tremor, all of the catecholamines tested as well as ATP antagonize the motor symptoms.   Further, if a beta-receptor blocking agent such as dichloroisoproterenol (DCI) or propranolol is injected into the caudate 15 minutes before an epinephrine injection, then the usual adrenergic inhibition of cholinergic tremor is prevented.   Each of these effects is depicted in Fig. 10-11.   A micro-injection of chlorpromazine or an alpha adrenergic antagonist such as phentolamine does not block the adrenergic inhibition of tremor.   Through the usage of vasoactive agents as controls, Connor *et al.* ensured that the local effects of the amines are not the result of local vascular

Fig. 10-11   Effect of local pretreatment with adrenergic blocking agents on the anti-tremor activity of epinephrine.   In each panel: upper tracing, caudate electrogram; lower tracing, foot movements.   Numbers in parentheses represent continuous time sequence in minutes from control.   Tremor initiated (B) by an intracaudate injection of carbachol.   Injection of a beta-receptor blocking drug (C) prevented subsequent epinephrine antagonism of tremor (D); thus, involuntary movements persist.   However, injection of an alpha-receptor blocking drug (E) into the contralateral caudate did not interfere with subsequent epinephrine antagonism of tremor (F).   The 50 μV calibration pertains to the gain setting for both the electrogram and tremor channels.   Phonocartridge output indicating foot activity is a resultant of both frequency and amplitude of movements.   (From Connor, J. D. *et al.*, 1967. *J. Pharmacol. Exptl. Ther.* **155**:545–551. The Williams and Wilkins Co., Baltimore)

dilatation or constriction within the caudate nucleus. That a balance exists between neurohumoral factors in the caudate nucleus that are involved in motor control is a reasonable supposition. In terms of the anti-tremor potency of the catecholamines and the results with the cholinergic blocking agents, this equilibrium seems to be between cholinergic and adrenergic systems. These two sets of systems are apparently mediated by muscarinic and beta receptors, respectively.

In a very extensive study in which a large number of compounds was injected into the caudate nucleus of the cat, Lalley *et al.* (1970) distinguished between pharmacological tremor produced by carbachol and endogenous tremor evoked by one of two classes of anticholinesterase: (1) reversible (eserine) or (2) irreversible (DFP or echothiophate). An intracaudate injection of a catecholamine or of a substance which blocks the synthesis of ACh or its release onto post-synaptic receptors attenuates two of the three stages of tremor. A residual tremor produced by the irreversible anticholinesterase and lasting for weeks or even months was generally resistant to a local injection of all tremor antagonists except hemicholinium, which prevents ACh synthesis. The development and progression of the stages of cholinergic tremor are presented in Fig. 10-12.

It would appear that local cholinesterase activity in the caudate nucleus contributes to the absence or presence of tremor. Further, on the basis of the catecholamine antagonism of cholinergic tremor, Lalley *et al.* have suggested that "increased levels of cholinergic activity mediate and directly release dopamine." Tremor would result only after the compensatory limit of dopamine release was exceeded. This interesting idea was modeled after the traditional Burn-Rand hypothesis that ACh acts to release NE from specific autonomic ganglia.

In the cat in which tremor had already been produced by eserine or carbachol injected into the caudate nucleus, Lalley *et al.* (1971) found that Ca^{2+}, Mg^{2+} or K^+ ions, in this order of potency, either abolished or reduced partially the motor discharges when the cations were also injected at the same site in the caudate. Na^+ was without effect. A prior injection of propranolol, a beta-receptor antagonist, into the caudate reduced the length of time that Ca^{2+} ions inhibited the tremor. Taken together, these results suggest that Ca^{2+} may exert a dual action: (1) in stabilizing the cholinoceptive neuronal membrane, and (2) in evoking the presynaptic release of dopamine. The effect of Na EDTA could be due to the reduction of endogenous Ca^{2+} ions through chelation which would exacerbate the condition of tremor.

By the clever use of the principle of a magnetic field to record the limb tremor of a rat, Dill *et al.* (1968a) confirmed that carbachol injected into the corpus striatum of the rat induces contralateral forelimb tremor. The rhythmic bursts of movement occurred within 2 to 3 minutes and continued irregularly for up to 1 hour. Little and Dill (1969) have also demonstrated that the injection of different O-methylated-β-phenylethylamines such as mescaline or dimethoxy-phenylethylamine into the caudate-putamen complex of the rat causes a variety

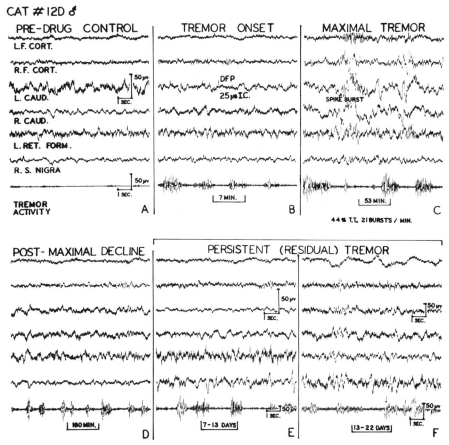

CAT # 12D ♂

PRE-DRUG CONTROL | TREMOR ONSET | MAXIMAL TREMOR

L.F. CORT.

R.F. CORT.

L. CAUD.

R. CAUD.

L. RET. FORM.

R. S. NIGRA

TREMOR
ACTIVITY

50 μν.
I SEC.

DFP
25 μ I.C.

SPIKE BURST

A | 7 MIN. | B | 53 MIN. | C

44 % T.T. 21 BURSTS / MIN.

POST- MAXIMAL DECLINE | PERSISTENT (RESIDUAL) TREMOR

50 μν
I SEC.

50 μν
I SEC.

50 μν
I SEC.

50 μν
I SEC.

| 180 MIN. | D | 7-13 DAYS | E | 13-22 DAYS | F

Fig. 10-12 Tremor and electrographic responses which characterize the development of endogenous cholinergic tremors following micro-injection of DFP (25 μg) into the left caudate nucleus. Spike bursts were initiated in the caudate and cortex during the maximal stage (C) but were more characteristic of late maximal and post-maximal stages (D).   Bracketed values in (B–D) represent continuous time sequence in minutes; responses in (E) and (F) are typical of the residual responses observed at regular intervals following a single micro-injection of DFP. (From Lalley et al., 1970)

of motor disturbances. These include forelimb tremor that is usually contralateral, salivation, chewing, facial spasms, contralateral head turning, and a hyperextension of the trunk which results in rearing-up on the hind feet (Little and Dill, 1969). The latency for these abnormal symptoms to appear is about 15 minutes and the motor effects last from ½ hour to 2 hours. Carbachol has much the same effect but differs quite markedly in terms of its short latency and limited duration of action. Thus, these compounds probably do not act as false cholinergic transmitters but could produce the disabling motor reactions in a number of ways: (1) reduction in acetylcholinesterase synthesis; (2) blockade of adrenergic receptor sites; (3) enhancement of ACh release; (4) inhibition of dopamine release; or (5) a combination of these responses.

B. Parkinsonian Symptoms

Cholinergic stimulation of the caudate-putamen complex of the rat also results in bursts of tremor in the forelimb contralateral to the site of injection (Dill *et al.*, 1968b). Facial muscles also twitch and the animal salivates and chews aimlessly. Reserpine given repeatedly in the same region of the neostriatum causes a contralateral hypokinesia which is characterized by flexion of the digits and subsequent disuse of the limb. Differences between the rat and cat are seen mainly in the unilaterality of these effects and the lower tremor frequency of 8.5 cps in the rat which corresponds to the rate seen in many Parkinsonian patients.

In the infrahuman primate, cholinergic stimulation of neostriatal structures produces a variety of severe dyskinesias. After carbachol is injected into the head of the caudate, globus pallidus or putamen of a squirrel monkey, tremor, choreoform movements, limb hyperextension and other profound motor anomalies develop (Murphey and Dill, 1972). Aspects of the remarkable clinical syndrome are shown in the pictures of Fig. 10-13. After carbachol is injected into the subthalamus, the monkey becomes hyperactive and circles around its cage. Unlike the Parkinsonian syndrome, these responses clearly did not represent an "at rest" disturbance to the extrapyramidal system.

A superlative account of the physiological response of a human to localized injection of a chemical was presented by Nashold (1959). In 110 Parkinsonian patients, tremor amplitude increased contralaterally during the first 5 to 10 minutes after acetylcholine was injected into the globus pallidus at a rate of 50 μl/minute. Although lasting only 1 to 2 minutes, episodes of focal twitches and spontaneous eye movements recurred for several hours. A variety of other conspicuous responses were recorded but none were nearly as astounding as those observed when a cholinergic blocking agent, oxyphenonium, was infused similarly. Parkinsonian rigidity was reduced in five patients and tremor was alleviated in two others. One man became soporific and "exclaimed that his head had gone to sleep." Several other persons complained of dryness of the mouth 15 to 30 minutes following this cholinergic blockade of their globus pallidus.

A rather extraordinary alleviation of the severe symptoms of Parkinsonian tremor and rigidity was achieved clinically by the unilateral or bilateral injection of procaine, mixed in a solution of oil and wax, into the globus pallidus (Narabayashi *et al.*, 1956). Since an intracaudate injection did not seem to ameliorate the involuntary movements, the globus pallidus seems to be a major anatomical element in human muscle hypertonus and rigidity. The long lasting

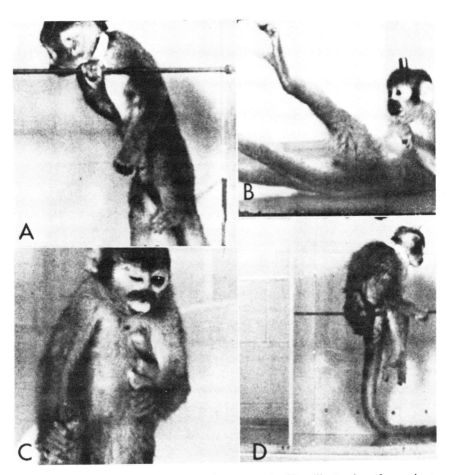

Fig. 10-13 Selected frames from 16-mm movie film illustrating the various dyskinesias. A. Choreiform movements in the left limbs and digits resulting from the injection of 4 μg of carbachol into the right caudate nucleus. B. Choreiform movements in the left forelimb and extension of the left hind limb in response to the injection of 5 μg of carbachol in the right caudate nucleus. This animal was approaching the convulsive state. C. Facial dyskinesia showing sialorrhea and blepharospasm on the right after the injection of 4 μg of carbachol into the right caudate nucleus. D. Hyperextension and akinesia of the left extremities after the injection of 2 μg of carbachol into the medial globus pallidus. Note that the left forelimb extended down behind the horizontal bar and in front of the tail. The hind limb is extended down in front of the bar. (From Murphey and Dill, 1972)

effects of procaine therapy are illustrated in the following case study taken from Narabayashi *et al.* (1956).

">.... Case 7 (Operation 15).–Businessman, aged 56.
Diagnosis: bilateral paralysis agitans.

The onset of his disease was at the age of 50. The first sign was slight rigidity and tremor of the fingers of the right hand, which became progressively severer, spreading to the other side. On admission, rigidity and tremor were so severe that he could not write, take meals by himself, dress himself, or even turn over in bed. Tremor of the hands was typical of paralysis agitans, of pill-rolling type, and about 6 or 7 cps, with marked tremulousness of the lips, chin and tongue. There was masking of faces, semiflexion of posture, hypersalivation, and hyperhidrosis of midgrade severity. Because of these difficulties, the patient had not been able to visit his office for more than two years, where he was the managing director of the company.

Operation.–On June 23, 1953, injection of 1 cc of 10% procaine

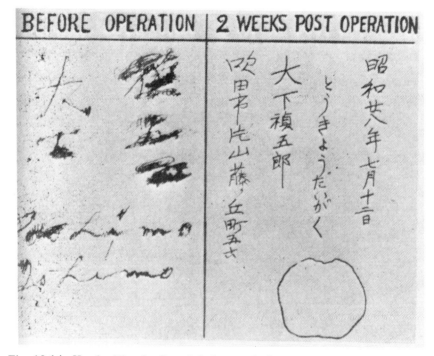

Fig. 10-14 Handwriting in Case 7 before and after the operation for infusing procaine into the globus pallidus. (From Narabayashi, H. *et al.*, 1956. *AMA Arch. Neurol. Psychiat.* **75:**36–48. Copyright 1956, the American Medical Association)

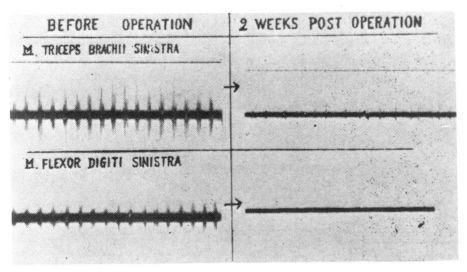

Fig. 10-15 Electromyogram in Case 7 before and after operation for infusing procaine into the globus pallidus. (From Narabayashi, H. *et al.*, 1956. *AMA Arch. Neurol. Psychiat.* **75**:36–48. Copyright 1956, the American Medical Association)

HCl in oil and wax was made into the left pallidum. On July 3 the same procedure was carried out on the right side. Effects were observed in both operations, not directly after operation, but in about 12 hours. Rigidity and tremor were practically absent by the following morning. This improvement was more impressive than we had anticipated. He became able to feed himself without help or to write far more easily and steadily."

Figure 10-14 shows the handwriting before and after.

"In three months there was reappearance of the symptoms, but their intensity was substantially far less than before this operation. Figure 10-15 shows the electromyogram before and after operation.

At present, about 20 months since operation, the symptoms remain markedly improved. His everyday living has been easier, and he is visiting the office several times a month."

The Spanish neurosurgeon, Obrador (1957), also used the method of bilaterally injecting procaine directly into the globus pallidus of the Parkinsonian patient. Figure 10-16 illustrates the temporal approach to the human pallidum. Postoperatively, the symptoms of tremor and rigidity were usually abolished. In some patients, the symptoms recurred within several days or a few weeks, but not usually with the intensity or discomfort seen before the surgical procedure. With the quite elegant technique of Obrador, great advances should have been

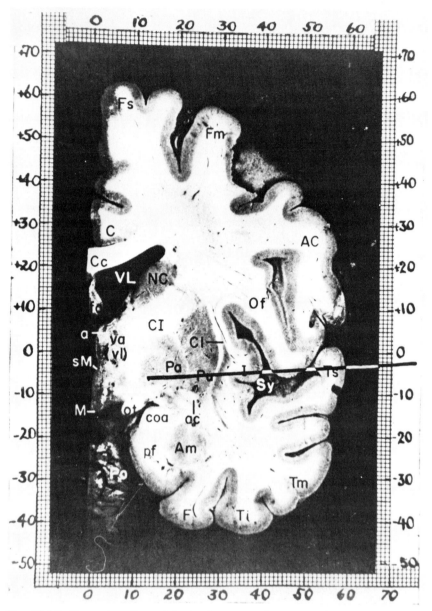

Fig. 10-16 Coronal section of brain showing path of cannula and site of lesion in the globus pallidus after the infusion of procaine in the Parkinsonian patient. (From Obrador, 1957)

possible in the alleviation of Parkinsonian symptoms, particularly in the long interval before the treatment with drugs became so widespread.

In another clinical study in which cortical procainization was attempted by infiltrating the anesthetic into the frontal lobe of the emotionally disturbed patient, a transitory slowing of EEG activity was observed in most cases (Walter et al., 1954). In other patients a long lasting electrical silence also followed. Short bursts of paroxysmal activity occurred in a few individuals. Some of these effects lasted weeks or even months.

V. SEIZURES AND EPILEPSY

A seizure can be defined by two major kinds of change: (1) the distinctive pattern of movement of certain muscle groups, and (2) the unique electrical disturbance recorded from cerebral sites which is characterized by high voltage, sharp spike activity in the EEG. The first type is seen clinically with respect to the well-known tonic and clonic seizures, and it can be monitored quantitatively by means of electromyographic recordings from the neck, pelvic or other muscles. The second type of change may be recorded from electrodes placed on the calvarium, on the surface of the cerebral cortex or directly in a subcortical structure.

A circumscribed focal discharge or so-called focus of abnormal electrical activity can be established permanently within a given cerebral structure simply by applying a chemical to the tissue. The physiological consequences of such a focus are often dramatic. Further, the chronicity of the preparation permits the examination of the morphological and neurochemical changes in the cells of the focus as well as the investigation of anticonvulsant drugs.

A. Focal Epilepsy: Cortical

As indicated by Wilder (1972) there are five major features of an epileptic focus in brain tissue: (1) the abnormal electrical potentials are self-regenerating and may be independent of other cerebral activity; (2) the local electrical perturbation is propagated to other regions including a contralateral structure; (3) the aberrant discharge frequency may suddenly become paroxysmal and sustained; (4) as the electrical disturbance progresses, a clinically manifest motor seizure will eventually develop; and (5) a secondary or mirror focus may arise whose discharge characteristics can often be temporally autonomous from the primary focus. The mirror focus is of great scientific interest because of its experimental virginity. The reason for this is that the primary epileptic focus induced artificially by a chemical lesion may be contaminated by nonspecific anatomical artifacts so that there is no resemblance to a pathological focus in clinical epilepsy.

1. Alumina Cream, Cobalt and Other Metals

In 1942, Kopeloff et al. discovered that a monkey would undergo a Jacksonian seizure after alum-precipitated egg white was applied to the surface of its cerebral cortex. What is more, the seizure activity was recurrent and could be evoked for months after the original deposition of alum. Since that time, the epileptiform effect of alumina cream, metals, and other substances on the surface of the cortex has been examined in terms of the differences in the genesis of the focus, its duration, the spontaneity of repetitive seizures, morphological specificity and the onset and nature of a mirror focus (Chusid *et al.*, 1955).

By injecting or applying epileptogenic compounds directly to the brain substance, a focus arises of varying intensity and often of differentiable features. For example, a chronically discharging epileptic focus is produced by the application of cobalt powder to the motor area of the cerebral hemisphere of the mouse or rat (Kopeloff, 1960) or cat (Dow *et al.*, 1962). On pathological examination of the cortical surface, the site of the cobalt lesion appears as a concave ulcer with coagulation necrosis; after one month, a severe toxicological gliosis appears (Henjyoji and Dow, 1965). Dawson and Holmes (1966) distinguished spatially the areas of the rat's sensorimotor cortex that are sensitive to cobalt powder. Just as electrical stimulation of the cerebellum can inhibit epileptic activity, the implantation of cobalt in the cerebellar hemispheres likewise reduces the convulsions elicited by the application of cobalt to the frontal lobe of the rat (Payan *et al.*, 1966).

In 1967, variations on the metallic powder technique were introduced. Either a small cobalt wire rod (Payan, 1967) or a cobalt-gelatin stick (Fischer *et al.*, 1967) placed in the superficial layers of the cortex evokes an epileptic focus in the rat. Holubář and Fischer (1967) also found that a cobalt stick inserted into the somatosensory cortex yielded a spontaneously spiking mirror focus on the rat's contralateral cortex. The same sort of secondary focus was observed in the rat by Klingberg *et al.* (1969). In the monkey, the focus can also be detected subcortically after the application of alumina cream to the motor cortex (Wilder *et al.*, 1969). Although the onset of the seizure activity of the rat seems to be correlated with the cytological formation of a glial-mesenchymal scar (Fischer *et al.*, 1968), cholinesterase and choline acetyltransferase activity decrease significantly in the cortical tissue adjacent to the cobalt implant (Goldberg *et al.*, 1972).

In the rhesus monkey, aluminum and beryllium powder are as epileptogenic as cobalt when injected or placed in the cortex (Chusid and Kopeloff, 1962; 1967). Of many other metals tested, most were not as active. Epileptic foci can also be induced by cobalt applied to the somatosensory cortex of the squirrel monkey (Grimm *et al.*, 1970 a and b). When the activity of single neurons in the monkey's focus is recorded, the units show autonomous, regular bursts of high frequency. Surprisingly, the unit activity seems to be locked together in synchronous rather than disparate discharges (Sypert and Ward, 1967).

B. Subcortical Seizure Foci

Ever since the work of Scherp and Church in 1937, it has been known that the intracerebral injection of an aluminum salt at an unspecified site causes ataxia, nystagmus and severe convulsions which ultimately terminate in death (Scherp and Church, 1937). However, the production of experimental epilepsy by a discrete subcortical injection of alumina cream was first demonstrated by Whittier *et al.* as early as 1949. In the rhesus monkey, 100 to $200\mu l$ volumes of alumina infused in the thalamus or putamen evoked motor convulsions and EEG seizures recorded from cortical leads (Kopeloff *et al.*, 1950). Strangely, the onset of the epileptic syndrome did not begin until 1 to 12 months after the injection. Using the same procedure, Faeth and Walker (1957) confirmed the alteration in EEG patterns but did not observe spontaneous clinical seizures during a 6-month period following a subcortical injection of alumina cream.

In the cat, Gastaut and his collaborators (Gastaut *et al.*, 1952; 1953; 1959) have produced seizures by injecting unspecified volumes of alumina cream into the amygdaloid complex. Unfortunately, the alumina spread throughout the ventricular system producing widespread ischemic lesions on its way. Therefore, in all of these studies, the crucial factor of diffusion, because of an enormous nonlocalizing injection volume, rules out the possibility of specifying any anatomical locus of action of the toxic metal (Shirao, 1969).

Guerrero-Figueroa and his colleagues have investigated extensively the epileptogenic properties of aluminum oxide in subcortical structures (Guerrero-Figueroa *et al.*, 1962; 1965). An experimental model of age-dependent petit mal epilepsy is probably capable of being developed. After the deposition of alumina powder in the thalamus or mesencephalon of the immature kitten, three-per-second spike and wave activity is seen in the EEG (Guerrero-Figueroa *et al.*, 1963a). The developmental significance of this observation is implicit since a cat 30 days of age or older did not develop these epileptic symptoms in response to thalamic penicillin. The so-called attentive factors produced by acoustic, tactile or visual stimuli directed toward the kitten inhibited the three-per-second spike waves as well as some of the paroxysmal discharges (Guerrero-Figueroa *et al.*, 1963b). As the cat watched a rat set before it or if it smelled a sardine placed under its nose, the spike-wave complex tended to flatten. An injection of acetylcholine either directly into the focus or into the mirror focus precipitated pronounced epileptiform activity (Guerrero-Figueroa *et al.*, 1964b). Figure 10-17 illustrates the intense spiking recorded from the secondary hippocampal focus after ACh had been injected into it.

While carbachol also activated trains of seizure discharges, GABA diminished the amplitude of spontaneous discharges and evoked responses but the suppression of the epileptogenic focus was brief. That a neurochemical change of a metabolic nature is, in fact, responsible for the focal epileptic activity has been adroitly demonstrated by Guerrero-Figueroa and his collaborators (1964a). By sectioning the interconnecting hemispheric fiber tracts, including the corpus callosum and the anterior commissure, before alumina was injected into the hippocampus, they were able to prevent the contralateral development of a secondary mirror focus. However, the total isolation of the hemisphere containing the primary focus by the same knife-cuts failed to modify an on-going mirror focus once established.

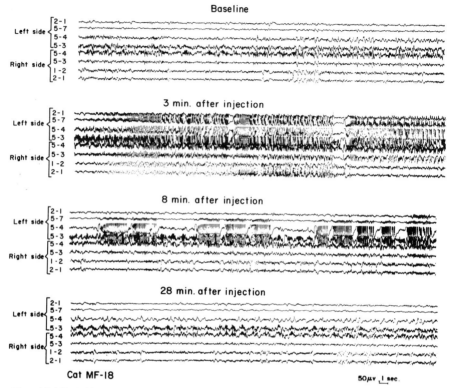

Fig. 10-17 Effect of injection of 145.3 μg acetylcholine into the secondary focus (left hippocampus). 1, left cortex (bipolar); 2, left amygdaloid nucleus– left septal region; 3, left ventral hippocampus–left amygdaloid nucleus; 4, left dorsal hippocampus (bipolar); 5, right dorsal hippocampus (bipolar); 7, right septal region–right cortex. (From Guerrero-Figueroa et al., 1964b)

This observation seems to validate the internal reliability of the technique in that the secondary focus was not generated simply by the unobstructed spread of the metallic powder by the way of the ventricles as was reported previously by Gastaut and his group.

Interestingly, Guerrero-Figueroa et al. (1964a) were able to suppress the amplitude of the focal discharges when they injected Dilantin directly into either the primary or the mirror hippocampal focus produced earlier by alumina. The protracted duration of the anticonvulsive effect of Dilantin on the abnormal EEG activity is shown in Fig. 10-18. A butyrophenone compound given systemically or the tricyclic antidepressants, imipramine or pinoxepin, will activate an alumina or penicillin focus (Guerrero-Figueroa and Gallant, 1967; Guerrero-Figueroa et al., 1969b). On the other hand, the systemic administration of diazepam or other benzodiazepine derivative attenuates petit mal episodes as well as the

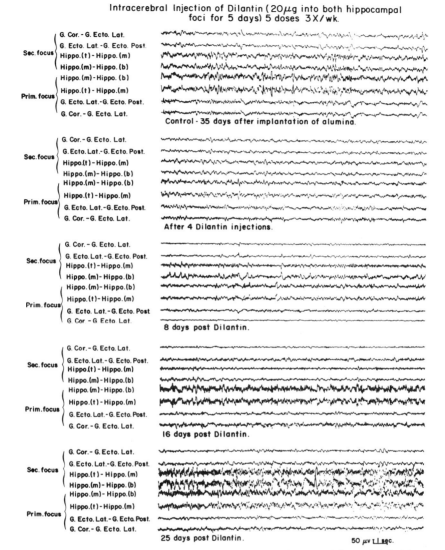

Fig. 10-18 Effect of injection of diphenylhydantoin into right and left hippo-campi. (From Guerrero-Figueroa *et al.*, 1964a)

secondary epileptiform discharge of a mirror focus (Guerrero-Figueroa *et al.*, 1967; 1969a; 1973).

Classical temporal lobe epilepsy occurs after the injection of tungstic acid into either the hippocampus, amygdala or lower brain-stem of the cat (Blum and Liban, 1960; 1963; Black *et al.*, 1967). During a hippocampal seizure, the cat retches or gags, salivates profusely, chews, turns its head ipsiversively, and its lips

a   b   c

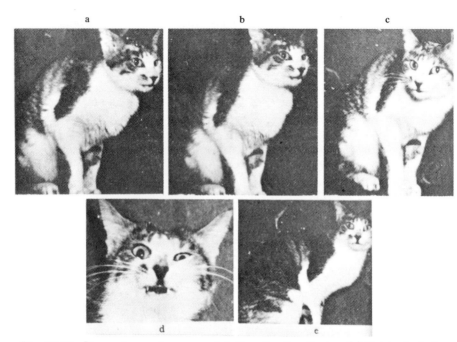

d   e

Fig. 10-19 Phases in a minor amygdaloid epileptic attack. (a) Cat is alerted, preoccupied, and staring, its pupils gradually dilating. (b and c) Twitching starts in the mouth region, spreading to other head regions, beginning contralaterally on the left side, sometimes remaining unilateral, and sometimes becoming also bilateral. (d) Chewing movements and twitching of left side of face (contralateral), causing palpebral narrowing on that side. (e) Abrupt termination of the attack, with disappearance of symptoms. Pupils reconstrict. No loss of pupillary reaction takes place during attack. (From Blum, B. and E. Liban. 1960. Reprinted from *Neurology*. **10**:546–554. Copyright The New York Times Media Company, Inc.)

twitch. Although Blum and Liban found that the EEG changes are very similar during the seizure following the injection of tungstic acid in the amygdala, the cat in the latter case rotates its head contraversively, and then tonic and clonic convulsions of the limbs and trunk develop. Figure 10-19 presents the stages of a developing amygdaloid epileptic attack.

A long-lasting status epilepticus is also caused in the rabbit by alumina cream when injected in enormous volumes into the general region of the pons or into the temporal lobe (Wiśniewski *et al.*, 1966). Pathological EEG patterns, motor seizures, paresis and ataxia are consonant with extensive histopathological changes in the brain. Neurofibrillary degeneration is widespread in neurons throughout many parts of the brain-stem.

1. *Penicillin Seizures*

In experiments with both the cat and monkey, Gloor and his colleagues (Gloor *et al.*, 1966; Gloor, 1969) deduced that because of the large 5 to 10 μl volume injected into some subcortical structures, the epileptiform activity could be due to the spread or transport of penicillin to the cortex, amygdala or brain-stem reticular formation. At any rate, penicillin does not have a ubiquitous epileptogenic action, as was thought previously, when it comes into contact with nervous tissue. The features of the spiking activity induced by penicillin acting on a

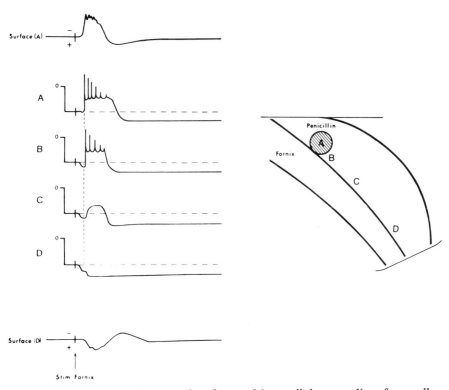

Fig. 10-20 Schematic diagram of surface and intracellular recordings from cells in and around a penicillin focus. On the right is a diagram of the exposed dorsal hippocampus and fornix with the corresponding areas indicated by the letters. A. Typical response from pyramidal cells within the penicillin focus illustrating the early depolarizing potential with action potentials, arising from a flat background, followed by long-lasting hyperpolarization. Successive action potentials of a burst would be smaller due to inactivation of the soma spike generating mechanism. B. Intermediate form consisting of early hyperpolarization, the depolarizing potential with action potentials, and finally a late hyperpolarization. C. Another intermediate form consisting of a more delayed and somewhat reduced depolarizing potential arising out of a hyperpolarization. D. Pure hyperpolarizing response characteristic of cells at the periphery of the focus. Often the IPSP appeared double—one arising from the fornix triggering and one due to the peripheral inhibition generated by the cells in the center of the focus during the paroxysmal discharge. In the focus (A) the surface discharge is negative-positive while at a distance from the focus (D) the surface discharge is positive-negative. (Intracellular traces: positive up.) (From Dichter and Spencer, 1969a)

subcortical structure that has been described by so many other investigators (Faeth *et al.*, 1955, 1956; Ralston and Ajmone-Marsan, 1956; Ralston and Langer, 1965; Walker and Udvarhelyi, 1965) is functionally identical to that produced when the antibiotic is infused into the cerebral ventricles. The phenomenon of dissemination of foci is certainly due in part to the gradual diffusion of the drug to structures sensitive to the epileptogenic properties of penicillin (Ralston and Langer, 1965).

Following up the findings of Gloor and his co-workers, Dichter and Spencer (1969a) investigated the large depolarizing potentials that they recorded from single cells in the penicillin-treated hippocampal focus of the cat. Figure 10-20 illustrates the shift in the type of potential, from depolarizing to hyperpolarizing, in the cells monitored at increasing distances from the site of the penicillin focus. The hyperpolarization of the neurons in the area surrounding the focus resembles a recurrent inhibitory postsynaptic potential in terms of temporal and other characteristics (Dichter and Spencer, 1969b). A ring of recurrent inhibition around the penicillin focus' could be the mechanism which helps to prevent the spatial spread of the local electrical discharges. The repetitive spiking of individual neurons progresses gradually into a repetitious firing until the cat finally develops a seizure.

Schmaltz (1971) also found that in the rat, crystalline penicillin deposited in the hippocampus in a high dose evoked focal epileptiform activity with spike discharges within 10 minutes after the implant. The local discharges could be recorded for up to a month.

That the thalamus could be the pacemaker of epileptogenic potentials is disputed by Voiculescu and Voinescu (1968). After an injection of penicillin into the thalamus of the anesthetized cat, a focus of paroxysmal EEG activity developed in the hippocampus in 22 of 28 animals, sometimes within one minute. Even though focal discharges could be recorded from thalamic sites in some cats, a generalized seizure was always preceded by hippocampal discharges. Somewhat similar results have been reported by Inutsuka (1969) who injected penicillin similarly into the thalamus of the cat.

2. Cobalt Seizures

Cobalt deposited in the pons or medulla of the cat causes irregular spikes in the EEG and myoclonic twitches of facial, cervical and forelimb muscles (Cesa-Bianchi *et al.*, 1967). A sudden noise or tapping of the animal brought about severe convulsions that sometimes led to death. The marked changes in the EEG which develop over several days are represented in Fig. 10-21. When the metallic powder is deposited in the mesencephalon, no generalized attack occurs; however, cobalt placed in the midline-thalamic nuclei provokes high voltage spikes, that can be recorded from any area of the cerebral cortex, as well as generalized epileptic episodes with myoclonic movements (Mancia and Lucioni, 1966).

An exceptionally active epileptic focus is produced in the amygdala of the cat

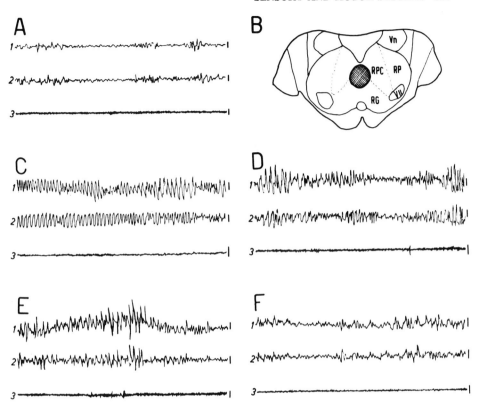

Fig. 10-21   Unrestrained cat before (A) and one (C, D), two (E) and four (F) days after the introduction of cobalt in the midline of the caudal pons as indicated by B.   1: right fronto-parietal EEG; 2: left fronto-parietal EEG; 3: posterior cervical EMG.   Calibration: 1 second, 200 μV.   (From Cesa-Bianchi, M. G. *et al.*, 1967.   *EEG Clin. Neurophysiol.* **22**:525–536. (Elsevier Publishing Co., Amsterdam, The Netherlands)

by cobalt powder deposited in this structure (Mutani, 1967a). Partial or generalized motor seizures are accompanied by typically intense EEG changes, all of which persist for about a month. Of special interest is the propagation within a week of the cobalt focus from the cat's amygdala to the contralateral temporal lobe. Similarly, Mutani and his co-workers (1967b and c; 1969) found that cobalt introduced into the hippocampus of the cat also produces a powerful epileptogenic focus that endures for over 2 months. Again, a mirror focus arises in the contralateral hippocampus but within only 1 to 2 days. The typical activity of a mirror focus is illustrated in Fig. 10-22. Although a large number of seizure discharges emanate just from the hippocampal electrode, epileptiform episodes spread to other recording loci. Still others are accompanied by the behavioral manifestations of seizure. Because the cobalt powder is confined to the region of

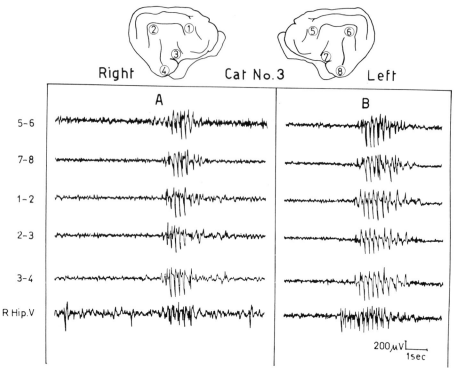

Fig. 10-22 Cobalt epileptogenic lesion in the right ventral hippocampus in a cat 7 days after cobalt introduction: paroxysmal, widespread and bilaterally synchronous projected EEG activity. In A the discharge begins simultaneously at hippocampal and cortical levels; in B the hippocampal and cortical discharges are displaced in time. (From Mutani, 1967a)

implant, Mutani proposed that the local action of cobalt is due to a neurochemical interference with oxidative metabolism of the neurons rather than to a purely mechanical effect of the metallic lesion.

Although Mutani found that a cobalt focus in the amygdala ordinarily requires several days to develop following the deposition of the metal powder, such a focus can be induced very rapidly (Thomalske and Lyagoubi, 1969). If aluminum phosphate precipitated in gel is mixed with the cobalt, and the combined powders are implanted in the amygdala, the latency of the epileptic attack is reduced drastically to an average of only 30 minutes.

The primary and secondary epileptiform foci created by depositing cobalt or aluminum hydroxide into the hippocampus or olfactory bulb are differentially affected by diazepam, a drug which has been used clinically in the treatment of petit mal and other episodic disorders (Guerrero-Figueroa et al., 1968). Diazepam inhibits only the secondary sites of local seizure and does not alter the discharge activity of the primary focus. This important observation shows quite rightly that the abnormal electrical activity in a secondary focus is not due to the spread of electrical activity from the primary focus or to the physical diffusion of cobalt or alumina to another part of the brain.

3. Anti-Brain Antibodies

Following the important observation that EEG changes are introduced when anti-caudate nucleus antibody is injected intraventricularly (Mihailović and Janković, 1961), an attempt was made by Mihailović and Cupić (1971) to delineate the locus of action of anti-brain antibodies. Anti-hippocampus or anti-caudate nucleus gamma globulin injected repeatedly in 8 µl volumes into the homologous sites in the monkey caused marked abnormalities in the EEG pattern. Long-lasting epileptiform seizures that were self-regenerative appeared in both the hippocampus and caudate nucleus of the monkey, with hippocampal convulsions persisting even after one month. Since irritative foci did not develop when anti-monkey liver gamma globulin was similarly infused, the specificity of action of anti-cerebral antibodies is assured. Although the mechanism is utterly obscure, conformational changes at the molecular level may be at the basis of the focal abnormalities of hyperexcitability and the perpetual depolarization of hippocampal neurons.

C. Convulsant Drugs

A convulsant drug that evokes epileptiform seizures when given systemically can also have a distinct local action on a subcortical structure (Jasper, 1969). For example, infiltrating a paste of strychnine into the cat's amygdala causes spiking of the EEG recorded from electrodes placed in the hippocampus, septum, thalamus and hypothalamus (Aida, 1956). Similarly, after strychnine is placed in the amygdala of the dog, the animal shows paroxysmal discharges and convulsive behavior which last for many weeks.

When micro-injected in a large volume into the hippocampus of the cat, picrotoxin or strychnine elicits sharply defined and gradually propagated discharge foci recorded within this structure (Baker et al., 1965). Although both compounds elicit a spike-wave complex, picrotoxin is far more potent. As illustrated in Fig. 10-23, the picrotoxin discharges persist to become actual seizures. On the other hand, Metrazol injected in a very high dose produces only a rapid and transitory local excitation of the hippocampal EEG pattern, with neither spike and wave characteristics nor overt seizures. From a consideration of the action of a convulsant drug on the spinal cord, it is possible that the local effect of Metrazol is strictly excitatory. The effects deriving from picrotoxin and strychnine probably stem from a local disinhibition of hippocampal neurons. Moreover, presynaptic inhibition is decreased by picrotoxin whereas strychnine reduces postsynaptic inhibition. Thus, the uniqueness in the quality of the foci generated by these drugs may be explained by the differences in their action on the synaptic membrane.

Tremorine given intraperitoneally blocks the abnormal EEG discharges pro-

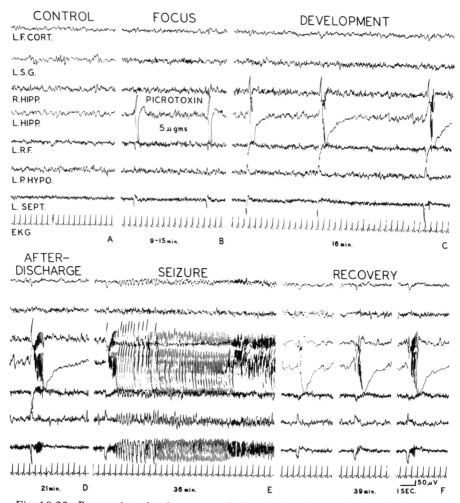

Fig. 10-23 Progressive development of picrotoxin foci and after-discharges subsequent to a single micro-injection of the drug into the left hippocampus. Recovery patterns from the seizure recapitulate the stages leading to the seizure. Time sequence of these events is indicated. (From Baker *et al.*, 1965)

duced by the local micro-injection of strychnine into the hippocampus of the cat (Baker, 1965). Since atropine fails to prevent the focal activity, tremorine probably acts generally on nicotinic or other non-muscarinic receptors. The mechanism again could be an enhancement of postsynaptic inhibition.

After a seizure focus is produced in the hippocampus by picrotoxin or strychnine injected there, either chlorpromazine or imipramine injected in a dose of

10 μg accentuates the electrical excitability of the region (Baker and Kratky, 1967). At a higher dose, either substance depresses the activity of the hippocampal focus. These psychotropic drugs and desipramine possess the same sort of dose-related efficacy on the intensity of focal hippocampal discharges established previously by DFP (Baker and Kratky, 1971). In comparison with scopolamine, these agents exert only a relatively weak cholinolytic action. Similarly, tetracaine injected in the same dose range into the hippocampus abolishes the epileptiform pattern evoked by a prior injection of DFP or carbachol (Baker and Kratky, 1968). However, a much higher dose of up to 550 μg of this local anesthetic is required to attenuate the focal discharge produced by d-tubocurarine injected at the same hippocampal site.

An important distinction between the blockade by an anesthetic as opposed to a cholinergic blocking agent of focal hippocampal after-discharges has been revealed by Baker and Benedict (1968a). A seizure focus induced by picrotoxin or d-tubocurarine is inhibited selectively by intravenous pentobarbital. A focus of carbachol or DFP origin is abolished selectively by intravenous scopolamine. Thus, the complex neurochemical makeup of a seizure focus is susceptible to suppression by different compounds according to the special chemical used in the genesis of a focus.

Using a 40 μl infusion into the amygdala or hippocampus, Tuttle and Elliott (1969) showed that a local anesthetic such as butacaine or lidocaine evokes EEG spike discharges and seizure activity. Metrazol and morphine have much the same effect, although Metrazol also produces convulsant activity when it is infused into the mesencephalon. Probably a localized action of each drug is intermingled with a diffuse effect because of the obvious seepage of each solution into the ventricular lumen of the cat.

In a well-controlled study in which a small micro-injection volume was used, Banerjee et al. (1970) localized the epileptogenic properties of several drugs. This was accomplished since the tip of the injector cannula, which was raised or lowered to a different depth, served also as the recording electrode. When injected into the gray matter of the cerebral cortex, picrotoxin, tubocurarine, strychnine or leptazol, in that order of potency and duration of action, produced foci of excitation that gave rise to synchronous firing of high voltage spikes. An injection into fiber tracts or other subcortical structures did not cause seizure effects. Typical spike discharges from discrete sites are shown in Fig. 10-24. Although each of the drugs except tubocurarine is considered to be a convulsant, all seem to share a common mechanism of action when acting centrally. Since these compounds may depress inhibitory potentials in the spinal cord, cortex or both, their mechanism of action could be one involving disinhibition in terms of an interference with either pre- or postsynaptic inhibition. However, one could assume that the firing of a neuron at a rate of two per second or faster is the result of a total disinhibition of cortical neurons rather than the result of an excitatory consequence of the drug.

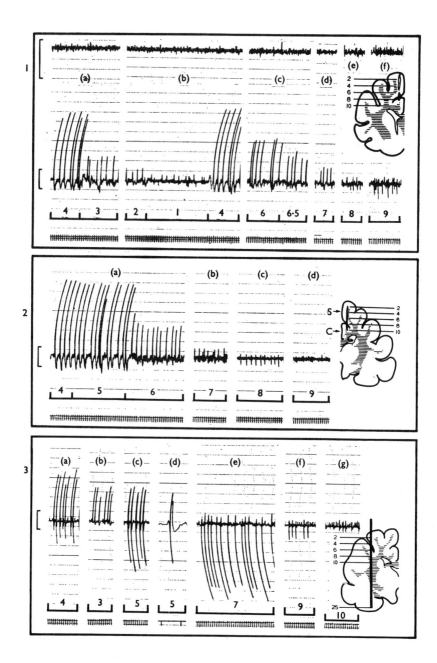

D. Transitory Epileptic Episodes

In 1954, MacLean described the first of his notable experiments in which seizure discharges appeared in the hippocampus of the curarized cat or monkey at the very site at which crystals of carbachol were deposited. This convulsive activity often continued for several hours, and there was some spread to the caudate nucleus without a discernible change in neocortical potentials (MacLean, 1954). A truly classical study by MacLean in 1957 (Chapter 2) described the stratagem for the use of crystals rather than solutions (MacLean, 1957a). Carbachol, ACh and methacholine implanted in the hippocampus evoked oscillatory potentials, intermittent spike activity, and seizure discharges in the anesthetized or unanesthetized cat. The typical effects portrayed in Fig. 10-25 were long-lasting and occurred almost continually for 45 to 60 minutes, reaching amplitudes of 1 to 2 mV. Generally, the effect of ACh was much less intense and, unless used in combination with the anticholinesterase, was of short duration. After an afterdischarge elicited by a brief electrical stimulation, a remarkable and prolonged recrudescence occurred often for 9 to 10 minutes. At that time, MacLean made the suggestion that because of the temporal features of the after-discharge, the action of electrical stimulation of the hippocampus was probably due to the sustained release of ACh after the stimulation has been discontinued.

1. *Cholinergic Discharges*

Recording from leads on the surface of the cat's cortex, Rakić *et al.* (1962) found that eserine injected in 50 to 100 μl volumes in the caudate nucleus, hippocampus or hypothalamus evoked spiking discharges characteristic of an electroconvulsive seizure. The precise localization of this effect of the anticholinesterase is not possible because the large amount injected passed into the ventricular fluid. Over and above carbachol's action on the caudate nucleus of evoking a marked change in the EEG, the cholinomimetic also synergizes with the effect of simultaneous electrical stimulation of this structure (Militello *et al.*, 1970).

Fig. 10-24 Electrical activity recorded from the tip of a micro-injection cannula after injection of tubocurarine 4 mm deep into the cerebral cortex and subsequently raising and/or lowering micro-injection cannula in three cats anesthetized with chloralose. Experiment 1: injection of 1 μg into right gyrus splenialis 10 minutes before beginning of record a. Upper records from surface of right occipital cortex. Experiment 2: injection of 10 μg into the left gyrus splenialis 35 minutes before beginning of record a. Experiment 3: injection of 10 μg into gyrus adjacent to left gyrus splenialis 15 minutes before beginning of record a. The figures below the records refer to the depth of the tip of the cannula in millimeters from the brain surface, and the diagrams on the right show the cannula track (experiments 1 and 2) or the position of the cannula (experiment 3). S, Gyrus splenialis; C, gyrus cinguli. Calibration 1 mV, negativity upwards. Time marker in seconds. (From Banerjee *et al.*, 1970a)

L.HIPPO. - R.

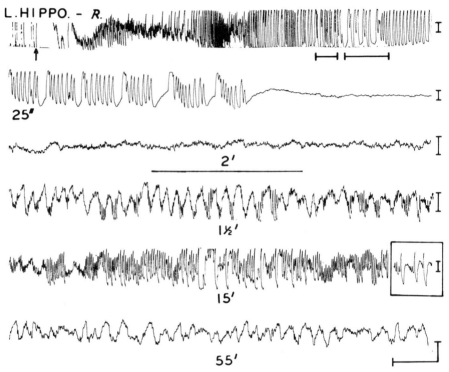

Fig. 10-25 Electroencephalographic records from an experiment in which crystalline acetylcholine and physostigmine were deposited in the hippocampus. Top three tracings illustrate injury discharge and subsequent flattening of the record that are typically seen when needles enter or impinge upon the hippocampus. Acetylcholine was ejected from the needle several minutes after physostigmine, sealing tip, was allowed to dissolve *in situ*. Tracings below solid line illustrate the changes that followed. Calibrations, 1 second and 200 μV; negativity upward. (From MacLean, P. D. 1957. *AMA Arch. Neurol. Psychiat.* 78:113–127. Copyright 1957, the American Medical Association)

An intrahippocampal injection of a cholinomimetic, as well as an anticholinesterase produces severe focal EEG discharges in the cat (Baker and Benedict, 1968b) as illustrated in Fig. 10-26. The most potent of each of these classes of compounds is carbachol and diisopropylfluorophosphate (DFP). Two observations indicate that the drugs affect muscarinic receptors. Nicotine and other related nicotinic agonists had no effect when injected into the hippocampus, and not one of the nicotinic blocking agents altered either the DFP or carbachol-induced discharges. In the primate, Delgado (1966) has found that ACh evokes high voltage spike activity at focal sites also in the cingulate gyrus in addition to the hippocampus. No behavioral changes were observed during the bursts of activity which lasted for 10 to 25 minutes. Thus, it would appear that a cholinergic

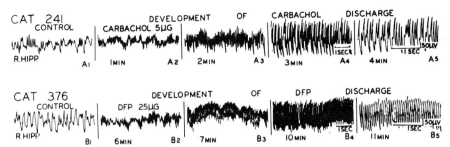

Fig. 10-26 Hippocampal discharges established by intrahippocampal micro-injections of either carbachol or diisopropylfluorophosphate (DFP). (From Baker, W. W. and F. Benedict. 1968b. *Int. J. Neuropharmacol.* 7:135–147. Pergamon Press, New York)

system in the hippocampus and other limbic structures is of paramount importance in the functioning of this system.

In a pertinent paper by Baker *et al.* (1965), EEG discharges of hippocampal foci in the cat were first established by a local micro-injection of one of two convulsants, picrotoxin or strychnine. Then the level of cholinergic activity at the same hippocampal locus was varied by a supplemental injection of a cholinomimetic or anticholinesterase. Carbachol enhanced the rate of seizure discharge and the duration of after-discharge, whereas DFP induced only a more rapid firing rate at the picrotoxin or strychnine focus. When scopolamine, which blocks muscarinic receptors, was given in the hippocampus, the cholinergic after-discharge component of the focus was eliminated (Baker and Benedict, 1970). Such a representative blockade is shown in Fig. 10-27 in which the action of 10 μg of scopolamine is demonstrated. These results clearly indicate that an increase in cholinesterase level or ACh metabolism is related to the epileptogenic features of a hippocampal focus. Again, a key role is suggested for the muscarinic side of the cholinoceptive mechanism with respect to psychomotor seizures and other functional disorders of the hippocampus.

Hippocampal theta rhythm which is elicited by electrical stimulation of the posterior hypothalamus or reticular formation of the cat is suppressed by hemicholinium injected into the posterior hypothalamus (Friedman and Wikler, 1970). On the basis of lesion experiments, this area is thought to contain synaptic connections to the hippocampus. The fact that the latency was 90 to 180 minutes fits in well with the known blocking mechanism of hemicholinium of preventing the synthesis of ACh by competing with the presynaptic uptake of choline. Since a cholinergic agonist reverses this blockade within only 15 minutes, it is not possible that the latency is due to the diffusion of hemicholinium to a distant site. The drug may also have some postsynaptic action in that the integrity of a pre- as well as postsynaptic mechanism seems to be necessary for an electrical current applied in the hypothalamus to evoke the theta pattern.

The transitory spiking activity in the cat's EEG superimposed on low voltage

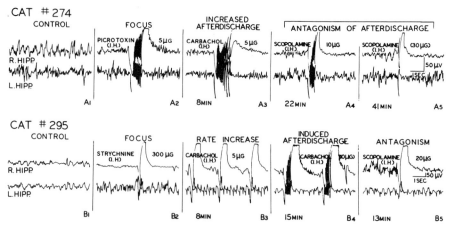

Fig. 10-27 Scopolamine antagonism of excitatory effects of carbachol on picrotoxin and strychnine foci. Against activated picrotoxin foci, scopolamine not only removed the potentiation resulting from carbachol (A4) but at slightly higher doses totally eliminated the after-discharge (A5). The spike-wave was resistant. Cumulative effects of carbachol on strychnine discharge reversed by scopolamine and restored to control levels of firing (B5). Although activating the focus, carbachol still potentiated the effects of scopolamine on total after-discharge component. Lapse of time after the administration of each agent is indicated. Doses in parentheses are cumulative. (From Baker, W. W. and F. Benedict. 1970. *EEG Clin. Neurophysiol.* 28:499–509. Elsevier Publishing Co., Amsterdam, The Netherlands)

fast waves after ACh is injected into the hippocampus has been confirmed (Rogozea *et al.*, 1971). Over and above the evocation of hippocampal theta activity, ACh does not prevent the cat from orienting toward an auditory stimulus and perhaps facilitates the habituation to such an arousing stimulus.

That the nonspecific thalamic nuclei of the cat may be involved in the cholinergic synapses mediating epileptogenic discharges has been proposed. When these nuclei are stimulated with carbachol, ACh and neostigmine, focal discharges develop in the anesthetized animal which may spread to other regions including the neocortex (Babb *et al.*, 1971).

Cholinergic stimulation of the amygdala reportedly induces permanent changes in the emotional behavior and regional electrical activity of the cat (Grossman, 1963). Crystals of ACh or carbachol applied directly to the amygdala evoke EEG changes, denoted by spike activity of high amplitude and low frequency which pass from the amygdala to the hippocampus and hypothalamus. Overt epileptiform seizures then occur within 10 to 15 minutes. Similar seizure episodes are also produced in the rat by carbachol implanted in the amygdala (Belluzzi and Grossman, 1969), and long-term effects are equally manifest. Further, crystals of carbachol deposited in the caudate-putamen complex of the rat may also cause EEG seizures that are recorded from the cerebral cortex (Deadwyler *et al.*, 1972).

Taken together, these results suggest that subcortical structures other than the hippocampus are involved in the anatomical system which mediates convulsive activity.

2. Toxicants and Other Substances

At the turn of this century, Delezenne (1900) demonstrated the exceptional sensitivity of the CNS to the direct application of toxic material. Serum taken from an eel was injected into the frontal pole of the rabbit in a volume of 2 to 5 μl/kg according to the intracerebral infusion technique of Roux and Borrel (1898). Within one-half hour the animal died of severe motor seizures terminating in clonic convulsions. In this memorable account, Delezenne also showed that duck serum infused similarly into the cortex of the dog produced the same toxic symptoms which were dependent upon the dose of serum given.

A small dose of the highly toxic fluorocitrate injected at nearly any site tested in the rat brain causes dose-dependent convulsions and death (Morselli et al., 1968). By the intracerebral route, fluoroacetate, which produces convulsions after its intraperitoneal injection, was much less toxic and produced convulsions only when at least 100 times the intraperitoneal dose was injected. Because of the large volume given, no localization of the action of the drug was possible; in fact, intraventricular fluorocitrate is equivalent in its effect to a tissue injection. In connection with their assay, Morselli et al. (1968) have substantiated the notion that the lethality of systemic fluoroacetate is probably due to its peripheral conversion to the metabolite fluorocitrate which then enters the brain and exerts its toxic action.

To trace the convulsant properties of other drugs when acting on a subcortical structure of the rabbit, Bergmann et al. (1970) implanted several crystalline substances into the hypothalamus. In order of decreasing potency, ouabain, digitoxin, ethacrynic acid and a mercury salt evoked intense seizure activity recorded within the hippocampus. For the most part, the abnormal discharges were confined particularly to this structure. Along with the intense spiking response, the rabbit often had an epileptic convulsion if the EEG discharge did spread to a superficial cortical recording site. An implant of ouabain in one of several other limbic structures revealed that the thalamus, geniculate body, caudate nucleus, septum and amygdala were also very sensitive to the application of the glycoside in mediating an epileptogenic response. Thus, the pathways subserving convulsive activity from the thalamus or hypothalamus to the hippocampus seem to be verified by pharmacological analysis. Although unknown, the convulsant mechanism of the drugs could be due to an increase in the level of intracellular Na^+ and release of cellular K^+, because each compound inhibits membrane ATPases which thereby block the active transport of Na^+ ions.

Other substances have a potent epileptogenic action on structures in the limbic system. For example, tetrodotoxin micro-injected in the hippocampus (or lateral geniculate) causes focal spiking in the EEG of the cat (Hafemann *et al.*, 1969). Cyclic AMP injected into the cat's hypothalamus, mesencephalon or amygdala evokes convulsions, contraversive movements, catatonia in some cases, and other motor effects (Gessa *et al.*, 1970). Xanthinol nicotinate, CDP-choline or caffeine-sodium benzoate infused into the mesencephalon or posterior hypothalamus of the cat produces EEG seizure patterns recorded from the hippocampus or neocortex (Yanagida and Yamamura, 1971). Cortisol infused in a large volume into the hippocampus, rostral or posterior hypothalamus of the cat also evokes transitory epileptogenic activity. Although there were temporal differences between hippocampal and hypothalamic sites in the high-voltage spike activity and the continuous repetitive discharge, the reason for the simultaneous appearance of the electrical disturbances is apparently due to the spill-over of cortisol into the CSF. Even so, the hippocampal discharge latency to the corticoid is much shorter than that seen when the steroid is infused directly into the ventricle. The mechanism of cortisol's local action is totally unknown (Feldman, 1971).

A large volume of lithium Cl solution injected into the hippocampus or amygdala of the monkey causes high-voltage, sharp biphasic waves followed by after-discharges within the region of injection (Delgado and DeFeudis, 1969). A similar application of glutamate or ACh re-triggered these waves once they had subsided. Since lithium acts as a cation substitute for Na^+ but can only be extruded from the intracellular compartment at about half the rate of Na^+, an altered distribution of Na^+ may have given rise to these waves. Because both glutamate and ACh may increase the permeability of the neuronal membrane to Na^+ and thus cause further depolarization, their rather immediate local effect in re-triggering the lithium waves would be expected.

EEG seizure activity has also been produced in the cat by Na glutamate injected into any part of the hippocampus, probably because of the enormous volume given (Knaape and Wiechert, 1970). In other areas including the amygdala, caudate nucleus, cortex or ventricle, seizures were also produced if a high dose was given. Even though the hippocampus seems to be most sensitive to this amino acid, a careful anatomical study is required because the diffusion may have been so extensive that the results may be spurious.

Localized perfusion of the dorsal hippocampus with a solution of excess cations shows that potassium enhances the magnitude of local evoked responses following the electrical stimulation of the fornix or commissural fibers in the rat (Izquierdo *et al.*, 1970). Further, seizure activity of the hippocampus elicited by electrical stimulation depends on the concentration of K^+ ions not only in terms of the latency of the seizure but also its intensity. These data support the idea of Izquierdo and his colleagues that the regulation of K^+ ion concentration is intimately linked with the specialized functions of the hippocampus. Whether or not K^+ ions do play some unique role as is proposed for Na^+ and Ca^{2+} in the posterior hypothalamus (Chapter 6) is not known at present.

E. Tubocurarine Seizures

Using a 6 μl volume, Kumagai et al. (1962a and b) were the first to demonstrate that tubocurarine injected subcortically in a high dose evokes a seizure in the hippocampus. When micro-injected at a large number of structures including the caudate nucleus, reticular formation, thalamus, amygdala and globus pallidus, focal discharges were generated. An analysis of the latency from the beginning of a seizure which could be recorded from any of these structures would seem to implicate the thalamus and reticular formation almost as much as the hippocampus as the site of origin of the electrical activity. Usually, however, the seizure discharge began in the hippocampus and then spread to the other structures. Endröczi et al. (1963b) employed somewhat lower doses in the 10 to 20 μg range to confirm the epileptogenic properties of tubocurarine acting locally on hippocampal neurons. In addition, they found that the rhythmic spike activity of the EEG could be inhibited by acetylcholine or a 2% KCl solution micro-injected into the same or contralateral site.

When d-tubocurarine was injected in an even larger volume into the hypothalamus of the cat, a focal hypersynchronous discharge consisting of a spike-wave complex usually developed in 10 to 20 minutes (Baker and Benedict, 1967). The amplitude and duration of the focal activity depended on the dose of this neuromuscular agent. Other curare-like agents such as gallamine triethiodide (Flaxedil) or dihydro-β-erythroidine failed to evoke a typical focal discharge. Decamethonium and succinylcholine, which block neuromuscular transmission by sustaining the depolarization at the myoneural junction, also did not produce the tubocurarine-type focus when injected similarly. Since d-tubocurarine may interfere with a presynaptic inhibitory regulatory mechanism, the drug could cause a central disinhibition within the hippocampus.

To identify the site of origin of the seizure-like, high-voltage spike discharges observed with ventricular perfusion of the cat's anterior horn, Feldberg and Fleischhauer (1967) micro-injected tubocurarine into the septum, into the anterior limbic area which forms the medial wall of the anterior horn just rostral to the septum, or into the gray matter of the cerebral cortex close to midline. Tubocurarine in a 25 μg dose produced abnormal EEG changes when injected into any of these structures but not in the caudate nucleus. When the injection was made into the corpus callosum and the solution leaked out into the subarachnoid space close to the cingulate gyrus, then the epileptiform response also occurred. Records of spike activity after tubocurarine infusion into the septum are shown in Fig. 10-28.

A micro-injection of tubocurarine into the hippocampus of the cat also causes a focus of local electrical activity which spreads to the occipital cortex (Feldberg and Lotti, 1970). The abnormal negative spike waves were supplemented by periods of fast activity or episodes. When injected into the cortex in the postsplenial area, a similar focus of excitation was set up in the hippocampus but not

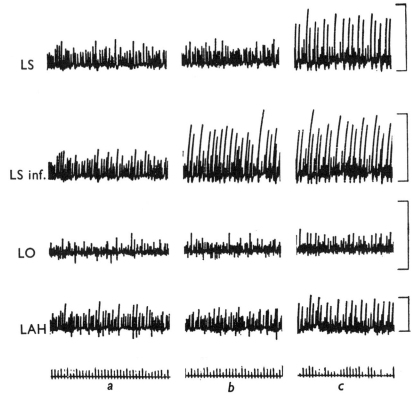

Fig. 10-28 Electrical activity recorded monopolarly from the bared tip of an insulated micro-injection cannula in left septum (LS inf.), from a needle electrode in left septum (LS) inserted 2 mm rostral to the micro-injection cannula, from an epidural electrode on the left occipital cortex (LO) and from the bared tip of the insulated perfusion cannula in anterior horn (LAH) during perfusion of the cerebral ventricles with artificial CSF in a cat anesthetized with chloralose. Record *a* before, and record *b* 25 minutes after micro-injection of 1 µl tubocurarine (3.6×10^{-2} *M*) (25 µg) into left septum. Record *c* 50 minutes after record *b* and 25 minutes after a second micro-injection of 25 µg tubocurarine. Calibration 1 mV, negativity upward. Time marker in seconds. (From Feldberg and Fleischhauer, 1967)

in the cortex. Feldberg and Lotti suggest that in the experiments of Kumagai *et al.* (1962b) the tubocurarine may have escaped into the ventricular lumen from the caudate nucleus. Thus, the entire surface of the hippocampus could have been activated without any direct pharmacological effect on the caudate nucleus *per se*.

VI. SUBCORTICAL SPREADING DEPRESSION

Spreading depression is a characteristic slow-potential change of 1 to 2 minutes duration that passes over the cortex at a rate of 2 to 3 mm/minute (Leao, 1972).

Within subcortical structures of the rat including the corpus striatum, spreading depression is induced by a direct micro-injection of KCl (Fifková and Bureš, 1964). Electrical recordings from the lateral septum also show some evidence of electrical depression as well. No slow potential change, however, is registered in the adjacent globus pallidus or in the internal capsule. This was prevented prob-- ably by the considerable density of myelinated fibers that would retard the movement of the wave. Typical records of the striatal wave of negativity recorded from several sites are shown in Fig. 10-29.

An extensive investigation of spreading depression in the rabbit has revealed that the injection of 25% of KCl solution into the amygdala, septum, thalamus or pyriform cortex evokes a strong wave of negativity (Fifková, 1966). Unlike the rat, the spreading depression does not pass across the rabbit's midline to the contralateral thalamic nuclei. Similarly, although spreading depression induced by KCl injected into the hippocampus of the rat invades the entire structure, the wave of negativity does not pass into the pyriform cortex (Fifková, 1964). However, localized spreading depression again produced by a micro-injection of a strong KCl solution into the rat's corpus striatum is carried to structures in the pyriform lobe (Fifková and Syka, 1964). A slow negative potential change can be recorded

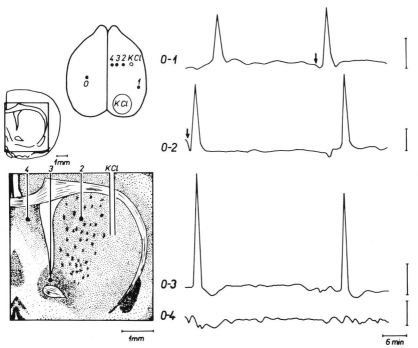

Fig. 10-29 Spread of striatal SD in rat 0-1 neocortex; 0-2 nucleus caudatus; 0-3 nucleus accumbens septi; 0-4 nucleus lateralis septi; calibration: 6 mV. KCl application indicated by arrow. (From Fifková and Bureš, 1964)

in the amygdala, claustrum and pyriform cortex. Neocortical spreading depression is bi-directional, passing to and from the striatum and these limbic structures.

Just as is seen in the surface recording of cortical neurons of the rat, spreading depression also affects all of the pigeon's neurons recorded individually in the corpus striatum (Burešová et al., 1963). After a solution of KCl is injected into the bird's striatum, the wave of negativity passes to all of the surrounding cells with none being unaffected.

When spreading depression is produced by KCl in specific relay nuclei of the rat's thalamus, a diffuse depression of spontaneous EEG activity is always seen in the cortex (Bureš et al., 1965). Acoustic, somatosensory and visual evoked potentials are blocked in specific areas of the cortex by this thalamic wave of spreading depression. Although the deficit of impulse transmission in the sensory pathway is transitory, lasting usually less than 2 minutes, the effect represents a reversible deafferentation of the cerebral cortex.

Evoked responses recorded on the somatosensory cortex from stimulation of peripheral nerves are inhibited by the spreading depression introduced by KCl in the caudate nucleus of the rat (Bureš et al., 1967). The cortical responses to antidromic electrical stimulation of the pyramidal pathway at the level of the pons are also impeded.

Mydriasis is another major symptom of thalamic spreading depression (Burešová et al., 1966). Maximal pupillary dilatation culminates in about 90 seconds after a micro-injection of KCl and slowly subsides after about 5 minutes. By correlating the time course of the process of spread with the intensity of mydriasis, Burešová et al. hypothesize that the structure probably affected is the Edinger-Westphal nucleus.

Following a micro-injection of saturated KCl into the caudate nucleus of the cat, Trachtenberg et al. (1970) found that a large slow potential change arises which consists primarily of a negative wave characteristic of classical spreading depression. This negativity was recorded initially from the region of injection, and is spread only to contiguous cellular sites at a rate exemplified by the tracings of Fig. 10-30. Unlike the rat, the wave of spreading depression in the cat cannot be recorded from the surface of the cortex. The reason is probably because the cat has a much larger basal ganglia, and the negative wave is thereby physically restricted. This corresponds to Fifková's (1966) finding with the rabbit. As in other studies, a burst of local unit activity also appears in the caudate of some cats at the onset of the wave of negativity. This is followed by a small decline in discharge frequency. From these results, one could argue for an interpretation that spreading depression does not really ablate the subcortical structure in a functional sense. Rather, an undifferentiated disorganization of the neurons occurs in terms of the sequence of firing patterns relative to one another.

Recently, a remarkable effort has gone into the question of the physical kinetics

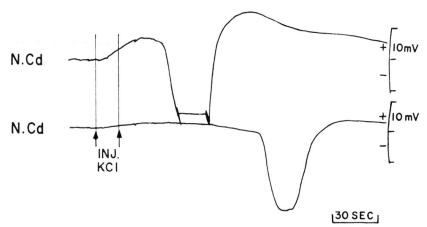

Fig. 10-30 SD waves at two different caudate sites in response to the same injection of 4 μl 27% KCl. Injection is made at a time indicated by arrows in lower trace. Upper trace recorded 4 mm closer to injection cannula than is lower trace. Positive, up; negative, down. Negative change in upper trace exceeded limit of pen excursion. (From Trachtenberg, M. C. *et al.*, 1970. *Brain Res.* **20**:219–231. Fig. 1. Elsevier Publishing Co., Amsterdam, The Netherlands)

of the phenomenon of potassium ion depression. Recording from glass capillary tubes fixed at different distances on the surface of the cortex, Matsuura and Bureš (1971) have determined that a minimum of one cubic millimeter of cortical tissue must be depolarized by KCl in order to trigger a supra-threshold wave of spreading depression. The threshold concentration of KCl required to initiate a negative wave is 3.4×10^{-8} M.

VII. CONCLUDING CONSIDERATIONS

What is particularly revealing about the findings in this chapter is the fact that every aspect of motor activity studied thus far can be chemically triggered or suppressed. The crucial evidence that has accumulated from the chemical stimulation experiments strongly underpins the concept that a focal aberration in a neurochemical mechanism within a given structure can account for a variety of pathological disturbances in motor function.

In spite of the modicum of information, sensory input likewise can be modified centrally by a chemical substance. As yet, only one of the somatosensory modalities has received concerted study with the drug stimulation technique—the central pathway serving the perception of pain.

A. Shift in Sensory Threshold

Why a cholinomimetic compound would subdue rather than enhance the responsiveness to sensory input is difficult to comprehend. With but one exception, the research indicates that the afferent signals that encode such a vital sensory stimulus as pain are inhibited by carbachol applied to subcortical structures. This is in the face of contradictory evidence based on studies employing the electrophoretic injection of ACh or on other experiments in which the release of ACh from the cerebral cortex has been examined (Chapter 13). In both instances, the interpretation can be made unreservedly that the presynaptic release of ACh along the afferent pathways mediates the transmission of a specific sensory impulse.

Although the limited pharmacological results favor the idea that the reaction to pain is attenuated by a set of cholinergic synapses, a methodological vagary of one sort or another may ultimately explain these results. For example, the large volume of a cholinomimetic ordinarily given may result in a nonspecific depolarization of the neurons in the sensory pathway or even a transient focus of spike activity. In either case, a blockade of the system occurs. Also, it is possible that if ACh were used instead of carbachol, quite an opposite effect could be seen (Yamaguchi et al., 1964).

The central site of action of a compound which is capable of modifying the sensory threshold of an animal also is not clarified. From their interpretation of ventricular studies viewed together with micro-injection experiments, Herz and Teschemacher (1971) hypothesize that there is one certain locus at which an anti-nociceptive compound exerts its effect—the periaqueductal gray matter. Based on an analysis of the dose and volume of morphine infused into various parts of the upper and lower brain-stem, they conclude that neurons in the mesencephalon are the target site for the analgesic action of an opiate drug. Parenthetically, the structures have not been identified whose metabolic features change with prolonged usage of an opiate until physical dependence and consequent addiction are manifest.

B. Cholinergic Mediation of Motor Activity

There is no question that ACh or one of several synthetic analogues can stimulate or activate movement of the muscles that control swallowing, turning, the movement of a limb, or even a convulsive episode. When ACh is tested in any of the structures comprising the basal ganglia, diencephalon or mesencephalon, it is likely that cholinoceptive synapses perhaps serve each of the separate parts of the motor system. Rather sound pharmacological results based on the elevation of the endogenous level of ACh by an anticholinesterase injected at any of several structures support this view. Moreover, experiments in which cholinolytics have been given locally in the same region indicate that the receptor sites are muscarinic in nature.

From every standpoint, one would conclude that a cholinergic mechanism is of pivotal importance in experimentally-induced tremor or in the pathological *sequelae* of Parkinsonism. This statement is based on the observations made across species including the rat, cat, monkey and human. These show that a cholinomimetic or an anticholinesterase applied to the caudate nucleus produces a variety of dyskinesias, including choreiform movements, facial spasms and twitching. As Lalley and his co-workers have proposed, this type of disabling motor dysfunction could have as its primary basis an interference with cholinesterase metabolism just as much as a perturbation in the release of ACh or its action on muscarinic receptor sites. The principal anatomical locus of the tremorogenic activity is generally acknowledged to be the caudate nucleus.

Although the cortical thalamic circuitry is more profuse than the caudate-thalamic connections, Bureš et al. (1964) have asserted that the caudate nucleus exerts, by the way of direct neuronal fiber systems, a similar motor influence on the thalamus as does the cortex. Some disagreement exists about the role of the lower brain-stem in the anatomical pathway for tremor activity; however, abnormal movements have been evoked by oxotremorine and carbachol injected into mesencephalic, pontine and other regions.

The clinical application of chemical stimulation for the relief of Parkinsonism and related diseases has been explored widely by a number of neurosurgeons (e.g., Nashold, 1961). For instance, Cooper (1954) found that a peripheral nerve blocker such as procaine reduces Parkinsonian symptoms within minutes after it is injected into the globus pallidus of the human. Unfortunately, the patient's tremor or rigidity returns within 3 to 48 hours. At the present time, therefore, the therapeutic value of this procedure is very limited, at least in terms of an acute injection. As we shall see (Chapter 11), this conclusion is also reached concerning the palliative efficacy of chemical stimulation in other disorders.

Neuropathological conditions may also ensue as a result of a defect in subcortical protein metabolism. As demonstrated by Mihailović and his colleagues, anti-brain antibodies deposited in the hippocampus or caudate nucleus evoke long-lasting, self-regenerative epileptic attacks. How the protein mechanism interacts with an intrinsic humoral system in the hippocampus or other structure that is able to synchronize the explosive potential change of many neurons is far from clear. Nevertheless, the vast bulk of evidence indicates that seizure activity originating anatomically in the hippocampus is driven by synapses that are cholinergic in nature. After a seizure focus is established either permanently by a local deposit of alumina cream or temporarily by picrotoxin, the injection of ACh into the focus enhances the abnormal electrical discharge with all of its components. In other words, whether the circumscribed seizure activity is acute or irreversible, the mechanism involved in its evocation has a feature common to both—the facilitation by ACh. The experiments in which anticholinergic compounds inhibit hippocampal seizures reinforce this viewpoint.

An ionic change in the extracellular environment of the hippocampus may be integrated with a disturbance in ACh activity. In addition to the experiments of Izquierdo and his colleagues, the studies reviewed by Glaser (1972) implicate potassium ions in the pathophysiology of electrical abnormalities of cerebral tissue. Of course other cations (Rozear et al., 1971) as well as amino acids

(Herz *et al.*, 1970b) may also contribute to the enhancement of focal potentials. Overall then, a derangement in the metabolism of protein, ACh, potassium or all of these could trigger and sustain epileptiform activity in the brain.

C. Monoamines and Sensorimotor Function

Considerable perplexity surrounds the issue of how dopamine and norepinephrine modify the neuronal elements in sensory and motor function. Generally, catecholamines are believed to exert an inhibitory action on subcortical structures involved in sensorimotor function. Yet this is certainly not a uniform conclusion (Ernst, 1969; Fog *et al.*, 1970).

On the one hand, the superb pharmacological analyses of Connor, Baker, Lalley and others reveal that tremor induced by a cholinomimetic injected into the caudate nucleus is attenuated by any catecholamine tested. What is more, a beta adrenergic blocking agent given at the same site prevents this attenuation. This is clear enough.

On the other hand, Spiegel and his group show that L-dopa injected into the caudate nucleus reinstates limb movement and enhances the running speed of an animal. Many other investigators (see Randrup and Munkvad, 1968) find that dopamine, L-dopa or amphetamine injected into the caudate nucleus arouse all sorts of motor activity including walking, biting, chewing, licking, turning and classical hyperkinesias. An anticholinergic drug may even enhance stereotypy behavior, not suppress it as one would expect.

The imprudent disregard of the relationship between dosage, volume and effect would help to contribute to the confusion about the actual role of these amines. For example, as little as 0.5 μg of norepinephrine is sufficient to evoke a change in body temperature in the cat or an ingestive response in the rat. Yet, to evoke an aberrant motor response, a dose well over 100 times this amount must be injected in the same diencephalic structure. This dissimilitude alone could cast doubt on the credibility of a catecholaminergic system involved in motor function. Vascular and other local functions undoubtedly are affected and a sufficiently high dose of any compound, whether given in the brain or gut, will exert a generalized effect systemically. The importance of the dose of a drug in locomotor behavior is documented by the fact that a difference of less than 3 μg of neostigmine injected into the hippocampus will determine whether an animal's motor activity is enhanced or suppressed (van Abeelen *et al.*, 1972).

Finally, a distinction must be made between the movements characteristic of stereotyped behavior and those of tremor (Randrup and Munkvad, 1968). Although there may be some physiological overlap, at least anatomically the caudate nucleus seems to mediate both of these dysfunctional conditions. Probably the most direct way to determine the function of the monoamines in the caudate nucleus would be to record simultaneously the motor responses defined as tremor and those as stereotypy. Then as the caudate nucleus is pharmacologically examined by the micro-injection of agonists and antagonists, the component parts of each of the motor responses could be gradually separated to the point of ultimate delineation.

VIII. Master Summary Table
Chemicals that Exerted an Effect when Given at a Specific Site in the Brain

Chemical	Dose	Volume	Site	State*	Species	Response	Reference
Acetylcholine (ACh)	?	crystal	Mesencephalic reticular formation	U	Rat	Stereotyped standing.	Davis et al. (1967b)
	≈ 25–50 µg	crystal	Caudate nucleus	U	Cat	Contralateral circling; drowsiness.	Stevens et al. (1961)
	≈ 25–50 µg	crystal	Hippocampus	A U	Cat	Localized high-voltage spike potentials, seizure activity.	MacLean (1957a)
	≈ 100–300 µg	crystal	Hippocampus	U	Cat	EEG fast activity, hippocampal theta activity.	Rogozea et al. (1971)
	2–8 µg	1 µl or crystals	Mesencephalic reticular formation	A U	Rat	Sensory hyper-reactivity, impairment of shock avoidance conditioning.	Grossman (1968a)
	?	crystal or liquid	Septum, caudate nucleus	A	Cat	Altered evoked potentials from trigeminal nerve.	Guerrero-Figueroa et al. (1966a)
	56.4 µg	3–6 µl	Caudate putamen	U	Rat	Tremor; forelimb twitching.	Dill et al. (1968b)
	1–11 µg	<10 µl	Hippocampus	A	Cat	Re-established seizure focus.	Baker and Kratky (1971)
	200 µg	10 µl	Hippocampus	A	Cat	EEG spike discharges.	Baker and Benedict (1968b)
	300–500 µg	1–10 µl	Caudate nucleus	C	Cat	Tremor.	Connor et al. (1966a)

*U = unanesthetized and unrestrained; C = constrained, confined or curarized; A = anesthetized.

VIII. Master Summary Table (Continued)

Chemical	Dose	Volume	Site	Species	State*	Response	Reference
Acetylcholine (ACh)	36.34–145.34 µg	10 µl	Hippocampus	Cat	U	Activated alumina focus or contralateral mirror focus	Guerrero-Figueroa et al. (1964b)
	2–5 µg	5–10 µl	Thalamus	Cat	A	Cortical EEG spindles.	Endröczi et al. (1963b)
	2–5 µg	5–10 µl	Reticular formation	Cat	A	Cortical and hippocampal desynchronization.	Endröczi et al. (1963b)
	50–500 µg	5 µl	Cingulate gyrus, hippocampus	Monkey	C	Evoked EEG spike activity.	Delgado (1966)
	1.45 mg	8 µl	Hippocampus, amygdala	Monkey	C	Local, sharp EEG waves with after discharges.	Delgado and DeFeudis (1969)
	1×10^5 µg	1000 µl	Globus pallidus	Human	U	Parasympathetic excitation.	Nashold (1959)
Acetylcholine + Neostigmine	2–10 µg	2 µl	Thalamic nuclei	Cat	A	Focal epileptiform seizures; neocortical discharges.	Babb et al. (1971)
Acetylcholine + Physostigmine	$\simeq 1$ µg and 1 µg	crystal	Amygdala	Cat	U	Local EEG seizures in amygdala, hippocampus and hypothalamus. Motor seizures, attack.	Grossman (1963)
Adenosine triphosphate (ATP)	92.5 µg	<10 µl	Caudate nucleus	Cat	C	Antagonized carbachol tremor.	Connor et al. (1967)
Alumina cream	?	100–500 µl	Pons, temporal lobe	Rabbit	U	Convulsions, ataxia, paresis, death.	Wiśniewski et al. (1966)
	?	?	Amygdala	Cat	U	Motor and EEG seizures.	Gastaut et al. (1959)

Compound	Dose	Volume	Structure	Species	U/A	Effect	Reference
	?	50 µl	Substantia nigra	Cat	U	EEG epileptic discharges, myoclonic seizures.	Shirao (1969)
	?	50–200 µl	Caudate nucleus	Cat	U	Vertical nystagmus.	Szekely and Spiegel (1963)
	?	200 µl	Caudate nucleus	Cat	A	Ataxia, catalepsy, catatonia, aphagia, adipsia.	Spiegel and Szekely (1961)
	?	100–200 µl	Thalamus, putamen	Monkey	U	Motor and EEG seizures.	Kopeloff et al. (1950)
	3600–5500 µg	200–250 µl	Thalamus, corpus striatum	Monkey	U	EEG seizures.	Faeth and Walker (1957)
Aluminum oxide	?	crystal	Thalamus, mesencephalic reticular formation	Cat	U	Focal spike activity.	Guerrero-Figueroa et al. (1963a)
	?	?	Thalamus, mesencephalon	Cat	U	EEG seizures, focus, reduced by sensory stimuli.	Guerrero-Figueroa et al. (1963b)
	?	crystal	Hippocampus	Cat	U	Secondary foci.	Guerrero-Figueroa et al. (1968)
Amphetamine	25–200 µg	1 µl	Globus pallidus	Rat	U	Stereotypy behavior.	Costall et al. (1972b)
	25–400 µg	5 µl	Caudate putamen	Rat	U	Stereotypy behavior.	Costall et al. (1972b)
	10–60 µg	10 µl	Caudate nucleus	Cat	U	Stereotyped behavior, turning, limb extension.	Cools and van Rossum (1970)
Apomorphine	≈ 100 µg	crystal	Caudate nucleus, globus pallidus (neostriatum)	Rat	U	Compulsive gnawing.	Ernst and Smelik (1966)
	10–50 µg	5 µl or crystal	Caudate putamen	Rat	U	Contralateral turning; asymmetric posture.	Ungerstedt et al. (1969)
	5 µg	5 µl	Corpus striatum	Rat	U	Walking.	Fuxe and Ungerstedt (1970)

VIII. Master Summary Table *(Continued)*

Chemical	Dose	Volume	Site	Species	State*	Response	Reference
Apomorphine	20 µg	5 µl	Corpus striatum	Rat	U	Stereotyped walking, intense biting.	Fuxe and Ungerstedt (1970)
Arecoline	70–120 µg	20 µl	Medulla	Rat	A	Inhibition of nociceptive "tail-flick" reaction.	Andreas and Oelssner (1969)
	100–200 µg	1 µl	Hippocampus	Rat Rabbit	U U	Raised pain (nociceptive) threshold.	Metyš et al. (1969a)
	100–400 µg	5 µl	Caudate putamen	Rat	U	Inhibited stereotypy behavior.	Costall et al. (1972b)
	85–125 µg	1–10 µl	Caudate nucleus	Cat	C	Tremor.	Connor et al. (1966a)
N-Methyl-aspartic acid (NMA)	10–100 µg	10 µl	Caudate nucleus	Cat	U A	Motor hyperactivity, EEG activation.	Baker (1972)
Atropine	≃ 6–18 µg	crystal	Hippocampus, septum	Rat	U	Increased locomotor activity.	Leaton and Rech (1972)
	2–12 µg	1 µl or crystal	Mesencephalic reticular formation	Rat	A	Suppressed response to external stimuli.	Grossman (1968b)
	30–60 µg	3 µl	Caudate nucleus	Rat	U	Tremor.	Cox and Potkonjak (1969)
	100–400 µg	5 µl	Corpus striatum	Rat	U	Potentiated amphetamine stereotypy.	Costall and Naylor (1972a)
	2–5 µg	1–3 µl	Preoptic area	Cat	U	Prevented cholinergic effects.	George et al. (1966)
	200–325 µg	1–10 µl	Caudate nucleus	Cat	C	Abolished carbachol tremor.	Connor et al. (1966a)

Drug	Dose	Volume	Site	Species	Effect		Reference
Barium (Ba)	6–12.5 µg	12.5 µl	Infundibular region	Rat	Toxic effects, disorientation, tremor.	U	Clöetta and Fischer (1930)
	200 µg	25 µl	Infundibular region	Cat	Convulsions.	U	Clöetta and Fischer (1930)
Benperidol	75 µg	5 µl	Corpus striatum	Rat	Blocked amphetamine stereotypy, catalepsy.	U	Fog et al. (1971)
Benztropin	75–110 µg	1–10 µl	Caudate nucleus	Cat	Abolished carbachol tremor.	C	Connor et al. (1966a)
Bethanechol	28 µg	10 µl	Hippocampus	Cat	EEG spike discharges.	A	Baker and Benedict (1968b)
	25–38 µg	1–10 µl	Caudate nucleus	Cat	Tremor.	C	Connor et al. (1966a)
	40 µg	3–10 µl	Posterior hypothalamus	Cat	Reinstated hemicholinium-blocked theta rhythm.	A U	Friedman and Wikler (1970)
Biperiden	80–125 µg	1–10 µl	Caudate nucleus	Cat	Abolished carbachol tremor.	C	Connor et al. (1966a)
Butacaine	3.8 µg	40 µl	Amygdala, hippocampus	Cat	EEG spike activity, searching, turning, twitching.	U	Tuttle and Elliott (1969)
Caffeine-sodium benzoate	200 µg	10 µl	Mesencephalon, posterior hypothalamus	Cat	Hippocampal and neocortical EEG seizures.	C	Yanagida and Yamamura (1971)
Calcium chloride ($CaCl_2$)	16–40 µg	<10 µl	Caudate nucleus	Cat	Inhibited cholinergic tremor.	C	Lalley et al. (1971)
	2.6–10.4 mM	perfusion 50 µl/min	Postero-lateral hypothalamus	Cat	Behavioral and EEG sleep; catatonia	U	Veale and Myers (1971)
	?	crystal	Hippocampus	Cat Monkey	Seizure discharges, excitation.	U C	MacLean (1954)
Carbachol	.3–6 µg	?	Mesencephalic reticular formation, hypothalamus	Rat	Suppressed nociceptive reactions.	U	Metyš et al. (1969b)
	.5–1.5 µg	?	Neostriatum	Rat	Contralateral forelimb tremor.	U	Dill et al. (1968a)

VIII. Master Summary Table (Continued)

Chemical	Dose	Volume	Site	Species	State*	Response	Reference
Carbachol	≈ .5–2 µg	crystal	Amygdala	Rat	U	Convulsions; prolonged deficit in acquisition of avoidance response.	Belluzzi and Grossman (1969)
	≈ 3 µg	crystal	Dorsal mesencephalon	Rat	U	Motor seizures.	Routtenberg and Olds (1966)
	1–25 µg	?	Caudate nucleus	Cat	A	Synergizes with electrical stimulation.	Militello et al. (1970)
	≈ 300 µg	crystal	Caudate nucleus, reticular formation, thalamic nucleus, hypothalamic areas, mesencephalon	Cat Rabbit	U U	Circling behavior, vertical and rotational head movements (when applied at a large number of diffuse sites).	Nashold and Gills (1960)
	≈ .1–2 µg	crystal	Amygdala	Cat	U	Attack; seizures.	Grossman (1963)
	≈ 25–50 µg	crystal	Hippocampus	Cat	A U	Localized high-voltage spike potentials, seizure activity.	MacLean (1957a)
	≈ 200 µg	crystal	Substantia nigra, red nucleus	Cat	U	Compulsive circling, limb hypertonicity, hind leg tremor.	Nashold et al. (1965)
	240–360 µg	crystal	Caudate nucleus	Cat	U	Vertical nystagmus.	Szekely and Spiegel (1963)
	1.5–2 µg	1 µl or crystal	Mesencephalic reticular formation	Rat	A U	Sensory hyper-reactivity; impairment of shock avoidance conditioning.	Grossman (1968b)
	?	crystal or liquid	Caudate nucleus, septum	Cat	A	Altered evoked potentials from trigeminal nerve.	Guerrero-Figueroa et al. (1966a)

Dose	Volume	Region	Species		Effect	Reference
?	1 µl	Septum	Rat	U	Inhibited nociceptive reactions.	Herz and Metyš (1968)
.25 µg	1 µl	Amygdala	Rat	U	Hyperactive, aggression, seizures.	Goddard (1969)
1.5–3 µg	3–6 µl	Caudate putamen	Rat	U	Tremor; forelimb twitching.	Dill et al. (1968b)
.5–3.5 µg	1–7 µl	Corpus striatum	Rat	A	Limb tremor, facial spasms, chewing, trunk rigidity, salivation.	Little and Dill (1969)
1.1–4.3 µg	.25–1 µl	Dorsal mesencephalon	Rat	U	Motor seizures.	Routtenberg and Olds (1966)
.3–10 µg	1 µl	Mesencephalic reticular formation, septum, thalamus, caudate nucleus	Rat / Rabbit	U / U	Raised pain (nociceptive) threshold.	Metyš et al. (1969a)
2–10 µg	2 µl	Thalamic nuclei	Cat	A	Focal epileptiform seizures; neocortical discharges.	Babb et al. (1971)
36.53 µg	10 µl	Hippocampus	Cat	U	Activated alumina focus or contralateral mirror focus.	Guerrero-Figueroa et al. (1964b)
.5–7 µg	10 µl	Hippocampus	Cat	C	Enhanced all aspects of discharge foci.	Baker and Benedict (1970)
3 µg	1–3 µl	Preoptic area	Cat	U	Tremor, growling, hissing.	George et al. (1966)
3 µg	1–3 µl	Tegmentum	Cat	U	Atonia, sleep, EEG desynchronization, tremor.	George et al. (1966)
2–5 µg	5–10 µl	Thalamus	Cat	A	Cortical EEG spindles.	Endröczi et al. (1963b)
2–5 µg	5–10 µl	Reticular formation	Cat	A	Cortical and hippocampal desynchronization.	Endröczi et al. (1963b)
1–5 µg	10 µl	Hippocampus	Cat	A	EEG spike discharges.	Baker and Benedict (1968b)

VIII. Master Summary Table (Continued)

Chemical	Dose	Volume	Site	Species	State*	Response	Reference
Carbachol	7 μg	<10 μl	Caudate nucleus	Cat	C	Tremor.	Lalley et al. (1970) and Connor et al. (1967)
	5–8 μg	1–10 μl	Caudate nucleus	Cat	C	Tremor.	Connor et al. (1966a)
	5–8 μg	1–10 μl	Caudate nucleus	Cat	C	Hind leg tremor, fever.	Connor et al. (1966b)
	5–10 μg	<10 μl	Hippocampus	Cat	A	Continuous focal discharges suppressed by scopolamine.	Baker and Benedict (1968a)
	5–10 μg	<10 μl	Hippocampus	Cat	A	Focal seizures.	Baker and Kratky (1968)
	10 μg	3–10 μl	Posterior hypothalamus	Cat	A U	Reinstated hemicholinium-blocked theta rhythm.	Friedman and Wikler (1970)
	60–120 μg	6 μl	Reticular formation	Cat	C	Localized seizure discharges.	Kumagai et al. (1962a)
	2 μg	2 μl	Subthalamus	Squirrel monkey	U	Circling, hyperactivity	Murphey and Dill (1972)
	1–5 μg	1–5 μl	Caudate nucleus, putamen, globus pallidus	Squirrel monkey	U	Hyperkinetic, choreoform movements, tremor, limb hypertension.	Murphey and Dill (1972)
	10–20 μg	10 μl	Caudate nucleus	Cat	U A	Mild motor hyperactivity and EEG activation.	Baker (1972)
Chlorpromazine	10 μg	5 μl or crystal	Caudate putamen	Rat	U	Contralateral turning; asymmetric posture.	Ungerstedt et al. (1969)

Drug	Dose	Volume	Site	Species	Class	Effect	Reference
	50 μg	1 μl	Corpus striatum	Rat	U	Antagonized amphetamine-induced stereotyped behavior.	Fog et al. (1968)
	10–25 μg	<100 μl	Hippocampus	Cat	A	Low dose enhanced focus; high dose inhibited focus.	Baker and Kratky (1967)
	25–200 μg	<10 μl	Hippocampus	Cat	A	Increased seizure focus at low dose; suppressed focus at high dose.	Baker and Kratky (1971)
Chlorprothixene	150 μg	1 μl	Corpus striatum	Rat	U	Antagonized amphetamine-induced stereotyped behavior.	Fog et al. (1968)
CDP-Choline	.5 mg	10 μl	Mesencephalon, posterior hypothalamus	Cat	C	Hippocampal and neocortical EEG seizures.	Yanagida and Yamamura (1971)
Cobalt	?	crystal	Olfactory bulb, hippocampus	Cat	U	Focal epileptic seizures.	Guerrero-Figueroa et al. (1968)
	≈10 mg	crystal	Amygdala, ventral hippocampus	Cat	U	Focal epileptic seizures, mirror focus.	Mutani (1967a and b)
	≈10 mg	crystal	Midline thalamic nuclei	Cat	U	High voltage spikes; generalized epileptic attack.	Mancia and Lucioni (1966)
	≈10 mg	crystal	Midline thalamic nuclei	Cat	U	High voltage spikes; generalized epileptic attack.	Mancia and Lucioni (1966)
	≈5–15 mg	crystal	Medial thalamus	Cat	U	Cortical spikes.	Cesa-Bianchi et al. (1967)
	≈5–15 mg	crystal	Pons, medulla	Cat	U	EEG spikes, seizure activity.	Cesa-Bianchi et al. (1967)
	≈10 mg	crystal	Hippocampus	Cat	U	Hippocampal after discharges.	Mutani et al. (1969)
Cobalt-aluminum phosphate gel	5–20 mg	40 μl	Amygdala	Cat	A	Rapidly developed EEG focus.	Thomalske and Lyagoubi (1969)

VIII. Master Summary Table (Continued)

Chemical	Dose	Volume	Site	Species	State*	Response	Reference
Copper	≃ 50–60 μg	crystal	Caudate nucleus	Cat	U	Foot treading, listlessness, cataleptic episodes.	Butcher and Fox (1968)
Cortisol	150 μg	100 μl	Hippocampus	Cat	A	Local convulsive discharges.	Feldman (1971)
Cyclic AMP	50–100 μg	5–10 μl	Hypothalamus, mesencephalic reticular formation, amygdala	Rat Cat	U U	Locomotor activity, catatonia, seizures.	Gessa et al. (1970)
Desipramine	1–400 μg	<10 μl	Hippocampus	Cat	A	Increased seizure focus at low dose; suppressed focus at high dose.	Baker and Kratky (1971)
Dichloroisoproterenol (DCI)	25 μg	<10 μl	Caudate nucleus	Cat	C	Antagonized carbachol tremor.	Connor et al. (1967)
Dihydro-β-erythroidine	?	crystal or liquid	Caudate nucleus, septum	Cat	A	Altered evoked potentials from trigeminal nerve.	Guerrero-Figueroa et al. (1966)
Digitoxin	≃ 10–20 μg	crystal	Hypothalamus	Rabbit	C	Hippocampal discharges and spike activity.	Bergmann et al. (1970b)
Diisopropylfluoro-phosphate (DFP)	3 μg	3 μl	Caudate nucleus	Rat	U	Tremor.	Cox and Potkonjak (1969)
	.1–320 μg	10 μl	Caudate nucleus	Rabbit	U	Contraversive circling.	White (1956)
	60–160 μg	10 μl	Caudate nucleus	Rabbit	U	Contralateral turning movements.	White and Himwich (1957)
	2–7.5 μg	10 μl	Hippocampus	Cat	C	Accelerated discharge rate.	Baker and Benedict (1970)

Drug	Dose	Volume	Site	Species		Effect	Reference
	25–50 µg	<10 µl	Hippocampus	Cat	A	Continuous focal discharges suppressed by scopolamine.	Baker and Benedict (1968a)
	25–50 µg	<10 µl	Hippocampus	Cat	A	Focal seizure.	Baker and Kratky (1968)
	25–60 µg	<10 µl	Caudate nucleus	Cat	C	Irreversible tremor with residual motor effects.	Lalley et al. (1970)
	50–100 µg	<10 µl	Hippocampus	Cat	A	Seizure focus.	Baker and Kratky (1971)
	25–125 µg	10 µl	Hippocampus	Cat	A	EEG spike discharges.	Baker and Benedict (1968b)
Dimethoxyphenyl-ethylamine (DIMPEA)	15–105 µg	1–7 µl	Corpus striatum	Rat	A	Limb tremor, facial spasms, chewing, trunk rigidity, salivation.	Little and Dill (1969)
Diphenylhydantoin	20 µg	10 µl	Hippocampus	Cat	U	Suppressed amplitude of focal discharges.	Guerrero-Figueroa et al. (1964a)
L-Dopa	≈ 100 µg	crystal	Caudate nucleus, globus pallidus (neostriatum)	Rat	U	Compulsive gnawing.	Ernst and Smelik (1966)
	80–160 µg	4–8 µl	Caudate nucleus	Rat	U	Increased locomotion after tungstic acid.	Spiegel et al. (1968)
	2–160 µg	10 µl	Caudate nucleus	Cat	U	Stereotyped behavior; turning, limb extension.	Cools and van Rossum (1970)
Dopamine (DA)	5–200 µg	5 µl or crystal	Caudate putamen	Rat	U	Contralateral turning; asymmetric posture.	Ungerstedt et al. (1969)
	59 µg	3 µl	Corpus striatum	Rat	U	Motor hyperactivity.	Benkert and Köhler (1972)
	100–500 µg	5 µl	Corpus striatum	Rat	U	Stereotyped biting and sniffing.	Fog and Pakkenberg (1971)
	99.7 µg	<10 µl	Caudate nucleus	Cat	C	Antagonized carbachol tremor.	Connor et al. (1967)

VIII. Master Summary Table *(Continued)*

Chemical	Dose	Volume	Site	Species	State*	Response	Reference
Dopamine (DA)	3–150 µg	<10 µl	Caudate nucleus	Cat	C	Antagonism of anticholinesterase or carbachol tremor.	Lalley et al. (1970)
	2–120 µg	10 µl	Caudate nucleus	Cat	U	Stereotyped behavior; turning; limb extension.	Cools and van Rossum (1970)
DA + Scopolamine	40–200 µg + 20–100 µg	1 µl	Caudate putamen	Rat	U	Sniffing, biting, catalepsy.	Fog et al. (1967)
Ecothiophate	15–30 µg	<10 µl	Caudate nucleus	Cat	C	Irreversible tremor with residual motor effects.	Lalley et al. (1970)
	30 µg	10 µl	Hippocampus	Cat	A	EEG spike discharges.	Baker and Benedict (1968a and b)
Epinephrine	10.3 µg	<10 µl	Caudate nucleus	Cat	C	Antagonized carbachol tremor.	Connor et al. (1967)
	2.5–20 µg	<10 µl	Caudate nucleus	Cat	C	Antagonism of anticholinesterase or carbachol tremor.	Lalley et al. (1970)
Eserine	≈ 300 µg	crystal	Caudate nucleus, reticular formation, thalamic nucleus, hypothalamic areas, mesencephalon	Cat Rabbit	U U	Circling behavior, vertical and rotational head movements (when applied at a large number of diffuse sites).	Nashold and Gills (1960)
	≈ 200 µg	crystal	Substantia nigra, red nucleus	Cat	U	Compulsive circling, limb hypertonicity, hind leg tremor.	Nashold et al. (1965)
	10 µg	5–10 µl	Thalamus	Cat	A	Cortical EEG spindles.	Endröczi et al. (1963b)
	10 µg	5–10 µl	Reticular formation	Cat	A	Cortical and hippocampal desynchronization.	Endröczi et al. (1963b)

Substance	Amount	Volume	Structure	Animal	Type	Effect	Reference
	25–100 µg	50–100 µl	Hippocampus, caudate nucleus, hypothalamus	Cat	A	Cortical spikes and seizure patterns.	Rakić et al. (1962)
	100–200 µg	<10 µl	Caudate nucleus	Cat	C	Reversible tremor.	Lalley et al. (1970)
Estradiol	?	crystal	Preoptic area	Rat	U	Increased locomotor activity.	Wade and Zucker (1970)
Ethacrynic acid	≃ 50–100 µg	crystal	Hypothalamus	Rabbit	C	Hippocampal discharges and spike activity.	Bergmann et al. (1970b)
Floropipamide	75 µg	5 µl	Corpus striatum	Rat	U	Blocked amphetamine stereotypy; catalepsy.	Fog et al. (1971)
Flupenthixol	100 µg	1 µl	Corpus striatum	Rat	U	Antagonized amphetamine-induced stereotyped behavior.	Fog et al. (1968)
γ-Aminobutyric acid (GABA)	?	crystal or liquid	Caudate nucleus, septum	Cat	A	Altered evoked potentials from trigeminal nerve.	Guerrero-Figueroa et al. (1966a)
	≃ 700–800 µg	crystal	Mesencephalic reticular formation	Cat	U	Seizure discharges.	Rogozea et al. (1969)
	20.6–30.9 µg	10 µl	Hippocampus	Cat	U	Inhibited primary or secondary local activity.	Guerrero-Figueroa et al. (1964b)
Gamma-globulin-anti-hippocampus antibody	41.5–93 µg	8.3 µl	Hippocampus, caudate nucleus	Monkey	U	Epileptiform seizures.	Mihailović and Čupić (1971)
Gamma-globulin-anti-caudate antibody	41.5–93 µg	8.3 µl	Hippocampus, caudate nucleus	Monkey	U	Epileptiform seizures.	Mihailović and Čupić (1971)
Glucose	?	crystal	Ventromedial hypothalamus	Rat	A	Inhibited VMH electrical activity.	Gliddon (1970)
L-Glutamate	4.2–21 mg	50–250 µl	Hippocampus	Cat	A	EEG seizure activity.	Knaape and Wiechert (1970)

VIII. Master Summary Table (Continued)

Chemical	Dose	Volume	Site	Species	State*	Response	Reference
L-Glutamate	.84–1.69 mg	5–10 µl	Hippocampus, amygdala	Monkey	C	Local, sharp EEG waves with after discharges.	Delgado and DeFeudis (1969)
	.51–25.4 mg	3–150 µl	Hippocampus, amygdala	Monkey	C	Desynchronized EEG; tremor; motor convulsions.	Delgado et al. (1971b)
Haloperidol	25–100 µg	5 µl	Caudate putamen	Rat	U	Inhibited stereotypy behavior.	Costall et al. (1972b)
	100 µg	5 µl	Corpus striatum	Rat	U	Blocked amphetamine stereotypy, catalepsy.	Fog et al. (1971)
Hemicholinium	12–200 µg	3–10 µl	Posterior hypothalamus	Cat	A U	Blockade of hippocampal theta rhythm.	Friedman and Wikler (1970)
	50–500 µg	<10 µl	Caudate nucleus	Cat	C	Antagonism of anticholinesterase or carbachol tremor.	Lalley et al. (1970)
p-Hydroxy-amphetamine	50–150 µg	5 µl	Corpus striatum	Rat	U	Stereotyped biting and sniffing.	Fog and Pakkenberg (1971)
6-Hydroxydopamine (6-OHDA)	10 µg	10 µl	Substantia nigra	Cat	U	Circling; limb extension, ataxia	Frigyesi et al. (1971)
	8 µg	4 µl	Substantia nigra	Rat	U	Ipsiversive rotation, amphetamine-evoked rotation.	Ungerstedt and Arbuthnott (1970)
	2–8 µg	1–4 µl	Substantia nigra	Rat	U	Ipsiversive turning; motor asymmetry.	Ungerstedt (1968)
5-Hydroxytryptophan (5-HTP)	≃ 19 µg	crystal	Lateral hypothalamus	Rat	U	Tremor, piloerection, stereotypic behavior.	Hadžović (1971)
	≃ 20–200 µg	crystal	Substantia nigra	Rat	U	Tremor.	Hadžović and Ernst (1969)

Drug	Dose	Volume	Site	Animal		Effect	Reference
Imipramine	10–25 µg	<100 µl	Hippocampus	Cat	A	Low dose enhanced focus; high dose inhibited focus.	Baker and Kratky (1967)
	25–250 µg	<10 µl	Hippocampus	Cat	A	Increased focus at low dose; suppressed focus at high dose.	Baker and Kratky (1971)
Isoproterenol	7.8 µg	<10 µl	Caudate nucleus	Cat	C	Antagonized carbachol tremor.	Connor et al. (1967)
Lidocaine	2.03 µg	40 µl	Amygdala, hippocampus	Cat	U	EEG spike activity, searching, turning, twitching.	Tuttle and Elliott (1969)
Lithium chloride (LiCl)	326.45–652.9 µg	50–100 µl	Hippocampus, amygdala	Monkey	C	Local, sharp EEG waves with after discharges.	Delgado and DeFeudis (1969)
Magnesium chloride ($MgCl_2$)	107–178 µg	<10 µl	Caudate nucleus	Cat	C	Inhibited cholinergic tremor.	Lalley et al. (1971)
Mecholyl	1–14 mg	10 µl	Caudate nucleus	Rabbit	A	Contralateral turning movements.	White and Himwich (1957)
Mercuric acetate	≃ 50–100 µg	crystal	Hypothalamus	Rabbit	C	Hippocampal discharges and spike activity.	Bergmann et al. (1970)
Mescaline	10–70 µg	1–7 µl	Corpus striatum	Rat	A	Limb tremor, facial spasms, chewing, trunk rigidity, salivation.	Little and Dill (1969)
Metatyramine	15 mg	300 µl/5 hr	Corpus striatum	Rat	U	Contralateral rotation.	Andén et al. (1970)
Methacholine	≃ 25 µg	crystal	Hippocampus	Cat	A U	Localized high-voltage spike potentials, seizure activity.	MacLean (1957a)
	≃ 25–50 µg	crystal	Caudate nucleus	Cat	U	Contralateral limb weakness.	Stevens et al. (1961)
	38 µg	10 µl	Hippocampus	Cat	A	EEG spike discharges.	Baker and Benedict (1968b)
	90–110 µg	1–10 µl	Caudate nucleus	Cat	C	Tremor.	Connor et al. (1966a)

VIII. Master Summary Table (Continued)

Chemical	Dose	Volume	Site	Species	State*	Response	Reference
3-Methoxytyramine (3-MT)	15–105 µg	1–7 µl	Corpus striatum	Rat	A	Limb tremor, facial spasms, chewing, trunk rigidity, salivation.	Little and Dill (1969)
Metrazol	2–6 mg	10 µl	Caudate nucleus	Rabbit	A	Contralateral turning movements.	White and Himwich (1957)
	25–100 µg	1 µl	Cingulate gyrus, gyrus splenialis, pyriform cortex	Cat	A	Local high-voltage discharge foci.	Banerjee et al. (1970)
	150–1000 µg	10 µl	Hippocampus	Cat	A	Transitory EEG excitation, no seizure foci.	Baker et al. (1965)
	1.3–3.7 µg	40 µl	Amygdala, hippocampus, mesencephalon	Cat	U	EEG spike activity, scratching, twitching, turning.	Tuttle and Elliott (1969)
Morphine	2.5–5 µg	?	Mesencephalic reticular formation, hypothalamus	Rat	U	Suppressed nociceptive reactions.	Metyš et al. (1969b)
	10 µg	2 µl	Periaqueductal and periventricular gray	Rabbit	U	Analgesia: loss of pain response.	Tsou and Jang (1964)
	20–40 µg	2.5 µl	Thalamus, hypothalamus, mesencephalon	Rabbit	U	Blocked nociceptive reaction to pain stimuli; sedation.	Herz et al. (1970a)
	3.03 µg	40 µl	Amygdala, hippocampus	Cat	U	EEG spike activity, turning, twitching.	Tuttle and Elliott (1969)
Muscarine	.99 µg	1 µl	Myelencephalon, diencephalon	Chicken	U	Motor activity.	Marley and Seller (1972)
	60–120 µg	6 µl	Reticular formation	Cat	C	Localized seizure discharges.	Kumagai et al. (1962a)
Nalorphine	10–50 µg	4 µl	Periaqueductal and periventricular gray	Rabbit	U	Reversed morphine analgesia.	Tsou and Jang (1964)

Drug	Dose	Volume	Brain region	Species		Effect	Reference
Neostigmine	.07–.14 µg	.8 µl	Hippocampus	Mouse	U	Diminished exploration.	van Abeelen et al. (1972)
	2–10 µg	2 µl	Thalamic nuclei	Cat	A	Focal epileptiform seizures; neocortical discharges.	Babb et al. (1971)
Norepinephrine (NE)	2–8 µg	1 µl or crystal	Mesencephalon, reticular formation	Rat	A	Reduction in startle response.	Grossman (1968b)
	2–10 µg	5 µl or crystal	Caudate putamen	Rat	U	Contralateral turning; asymmetric posture.	Ungerstedt et al. (1969)
	65 µg	3 µl	Hypothalamus	Rat	U	Motor hyperactivity.	Benkert and Köhler (1972)
	100–200 µg	5 µl	Corpus striatum	Rat	U	No stereotyped compulsive and repetitive responses.	Fog and Pakkenberg (1971)
	51.5 µg	<10 µl	Caudate nucleus	Cat	C	Antagonized carbachol tremor.	Connor et al. (1967)
	10–60 µg	10 µl	Caudate nucleus	Cat	U	Drowsy, loss of tonus.	Cools and van Rossum (1970)
Orphenadrine	100–400 µg	2 µl	Globus pallidus	Rat	U	Potentiated amphetamine stereotypy.	Costall and Naylor (1972a)
Ouabain	≃ 1–100 µg	crystal	Hypothalamus	Rabbit	C	Hippocampal discharges and spike activity.	Bergmann et al. (1970b)
Oxotremorine	?	1 µl	Septum	Rat	U	Inhibited nociceptive reactions.	Herz and Metyš (1968)
	.28–2.4 µg	10 µl	Reticular formation, anterior hypothalamus, ventral thalamic nucleus, caudate nucleus	Rat	U	"Tail-flick" reaction suppressed.	Andreas and Staib (1971)
	1.25–10 µg	1 µl	Hippocampus	Rat / Rabbit	U / U	Raised pain (nociceptive) threshold	Metyš et al. (1969a)

VIII. Master Summary Table (Continued)

Chemical	Dose	Volume	Site	Species	State*	Response	Reference
Oxotremorine	3 µg	3 µl	Globus pallidus, caudate nucleus, substantia nigra, red nucleus	Rat	U	Tremor.	Cox and Potkonjak (1969)
	28–49 µg	20 µl	Medulla	Rat	A	Inhibition of nociceptive "tail-flick" reaction.	Andreas and Oelssner (1969)
	2–10 µg	1–3 µl	Tegmentum	Cat	U	Atonia, sleep, EEG desynchronization, tremor.	George et al. (1966)
	12–18 µg	1–10 µl	Caudate nucleus	Cat	C	Tremor.	Connor et al. (1966a)
Oxypertine	25 µg	5 µl	Corpus striatum	Rat	U	Blocked amphetamine stereotypy; catalepsy.	Fog et al. (1971)
Oxyphenonium	2 mg	1000 µl	Globus pallidus	Human	U	Blockade of parasympathetic response.	Nashold (1959)
Penicillin	?	crystal	Hippocampus	Cat	A	Focal spike discharges.	Dichter and Spencer (1969a and b)
	?	crystal	Hippocampus	Cat	A U	Random EEG spikes.	MacLean (1957a)
	?	2–10 µl	Thalamus	Cat	U	Propagated focal seizures.	Inutsuka (1969)
	260–300 µg	50–200 µl	Caudate nucleus	Cat	U	Vertical nystagmus	Szekely and Spiegel (1963)
	400–1800 units	10–20 µl	Thalamus	Cat	A	Seizure focus propagated to hippocampus.	Voiculescu and Voinescu (1968)

Drug	Dose	Volume	Site	Species		Effect	Reference
	2500–15,000 units	2–15 μl	Thalamus	Cat	A	Synchronized EEG spindles.	Ralston and Ajmone-Marsan (1956)
	3800–15,000 units	4–15 μl	Midbrain, pons, medulla	Cat	A	Cortical epileptiform discharge.	Ralston and Langer (1965)
	1000–10,000 units	5–10 μl	Neocortex, hippocampus, amygdala, thalamus, lentiform nucleus, reticular formation	Cat, Monkey	A, A	Epileptiform foci.	Gloor et al. (1966)
	1000 units	?	Caudate nucleus, thalamus	Monkey	A	Seizure discharges.	Walker and Udvarhelyi (1965)
	10,000 units	30 μl	Caudate nucleus, globus pallidus, putamen, thalamus	Monkey	U	Generalized psychomotor seizures, EEG spikes.	Faeth et al. (1955; 1956)
Pentobarbitone	60–360 μg	<10 μl	Caudate nucleus	Cat	C	Antagonism of anticholinesterase or carbachol tremor.	Lalley et al. (1970)
Perphenazine	100 μg	1 μl	Corpus striatum	Rat	U	Antagonized amphetamine-induced stereotyped behavior.	Fog et al. (1968)
Phenglutarimide	100–400 μg	2 μl	Globus pallidus	Rat	U	Potentiated amphetamine stereotypy.	Costall and Naylor (1972a)
Phenobarbital	50 μg	10 μl	Hippocampus	Cat	U	Slight inhibition of focal discharges.	Guerrero-Figueroa et al. (1964a)
Phenol	600–700 mg	10–13 ml	Frontal lobe	Human	A	Relief of carcinogenic pain.	Mandl (1951)
Phenoxybenzamine	2–16 μg	1 μl or crystals	Mesencephalic reticular formation	Rat	U	Enhanced lever responding.	Grossman (1968b)
Physostigmine	≃ 30 μg	crystal	Substantia nigra	Rat	U	Compulsive gnawing.	Smelik and Ernst (1966)

VIII. Master Summary Table (Continued)

Chemical	Dose	Volume	Site	Species	State*	Response	Reference
Physostigmine	60 μg	10 μl	Hippocampus	Cat	A	EEG spike discharges.	Baker and Benedict (1968b)
	70–100 μg	1–10 μl	Caudate nucleus	Cat	C	Tremor.	Connor et al. (1966a)
Picrotoxin	.02–2 μg	1 μl	Cingulate gyrus, gyrus splenialis, pyriform cortex	Cat	A	Local high-voltage discharge foci	Banerjee et al. (1970)
	.5–5 μg	10 μl	Hippocampus	Cat	A	Focal EEG spike discharges.	Baker et al. (1965)
	2.5–7.5 μg	<100 μl	Hippocampus	Cat	A	Epileptic focus.	Baker and Kratky (1967)
	3–10 μg	<10 μl	Hippocampus	Cat	A	After discharges suppressed by pentobarbital.	Baker and Benedict (1968)
Pilocarpine	5 μg	3–10 μl	Posterior hypothalamus	Cat	A, U	Reinstated hemicholinium-blocked theta rhythm.	Friedman and Wikler (1970)
Potassium chloride (KCl)	125 μg	.5 μl	Striatum	Pigeon	A	Spreading depression.	Burešová et al. (1963)
	250 μg	?	Hippocampus	Rat	A	Spreading depression.	Fifková (1964)
	1.25 mg	5 μl	Caudate nucleus	Rat	A, C	Reduction of cortical recruiting responses, decrease in firing rate of thalamic neurons.	Bureš et al. (1964)
	50–125 μg	.2–.5 μl	Caudate nucleus	Rat	A	Blocked cortical somatosensory evoked response.	Bureš et al. (1967)
	75–125 μg	.3–.5 μl	Thalamus	Rat	A	Blocked cortical response to sensory stimuli.	Bureš et al. (1965)

Drug	Dose	Volume	Structure	Species	Route	Effect	Reference
	125 µg	.5 µl	Corpus striatum	Rat	A	Spreading depression to amygdala, claustrum and pyriform cortex.	Fifková and Syka (1964)
	50–250 µg	.2–1 µl	Thalamus	Rat	A	Mydriasis	Burešová et al. (1966)
	375.5–1125.5 µg	1.5–4.5 µl	Caudate nucleus	Rat	U	Contralateral circling behavior.	Weiss and Fifková (1963)
	.22–2.91 mg	perfusion	Hippocampus	Rat	A	Enhanced evoked response; lowered focal seizure threshold.	Izquierdo et al. (1970)
	125–250 µg	.5–1 µl	Corpus striatum	Rat	A	Spreading depression in caudate-putamen complex.	Fifková and Bureš (1964)
				Rabbit	A		
	125–250 µg	.5–1 µl	Amygdala, pyriform cortex, septum, thalamus, superior colliculus	Rabbit	A	Spreading depression.	Fifková (1966)
	375.5–1125.5 µg	1.5–4.5 µl	Caudate nucleus	Rabbit	U	Contralateral circling behavior.	Weiss and Fifková (1963)
	.22–2.91 mg	<10 µl	Caudate nucleus	Cat	C	Inhibited cholinergic tremor.	Lalley et al. (1971)
	540–1080 µg	2–4 µl	Caudate nucleus	Cat	A	Focal slow potential changes; increase in unit activity.	Trachtenberg et al. (1970)
Procaine	300 µg	1–10 µl	Caudate nucleus	Cat	C	Abolished tremor.	Connor et al. (1966b)
	?	?	Frontal lobe (white matter)	Human	A	EEG slowing coma, isoelectric state.	Walter et al. (1954)
	1540 µg	308 µl	Globus pallidus	Human	C	Alleviation of tremor and rigidity.	Cooper (1954)
	20–100 mg	1000 µl	Globus pallidus	Human	A	Cessation of Parkinsonian tremor and rigidity.	Narabayashi et al. (1956)

VIII.   Master Summary Table   (Continued)

Chemical	Dose	Volume	Site	Species	State*	Response	Reference
Procaine	100–130 mg	10–13 ml	Frontal lobe	Human	U	Relief of carcinogenic pain.	Mandl (1951)
	500–1000 mg	250–500 μl	Globus pallidus	Human	A	Attenuated Parkinsonian symptoms.	Obrador (1957)
Propranolol	25 μg	<10 μl	Caudate nucleus	Cat	C	Antagonized carbachol tremor.	Connor et al. (1967)
	45 μg	<10 μl	Caudate nucleus	Cat	C	Reduced calcium tremor inhibition.	Lalley et al. (1971)
Pyridine-2-aldoxime methiodide (2-PAM)	50 μg	10 μl	Hippocampus	Cat	A	Suppressed DFP discharges.	Baker and Benedict (1968b)
Reserpine	≈ 200 μg	crystal	Substantia nigra, red nucleus	Cat	U	Compulsive circling, limb hypertonicity, hind leg tremor.	Nashold et al. (1965)
	≈ 300 μg	crystal	Caudate nucleus, reticular formation, thalamic nuclei, hypothalamic areas, mesencephalon	Cat Rabbit	U U	Increase in locomotor activity and excitability.	Nashold and Gills (1960)
	10 μg	3–6 μl	Caudate putamen	Rat	U	Contralateral hypokinesia of forelimb.	Dill et al. (1968b)
Scopolamine (Hyoscine)	7–10 μg	.8 μl	Hippocampus	Mouse (C57BL/6)	U	Reduced exploration.	van Abeelen et al. (1972)
	7–10 μg	.8 μl	Hippocampus	Mouse (DBA)	U	Increased exploration.	van Abeelen et al. (1972)
	80–400 μg	1 μl	Caudate putamen	Rat	U	Sniffing, biting, catalepsy.	Fog et al. (1967)
	18–31 μg	1–10 μl	Caudate nucleus	Cat	C	Abolished carbachol tremor.	Connor et al. (1966b)
	5–50 μg	10 μl	Hippocampus	Cat	A	Antagonized cholinergic spike discharges.	Baker and Benedict (1968b)

Substance	Dose	Volume/Form	Region	Species	Code	Effect	Reference
	20–120 µg	<10 µl	Caudate nucleus	Cat	C	Antagonism of anticholinesterase or carbachol tremor.	Lalley et al. (1970)
	75 µg	10 µl	Caudate nucleus	Cat	U / A	Failed to block motor hyperactivity and EEG activation caused by NMA.	Baker (1972)
	10–200 µg	10 µl	Hippocampus	Cat	C	Eliminated cholinergic after-discharges.	Baker and Benedict (1970)
Serotonin (5-HT)	≃ 19 µg	crystal	Lateral hypothalamus	Rat	U	Tremor, piloerection, stereotypic behavior.	Hadžović (1971)
	≃ 20–200 µg	crystal	Corpus striatum	Rat	U	Gnawing behavior.	Hadžović and Ernst (1969)
	≃ 20–200 µg	crystal	Substantia nigra	Rat	U	Tremor.	Hadžović and Ernst (1969)
Sodium (Na$^+$)	200–1000 µg	25 µl	Infundibular region	Rat	U	Paralytic-like condition, agitation.	Clöetta and Fischer (1930)
Na$_2$EDTA	110–165 µg	<10 µl	Caudate nucleus	Cat	C	Increased cholinergic tremor.	Lalley et al. (1971)
Na fluoroacetate	10–100 µg	10–20 µl	Thalamus, septum, frontal lobe	Rat	A	Convulsions, no death.	Morselli et al. (1968)
Na fluorocitrate	.115–3.1 µg	10–20 µl	Thalamus, septum, frontal lobe	Rat	A	Convulsions, death.	Morselli et al. (1968)
Strontium (Sr)	20–50 µg	?	Infundibular region	Cat	U	Toxic effects, motor impairment, agitation.	Clöetta and Fischer (1930)
	125–750 µg	12.5 ml	Infundibular region	Rat	U	Toxic effects, motor impairment, agitation.	Clöetta and Fischer (1930)
Strychnine	?	?	Amygdala	Cat	A	EEG spikes.	Aida (1956)
	≃ 200 µg	crystal	Substantia nigra, red nucleus	Cat	U	Compulsive circling, limb hypertonicity, hind leg tremor.	Nashold et al. (1965)
	≃ 300 µg	crystal	Caudate, reticular formation, thalamic nuclei, hypothalamic areas, mesencephalon	Cat Rabbit	U / U	Circling behavior, vertical and rotational head movements (when applied at a large number of diffuse sites).	Nashold and Gills (1960)

VIII. Master Summary Table (Continued)

Chemical	Dose	Volume	Site	Species	State*	Response	Reference
Strychnine	299.9 µg	10 µl	Hippocampus	Cat	A	Focal spike discharges.	Baker (1965)
	5–20 µg	1 µl	Cingulate gyrus, gyrus splenialis, pyriform cortex	Cat	A	Local high-voltage discharge foci.	Banerjee et al. (1970)
	25–100 µg	10 µl	Hippocampus	Cat	A	Focal EEG spike discharges.	Baker et al. (1965)
	300–600 µg	<100 µl	Hippocampus	Cat	A	Epileptic focus.	Baker and Kratky (1967)
	?	?	Amygdala	Dog	U	Paroxysmal discharges; convulsive behavior.	Aida (1956)
Tetracaine	20–60 µg	10 µl	Hippocampus	Cat	A	Antagonized cholinergic spike discharges.	Baker and Benedict (1968b)
	10–550 µg	<10 µl	Hippocampus	Cat	A	Suppressed focal seizure.	Baker and Kratky (1968)
	100–500 µg	10 µl	Caudate nucleus	Cat	U	Failed to block	Baker (1972)
					A	NMA effects on motor hyperactivity and EEG activation.	
Tetrodotoxin	.005–.25 µg	.5 µl	Hippocampus	Cat	C	EEG seizures.	Hafemann et al. (1969)
					U		
	.005–.25 µg	.5 µl	Lateral geniculate body	Cat	C	Reduced visual-evoked potentials, nystagmus.	Hafemann et al. (1969)
					U		
Tremorine	60 µg	3 µl	Globus pallidus, caudate nucleus, substantia nigra, red nucleus	Rat	U	Tremor.	Cox and Potkonjak (1969)
d-Tubocurarine	.2–10 µg	1 µl	Cingulate gyrus, gyrus splenialis, pyriform cortex	Cat	A	Local high-voltage discharge foci.	Banerjee et al. (1970)

	Dose	Volume	Region	Species	Class	Effect	Reference
	1.8–9 µg	6 µl	Reticular formation	Cat	C	Hippocampal spike activity.	Kumagai et al. (1962a)
	10–20 µg	5–10 µl	Hippocampus	Cat	A	Rhythmic spike discharges.	Endröczi et al. (1963b)
	4–20 µg	10 µl	Hippocampus	Cat	A	Local electrical discharges.	Baker and Benedict (1967)
	7–20 µg	<10 µl	Hippocampus	Cat	A	After-discharges suppressed by pentobarbital.	Baker and Benedict (1968a)
	7.5–20 µg	<10 µl	Hippocampus	Cat	A	Focal seizure.	Baker and Kratky (1968)
	20 µg	1 µl	Hippocampus	Cat	A	Shivering, focal spike discharges, cortical synchrony.	Feldberg and Lotti (1970)
	18–180 µg	6 µl	Reticular formation, hippocampus, thalamus, caudate nucleus	Cat	A	Seizure discharges.	Kumagai et al. (1962b)
	18–180 µg	6 µl	Reticular formation, caudate nucleus, thalamus, amygdala, globus pallidus	Cat	C	Seizure discharges in hippocampus.	Kumagai et al. (1962a)
	25–50 µg	1 µl	Cortex (gray), septum, anterior limbic area	Cat	A	Spike discharges.	Feldberg and Fleischhauer (1967)
Tungstic acid	?	4–8 µl	Caudate nucleus	Rat	U	Bradykinesia.	Spiegel et al. (1965)
	?	10 µl	?	Cat	?	Seizures.	Black et al. (1967)
	?	25–30 µl	Hippocampus, amygdala	Cat	U	Epilepsy.	Blum and Liban (1960)
Xanthinol nicotinate	1.5 mg	10 µl	Mesencephalon, posterior hypothalamus	Cat	C	Hippocampal and neocortical EEG seizures.	Yanagida and Yamamura (1971)

11
Emotional Behavior

I. INTRODUCTION

The enormous amount of laborious research conducted during the first five decades of this century on the problem of emotion has delimited many of the general anatomical and functional facts concerning emotional behavior. Detailed studies such as those carried out by Sherrington, Cannon, Bard and Dusser de Barenne, involving total or partial decerebration[1] or a more selective subcortical ablation, have given great insight into the general morphology of the regions required for the manifestations of emotional behavior (see review of Masserman, 1941). The concurrent investigations of many famous physiologists including Karplus, Hess, Ranson, Masserman and their colleagues have helped to identify most all of the recognized pathways and loci within structures serving emotional reactivity and autonomic processes.

Today there are over 20 theories of emotion which can be categorized according to their approach and their scope; naturally there is considerable overlap among many of these (Strongman, 1973). Only a few of the theories currently held in some favor by psychologists have any basis in neuroanatomical or neurophysiological fact, most being founded on black-box inference and logical (or illogical) speculation (see Arnold, 1970). Of central importance to the investigations described in this chapter is the research impetus given by Hess and by Papez toward an understanding of the role played by hypothalamic and limbic structures, respectively.

Between the two World Wars, Hess and his collaborators employed the method of electrical stimulation to delineate the zones in the hypothalamus and other diencephalic areas of the cat from which all the components of an affective rage response with its concomitant autonomic effects can be elicited (see Hess, 1954, 1957). Other workers have since found that an attack response could be dissoci-

---

[1]The word "decortication" is an anatomical misnomer. No one has ever succeeded in aspirating the differentiated mantle layers of the cerebrum defined cytologically as the cortex.

ated from an escape response as a result of the locus and parameters of an electrical stimulus (see Black, 1970).

The well known emotional condition of sham rage is observed when a decerebrate animal makes nondirected and aimless aggressive responses to itself or even to an inanimate object in the environment. At the other extreme of this remarkable phenomenon are the observations of Flynn and his colleagues (e.g., MacDonnell and Flynn, 1964; Bandler et al., 1972) who have pinpointed several distinct regions in the diencephalon and mesencephalon which, when stimulated electrically, mediate a purposeful biting attack. In this case, a cat stalks and attacks a given stimulus object in the environment with or without the typical autonomic manifestations of rage such as growling, hissing, or piloerection which usually herald a cat's assault. Thus, affective aggression or escape behavior can be clearly differentiated from a predatory kind of attack which may be entirely related to the animal's requirement for food.

The impact of the concept of Papez (1937) concerning the part played by the limbic system in the elaboration of emotional expression has been felt by numerous investigators. For example, MacLean (1970a; 1970b) has provided evidence that because of their rich anatomical interconnections, the structures in the limbic system act to integrate emotional experience. The visceral and olfactory representation in each of the limbic structures is conceivably required for the sensory and autonomic elements inherent in any emotional reaction. Figure 11-1 illustrates schematically, the exceptional complexity of the functional relationships between many of the structures implicated in the afferent and efferent pathways serving emotional behavior.

A. Chemical Evocation of Emotion

Unlike the studies done in the past with electrical stimulation or ablation, the main purpose of using chemical stimulation to elicit or suppress an emotional state is to differentiate the possible humoral substrates involved in the various types of emotional response. Although in its infancy, the method has exceptional value in the matter of chemically tracing the pathway in the limbic system underlying directed attack or its suppression. Of course, the possible coding of emotional reactivity on the basis of the activation of a given class of receptors has yet to be demonstrated. As in the case of the epileptogenic focus and other circumscribed morbidities associated with motor dysfunction (Chapter 10), a pathological emotional state may also have a chemical basis that revolves about some sort of local metabolic abnormality within a given subcortical structure. In this connection, another aim of chemically stimulating a subcortical area is to mimic a particular emotional or autonomic state.

Whether or not a chemical substance does reproduce the synaptic condition that triggers actual fear, rage or other manifestation of emotionality cannot be specified. However, conditioning studies and the prolonged retention of some

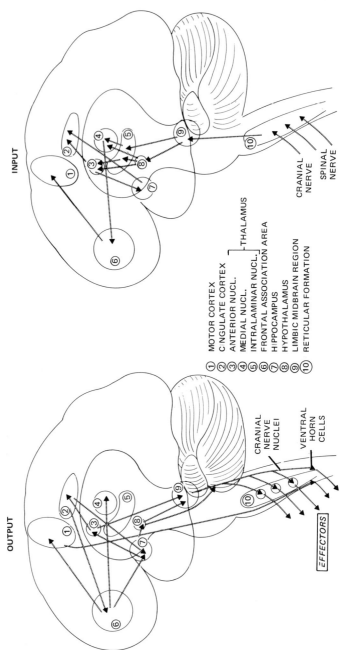

Fig. 11-1 Circuitry in emotional brain. Right, input; left, output. (From Jacobson, 1972)

aspects of the response would indicate that the chemically-induced emotional state mimics an endogenous or true response. Even though promising, this level of analysis is nevertheless subject to the same sort of problem of imprecise definition and difficulties that are encountered in other approaches in terms of measuring incisively the response of an animal.

B. Measuring a Change in Emotion

How an emotional change is annotated in a free-moving animal varies considerably from study to study. Intense experimental interest has dwelt on the reflexive-like responses that are easily elicited during an emotional crisis in an animal such as the cat. These include: meowing, howling, hissing, spitting, growling, ear retraction, salivation, sniffing, claw extension, piloerection, pupillary dilatation, nystagmus, cutaneous vasodilatation, tachypnea, tachycardia, defecation, micturition, hyperasthesia, vomiting, retching, crouching, arching of the back, agitation, gnawing, hyperactivity, trembling, tremor, twitching of vibrissae, pressor response, postural shift, furtive searching, flight, clawing, running, attack, scratching, biting, and killing.

When a given stimulus causes an emotional disturbance, one of the first consequences is a change in the muscular activity of the animal. This may take one of two forms. First, the animal may freeze on the spot and as a result, its motor response is drastically curtailed. If one is investigating the effect of a chemical on a particular limbic structure in a specific performance task, a rather ludicrous deduction could easily be made. For example, impairment in the acquisition of shuttling behavior in a two-way shock avoidance problem might be taken as an interference by the chemical with the learning process. Similarly, a decline in the bar-pressing rate for a water reward could be readily mistaken for an inhibitory action of the chemical on a so-called thirst center. Quite clearly, an adequate control is required which separates responses related to fear or aggression from those due to a transient motor dysfunction.

Second, a state of hyperactivity is as common a corollary of emotional excitation as is immobilization. If the chemical that is applied to a limbic structure simply triggers the central component of the autonomic nervous system so that other control mechanisms are overridden, the anticipated response of the animal may appear to be deranged. In fact, ongoing behavior such as lever pressing for an appetitive reinforcement or performance on a discrimination task would simply become desultory.

To assess objectively the internal changes that arise during an emotional response is a very difficult task. For example, a person may be able to disguise or suppress his own emotional state to a degree sufficient to confuse the recording of a GSR. One would never suspect that this state of affairs may also exist in the animal kingdom. However, after chemical stimulation of the hypothalamus, a rat that appears normal superficially may suddenly become a killer if presented with an appropriate prey.

Ordinarily, a state of evoked rage is readily apparent to any observer, particularly if the individual crosses the path of the incensed animal. Even so, this state is often difficult to quantify in numerical terms. Usually some sort of three or five category rating scale is used to define the magnitude of the behavioral responses. Of course, the duration of the reaction and the variety of symptoms can be tabulated somewhat more readily. Even more complex is the experiment in which aggressive behavior is examined. Great care must be taken to assure that an attack is either species-specific or nonspecific, since some animals will not attempt to kill a member of its own genus and species, but rather one which is lower or higher on the phylogenetic scale.

II. HYPOTHALAMIC MECHANISMS OF EMOTION

Because of its pivotal function in the mediation of every aspect of emotional behavior, the hypothalamus has been investigated more extensively with the technique of chemical stimulation than any other structure.

A dramatic account of the earliest report of chemically-incited rage was given by Masserman (1938b) who showed that the convulsant, strychnine, acted centrally to produce all of the symptoms of autonomic and behavioral excitation so well known from classical studies with electrical stimulation. After the powerful convulsant was injected in a volume of up to 100 μl into the hypothalamus of the cat, nearly all of the physiological components of the response observed in later investigations with more localized injections were described. These included the tremor and panting characteristic of a shift in temperature, cardiovascular changes seen after posterior hypothalamic stimulation, and the aggressive-defense reaction which follows lateral hypothalamic stimulation. In Masserman's experiment, the strychnine solution reached the ventricle and refluxed bilaterally over the surfaces of the third and fourth ventricles, thereby bathing the medial portions of the hypothalamus, thalamus, aqueduct and other structures that form the ventricular lumen.

In some cats, ethanol injected in a large volume seemed to enhance rather than depress the usual rage and fear response produced by electrical stimulation of the hypothalamus (Masserman, 1940b). Although the intrahypothalamic injection of ethanol had no effect on its own, these early data suggested that at a "strength well below toxic levels," alcohol enhances the reactivity of the CNS. Thus, in low doses it may possess a direct stimulating effect on the diencephalon.

From the results of another early study in which an enormous dose of Metrazol was injected, again in a huge volume, into the cat's hypothalamus, Masserman (1939) concluded that in contrast to strychnine's effect on the sensory system, Metrazol acts on the motor side of the diencephalic reflex arc. In a dose of 5 to 10 mg, Metrazol evoked vocalization, autonomic effects and rage. Obviously, systemic involvement of the convulsant cannot be ruled out in view of the absence of any localization of the action of the drug.

A. Cholinergic Rage

The initial observation of a hypothalamically-induced change in emotional behavior produced by stimulation with a presumed neurotransmitter (Myers, 1961) has been verified many times. Myers (1964) found that ACh or carbachol injected in a 1 μl volume or as crystals elicits all of those changes associated with a full-blown affective defense reaction. Elevated heart and respiratory rates, vocalization, salivation, pupillary dilatation, piloerection, fear and withdrawal were evoked by cholinergic stimulation. A remarkable attack by the cat upon either an inanimate object as shown in Fig. 11-2, or on the experimenter was not an uncommon occurrence.

The intensity of each of these reactions depends on the concentration of ACh or carbachol injected into the cat's diencephalon (Myers, 1964). Surprisingly, there is a noteworthy lack of localization of these responses within the hypothalamus; however, stimulation of sites in the thalamus, preoptic area, and mesencephalon or injections into the cerebral ventricle evoke other effects such as exploration, hyperactivity or a disturbance to the animal's motor function. Thus, Myers presumed that these effects are not due to diffusion of the cholinergic substance to a structure outside of the hypothalamus.

A micro-injection of epinephrine at homologous sites in the hypothalamus generally has the opposite action on behavior. The catecholamine produces a slight impairment of motor coordination, weakness, stupor, a fall in respiration, sedation, drowsiness and in some cats a compulsive or anesthetic-like sleep. The picture of such a response is exemplified in Fig. 11-2. No ingestive behavior is produced nor is sleep evoked by either ACh or carbachol.

Várszegi and Decsi (1967) have also reported that the rage reaction could be evoked by carbachol at any number of sites in the hypothalamus of the cat. Unfortunately, the volume of 5 to 20 μl that was used by the Hungarian researchers would render any sort of localization impossible. A large dose of one of several drugs that block either muscarinic or nicotinic receptors attenuated nonselectively the emotional display and the autonomic signs. Of several tranquilizers given systemically, however, none seemed to inhibit the cat's rage induced 30 minutes later by intrahypothalamic carbachol.

In an extension of Myers's (1964) earlier observations, Baxter (1967) confirmed the findings with cholinergic stimulation of the cat's hypothalamus. In addition, tests were carried out to determine whether crystals of carbachol deposited in the ventromedial hypothalamus would elicit a spontaneous attack on the experimenter. Even at the higher doses, Baxter could see no evidence of spontaneous attack in response to a glove as long as the cat was ". . . given the opportunity to retreat. These previously docile cats, however, savagely resisted being handled and vigorously clawed and bit the experimenter when attempts were made to pick them up." Electrical stimulation of the same site did elicit a well-directed strike and the cat did attack in response to Baxter's glove. The cat

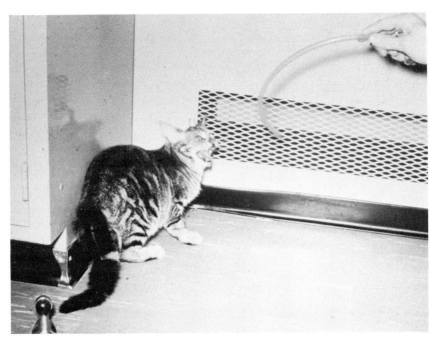

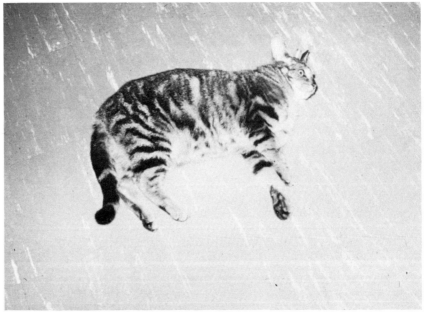

also captured and killed a mouse that was placed in its test cage. These data were presumed to indicate that different neural systems are activated by the two types of stimuli.

Electrical stimulation encompasses the entire continuum of an emotional response embodying both escape and attack, whereas cholinomimetic stimulation activates only the escape component. Baxter also found that carbachol crystals implanted in the third ventricle evoke the emotional reaction with a far shorter latency than in tissue, thus giving some support to a ventricular hypothesis. These latency results do not correspond to those of other investigators. Further, the sites where carbachol could exert a greater action than on the hypothalamic neurons is not known. It may be, of course, that simply more of the cells in the ventromedial hypothalamic region on both sides of the ventricle are being simultaneously stimulated, whereas a crystalline deposit in tissue may require some time for the recruitment of a large enough population of neurons to activate an emotional display.

1. *Arousal Versus Suppression*

Macphail and Miller (1968) repeated the experiments on cholinergic stimulation in an attempt to reconcile the conflicting reports that a cholinomimetic applied at homologous sites in the hypothalamus produces sleep (Hernández-Peón *et al.*, 1963; Hernández-Peón, 1965) instead of rage and a full-blown affective defense reaction (Myers, 1964). Examining sites similar to those purported to be part of the hypnogenic sleep circuit of Hernández-Peón, the results of Myers were generally verified in that the cat never showed signs of sleep but rather the manifestations of autonomic arousal and the rage reaction. Again, these responses could not be specifically localized by Macphail and Miller to any particular part of the hypothalamus. One explanation offered to account for the discrepancy was the use of crystals as opposed to a solution. However, this can be rejected since Myers (1964) used cholinomimetics in both forms. Since a cat may fall asleep in a quiet environment, it may be that adequate control procedures were not exercised. Unfortunately, the work of Hernández-Peón has never been replicated in its entirety with the completion of a thorough anatomical mapping of the responses. However, isolated reports such as those of Hull *et al.* (1967) and Vahing and Allikmets (1970) suggest that the injection of ACh into the hypothalamus of a cat can elicit sleep.

Fig. 11-2 Top: Cholinergic stimulation (10 µg carbachol) of lateral hypothalamus. Note pupillary dilation, piloerection, spitting, and a fear-like withdrawal to a piece of tubing. Pronounced hissing and spitting accompanied the eventual attack of the tubing. Bottom: Adrenergic stimulation at the same locus (10 µg epinephrine) results in proneness, pupillary constriction, and absence of emotional behavior. A sleep-like state persisted for nearly 1 hour following the 1 µl injection of the drug. (From Myers, 1964a)

What is particularly perplexing is the fact that Hernández-Peón *et al.* (1963) did observe signs of emotional behavior after ACh or carbachol was applied at some sites extending all the way from the septum to the mesencephalon. In a most significant but brief account, Yamaguchi *et al.* (1964) also found that ACh crystals produce sleep when implanted in the preoptic area of the cat. After carbachol is deposited at the same site, the cat becomes enraged even though the dose used was one-sixth that of ACh. Of course, these inexplicable results may have been obtained as a result of some sort of technical or experimental difficulty; or they may signify a very important difference between the cholinomimetic and the endogenous analogue.

2. Hypothalamic Localization

A similar replication by Vahing and Allikmets (1970) showed also that in the Russian cat ACh injected in widespread areas of the hypothalamus produces emotional-affective reactions. Quite surprisingly, they also found evidence of behavioral inhibition and sleep when ACh was infused in the dorsal preoptic area or in the lateral septal region, a finding contradictory to most others. Norepinephrine had significantly "weaker visceral effects."

In terms of the affective defensive behavior, Vahing *et al.* (1971) have demonstrated lucidly the considerable overlap in sites stimulated either electrically or by a micro-injection of acetylcholine. In an elegant anatomical mapping study, they showed, as indicated in Fig. 11-3, that the region incorporating the rostral and medial hypothalamus mediates growling, hissing and escape behavior. Cholinergic stimulation of the central gray of the midbrain and caudal hypothalamus elicits directed attack together with aggressive vocalizations. At some sites in the lateral hypothalamus, Vahing *et al.* again found that ACh causes behavioral inhibition and a diminution in the level of arousal.

Other corroborating observations on chemically-induced emotional behavior in the cat have been presented in a number of reports. Nashold and Gills (1960) described the severe autonomic signs such as decerebrate rigidity, hissing, growling, salivation and pupil dilatation after approximately 300 μg of crystalline carbachol were applied between the habenular nuclei of the cat. Neither sleep

---

Fig. 11-3 Top: Map of frontal section of cat brain at the level of hypothalamus. A—section across the anterior hypothalamic region (AP 13.0); Б, B and Г— corresponding to 1, 2 and 4 mm caudally. Illustration of sites in which stimulation elicits different behavioral responses. Left of midline (3rd ventricle)—effect of electrical stimulation; right—effect of micro-injection of acetylcholine in the same site; ●—affective posture and vocalization; ■—attack; ▲—flight with vocalization; ▲—flight without vocalization; Δ—orienting response; +—inhibition of behavioral response, sleep. Bottom: Schematic portrayal of frontal section of an average brain (AP 3.0) with localization of sites of electrical and cholinergic stimulation. Left of midline—effect of electrical stimulation; right—effect of micro-injection of acetylcholine (300 μg) in the same site. Symbols same as in top. (From Vahing *et al.*, 1971)

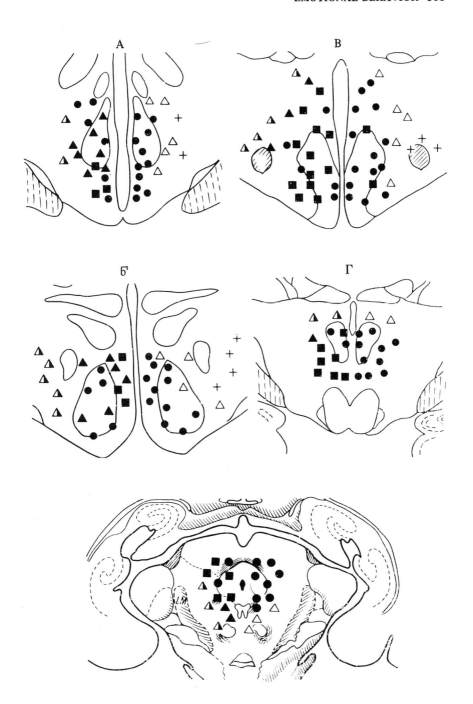

nor ingestive responses were noted. Similarly, Endröczi *et al.* (1963a), George *et al.* (1966) and Rudy and Wolf (1972) have noted one or more of the various symptoms typical of an emotional defense reaction after stimulation of the hypothalamus or other area with a cholinomimetic substance. In addition, Baker (1972) has found that N-methyl-aspartic acid is even more potent than carbachol when applied to the caudate nucleus.

In a succinct but carefully done study with the ring dove, Macphail (1969) has described a variety of unusual emotional responses that are evoked by carbachol injected in different doses into sites in the fowl's diencephalon. The bird cackles, pants, basks, vomits or attempts to flee from its test environment. Again, drinking, eating or sleeping does not occur. On this basis, one could surmise that a dove's cholinergic circuitry, at least in the diencephalon, is more like that of a cat than a rat (Chapters 7 and 8).

B. Blockade of Cholinergic Rage

Using the conscious cat, Decsi and his Hungarian co-workers have characterized very thoroughly the phenomenon of cholinergic rage, its dose dependency, pharmacological features and the highly consistent reproducibility of the response (Decsi *et al.*, 1969). Norepinephrine or isoproterenol given before carbachol at the same hypothalamic site partially abolishes the rage reaction; GABA applied similarly has no significant inhibitory effect. Thus, substances that occupy both alpha and beta adrenergic receptors seem to suppress the emotional reaction, and, in fact, may produce a taming of the laboratory cat similar to what Myers (1964) described as sedation. In contrast to the cat's attack on an experimenter following an intrahypothalamic injection of carbachol, tubocurarine injected at the same locus causes the cat to become fearful, crouch and then try to escape from the test situation. The idiosyncratic posture of such a cat is illustrated in Fig. 11-4. Curiously, this flight response can be partially or fully inhibited by the simultaneous administration of carbachol and tubocurarine. Quite surprisingly, Decsi *et al.* find that these two potent stimulators of emotional behavior are mutually antagonistic, and given together, they evoke only minimal autonomic signs. By a prior injection of norepinephrine or eserine, the tubocurarine induced fear-escape reaction also can be inhibited. Further, as shown in Fig. 11-5, carbachol itself can suppress carbachol-induced rage if the cholinomimetic is given at a discrete site in the hippocampus or amygdala before it is injected into the hypothalamus. These important observations serve to illustrate the astounding complexity of the receptor system that mediates these autonomic and emotional responses. They further suggest that anatomically independent ACh systems are capable of functionally suppressing or switching on the state of enraged behavior.

The cat's emotional threat reaction of spitting and growling provoked by an injection of ACh into the hypothalamus can be blocked by the systemic ad-

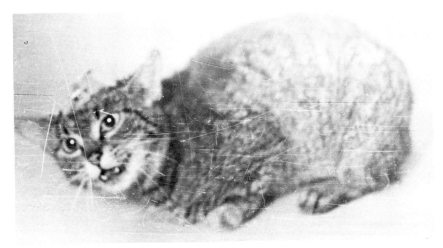

Fig. 11-4 Fear-and-escape reaction evoked by the intrahypothalamic injection of *d*-tubocurarine. (From Decsi and Várszegi, 1971)

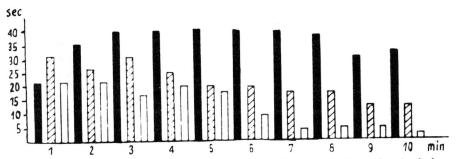

Fig. 11-5 Inhibition of the hypothalamic rage reaction by injection of carbachol into the central amygdaloid nucleus, measured at one minute intervals. Black columns, 2.5 μg carbachol injected into the hypothalamus; striated columns, 2.5 μg carbachol injected into the central amygdaloid nucleus + 2.5 μg carbachol injected into the hypothalamus; white columns, 5 μg carbachol injected into the central amygdaloid nucleus + 2.5 μg carbachol injected into the hypothalamus. Abscissa: time in minutes after the injection. Ordinate: duration of the rage reaction. (From Decsi and Várszegi, 1971)

ministration of either benactyzine or atropine (Kurochkin and Burov, 1971). A corresponding dose of other drugs given similarly, such as chlorpromazine, haloperidol, meprobamate, morphine or chlordiazepoxide, is without effect. Pharmacologically, the cholinergic rage response thus appears to be mediated through a pathway involving muscarinic receptors.

A prior systemic injection of atropine, scopolamine or phentolamine also antagonizes the cholinergic emotional reaction induced by a high dose of acetyl-

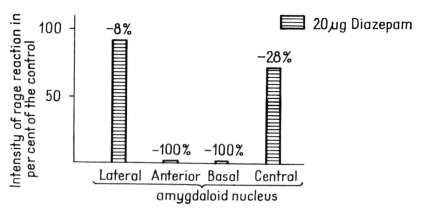

Fig. 11-6 Inhibition of the rage reaction by injections of diazepam into the amygdaloid nucleus. (From Decsi and Várszegi, 1971)

choline in the 200 to 300 μg range (Allikmets, 1972). This affective defense reaction, aggressive growling and escape behavior, produced in the cat when ACh is micro-injected into the anterior or central part of the hypothalamus, is not significantly diminished by systemic propranolol, methysergide or haloperidol. Part of the hypothalamic trigger mechanism for rage that may be mediated through a muscarinic receptor is again confirmed. In addition, an alpha adrenergic system could be responsible for part of the motor component or afferent manifestations of this behavior.

Although Decsi and Várszegi (1971) have found that most major tranquilizers given systemically to the cat are not capable of preventing the carbachol-induced rage reaction, they did discover that one of the minor tranquilizers has a mollifying effect. When diazepam is infused into either the hypothalamus or amygdala, the carbachol rage reaction is attenuated in a dose-dependent fashion. Thus, diazepam possesses the action of two classes of compounds in mimicking cholinergic stimulation of the amygdala on the one hand and adrenergic stimulation of the hypothalamus on the other. Figure 11-6 shows the remarkable anatomical specificity of diazepam's action in terms of the magnitude of rage suppression when the drug was injected into different nuclei of the amygdala.

Other compounds given systemically can also suppress the emotional display evoked by acetylcholine injected either into the hypothalamus or mesencephalon. Two tricyclic antidepressants, imipramine or amitriptyline, as well as related psychotropic drugs such as benactyzine, chlorprothixene or levomepromazine are effective to some degree when given systemically (Vahing et al., 1972).

C. Curare and Other Substances

As described in the previous section, fear and flight reactions are produced by an injection of d-tubocurarine into the hypothalamus of the cat (Decsi and

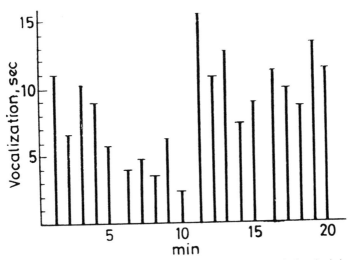

Fig. 11-7 Abscissa: time in minutes after the intrahypothalamic injection of 5 μg of d-tubocurarine. Ordinate: duration of vocalization at one minute intervals (Cat). (From Decsi and Várszegi, 1969)

Várszegi, 1969). The escape behavior is never accompanied by an aggressive reaction which is quite dissimilar to that produced by stimulation of a similar area with a cholinomimetic (Myers, 1964). As shown in Fig. 11-7, persistent vocalizations characterize the symptoms of tubocurarine-induced emotional behavior. Although the region of maximal sensitivity to tubocurarine is purportedly the anteromedial hypothalamus, the large volume injected would preclude precise localization. In fact, Decsi and Várszegi found that tubocurarine also evokes the flight response when injected into the posterior region of the hypothalamus. The marked tachypnea observed could be due to tubocurarine's local swamping of receptor sites. This in turn would block the cat's anterior or posterior hypothalamic mechanisms for heat production, which are probably cholinergic, and activate subsequently one of the most effective physiological means of dissipating heat—hyperventilation.

Hypothalamic stimulation of isolated sites with a solution containing an excess in sodium ions produces emotional and autonomic changes in the cat (Veale and Myers, 1971). Most of the sites are localized in the posterior portion of the hypothalamus as designated in Fig. 11-8. A description of these striking changes is as follows:

"... . Typically, the emotional response began about 4-6 minutes after the start of the perfusion with sodium. At this time, the pupils began to dilate and a few minutes later the cat began to lick and swallow repeatedly. Then, the animal became alert and alternated between periods of extreme excitability and complete motionless-

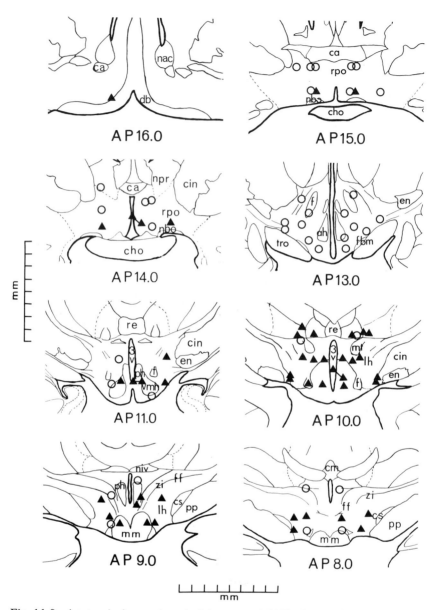

Fig. 11-8 Anatomical mapping at eight coronal (AP) planes of sites within the hypothalamus of the cat at which sodium ions, perfused by means of push-pull cannulae, 34.0 to 88.0 mM in excess of the concentration of extracellular fluid, produced signs of the affective defense reaction (▲). The sites at which excess sodium failed to elicit signs of autonomic or emotional responses are represented by (○). The scales are in millimeters. ah, anterior hypothalamic area; ca, anterior commissure; cho, optic chiasm; cin, internal capsule; cm, central medial nucleus

ness, the latter becoming less frequent as the perfusion continued. At this point, the ears became warm, reflecting vasodilatation, the respiratory rate increased unusually from 30-40 per minute to 80-100 per minute and the cat sometimes urinated and defecated. During several of these experiments, the cat had to be restrained or returned to its transport cage as shown in Fig. 11-9, because of the extreme difficulty in holding the hyperactive animal and retaining the push-pull cannula assemblies within the guide tubes. Then the perfusion was terminated immediately. Clawing, meowing and piloerection were regularly elicited during the latter stages of this defense reaction.

At the end of the perfusion period, the respiratory rate frequently reached 140-170 per minute, but in a few experiments, increased to 240 per minute to become indistinguishable from panting. The cat circled around the cage, hissing and growling, and appeared to search for a way to escape from the cage. If approached, the cat would attempt to attack the experimenter's hand, arm or even a glove. Ataxia, salivation, nystagmus, constant meowing, crouching and persistent searching behavior were also characteristic of this reaction. The maximum change in emotional behavior was usually reached approximately 5-15 minutes after the end of the perfusion, and then the response gradually subsided over the next 30-60 minutes. During a fully developed defense reaction, body temperature fell by as much as 2.0-2.5°C due to profound dilation of the ear vessels and a marked tachypnea. Then the ear vessels became constricted and strong shivering often accompanied the return of body temperature to its base-line level. When all signs of the sodium-induced rage response had abated, the cat usually curled up and began to sleep."

As in the case of the temperature responses following a localized alteration of the ratio of sodium to calcium (Chapter 6), the neuronal specificity of these cation-induced changes has not as yet been fully documented.

An injection of a large volume of L-glutamate into the hypothalamus of a cat causes the same responses as those produced by electrical stimulation of the same sites: hissing, an attack of a rat and escape or flight behavior (Brody *et al.*,

---

of the thalamus; cs, subthalamic nucleus; db, diagonal band of Broca; en, endopeduncular nucleus; f, fornix; fbm, medial forebrain bundle; ff, fields of Forel; lh, lateral hypothalamic area; mm, medial mammillary body; mt, mammillothalamic tract; nac, nucleus accumbens; nbo, supraoptic nucleus; niv, interventricular nucleus of the thalamus; npr, prothalamic nucleus; ph, posterior hypothalamic area; pp, cerebral peduncle; re, nucleus reuniens; rpo, preoptic tract; vmh, ventromedial nucleus; zi, zona incerta; 3v, third ventricle. (From Veale and Myers, 1971)

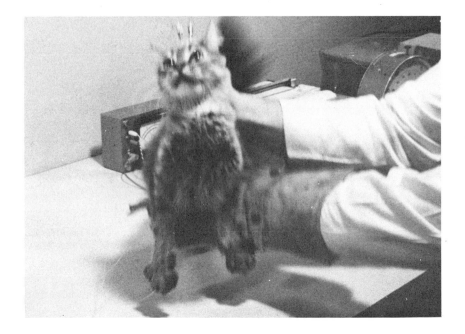

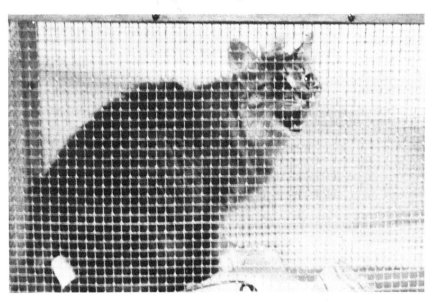

Fig. 11-9 Emotional behavior exhibited by a cat during (top) and after (bottom) the posterior hypothalamus was perfused with sodium 34.0 mM above that of the normal value. Restraint was necessary as the animal attempted to escape. (From Veale and Myers, 1971).

1969). GABA injected similarly reduced such an electrically elicited emotional display and the consequent attack. The relationship to a cholinergic emotional response or the specificity of the injection in terms of a control for mechanical disturbance is unknown.

D. Hypothalamic-Mesencephalic Emotional Axis

As is well known from the classical anatomical studies of Hilton and his colleagues (Abrahams et al., 1962; Hilton and Zbrożyna, 1963), the pathways for the affective defense reaction project from the limbic system caudalward through the mesencephalon. To answer partially the question of whether other areas in the brain-stem are sensitive to a cholinomimetic insofar as the evocation of the rage response, Baxter (1968) has examined the effect of cholinergic stimulation of the periaqueductal gray. After crystals of carbachol are implanted in the mesencephalon of the cat, the typical emotional behavior and autonomic responses appear. The anatomical sites sensitive to cholinergic stimulation are shown in Fig. 11-10. Interestingly, the latency of 5 minutes was shorter compared to Baxter's (1967) previous study of hypothalamic stimulation, but similar to Myers's (1964a) latencies after crystals of carbachol were placed in the hypothalamus. Electrical stimulation of the same loci also evokes similar responses including hissing, growling and retreat. Therefore, it is difficult to know whether the medial mesencephalon is one of the primary anatomical loci containing cholinergic receptors that mediate aggressive behavior in the cat.

Deposited in an area along the edge of the central gray matter of the cat's mesencephalon, a high dose of crystalline carbachol also elicits the customary changes in emotional behavior including hissing, growling and escape responses (Baxter, 1969). At these periaqueductal sites, the carbachol-elicited emotional behavior is followed by an intense burst of REM sleep from which the animal reportedly cannot be aroused even by strong tactile or other sensory stimuli. However, if an electrical pulse is delivered to the site at the tip of the cannula, the carbachol-induced REM sleep can be reversed. These results suggest that carbachol acts in the first instance to excite the neurons within the local region of the crystalline implant. Secondly, the activity of the cells is totally blocked probably because of the high dose given; this blockade can be overridden or circumvented by the electrical current. Information on a dose response, pharmacological antagonism and other controls would help to clarify the role of this part of the mesencephalon in the cholinergic emotional pathway.

III. LIMBIC MECHANISMS IN EMOTIONAL BEHAVIOR

Of acknowledged significance to the protection of the animal is the unique capacity of the limbic system to integrate the disparate inputs to each of its parts so that a unified emotional response can emerge. Not unexpectedly, several

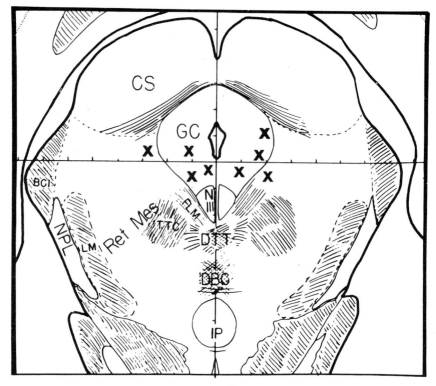

Fig. 11-10 Mesencephalic chemitrode placements from which emotional behavior was elicited by the application of either electric current or carbachol. For the sake of brevity all placements are shown at frontal 2, although some chemitrodes were slightly (up to 1 mm) anterior or posterior to this plane. (From Baxter, 1968)

structures in the limbic lobe are exceptionally sensitive to a chemical substance in relation to the emotional demeanor of an animal or human (this chapter, Section VI).

A. Hippocampus

In an early analysis of the effect of chemical stimulation of the hippocampus, MacLean and Delgado (1953) described perspicuously the fierce rage of a cat and its subsequent attack when ACh was injected in a large volume of a high dose into the hippocampus. After being scratched, the experimenter had to release his hold on the cat. However, within 7 minutes, the animal became friendly again and showed no residual aggression. The short duration of the emotional display probably corresponds to the rapid hydrolysis of ACh.

The behavioral manifestations of cholinergic stimulation of the cat's hippocampus do not necessarily parallel the electroencephalographic recordings

(MacLean, 1957b). As a focal EEG seizure induced by carbachol reaches the stage of culmination, the animal may appear stuporous and assume a cataleptic position without showing any signs of autonomic disturbance. The animal then displays evidence of extreme pleasure including the reactions of sustained grooming and penile erection on genital stimulation. In contrast to these findings, if carbachol crystals escape from the hippocampal site of implantation and diffuse into the lateral ventricle, the cat then becomes angry, circles and growls as in the typical hypothalamic reaction to the cholinomimetic. If approached, the cat sometimes makes a ferocious and directed attack upon the experimenter. Salivation, shivering and panting often accompany this bizarre perturbation in behavior.

B. Amygdala

Cholinergic stimulation of the amygdala may induce a relatively permanent change in the emotional state of the animal (Grossman, 1963). Moreover, the local application of crystals of ACh or carbachol to the amygdala evokes irreversible focal changes in the electrical activity of this structure similar to those described in Chapter 10. High amplitude, low frequency spike activity also spreads from the amygdaloid focus to the hippocampus and to the hypothalamus, and overt epileptiform seizures may occur within 10 to 15 minutes. After the cat exhibits signs of hypersensitivity and starts to salivate, a well-coordinated purposeful assault on another cat or on the experimenter frequently follows the seizure episode. Although this aggressive activity is similar to that found after hypothalamic stimulation with a cholinergic compound, carbachol's effect is much more intense than ACh and, in fact, can persist for up to 5 months. An attempt made by Grossman to tame such a cat has failed in that the animal is completely refractory in response to normal handling; however, there is no permanent interference with feeding, exploratory or other behavior. There is some evidence for the neurochemical specificity of the cholinomimetic's action since a control implant of other centrally active substances is without effect.

Different parts of the amygdala mediate different aspects of emotional and autonomic responses. Using surprisingly large volumes, Allikmets et al. (1969) have found that serotonin injected in the ventrolateral amygdala evokes salivation and vomiting, but at dorsomedial points, an exploratory-motor reaction. Although ACh injected into the same area has a somewhat similar effect, ACh also evokes emotional behavior including aggressiveness and vocalization. At three stimulation sites ACh can also cause an inhibition of behavior, EEG synchronization and sleep. The anatomical points at which serotonin and ACh elicited the responses are given in Fig. 11-11. Neither norepinephrine nor amphetamine injected in doses of 200 or 400 μg, respectively, has an observable action on the function of the amygdala. The prior pretreatment with systemically given antidepressants, imipramine and benactazine, or a tranquilizer, promazine, had virtually the same general inhibitory effect on the ACh-induced emotionality. After pretreatment with imipramine, serotonin evoked vomiting.

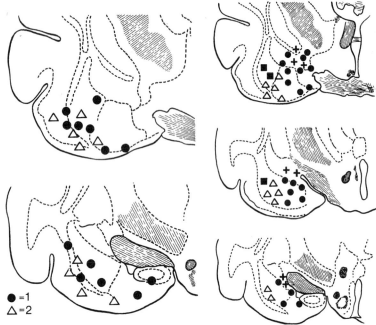

Fig. 11-11 Left panel—Frontal sections through the temporal lobe tip of the cat brain. Localization of regions in the amygdala where micro-injections of serotonin elicited exploratory motor reaction (1) and salivation-vomiting (2). Right panel—Localization of the effects elicited by micro-injection of acetylcholine into amygdaloid complex: ● attention response, + aggressiveness (emotional reactions), △ salivation, vomiting, ■ inhibition of behavior, sleep. (From Allikmets *et al.*, 1969)

Generally speaking, the amygdala would seem to mimic several of the functional aspects of the hypothalamus, at least in respect to those factors involved in the activation of emotional behavior.

C. Caudate Nucleus

When injected into the caudate nucleus of the cat in a dose of less than 4 µg, carbachol interferes with the ongoing performance of a learned bar-pressing response for milk (Hull *et al.*, 1967). This interference could be analogous to the inhibition of ingestive behavior produced by the cholinomimetic applied to the hypothalamus of the monkey; alternatively, the cholinomimetic may simply block select motor responses (Myers, 1969b). At a higher dose, an injection of carbachol into the caudate nucleus and several other sites, depicted in Fig. 11-12, including the anterior hypothalamus and thalamus evokes intense rage and the usual autonomic responses. A secondary effect is a fall in temperature due probably to hyperventilation, since the caudate nucleus is not a principal struc-

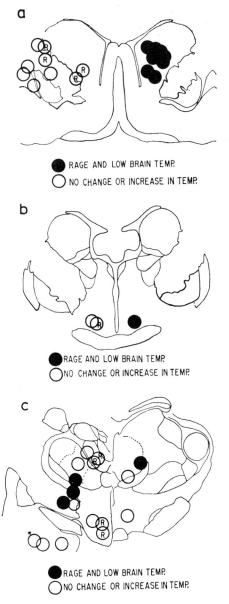

Fig. 11-12 Location of cannula placements tested for temperature and rage responses to "high dose" injections of carbachol. a, Section through caudate nucleus. b, Section through optic chiasm. c, Section through thalamus (right side of figure is rostral to left). ●, indicates rage and brain temperature decrease. ○, indicates neither rage nor brain temperature decrease. R, indicates rage but no decrease in brain temperature. (From Hull, C. D. *et al.*, 1967. *Brain Res.* **6**:22–35, Fig. 5. Elsevier Publishing Co., Amsterdam, The Netherlands)

ture involved in the mediation of hypothermia (Chapter 6). A ventricular hypothesis was first considered by Hull *et al.* to explain their results but they rejected this notion since sites at which the cholinomimetic evoked a behavioral change were often a considerable distance from the ventricular lumen, as indicated in Fig. 11-12. Since electrical stimulation of both the caudate and thalamic sites had the same general effect as an injection of carbachol, both procedures of cellular excitation could act on the same pool of neurons to inhibit or excite motor, autonomic and other pathways.

IV. KILLING BEHAVIOR

The upsurge in world concern about the violent outbursts of human aggression, which recently have had political as well as personal consequences, has led to the unquestionable desideratum of understanding the neurochemical nature underlying such an act. Many investigations are focusing currently on drugs which may inhibit homicidal tendencies as well as on the synaptic mechanisms in the brainstem which may possibly mediate the motivation to kill. Generally, the behavior that has been discussed to this point is referred to as affective rage or an affective defense reaction. In the animal kingdom, visible symptoms of irritability and drastic autonomic changes arise. The characteristics of predatory aggression are very different indeed. Autonomic responses ordinarily are not seen. In fact, the animal is usually quiet, stalking stealthily before it makes the kill, with the intention of consuming its prey. Whereas affective or defensive aggression may have negative emotional properties, predatory aggression probably is associated with a pleasurable or rewarding condition.

A. Chemically-Induced Muricide

On logical grounds alone, one would assume from the information in the preceding sections that ACh could certainly be a link in this exaggerated form of emotional behavior, that of predatory aggression. In fact, Bandler (1969) reported briefly that crystalline carbachol deposited in the rat's hypothalamus either evokes drinking or reduces the interval taken by a rat to kill a mouse or frog placed in its cage. Since both responses do not occur simultaneously, some specificity of the site of the cholinomimetic's action is possible. Because norepinephrine implanted in the same way generally increases the time interval required for the killing behavior to occur, a cholinergic rather than adrenergic link would seem to mediate the predatory behavior. Extending this study, Bandler (1970) showed that crystals of ACh mixed with physostigmine, or neostigmine crystals alone placed in the rat's hypothalamus again lower the latency for the rat to attack as well as to kill a frog. An intraperitoneal injection of atropine sulfate suppresses the predatory killing whereas methyl atropine is not nearly as effective. Thus, Bandler hypothesized that the stimulation with carbachol, although it evokes drinking when deposited at many of the same sites, is affecting a cholinergic mechanism in the hypothalamus involving predatory aggression.

1. *Anatomical Localization*

An anatomical mapping of the sites of carbachol or ACh-physostigmine action revealed a region of maximum sensitivity localized to an area ventral to the fornix (Bandler, 1970). Locally applied crystals of atropine failed in most cases to inhibit predatory aggression. This is not only difficult to explain in terms of the findings of Smith *et al.* (1970) but somewhat unique in the chemical stimulation literature. Although peripherally administered atropine obviously acts at cholinoceptive sites throughout the body, pharmacological controls are needed to account for a general excitation of the given site.

The dorsomedial thalamus is an area that has been implicated in aggressive behavior by experiments in which this structure was lesioned or electrically stimulated. In moving the sites of cholinergic stimulation to the thalamus, Bandler (1971a) found that crystals of carbachol facilitated frog-killing but not necessarily mouse-killing in a non-mouse killer rat. Although crystals of norepinephrine, serotonin, strychnine or Dibenzyline deposited similarly failed to alter the aggressive behavior, methyl atropine applied at the same sites suppressed killing of the frog. In some rats in which a hypothalamic cannula had been similarly implanted, atropine deposited in the thalamus also blocked the killing evoked by carbachol implanted in the hypothalamus; on the other hand, a hypothalamic implant of atropine did not prevent the thalamically-elicited killing. An anatomical summary of the sites designated in the cholinergic facilitation of muricide is presented in Fig. 11-13. Although confusing on the surface, these observations probably reflect some differences in the behavior that is actually mediated by an individual portion of the thalamus or hypothalamus, or alternatively demonstrate that thalamic signals can modify the hypothalamically mediated activity.

When sites in the rat's mesencephalon are stimulated by crystalline carbachol, predatory killing is facilitated particularly when the cholinomimetic is administered in the ventral tegmental area of Tsai (Bandler, 1971b). An astonishing finding was that a norepinephrine implant in the same mesencephalic area is reportedly as effective as carbachol in reducing the latency of the rat's attack or killing activity. This does not correspond with Bandler's earlier results in which norepinephrine was deposited in the thalamus or hypothalamus. When atropine crystals are placed in these hypothalamic sites that are sensitive to both norepinephrine and carbachol, the predatory aggression produced by carbachol applied similarly is attenuated. Although these data are suggestive of a cholinergic-noradrenergic system in the mesencephalon that carries the impulses for aggressive behavior, there are too many pharmacological and anatomical loose ends that require clarification before a definitive conclusion can be reached.

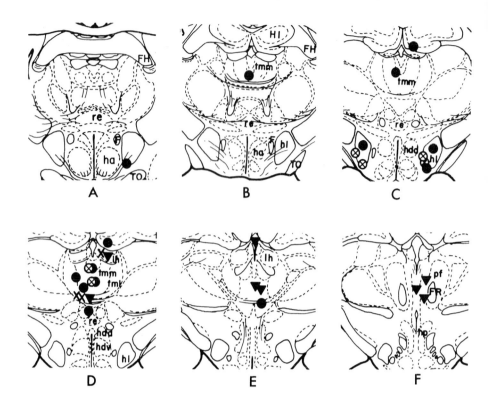

Fig. 11-13 Thalamic and hypothalamic cannula tip locations for cholinergic facilitation of aggression (closed circle), drinking (X), aggression and drinking (open circle with X) and no effect (triangle). Abbreviations: ha, nucleus anterior (hypothalami); hdd, nucleus dorsomedialis (hypothalami) pars dorsalis; hdv, nucleus dorsomedialis (hypothalami) pars ventralis; hl, nucleus lateralis (hypothalami); hp, nucleus posterior (hypothalami); lh, nucleus habenulae lateralis; pf, nucleus parafascicularis; re, nucleus reuniens; tml, nucleus medialis thalami, pars lateralis; tmm, nucleus medialis thalami, pars medialis; F, columna fornicis; FH, fimbria hippocampi; FR, fasciculus retroflexus; HI, hippocampus; TO, tractus opticus. (From Bandler, R. J., 1971a. *Brain Res.* 26:81–93, Fig. 1. Elsevier Publishing Co., Amsterdam, The Netherlands)

B. Pharmacological Blockade of Killing

The cholinoceptive mechanism for killing behavior in the rat has been examined in terms of pharmacological specificity (Smith *et al.*, 1970). In a normally non-killer rat, crystals of carbachol in very high doses of approximately 50 μg implanted bilaterally in the lateral hypothalamus evoke the killing of a mouse. Unfortunately, the protracted latency of 45 minutes to attack raises the possibility that carbachol causes a lesion, swamps the cholinergic receptor sites, interferes

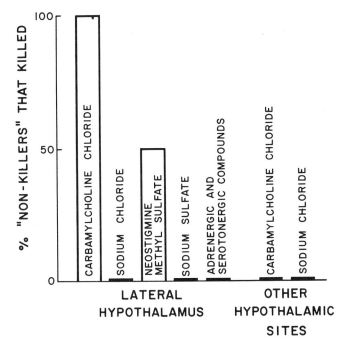

Fig. 11-14 Killing elicited after lateral hypothalamic injection of carbachol or neostigmine. Each bar represents data from at least five rats. (From Smith, D. E. *et al.*, 1970. *Science*. **167**:900–901. Copyright 1969, by the American Association for the Advancement of Science)

with the local blood supply or has other effects. As illustrated in Fig. 11-14, neostigmine given in the same high dose exerted the same effect, but with an even greater average latency of 165 minutes.

Contrary to the report of Bandler (1970), when crystals of methyl atropine were implanted in the rat's lateral hypothalamus before carbachol, the typical mouse killing response of a killer-rat was prevented for 12 to 60 minutes which contrasts with the usual 2 minute latency to kill. This difference is depicted in Fig. 11-15. Carbachol did not elicit killing when applied at sites in the ventromedial or dorsal parts of the hypothalamus. Surprisingly, the rat increased food but not water intake after a carbachol implant. Norepinephrine, amphetamine, 5-HT or 5-HTP injected similarly into the lateral hypothalamus did not affect aggressive behavior. This important study raises several important points, including the question of pharmacological specificity of the hypothalamic receptor sites, that are in contradistinction to Bandler's supposition. Again a dose-response curve would seem to be essential since injections of carbachol in a fraction of the dose used in these studies may produce an intense focal seizure (see Chapter 10).

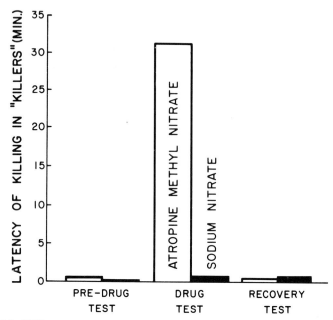

Fig. 11-15 Killing suppressed in five killer rats following lateral hypothalamic injection of methyl atropine. (From Smith, D. E. *et al.*, 1970. *Science.* **167**:900–901. Copyright 1969, by the American Association for the Advancement of Science)

By a blockade of cholinesterase activity and the concomitant endogenous accumulation of ACh at certain limbic sites, an aggressive response is also evoked. When amitone, an anticholinesterase, is injected into the septum of a non-killing rat, the animal becomes increasingly more irritable (Igić *et al.*, 1970). In 4 of 18 experiments, the rat killed a mouse. This change in emotional behavior is not so intense when amitone is injected into the basal amygdala and it could be suppressed by systemic injections of atropine. Just as we have seen with carbachol-induced drinking, it would appear that other structures in the limbic system may mediate a cholinergically activated system for aggression and killing behavior (Igić *et al.*, 1970).

Testing rats known to be innately muricidal, Horovitz (1966) found that either of two antidepressant drugs could prevent the killing of a mouse. Injected in a large 20 µl volume into the rat's amygdala, imipramine or thiazesim blocked muricide immediately for a period of up to 2 to 3 hours. The central efficacy of these two compounds is shown in Fig. 11-16. Chlorpromazine had no effect until after an hour and the inhibition of mouse-killing by this phenothiazine could have been due to the accompanying ataxia and generalized sedation. Since the antidepressants had little or no effect when injected into the hypothalamus or septum, the amygdala seems to be a focal region of significance in the intensely aggressive reaction.

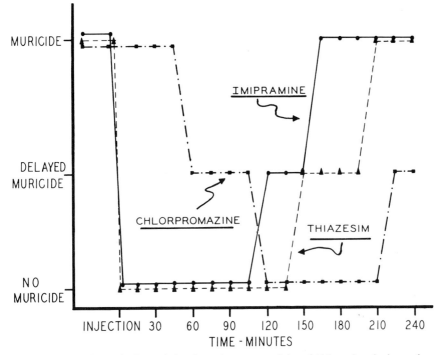

Fig. 11-16 Effect of direct injections into amygdala of thiazesim, imipramine and chlorpromazine on muricide. (From Horovitz, 1966)

The inhibition of mouse-killing can also be accomplished by the local elevation of a catecholamine in the amygdala (Leaf *et al.*, 1969). When norepinephrine or amphetamine is injected into the rat's amygdala, the latency to kill is protracted and the frequency of muricide is reduced. Amphetamine, which is thought to release catecholamines from endogenous stores, was more potent in preventing the rat's aggressive response. Again the neuroanatomical participation of the amygdala in attack behavior is apparent, with the synapses in this structure modifiable by an aminergic substance.

Ordinarily an intracisternal injection of 6-OHDA into the rat or an anatomically nonspecific intercerebral injection of 6-OHDA into the mouse produces lethargy and sedation (Scotti de Carolis *et al.*, 1971). However, a similar depletion of catecholamines by intracisternal 6-OHDA causes a marked and persistent increase in the number of attacks which one rat makes upon another when both are subjected to foot shock delivered to the floor of the cage (Eichelman *et al.*, 1972). An important side observation was the significant depletion simultaneously of 5-HT. Thus, an imbalance in monoamine activity in the limbic system as well as in ACh release in the brain-stem could be critical factors in the actual manifestation of aggression behavior.

V. TRANQUILIZERS AND OTHER DRUGS

The search for the anatomical site of action of a large number of tranquilizers and other compounds is usually carried out with the traditional techniques of lesioning or the recording of the electrical activity at different structures. One reason for this is that a tranquilizer given directly in the CNS in its synthetic form may have an irritative rather than specific effect on nerve tissue. Notwithstanding this possibility, several experimenters have investigated the effects of these substances injected into the brain.

To study the complex social behavior of a group of rhesus monkeys, Delgado (1962) has used a method of remote chemical stimulation by means of a radio-controlled gas-driven infusion pump mounted on the primate's neck collar. In one monkey, an infusion into the subthalamus of procaine in a large 4 mg dose and 20 μl volume did not inhibit the animal's aggressive search for a fight with another monkey. Even though some contralateral turning was induced by this local anesthetic, the monkey nevertheless jumped away from Delgado and consumed food avidly.

An antidepressant such as imipramine or amitriptyline, a neuroleptic such as promazine or chlorprothixene, and a local anesthetic all have the capacity to raise the threshold for EEG after-discharges in the amygdala of the rhesus monkey that are evoked by electrical stimulation of the site at which an injection of these compounds is given (Allikmets and Delgado, 1968). The attention responses of licking, searching and head turning are also modified by each of these drugs, but imipramine has the most powerful effect and procaine the least. Thus, the inhibitory effect of an antidepressant on a structure in the limbic system is not necessarily due to some sort of local anesthetizing effect but probably to a specific action on the metabolism or other chemical activity of the neurons in the amygdala.

Using a continual 3 hour drug infusion of a given antidepressant at the rate of 1.6 μl/minute, Allikmets et al. (1968) found that the electrical stimulation threshold shifts in a monkey in terms of the elicitation of affective emotional reactions that consist of agitation, vocalization and threat behavior. When injected into the mesencephalon or pons, three tricyclic compounds exert similar effects on attention and aggression, as shown in Fig. 11-17. Procaine exerts a much weaker action. The threshold for the motor reactions of the monkey including grimacing, turning of the head, or movement of the hands and limbs remained essentially unchanged by the infusion. Although it is possible, as the authors assume, that these large volumes are absorbed systemically, the similarity between the effect of an amygdaloid infusion of an antidepressant drug on the amygdala and on the pons or mesencephalon raises the question immediately of whether the solution escaped into the ventricular space and exerted the effect by this route. An equimolar dose of each drug given in the ventricle would resolve this issue.

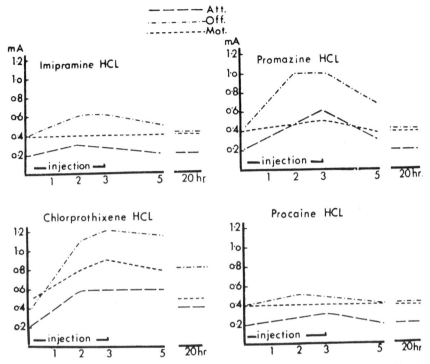

Fig. 11-17 Effects of local injection of imipramine, promazine, chlorprothixene and procaine on excitability of pretectal area. The effects tested were: attention (Att.), offensive-defensive responses (Off.), and motor reactions (Mot.). (From Allikmets, L. *et al.*, 1968. *Int. J. Neuropharmacol.* 7:185–193. Pergamon Press, New York)

Following the superficial application of pentobarbital sodium to the exposed surface of the hippocampus, the components of the hippocampal slow wave became depressed and eventually disappeared (Green and Adey, 1956); conversely, strychnine applied similarly potentiated hippocampal activity until spiking of the EEG waves occurred. After injecting a local anesthetic such as dibucaine into the hippocampus of the monkey at a rate of 8 to 14 μl/hour for 1 to 4 days, Delgado and Kitahata (1967) observed a number of changes in the electrical activity of this structure. For instance, the spontaneous pattern of EEG activity of the region of injection was silent or reduced for up to 4 weeks. The threshold for producing an EEG after-discharge by electrical stimulation of the site was raised up to 10-fold; the threshold returned to a normal level only after 2 to 4 weeks. Appearing in the hippocampus soon after the conclusion of a dibucaine injection was a spontaneous train of epileptiform discharges lasting up to 105 seconds. These locally recorded discharges did not propagate to other cerebral

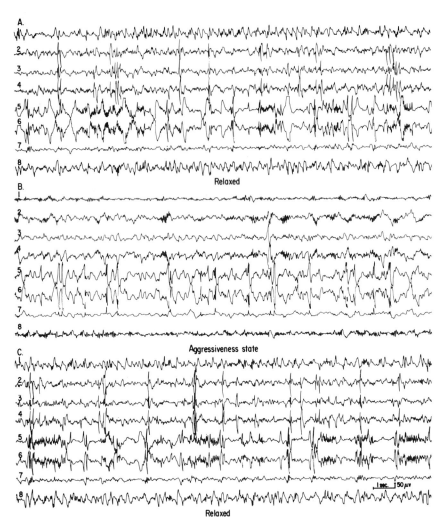

Fig. 11-18   A and C, tracings obtained during relaxed wakefulness from an animal after sectioning of interhemispheric communication and sectioning of reticular formation ascending influences to the right hippocampus. B, note the suppression effect produced on left hippocampal epileptiform discharges while the cat was attacked by a dog. 1, left sensory-motor cortex; 2, left septal region and left amygdala; 3, left hippocampus (bipolar); 4, left hippocampus and left amygdala; 5, right hippocampus (bipolar); 6, right hippocampus (bipolar); 7, right septal region (bipolar); and 8, right sensorimotor cortex. (From Guerrero-Figueroa *et al.*, 1966b)

areas and caused little change in the monkey's emotional behavior. This fact suggests that the area of stimulation does in fact possess a degree of functional independence. Surprisingly, after such large volumes were infused even at slow rates, a control NaCl solution did not affect the hippocampal electrical activity. When Delgado and Kitahata tested the behavioral reactivity of each monkey by presenting food, threatening the animal or striking its face lightly with a glove, the following clinical description gives a clear picture of the result:

> ... "After injection of 2.5–10% dibucaine, as well as with sodium pento-barbital and xylocaine, there was no change in interest in food, but there was a decrease in aggressiveness in all five monkeys, and the animals did not open the mouth, show the teeth, or bite the glove as was usual during control tests, and for several days after injection the animals reacted to threats simply by turning the head away."

The old concept of Hughlings Jackson that a violent aggressive attack made by an epileptic patient is related to a discharging seizure focus in the temporal lobe has been explored experimentally (Guerrero-Figueroa *et al.*, 1966b). Aluminum oxide was first deposited in the hippocampus of a cat so that both a primary and subsequent mirror focus developed. During any sort of emotional expression the spontaneous epileptiform EEG activity diminished substantially. Several types of emotional arousal were able to reduce markedly the episodic EEG discharges: sexual excitation of a male cat provoked by contact with a female cat; an attack by a dog; or the attack behavior necessary to catch a rat. As shown in Fig. 11-18, this attenuation of focal EEG activity occurred even following the sectioning of either the interhemispheric fiber connections or the ascending reticular pathway. It would appear that a diminution rather than an enhancement of convulsive electrical activity in the temporal lobe accompanies aggressive and other forms of emotional behavior. Thus, the clinical assumption relating an epileptogenic attack to assaultive behavior may be entirely erroneous.

VI. THERAPEUTIC APPLICATION IN THE HUMAN

Several fascinating avenues of approach have taken clinical advantage of the possibilities offered by the method of local chemical stimulation. Nearly all therapeutic measures used today for the emotionally disturbed individual revolve about the systemic administration of a psychopharmacological agent. However, several physicians have treated hospitalized patients for severe symptoms of psychosis and other disorders by the control injection of a drug.

A. Procainization of the Cerebrum

As a therapeutic alternative to frontal lobotomy, several neurosurgeons have attempted to block the functional activity of the white matter in the rostral cortex by the local application of an anesthetic. For example, Van Wagenen and Liu (1952) treated a violently assaultive, schizophrenic male with bilateral injections of procaine into the frontal lobes. The patient's usually fractious demeanor, including obscene speech and loquaciousness subsided into a quite calm, pleasant and cooperative manner. Shortly thereafter, however, the patient regressed and subsequent procaine infiltrations failed to effect a change. The result of a series of clinical trials with 20 psychotic patients was less than encouraging. Generally, procainization of the cerebral cortex and adjacent subcortical matter was only transitory in ameliorating the symptoms of severe schizophrenia. Hence, the technique would probably be useful only as a screening device for predicting the efficacy of a lobotomy if such a radical surgical procedure was called for.

In an unusually thorough clinical report based on only one patient, Myers *et al.* (1953) showed that an injection of 1% procaine in a 5 cc volume at 4 sites in the right and 5 sites in the left frontal lobe produced such marked improvement in a patient's obsessive compulsive disease that he was discharged within a month. There were none of the regressive signs usually observed in a patient following a prefrontal loboiomy. However, in nine other mental patients the response to this therapy of cerebral injection ranged from what was described as clinically "recovered" to "unchanged."

B. Chemical Transformation of Mood

In the severely ill human fitted neurosurgically with cannulae placed bilaterally in structures in the limbic system, Heath (1964, 1972) and Heath and De Balbian Verster (1961) have examined clinically the behavioral and EEG changes associated with local chemical stimulation. For example, in a woman afflicted with intractable psychomotor epilepsy accompanied by grand mal seizures, an injection into the septum of 400 μg of ACh or 140 μg of norepinephrine, both in a volume of 70 μl, elicited a dramatic change in her behavior (Heath, 1972). Within 1 to 2 minutes after the injection of either compound, the patient's mood began to alter. Her level of awareness increased and gradually she became euphoric. The elevation of mood into sexual responses culminated in repeated orgasms within 10 to 15 minutes after the intra-septal injection. Although concomitant spike and slow wave activity characterized the EEG pattern during the orgastic episode, the patient's personal reports were distinguished all in all by feelings of intense pleasure. One perplexing element in these protocols is the identical nature of the pleasurable experience evoked in the human by either the cholinergic or adrenergic substance infused into the septum. Pharmacological and other controls hopefully are in the offing.

An injection of ACh or norepinephrine into the caudate nucleus, hypothalamus or globus pallidus of a patient diagnosed as a schizophrenic was without any effect on the person's demeanor (Heath, 1964). However, atropine in a dose of

25 to 100 μg introduced into the septum or hippocampus exacerbated the patient's psychotic symptoms. The male became depersonalized, highly agitated and very irritable. In essence, pleasurable responses to chemical stimulation are produced consistently only in the human who is not schizophrenic, whereas the undesirable effect of an intra-septal infusion of atropine appears in nearly all of the individuals examined.

In a psychotic patient who, in addition, was plagued with uncontrollable psychomotor epilepsy, ACh injected into the septum promptly altered the patient's mood (Heath and Guerreo-Figueroa, 1965). The person's dysphoria and despair shifted consistently to euphoria and pleasure with each successive cholinergic stimulation. GABA injected similarly had no reproducible effect on the patient's behavior. The duration of these effects varied from patient to patient, but in each instance the palliative properties of an ACh injection into the septum were not permanent.

VII. CONCLUDING CONSIDERATIONS

Stemming from the very earliest observation of rage induced in a cat by ACh injected into the hypothalamus, it is very likely that a cholinergic pathway transmits the impulses for this striking aspect of the affective behavior. Cholinoceptive synapses seem to serve the autonomic storm of responses which are triggered by the artificial elevation of the level of ACh in the diencephalon. Similarly, the synaptic pathway delegated to a predatory, death-dealing attack seems also to have an unequivocal cholinergic component. An aberration in the level of ACh activity provided by a cholinomimetic can, in fact, transform a non-killer into a savage animal.

A. Cholinergic Emotional Circuit

The anatomy of the cholinergic pathway for the affective defense reaction as well as for predatory aggression may coincide precisely or at least run parallel with the amygdalo-fugal trajectory which has been delineated classically with electrical stimulation by Hilton and his associates and by Chi and Flynn (1968). Although the information is patchy, it is probable that the neuronal system of cholinergic synapses underlying emotional behavior traverses the hypothalamus and extends through the mesencephalon all the way to the spinal cord via pontine-medullary neurons. From the impressive findings of the Hungarian as well as Russian workers, the salient parts of the emotional circuit can be specified that course through and connect the hippocampus, septum, amygdala, thalamus, hypothalamus and mesencephalon. The fornix is ostensibly one of the key fiber pathways in the limbic-forebrain, diencephalic emotional circuit utilizing a cholinergic mechanism. In addition, sites in the fornical system are closely related to the cholinergic evocation of predatory attack.

Of notable importance is the possibility that the amygdala and hippocampus may possess definable nuclei or sub-portions in which a balanced release of ACh itself may act to suppress its own spontaneously-induced aggression. That is, ACh in other parts of these two limbic structures or in the lateral hypothalamus may contain anatomically independent cholinoceptive elements that inhibit arousal and subjugate an emotional outburst. Part of the mesencephalon in the vicinity of the periaqueductal gray seems also to possess important cholinoceptive elements. Interestingly, this particular region in the midbrain of the cat is relatively homologous to the one in which Adams (1968) identified single neurons that fire when the animal is attacked by another cat.

On the technical side of the fence, there is certainly no doubt from the work of MacLean, Baxter and others that ACh or a cholinomimetic agent injected into the cerebrospinal fluid may evoke rage by its action on neurons comprising those limbic structures that form the ventricular walls. However, two lines of evidence authenticate in a convincing way the anatomical specificity of a cholinergic affective mechanism. First, Hull and his collaborators were able to show that electrical stimulation of the same cholinoceptive sites produces nearly an identical emotional response. Obviously, electrical stimulation of the ventricular fluid would in itself be ineffectual. Second, the anatomical mapping analyses of Vahing and others attest to the unambiguous morphological segregation of sites that mediate at least three different affective reactions to cholinergic stimulation. Such a clear differentiation of each type of emotional response has begun to establish an anatomical groundwork for these respective changes in behavior.

1. *Receptor Specificity*

The characterization of the class of cholinergic receptors which mediate this behavior has not been accomplished to any degree of certainty. Yet from the studies demonstrating the peripheral and central pharmacological blockade of the emotional defense reaction, the muscarinic receptor is perhaps the most promising of the candidates. Preliminary findings on the prevention of muricidal behavior by drugs also suggest that the cholinoceptive receptor type that underlies killing again is muscarinic.

With clever insight and a break from sacrosanct viewpoints, Decsi and his colleagues have quite rightly proposed that *at least three* cholinergic-receptor types probably exist: nicotinic, muscarinic and tubocurarinic.[2] On the basis of their extensive experiments with agonists and antagonists, the muscarinic (M-receptor) sites are delegated primarily to rage; the nicotinic (N-receptor) sites mediate the autonomic elements of the defense reaction; and the tubocurarinic (T-receptor) sites are those that mediate responses for escape and fear. Three distinguishable functional systems are therefore subserved by three correspondingly distinct types of cholinoceptive mechanism.

The receptors in the pathways that are capable of assuaging or moderating the

[2] My terminology.

rage reaction may be alpha and possibly beta adrenergic in nature. All three of these cholinoceptive systems are antagonized in a similar fashion in that norepinephrine injected into the hypothalamus of the cat blocks rage, escape and the autonomic responses.

Which of the receptor types in the amygdala or hypothalamus is occupied when diazepam attenuates the cholinergic rage response is uncertain. Similarly, we do not know the endogenous humoral mechanism through which a tricyclic antidepressant, amino acid or anesthetic can act to alter the threshold of emotional arousal. In contrast to the local effect of a tranquilizer of the phenothiazine class, an antidepressant injected into the amygdala also suppresses an animal's killing behavior.

B. Catecholaminergic Mechanisms

What is the role of the catecholamine neurons in the affective defense reaction or in the manifestations of predatory aggression? Biochemical assays done by Reis and his co-workers (Reis *et al.*, 1970) of samples of whole brain or large fragments of cerebral tissue indicate that the level of one of these monoamines, norepinephrine, declines sharply during sham rage elicited by electrical stimulation of the amygdala or hypothalamus. Further, the results of several psychopharmacological investigations indicate that certain drugs including L-dopa and MAO inhibitors that can alter central catecholamine levels when administered peripherally facilitate affective aggression. As a result of these findings, a generalization has been made that a catecholamine may be released from diencephalic and other synapses to switch on the autonomic and emotional aspects of the rage response (Reis and Fuxe, 1969). Such an interpretation of these important observations may be false.

For some time now, it has been known that the elevation by micro-injection of the level of catecholamines in the hypothalamus suppresses emotional behavior (Myers, 1964) and may even tame an otherwise unruly cat (Decsi *et al.*, 1969). Furthermore, a micro-injection of an adrenergic substance or agonist into the hypothalamus inhibits the cat's rage induced by ACh. Just as important is the fact that killing is attenuated by norepinephrine injected into the amygdala. How then can we account for a downward shift in the norepinephrine level during rage? One possibility is that the content of norepinephrine declines as a reflection of some sort of compensation, in a humoral sense, of the monoamine in the neuronal network. This compensatory mechanism would be brought into play to offset or to temper the autonomic responses so that a balance in amine activity is maintained. In other words, norepinephrine may be utilized neuronally not to trigger the affective response but rather to attenuate or moderate the emotional behavior. Since the cerebral content of other amines remains reasonably constant during an emotional display, there is some evidence of noradrenergic specificity in the response.

In those scattered instances in which an intracerebral injection of a catecholamine has been reported to cause an emotional response rather than suppress it, the excitation of peripheral organs due to a large dose and/or volume injected into the brain cannot as yet be excluded.

C. Clinical Application

The praiseworthy achievements of Heath aimed toward the psychiatric usage of intracerebral chemotherapy to treat the deeply disturbed individual deserve special mention. A somewhat unconventional approach has been taken by Heath and his colleagues to alter the chemical function of certain structures in the limbic system so as to modify a patient's behavior. Essentially, the purpose of this endeavor is to (a) bring about an immediate improvement in the mental health of the patient and to (b) extricate whatever condition of momentary awareness is possible for the purpose of psychotherapy. As we have seen in Chapter 10, so many of the therapeutic procedures involving direct chemical stimulation provide only a temporary remission of the person's clinical symptoms. At the moment, therefore, the technique is useful primarily as a diagnostic tool for screening the profile of the symptoms of the patient so that another treatment can be undertaken.

In the future, these singular applications need not be so limited, particularly if the clinician would consider some revolutionary research ideas in addition to the traditional methods. To illustrate, a psychotropic compound that can elevate one's mood and prevent severe depression could be implanted in one of several structures such as the septum or hypothalamus. Long-term efficacy that is so imperative may be achieved by impregnating the compound in a slowly dissolving plastic material such as Silastic that is used as the carrier medium. In this way, a sustained release of the compound would occur. Naturally, there are many unresolved problems that offer a great challenge in this field. For example, the organic compound would of necessity have to be stable at a temperature of 37°C, which would rule out the usage of many substances that are potentially beneficial. Hopefully, the successful humanitarian usage of such a procedure outlined here is forthcoming.

VIII. Master Summary Table
Chemicals that Exerted an Effect when Given at a Specific Site in the Brain

Chemical	Dose	Volume	Site	Species	State*	Response	Reference
Acetylcholine (ACh)	?	crystal	Limbic structures, hypothalamus and mesencephalon, pons	Cat	U	Rage, convulsions, polypnea.	Hernández-Peón et al. (1963)
	?	crystal	Preoptic area, interpeduncular nucleus, tegmentum	Cat	U	Rage.	Velluti and Hernández-Peón (1963)
	≈25–50 μg	crystal	Hippocampus	Cat	U	Stupor, catalepsy, EEG seizure activity, grooming.	MacLean (1957b)
	1–50 μg	1 μl and crystal	Hypothalamus	Cat	U	Defense reaction, vocalization, attacks, flight, piloerection.	Myers (1964a)
	300 μg	10–20 μl	Hypothalamus, central gray	Cat	U	Attack, growling, escape.	Vahing et al. (1971)
	300 μg	150 μl	Hypothalamus, mesencephalon	Cat	U	Aggressive defense reaction.	Vahing et al. (1972)
	.12 μg	10 μl	Hypothalamus	Cat	U	Rage blocked by systemic atropine or benactyzine.	Kurochkin and Burov (1971)
	50–400 μg	5–10 μl	Amygdala	Cat	U	Autonomic responses, emotional behavior, aggression, sleep; seizures.	Allikmets et al. (1969)
	200–300 μg	1 μl	Anterior hypothalamus	Cat	U	Rage, vocalizing.	Allikmets (1972)
	500–2000 μg	20 μl	Hippocampus	Cat	U	Rage, attack.	MacLean and Delgado (1953)
	72.7 μg	40 μl	Septum	Human	U	Focal EEG seizures, contentment, euphoria.	Heath and Guerrero-Figueroa (1965)

*U = unanesthetized and unrestrained; C = constrained, confined or curarized; A = anesthetized.

VIII. Master Summary (Continued)

Chemical	Dose	Volume	Site	Species	State*	Response	Reference
Acetylcholine (ACh)	200–400 μg	70 μl	Septum	Human	U	Pleasurable feelings.	Heath (1964)
	400 μg	70 μl	Septum	Human	U	Euphoria; heightened awareness, orgasm.	Heath (1972)
Acetylcholine and Physostigmine	?	crystal	Lateral hypothalamus	Rat	U	Reduced latency for predatory aggression.	Bandler (1970)
Alcohol	100 μg	100 μl	Hypothalamus	Cat	U	Enhanced emotionality of electrical stimulation.	Masserman (1940b)
Aluminum oxide	?	crystal	Hippocampus	Cat	U	Mirror focus.	Guerrero-Figueroa et al. (1962)
	?	crystal	Hippocampus	Cat	U	Primary and secondary focus suppressed by emotional behavior.	Guerrero-Figueroa et al. (1966b)
Amitone	30 μg	1 μl	Septum and amygdala	Rat	U	Aggression, irritability, mouse-killing.	Igić et al. (1970)
Amitriptyline	500 μg	100 μl/hr	Amygdala	Monkey	C	Raised thresholds for behavioral attention and electrical after-discharges.	Allikmets and Delgado (1968)
Amphetamine	≃20–30 μg	crystal	Thalamus	Cat	U	Excitement and EEG activity.	Yamaguchi et al. (1964)
N-Methyl-aspartic acid (NMA)	10–100 μg	10 μl	Caudate nucleus	Cat	U A	Rage.	Baker (1972)
Atropine	?	crystal	Lateral hypothalamus	Rat	U	Suppressed predatory aggression.	Bandler (1970)
	?	crystal	Midbrain	Rat	U	Blocked hypothalamic induced killing.	Bandler (1971b)
	25–100 μg	70 μl	Septum, hippocampus	Human	U	Agitation, irritability, psychotic symptoms.	Heath (1964)
Methyl atropine	≃3–10 μg	crystal	Dorsomedial thalamus	Rat	U	Suppressed killing.	Bandler (1971a)

Drug	Dose	Form	Location	Animal	U	Effect	Reference
	≈20 μg	crystal	Lateral hypothalamus	Rat	U	Blocked killing in "mouse-killers."	Smith et al. (1970)
Carbachol	.3–2.7 μg	1 μl	Diencephalon	Ring dove	U	Emotional (fear) responses, panting, vomiting.	Macphail (1969)
	.25 μg	1 μl	Amygdala	Rat	U	Hyperactive, aggressive, seizures.	Goddard (1969)
	3–10 μg	?	Lateral hypothalamus	Rat	U	Drinking, reduced killing (mouse or frog) latency.	Bandler (1969)
	≈1–10 μg	crystal	Dorsomedial thalamus	Rat	U	Facilitated frog- or mouse-killing.	Bandler (1971a)
	≈1–10 μg	crystal	Lateral hypothalamus	Rat	U	Drinking or predatory killing or both.	Bandler (1970)
	≈3–10 μg	crystal	Midbrain	Rat	U	Frog- or mouse-killing.	Bandler (1971b)
	≈50 μg	crystal	Lateral hypothalamus	Rat	U	Mouse-killing in "non-killers."	Smith et al. (1970)
	?	crystal	Mesencephalon	Cat	U	Emotional behavior, growling, piloerection.	Baxter (1968)
	?	crystal	Limbic structures, hypothalamus, mesencephalon, pons	Cat	U	Rage, convulsions, polypnea.	Hernández-Peón et al. (1963)
	≈5 μg	crystal	Preoptic area	Cat	U	Defense reaction, rage, autonomic effects.	Yamaguchi et al. (1964)
	≈10 μg	crystal	Mesencephalon	Cat	U	Hissing, growling and retreat.	Baxter (1969)
	≈30 μg	crystal	Habenular nucleus	Cat	U	Growling and hissing.	Nashold and Gills (1960)
	≈4–24 μg	crystal	Hypothalamus, amygdala, hippocampus, septum, fornix, thalamus	Cat	U	Sham rage.	Krieger and Krieger (1970b)
	≈10–40 μg	crystal	Ventromedial hypothalamus	Cat	U	Autonomic and rage signs.	Baxter (1967)
	≈25–50 μg	crystal	Hippocampus	Cat	U	Stupor, catalepsy, EEG seizure activity, grooming.	MacLean (1957b)

VIII. Master Summary Table (Continued)

Chemical	Dose	Volume	Site	Species	State*	Response	Reference
Carbachol	.6–2.5 μg	5–20 μl	Hypothalamus	Cat	U	Rage reaction.	Várszegi and Decsi (1967)
	.14–3.9 μg	1 μl	Hypothalamus	Cat	U	Defense reaction, rage.	Macphail and Miller (1968)
	.6–10 μg	5–20 μl	Hypothalamus	Cat	U	Rage reaction, autonomic responses.	Decsi et al. (1969)
	3 μg	1–3 μl	Preoptic area	Cat	U	Growling and hissing.	George et al. (1966)
	5 μg	10 μl	Mesencephalon	Cat	U	Autonomic reactions, rage, fear, motor activity and escape.	Endröczi et al. (1963a)
	4–10 μg	1–4 μl	Thalamus, caudate nucleus, other limbic structures	Cat	U	Rage, autonomic effects, hypothermia.	Hull et al. (1967)
	5–10 μg	5–20 μl	Amygdala, hippocampus	Cat	U	Inhibited rage after hypothalamic carbachol.	Decsi et al. (1969)
	10–20 μg	10 μl	Caudate nucleus	Cat	U A	Rage.	Baker (1972)
	1–50 μg	1 μl and crystal	Hypothalamus	Cat	U	Defense reaction, vocalization, attack, flight, piloerection.	Myers (1964)
	≃300 μg	crystal	Habenular nuclei	Cat Rabbit	U U	Autonomic signs, hissing, growling, pupil dilation.	Nashold and Gills (1960)
Chlorprothixene	500 μg	100 μl/hr	Amygdala	Monkey	C	Raised thresholds for behavioral attention and electrical after-discharges.	Allikmets and Delgado (1968)
	940 μg	188 μl	Mesencephalon and pons	Monkey	C	Raised electrical stimulation threshold for attention, affective reactions and muscle responses.	Allikmets et al. (1968)

Drug	Dose	Volume	Site	Species		Effect	Reference
Diazepam	10–50 μg	?	Hypothalamus antero-central amygdala	Cat	U	Blocked carbachol-induced rage.	Decsi and Várszegi (1971)
Dibucaine	2.4–21 mg (slow infusion over 1–4 days)	210–768 μl	Hippocampus and amygdala	Monkey	C	Reduced aggressiveness, depressed local electrical activity, raised electrical stimulation thresholds.	Delgado and Kitahata (1967)
Eserine	?	crystal	Preoptic area, interpeduncular nucleus, tegmentum	Cat	U	Rage.	Velluti and Hernández-Peón (1963)
	5–10 μg	10 μl	Septum, anterior hypothalamus	Cat	U	Autonomic reaction, rage, motor activity, fear and escape.	Endróczi et al. (1963a)
γ-Aminobutyric acid (GABA)	?	7 μl	Hypothalamus	Cat	U	Elevated threshold for electrically elicited attack.	Brody et al. (1969)
L-Glutamate	1.8–7.61 mg	7–45 μl	Hypothalamus	Cat	U	Attack and flight behavior.	Brody et al. (1969)
Hexamethonium	50 μg	10 μl	Hypothalamus	Cat	U	Reduced carbachol-induced rage.	Várszegi and Decsi (1967)
Imipramine	50 μg	20 μl	Amygdala	Rat	U	Blocked killing behavior.	Horovitz (1966)
	500 μg	100 μl/hr	Amygdala	Monkey	C	Raised thresholds for behavioral attention and electrical after-discharges.	Allikmets and Delgado (1968)
	940 μg	188 μl	Mesencephalon and pons	Monkey	C	Raised electrical stimulation threshold for attention, affective reactions and muscle responses.	Allikmets et al. (1968)
Isoproterenol	25 μg	5–20 μl	Hypothalamus	Cat	U	Inhibited carbachol rage.	Decsi et al. (1969)
Mecamylamine	50 μg	10 μl	Hypothalamus	Cat	U	Reduced carbachol-induced rage.	Várszegi and Decsi (1967)
Methacholine	≃25–50 μg	crystal	Hippocampus	Cat	U	Stupor, catalepsy, EEG seizure activity, grooming.	MacLean (1957b)
Metrazol	5–10 mg	50–100 μl	Hypothalamus	Cat	A U	Vocalization, autonomic response, defense reaction.	Masserman (1939)

VIII. Master Summary Table (Continued)

Chemical	Dose	Volume	Site	Species	State*	Response	Reference
Metrazol	60 mg	600 μl	Hypothalamus	Cat	A U	Convulsions, apnea.	Masserman (1939)
Neostigmine	?	crystal	Lateral hypothalamus	Rat	U	Reduced latency for predatory aggression.	Bandler (1970)
	≈50 μg	crystal	Lateral hypothalamus	Rat	U	Mouse-killing in "non-killers."	Smith et al. (1970)
Nicotine	25–50 μg	5–20 μl	Hypothalamus	Cat	U	Autonomic effects.	Decsi et al. (1969)
Norepinephrine (NE)	3–10 μg	?	Lateral hypothalamus	Rat	U	Increased killing latency.	Bandler (1969)
	≈3–10 μg	crystal	Midbrain	Rat	U	Frog- or mouse-killing.	Bandler (1971b)
	?	crystal	Limbic structure, hypothalamus, mesencephalon, pons	Cat	U	Arousal and rage.	Hernández-Peón et al. (1963)
	25–50 μg	5–20 μl	Hypothalamus	Cat	U	Inhibited carbachol rage.	Decsi et al. (1969)
	140 μg	70 μl	Septum	Human	U	Euphoria, heightened awareness, orgasm.	Heath (1972)
	150–500 μg	70 μl	Septum	Human	U	Pleasurable feelings.	Heath (1964)
Phenobarbital	50–56 mg (slow infusion over 1–4 days)	500–560 μl	Hippocampus and amygdala	Monkey	C	Reduced aggressiveness; depressed local electrical activity; raised electrical stimulation thresholds.	Delgado and Kitahata (1967)
Procaine	500 μg	100 μl/hr	Amygdala	Monkey	C	Raised thresholds for behavioral attention and electrical after-discharges.	Allikmets and Delgado (1968)
	940 μg	188 μl	Mesencephalon and pons	Monkey	C	Raised electrical stimulation threshold for attention, affective reactions and muscle responses.	Allikmets et al. (1968)
	4000 μg	20 μl	Subthalamus	Monkey	U	Failure to block aggressive behavior, motor symptoms.	Delgado (1962)

Drug	Dose	Volume	Site	Species		Effect	Reference
	25 mg	2.5 ml	Frontal lobe	Human	U	Temporary calming effect.	Van Wagenen and Liu (1952)
	450 mg	45 ml	Frontal lobe	Human	C	Alleviated obsessive-compulsive psychosis.	Myers et al. (1953)
Promazine	500 µg	100 µl/hr	Amygdala	Monkey	C	Raised thresholds for behavioral attention and electrical after-discharges.	Allikmets and Delgado (1968)
	940 µg	188 µl	Mesencephalon and pons	Monkey	C	Raised electrical stimulation threshold for attention, affective reactions and muscle responses.	Allikmets et al. (1968)
Scopolamine	50 µg	10 µl	Hypothalamus	Cat	U	Reduced carbachol-induced rage.	Várszegi and Decsi (1967)
	75 µg	10 µl	Caudate nucleus	Cat	U A	Failed to block rage caused by N-methyl-aspartic acid.	Baker (1972)
Serotonin (5-HT)	50–400 µg	5–10 µl	Amygdala	Cat	U	Salivation, exploration.	Allikmets et al. (1969)
Sodium	39.07–101.1 µg/min	50 µl/min (perfusion)	Hypothalamus, ventral thalamus	Cat	U	Arousal, rage.	Veale and Myers (1971)
Strychnine	70–250 µg	50–100 µl	Hypothalamus	Cat	U	Generalized excitation, tremor, panting, escape behavior, salivation, vocalization, attack.	Masserman (1938b)
Tetrocaine	100–500 µg	10 µl	Caudate nucleus	Cat	U A	Failed to block rage caused by N-methyl-aspartic acid.	Baker (1972)
Tetraethyl-ammonium	50 µg	10 µl	Hypothalamus	Cat	U	Reduced carbachol-induced rage.	Várszegi and Decsi (1967)
Thiazesim	50 µg	20 µl	Amygdala	Rat	U	Blocked killing behavior.	Horovitz (1966)
d-Tubocurarine	5–10 µg	5–20 µl	Hypothalamus	Cat	U	Fear and escape responses.	Decsi et al. (1969)
	5–40 µg	5–10 µl	Hypothalamus	Cat	U	Vocalization, fear, escape, piloerection, tachypnea.	Decsi and Várszegi (1969)
Xylocaine	10.4 mg (slow infusion over 1–4 days)	260 µl	Hippocampus and amygdala	Monkey	C	Reduced aggressiveness; depressed local electrical activity; raised electrical stimulation thresholds.	Delgado and Kitahata (1967)

12 Learning and Memory

I. INTRODUCTION

How an organism acquires and then retains within its nervous system a new bit of information, regardless of its nature, represents today one of the most intricate puzzles in all of the neurosciences. In fact, the miniscule biochemical events that transpire as a stimulus complex from the environment impinges upon an individual set of neurons and an associated network of cells almost defy the contemplative resource of man's own brain.

The learning process, the motivational force behind it, if present at all, and the synaptic nature of perceived reward are three phenomena which are extraordinarily difficult to submit to a chemical analysis. Even less amenable to neurochemical quantitation are the mechanisms of experiential storage and retention, which are lumped customarily into a single term called memory. The reason for this is that the separate stages of memory formation as well as the events leading to the consolidation of a memory trace undoubtedly involve both transcellular and intracellular elements in many regions throughout the brain (Glassman, 1969).

A. Neuronal Processes

What can be learned by an injection of a certain chemical into a cortical or subcortical structure? How can this procedure help to unravel the intricate mechanisms of the learning and memory processes? To grasp the implication of these questions, let us first examine some of the essential points taken from a variety of learning hypotheses and memory models (e.g., Rose, 1969; Glassman, 1969; Ilyutchenok, 1969; Essman, 1970). Each of these points sets forth one or more of the functional attributes believed by most theoreticians to be requisite for the acquisition and retention of new information.

1. *Environmental Stimulus*

Sensory input from the environment must flow via an afferent pathway to a part of the brain specifically capable of processing such input. Unlike a retinal element or a muscle spindle, the area wherever it is located must contain cells capable of passing on or translating the environmental stimulus into a permanent rather than ephemeral modification.

2. *Cellular Events*

Within a finite number of cells, a biochemical trigger could initiate the gradual synthesis of new messenger RNA that is followed by the synthesis of new protein. The metabolism of protein molecules, therefore, is presumably dependent on the state of the animal. The protein may be of a new variety or it may simply be produced in a relatively greater quantity. Although the rate and cerebral localization of this protein synthesis are uncertain at this time, the new protein constituents could serve as the chemical code for a given memory.

3. *Protein Utilization*

To evoke a memory trace or perhaps inhibit its evocation, the intracellular protein code would have to be transformed into a synaptic event. This requires micro-tubular or other transport of the molecular species via axoplasmic flow, known now to be bidirectional, to the nerve ending itself. Here a mitochondrial or other interaction with the synpatic vesicles must take place in order to unleash a transmitter or other humoral material. This reaction alone is of primary, not secondary importance, because it is the key to the interneuronal recognition and subsequent communication with the very next neuron in a chain of neurons.

4. *Synaptic Reaction*

The presynaptic release of a neurotransmitter or neural factor into the sub-synaptic cleft would have one of several effects. Considering the polysynaptic nature of dendritic architecture, the next neuron or set of neurons in the chain may be depolarized; or their depolarization may be inhibited; or a reciprocal synchrony of both postsynaptic excitation and inhibition may happen simultaneously.

Several distinct possibilities surround the way a synaptic modification may take place. There may be: (a) a change in the activity of a particular enzyme; (b) an anatomical change that provides for a greater surface area of axo-somatic or axo-dendritic contact; (c) an alteration in the threshold for the release of a transmitter factor; (d) a lowering of the threshold of the postsynaptic membrane in relation to a reduction in the number of receptor sites that are ordinarily occupied before a neuron is discharged; (e) an alteration in receptor chemosensitivity; (f) or a combination of two or more of these alternatives.

5. *Transneuronal Circuitry*

The replication of a specific behavior requires the integrity of a well-defined system of neurons. Otherwise, a behavioral response would emerge haphazardly in a most random fashion. The registration of a learned bit of information or some sort of motor activity would seem to involve not only a conformational change in intraneuronal RNA but also a modification in the relationship between a spatially contiguous set of neurons within a given cortical or subcortical structure.

B. Local Action of a Chemical on Learning

When a chemical substance is applied to a subcortical structure, there are a number of ultrastructural sites upon which it can act (Chapter 1). If a collection of neurons is inundated with a chemical, one or more of the processes outlined in the preceding section could be significantly altered. Some of the sites and mechanisms of action of a chemical on neurons involved in the learning and retention of a task are: (a) the surface of the cell membrane which could change the temporal pattern of its firing rate; (b) the nucleus which could affect the level of nucleoprotein; (c) the cytoplasm which might alter the activity of messenger RNA, the synthesis of new protein, and the function of membrane-bound enzymes; (d) micro-tubules, microsomes or the process of axoplasmic transport; (e) the nerve terminal and its re-uptake, release or turnover of a substrate; (f) specific receptor sites, receptor binding and the catabolism of newly bound material.

Any of these mechanisms could have the net effect of modifying the activity of the neuron in an inhibitory or excitatory manner. One excellent example of this is the striking phenomenon of retrograde amnesia (or other form of memory loss). A logical possibility is that a set of cholinergic synapses in a vital pathway that serves a memory trace is inhibited (Ilyutchenok, 1969). In such a case, the basic pattern of a learned behavior is still retained within an intracellular chemical matrix. However, the trans-synaptic expression of this coded material is prevented temporarily, simply because the transmission of neuronal impulses across the synaptic membrane is blocked in a specific memory circuit or pathway.

C. Quantification of a Change in Learning

Probably a motor response that is being conditioned classically or instrumentally is exceptionally sensitive to any sort of central chemical manipulation, even more so perhaps than a vegetative function. Frequently there is no observable behavioral or physiological change after a chemical is injected into a subcortical structure. One reason for this is that the measurements which are taken may not be sufficiently sensitive to reflect what would appear to be an inappreciable action of a compound applied to brain tissue. However, when an animal is attempting to learn a difficult maze or other complex task, a subtle change in behavior following chemical stimulation can often be quantified.

1. *Anatomical Considerations*

Certainly many cortical and subcortical regions are intimately involved in the learning process. In evaluating the research described in the following sections of this chapter, it is necessary to consider the ever present possibility that a local chemical stimulus has either blocked or facilitated the passage of the sensory or motor impulse. Obviously, peripheral stimuli must arrive at a critical pool of neurons via an afferent route. By the same token, the expression of the learned response must transmigrate to an effector system via an efferent pathway.

A given compound may increase the sensibility of an aversive stimulus such as foot shock, or it may enhance the positive gustatory quality or particular odor of a food pellet. Should a neuromuscular deficit be produced by a drug micro-injected centrally with the result that the animal's movement is retarded or impeded, it would be very difficult to make a statement about the animal's subsequent inability to learn and just as difficult to describe an impairment of its ability to retain new information. Therefore, a control is always essential in order to be certain that the sensory and motor systems are functionally intact. In any case, the difficulty is always profound in distinguishing the effect of a chemical on an overlapping anatomical circuit underlying a particular sensory or motor system from a circuit involved in the solution of a problem and the registration of its solution.

2. *Behavioral and Pharmacological Controls*

The progression of learning a response ordinarily is measured by an improvement in the animal's performance, whereas the memory of the response is assessed by the subsequent duplication of that performance or relearning to that level. Regrettably, the absolute separation of one from the other is an age-old dilemma that has plagued the psychologist ever since Ebbinghaus. The control that is necessary to equate for a motivational state, in fact, goes hand in hand with the requisite pharmacological controls. The level of the animal's drive state is often varied, just as is the dose to be administered of the particular drug under investigation. Two normally motivating conditions can be contrasted experimentally to one another. That is, a natural appetitive response brought about by food deprivation can be differentiated with respect to an artificial one such as electric shock to the foot pad.

In a similar vein, the biogenic amines, amino acids and other substances are capable of altering synaptic function, no matter how complex. Therefore, at least two classes of drugs or chemical compounds should likewise be compared with one another and with a corresponding pharmacological antagonist. In the extreme, only a simplistic notion can be derived from an observation in which one dose of a specific drug is applied to a given forebrain structure during a single conditioning experience. In this case, a contribution to any sort of theory of reinforcement, conditioning process or memory mechanism would be irrefutably remote.

II. DRIVE AND REWARD MECHANISMS

It is almost a truism that the learning of a task is facilitated by some kind of a direct reward or a rewarding consequence of one type or another. The former may be as simple as a pleasurable sensation while the latter may take the more complex form of absence of punishment. From a chemical standpoint, we shall examine first the investigations which attempt to dissect the reward mechanism and then second, those that involve the punishment of behavior.

Perhaps the most powerful physiological tool ever used for studying the diencephalic substrate of reward is the method by which an animal delivers an electrical pulse to its own hypothalamus or septum simply by making some sort of instrumental response such as pressing a lever (Olds and Milner, 1954). The resultant activity could be regarded quite rightly in the category of emotional behavior (Chapter 11) particularly in view of the reports of the human patient. Each person who has perceived the pleasurable feeling associated with the self-delivery of electric current to his own septal nucleus describes the phenomenon as an ecstatic emotional experience. In this chapter, however, the behavior will be arbitrarily considered as a part of the functional substrate for reward.

A. Self-Stimulation

The interaction of rewarding self-stimulation with feeding and other behavior elicited by electric current (e.g., Hoebel and Teitelbaum, 1962; Krasne, 1962) has given rise to the possibility that a condition of generalized drive is engendered by the rewarding stimulus. This view is held in spite of the fact that the state of hunger is a highly negative one. Bearing on this question is the important study of Olds *et al.* (1971) who found that both a drive effect as reflected in the rat's eating and drinking, and a reward effect as indicated by self-stimulation behavior were produced simultaneously by electrical stimulation. The anatomical site of the intermingled reactions is illustrated in Fig. 12-1 and encompasses the medial forebrain bundle where it is crossed by perpendicular fibers from the ventromedial hypothalamus and basal ganglia. The drive responses alone were evoked by stimulation of the region dorsal to the medial forebrain bundle (Fig. 12-1), whereas the reward effect was localized to other parts of this fiber system.

Based on experiments on the peripheral action on self-stimulation behavior of agonists and antagonists of acetylcholine, the view could be adopted that the cholinergic synapse or pathway generally inhibits this behavior (Olds and Domino, 1969). For example, self-stimulation of the postero-lateral hypothalamus is suppressed by drugs such as arecoline or physostigmine given systemically. Of course, there is the possibility that raising the endogenous level of ACh in

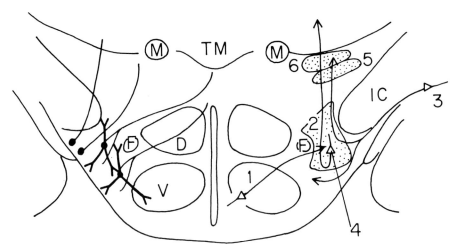

Fig. 12-1 Schematic drawings of fiber systems possibly involved in the mixed reward-and-drive effects and in pure drive effects. Fiber systems in mixed area = 1: medial-to-lateral hypothalamic fibers; 2: descending medial forebrain bundle (mfb) fibers; 3: basal ganglia-to-lateral hypothalamic fibers from globus pallidus and amygdala; 4: axons of mfb path neurons. Fiber systems in pure area = 3: basal ganglia-to-lateral hypothalamic fibers; 4: axons of mfb path neurons; 5: ascending reticular axons; 6: descending extrapyramidal fibers. Although fornix (F) is interdigitated with some mixed area fibers, it is probably not involved; and although mammillo-thalamic tract (M) is near pure set, it is probably not involved. TM, medial thalamus; D, dorsomedial nucleus of hypo-thalamus; V, ventromedial nucleus of hypothalamus. Drawing is based on that of Millhouse (1969) and some configurations of mfb path neurons suggested by him are indicated on left. (From Olds et al., 1971)

the CNS super-sensitizes the neurons so that a previously reinforcing electrical pulse is transformed into an aversive one.

Although taking no precautions against the effect of an immense volume, Olds and Olds (1958) carried out an important early study which showed that an MAO inhibitor, iproniazid, is apparently reinforcing to neurons in the posterior part of the hypothalamus. Each rat in their study depressed a lever to obtain an injection of 1.4 μl of 0.1% solution of iproniazid. In the course of a 20 minute test session, one rat responded nearly 300 times, thereby receiving 400 μl in its hypothalamus. For the next 20 minute extinction period during which time a lever press failed to cause an iproniazid injection, the rat nevertheless continued to emit operant responses at about the same rate. Solutions of saline, ATP or epinephrine self-injected again in the same huge volume had no such reinforcing effect. With this investigation, the first instance of behavior rewarded by a chemical infused into the brain-stem was demonstrated. Later, Morgane (1962) and Myers (1963) both reported very briefly that the self-injection of a cholinergic substance into the hypothalamus of a rat that was contingent on a lever press was rewarding; unfortunately, quantitative data were not given by either worker.

In a later more extensive study, Olds *et al.* (1964) employed an enormous number of animals, chemicals and conditions. A variety of chemicals self-injected into the hypothalamus when the rat depressed a lever were found to reinforce or attenuate the operant responding of the animal. When a tiny volume of 0.003 μl was injected into the postero-lateral hypothalamus after each lever press, carbachol and substances that chelate calcium such as NaEDTA evoked the highest self-stimulation rates. Records of carbachol-induced self-stimulation are illustrated in Fig. 12-2. A number of neurohumoral substances including epinephrine, norepinephrine, serotonin and GABA counteracted the excitatory effect of the NaEDTA and the other chelating salts. Although no pharmacological blocking agents were used, the findings of Olds *et al.* suggest that a cholinergic substrate underlying rewarded behavior does exist at the level of the hypothalamus. Contrary to the hypotheses pertaining to the cholinergic inhibition of the reward mechanism, ACh seems to possess an excitatory property in the reward system since the rat would self-inject a trivial amount of carbachol into its lateral hypothalamus. Surprisingly, both the catecholamines and indoleamines which have been found to have opposing effects on other functions, acted similarly to depress self-stimulation behavior when they were self-injected again into the lateral hypothalamic area in minute quantities.

When crystalline carbachol is implanted in the mesencephalon in the region of the dorsal tegmentum, electrical self-stimulation of the hypothalamus is suppressed by 90%, whereas self-stimulation of the septal area is reduced by only 30% (Routtenberg, 1965). Although the locally toxic properties of carbachol crystals could be responsible for attenuating or overriding the effect of electrical

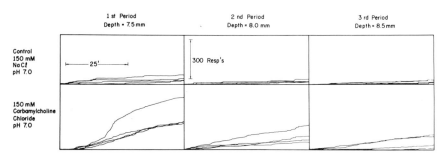

Fig. 12-2 Cumulative recorder tracing in which the slope of curve indicates response rate. In the upper tracings are curves generated by four rats self-injecting NaCl; in the lower tracing are curves generated by four different rats self-injecting carbamylcholine chloride. All rats were run three times during three successive hours with probes at 7.5, 8, and 8.5 mm of depth, respectively. Cumulative recorder tracing for the final 50 minutes of each hour is shown. In this case the concentration of carbamylcholine was 28 μg/μl, similar results were obtained with concentrations of 14 μg/μl. (From Olds *et al.*, 1964)

stimulation, it appears that there is an anatomical differentiation of cholinoceptive sites in the reward system. In an extension of this experiment, the stimulation of the dorsal mesencephalon of the rat by either electric current or a seizure-inducing dose of crystalline carbachol reduces the rate of self-stimulation applied to the posterior hypothalamus or septum.   Once again, the response to the chemical or electrical stimulation of hypothalamic sites was less than that to septal stimulation (Routtenberg and Olds, 1966). Although carbachol produces a motor seizure and therefore would be expected to suppress the behavior of the rat in a global sense, the anatomical separation between the effect on the hypothalamus and the septum would suggest that the two limbic structures relate neurophysiologically to the dorsal mesencephalon in a distinct way.   In any event, a dose response curve and pharmacological controls are necessary in order to determine whether a blockade of cholinergic receptors or a nonspecific action of the drug can account for these results.

The Russian workers, Kraus and Lapina (1972) have demonstrated that self-stimulation of the hypothalamus with electrical stimulation is inhibited in the dog by systemic metamyzil. Acting principally on muscarinic receptors, this cholinolytic attenuates self-stimulation when it is infused in a 1 to 7 μl volume into the fields of Forel. Kraus and Lapina interpret this significant finding as follows. Electrical stimulation of neurons in the reinforcement system evokes the local release of ACh from neurons in the reward pathway. This serves to sustain the self-stimulation responses that are reinforcing to the dog. Thus, metamyzil would block self-stimulation by preventing the liberated ACh from occupying muscarinic receptors.   If this is correct, a cholinergic link is present in the mesencephalic part of the reward system.

To test the idea that the entire medial forebrain bundle-lateral hypothalamic complex participates in the mediating of the rewarding properties of self-stimulation, Madryga and Albert (1971) injected procaine in a large dose into the hypothalamus at the same time that the rat was lever-pressing to deliver electrical stimulation to its septum or preoptic area. As shown in Fig. 12-3, a unilateral injection of procaine on the side of the stimulating electrode strongly suppresses self-stimulation behavior, whereas an injection on the side contralateral to the electrode has a somewhat reduced effect. Even though a unilateral injection of procaine also inhibits the rat's bar-pressing for food pellets in the interval immediately after the injection, this result nevertheless was assumed to indicate that procaine does not act simply as a result of a general neural blockade of the motor pathway or other efferent system. In spite of the fact that an animal which showed any overt sign of behavioral disruption was not included in the data analysis, part of the pathway associated with the reward system that is sensitive to a chemical disturbance apparently courses through the lateral hypothalamic area.

That the rewarding effect of hypothalamic self-stimulation in the rat depends on the integrity of both the medial forebrain bundle and ventral tegmental

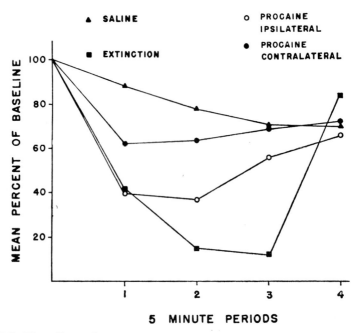

Fig. 12-3 The effect of stopping the stimulating current (extinction), injecting procaine, or injecting isotonic saline into the MFB-LHA on the rate of bar-pressing in the self-stimulation situation. Data from ipsilateral and contralateral sites for the saline and for the extinction treatments are combined into single curves. (From Madryga and Albert, 1971)

system is another reasonable supposition. Nakajima (1972a) has shown that the blockade of either the midbrain tegmentum or lateral hypothalamus by a micro-injection of procaine attenuates the self-stimulation of the lateral hypothalamus. On the other hand, the neural excitant L-glutamate elevates the rate of self-stimulation when it is injected into the lateral hypothalamus; however, this amino acid reduces the rate of stimulation only partially when given in the tegmentum. The time course of these changes in response to an ipsilateral injection of the two compounds is shown in Fig. 12-4. Concurrent observations of motor activity rule out the possibility that the drugs produce a nonspecific interference of hypothalamic function. Overall, these findings agree with the notion that ascending and descending components of the midbrain and basal forebrain pathways comprise an integrated anatomical system for reward.

B. Punishment Versus Reward

From the preceding discussion it is apparent that the humoral substrate in the brain underlying the anatomical circuitry for the reward system is far from being understood. Electrical pulses to structures which yield high rates of self-

A. Ipsi. VT Injections

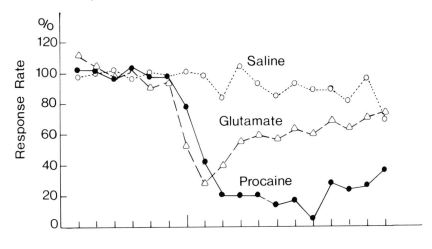

B. Ipsi. LH Injections

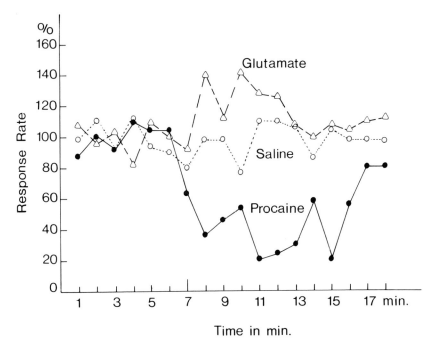

Time in min.

Fig. 12-4 Effects of ipsilateral injections on self-stimulation. A. Hypothalamic self-stimulation with tegmental injections. B. Tegmental self-stimulation with hypothalamic injections. Each point in the graph represents the mean of five animals. Injections were made during the 7th minute. (From Nakajima, 1972a)

stimulation may release acetylcholine, norepinephrine, serotonin, and probably other substances if adequate measures would be taken. For years the experiments in which a drug is applied systemically and then presumed to have a specific central action have reaped conflicting results at least in terms of the function of a biogenic amine in rewarded behavior (Margules, 1969a).

A neurochemical model of rewarded activity put forth by Carlton (1963; 1969) proposes that a cholinergic mechanism is involved in the inhibition or suppression of a behavior pattern that is not reinforced. Thus, a cholinolytic should exert its action mainly by disinhibiting a response pattern that was previously extinguished and hence restore the animal's behavior. In contrast to a cholinergic inhibitory mechanism, an excitatory adrenergic system is hypothesized which functionally opposes the cholinergic system. Thus, a sympathomimetic compound such as amphetamine would have the same effect as a cholinergic blocking agent in disinhibiting or releasing the inhibited behavior. By such a mechanism the stimulating properties of an amphetamine-like compound could be explained.

Based on the anatomical findings of Olds, Nauta, Sutin and others, Stein (1968) has postulated that two mutually reciprocal mechanisms function in the phenomena of reward and punishment. As shown in Fig. 12-5 (Sutin, 1966), one signals and thus controls punishment via a periventricular pathway. This is thought to be mediated by a collection of cholinergic synapses in the ventromedial hypothalamus. The second mechanism signals and thereby mediates reward via the medial forebrain bundle (Fig. 12-5). This is believed to be served by a system of adrenergic synapses in the limbic-midbrain circuit.

A preliminary study was reported by Margules and Stein (1966) who tamped crystals of carbachol and other substances into the ventromedial hypothalamus of the rat. A situation was utilized in which the punishment of foot shock was simultaneously paired with a milk reward, both delivered at once when the animal pressed a lever in its test chamber (Geller and Seifter, 1960).

Cholinergic stimulation of the ventromedial hypothalamus suppressed the lever-pressing, whereas a cholinergic antagonist did not reduce the responding. When crystalline atropine was applied to the rat's ventromedial hypothalamus, this cholinolytic had the same effect as a lesion in producing a deficit in passive avoidance (Margules and Stein, 1969a). That is, the animal accepted more shocks as it pressed a lever which resulted again in the simultaneous delivery of a droplet of milk together with shock to the floor of the rat's cage. The cholinergic blocking agent also did not increase the drinking of milk after the rat had been artificially satiated with milk, although the bar-pressing continued anyway. Thus, in addition to functioning in a satiety mechanism (Chapter 7), it would appear that the ventromedial region is also part of a reward-punishment system. The local application of either of two anticholinesterases, neostigmine or eserine, to the ventromedial hypothalamus completely blocked all operant behavior. This makes it difficult to interpret the synaptic specificity of atropine in increasing the operant behavior but not the drinking response.

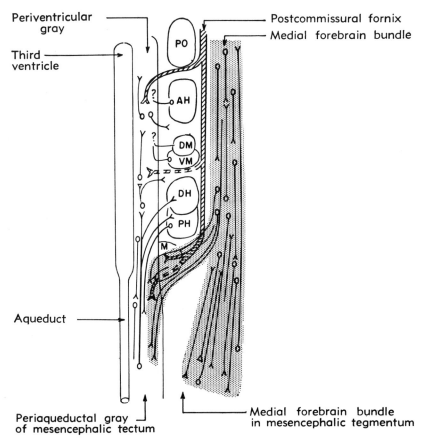

Fig. 12-5 Schematic representation of the fiber bundles forming the periventricular stratum based upon the results of degeneration studies in several species. Stippling indicates the medial forebrain bundle. The tegmental component contains both ascending and descending axons whereas the periaqueductal component is mainly descending. Oblique lines denote the fornix system. Its anterior and tuberal periventricular connections are found only in the rodent. Fornix fibers extending to the central gray are most numerous in rodents, but some are also seen in carnivores. The posterior division of the periventricular stratum contains mostly ascending fibers. AH, anterior hypothalamic area; DH, dorsal hypothalamic area; DM, dorsomedial nucleus; M, mammillary nuclei; PH, posterior hypothalamic area; PO, preoptic region; VM, ventromedial nucleus. (From Sutin, 1966)

In contrast to the cholinergic blocking effect on avoidance behavior of atropine and scopolamine shown in Fig. 12-6, the application of crystals of carbachol, muscarine or physostigmine to the ventromedial hypothalamus partially enhanced passive avoidance responding in that the number of shocks were reduced that the rat would accept while it attempted to obtain milk (Margules and Stein,

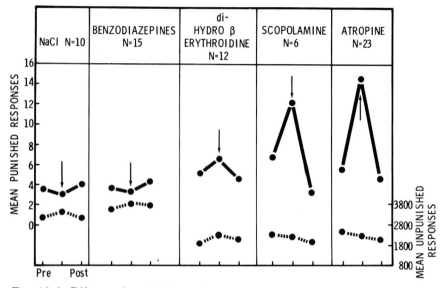

Fig. 12-6   Effects of medial hypothalamic application of drugs on punished (solid lines) and unpunished (dashed lines) responses of rats without cannula-induced passive-avoidance deficits.   N = number of administrations.   (From Margules and Stein, 1969b)

1969b).   The actual lever responding for the milk reward, termed "unpunished behavior," however, was also somewhat suppressed.   Control substances and other compounds including norepinephrine did not have this effect.   As shown in Fig. 12-7, cholinergic stimulation of the ventromedial region with four different compounds does maintain passive avoidance behavior or restores it following a lesion.   Taken together with the earlier experiments with atropine and scopolamine, the results parallel those of electrical stimulation and lesioning of the ventromedial hypothalamus in that the cholinergic synapses in the ventromedial hypothalamus seem to have an excitatory rather than inhibitory component.

If crystals of carbachol are tamped in the lateral hypothalamus or atropine is placed in the ventromedial region, the approach-avoidance conflict produced when both food and shock are delivered in a lever-pressing situation is reduced to some extent (Sepinwall and Grodsky, 1969).   When carbachol is applied to the ventromedial hypothalamus, both types of responses are suppressed in the same situation. In this behavioral task, cholinergic stimulation of the lateral hypothalamus is, therefore, tantamount to a cholinergic blockade of the ventromedial region.

Noradrenergic inhibitory synapses located in the amygdala may also be involved in the control of punishment.   In the same passive avoidance task in which a lever-press for milk causes the simultaneous delivery of an aversive foot shock, norad-

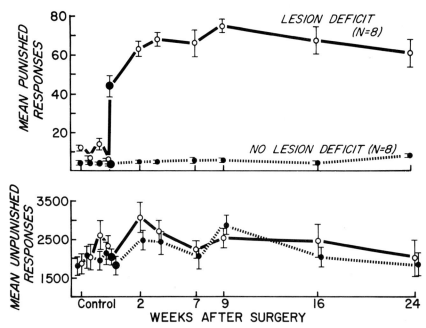

Fig. 12-7 Effects of cannula-induced lesions on punished and unpunished responses. Large circles indicate day of surgery, bars indicate standard errors. (From Margules and Stein, 1969b)

renergic stimulation of the amygdala increases the amount of punishment in terms of the number of shocks that a rat will accept in order to continue to obtain a milk reward (Margules, 1968). That is, the local application of crystals of norepinephrine to the amygdala has virtually the same net effect on the animal's acceptance of shock as a lesion to the same structure. The action of this catecholamine may be pharmacologically specific since crystalline atropine applied in the same way does not cause the rat to increase the amount of punishing responding. The complexity of an interpretation of this result is amplified by the fact that stimulation of the amygdala with norepinephrine also increases the magnitude of feeding in the fasted rat but not in the satiated rat. Therefore, it would appear that there must be some sort of reciprocal inhibition at the neurochemical level between reward and punishment (Stein, 1964).

The effect of norepinephrine on the amygdala in ameliorating the inhibitory effect of punishing shock every time the rat presses the lever for milk reward is antagonized by pretreating the amygdala with crystals of either the alpha or beta receptor blockers, phentolamine and dl-4-(2-hydroxy-3-isopropylaminopropoxy)-indole (LB-46), respectively (Margules, 1971a). As indicated in Fig. 12-8, however, phentolamine is much more potent in reversing the effect. At a low intensity of foot shock, the deposit of the beta receptor agonist, isoprotere-

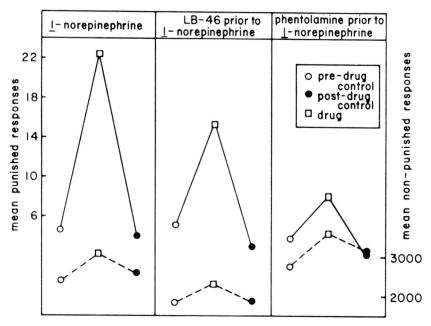

Fig. 12-8 Effects of direct bilateral placement of drugs in the amygdala on punished and non-punished operant responses. All doses were 10 μg. Punished responses are indicated by the solid lines, non-punished responses are indicated by the dashed lines. (From Margules, 1971a)

nol, into the amygdala reduces substantially the acceptance of punishing foot shock but at the same time abolishes lever-pressing for milk. The magnitude of these responses is presented in Fig. 12-9. Thus, it would appear that the alpha and beta receptor sites in the amygdala oppose one another in the mediation of the rat's ultimate response to punishing foot shock, that is whether the rat accepts a greater or lesser number of shocks than normally taken.

The so-called anti-punishment effect of norepinephrine has been localized by Margules (1971b) in an anatomical mapping study to the dorsal, corticomedial portion of the amygdala as shown in Fig. 12-10. When crystalline norepinephrine is applied to this region, the rat accepts far more shocks than during a control trial. If atropine is implanted similarly in the internal capsule particularly in the region of the entopeduncular nucleus, the effect of shock punishment on the rat again is much weaker in that the number of shocks taken by the rat increases. This area of the amygdala may represent a termination of the ascending noradrenergic component of the medial forebrain bundle which inhibits punishment and thereby would facilitate reward. The cholinergic receptors may be part of the ascending ventral tegmental pathway involved only in reducing the overall suppression of behavior occasioned by a punishing stimulus such as that of shock. The latter could represent anatomically a part of a cholinergic inhibitory mechanism (Carlton, 1963).

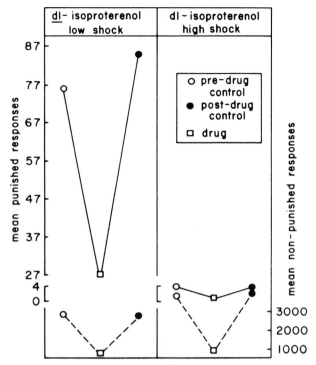

Fig. 12-9 Effects of direct bilateral placement of 20 μg *dl*-isoproterenol hydrochloride in the amygdala on moderately punished (low shock), intensely punished (high shock), and non-punished operant responses. Punished responses are indicated by the solid lines, non-punished responses are indicated by the dashed lines. (From Margules, 1971a)

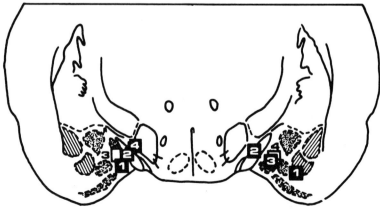

Fig. 12-10 The squares on this frontal section from the atlas of König and Klippel (1963) represent the sites immediately below the cannula tips in four rats with isoproterenol-induced intensification of punishment. (From Margules, 1971a).

With the squirrel monkey, a result somewhat similar to that of the rat is obtained using the Geller-Seifter (1960) conflict paradigm. Crystalline atropine implanted in the ventromedial hypothalamus increases the amount of punishing shock to the tail that the monkey will accept as it presses a lever for food pellets or dextrose solution (Miczek and Grossman, 1972). However, the rate of non-punished responding when shock was not given also increases. Although eserine implanted similarly has little or no effect, carbachol has the expected opposite action of atropine in reducing substantially both punished and non-punished lever-pressing for food reinforcement. Interestingly, the enhanced responding evoked by atropine is apparently situation-dependent since the manipulation of the schedule of reinforcement attenuates atropine's potency. Overall, the cholinolytic seems to exert a paradoxical effect, since it does enhance avoidance conditioning when applied to the ventromedial hypothalamus of the rat (Grossman, 1966a).

III. CHOLINERGIC MECHANISMS AND LEARNING

How a rat learns to avoid an electric shock to its feet delivered in one or more of a myriad of ways has been used in the vast majority of the studies in this field to evaluate the role of a presumed transmitter or other neurohumoral substance within a specific anatomical region. What is the principal reason for this? In terms of the frequent vagaries in the motivational state, it is ordinarily easier to bring the animal's behavior under stimulus control during the acquisition of a shock avoidance response than by any other procedure. For example, when an ordinary laboratory chow or tap water is used as an incentive in a given learning task, some sort of period of deprivation is always required. However, this signifies a different drive level in each animal. Even when a highly palatable reinforcer such as sugar water or milk constitutes the goal object, a variation from one animal to the next in the value of the incentive presents lamentable difficulties.

Of great significance to this type of experimental analysis is perhaps the most important consideration of all: the mechanisms for hunger, thirst and emotion may have a similar neurohumoral representation within the limbic system (Chapters 7, 8, 11) as those implicated in the learning of a given task.

A. Avoidance Learning

Following the original paper of Stevens et al. (1961), a number of investigators have tried to determine whether a conditioned avoidance response is impaired or its performance is enhanced by varying the chemical nature of a cerebral structure. In the following sections, the role of a cholinergic mechanism is examined in respect to different anatomical regions of the limbic system.

1. *Mesencephalon*

A small lesion produced by a cannula implanted in the mesencephalon depresses avoidance performance in the rat (Grossman, 1966b). This deficit in the shock-induced escape behavior is exaggerated further by a mesencephalic deposit of crystalline carbachol or ACh but not other drugs tested including norepinephrine, serotonin or GABA. Repeated cholinergic stimulation of the mesencephalon at 24-hour intervals seems to improve the rat's performance but only after the rate of avoidance responding approaches an asymptote. Although the behavioral deficits do not appear to be due to a nonspecific loss in sensory or motor function in that the rat reacts to shock in a normal fashion, it is not clear which system of arousal or motivation is altered or how it is affected by the chemical stimulus.

An enhancement of sensory input in the rat is brought about by cholinergic stimulation of the mesencephalic reticular formation. Light, noise or gentle tactile stimulus evokes abnormal startle reactions for up to an hour after a carbachol implant (Grossman, 1968b). A frantic reaction to an electric shock to the feet impairs in itself the rat's learning of a simple conditioned avoidance task. However, when the shock intensity is lowered to near threshold level for the normal animal, the carbachol-treated rat acquires the avoidance response even more rapidly than a paired control. The relationship between three levels of shock and the rapidity of acquisition of the avoidance response is presented in Fig. 12-11. Injected at the same mesencephalic site, atropine suppresses somewhat this sensory facilitation, but norepinephrine lowers the reactivity to the environmental stimuli. Under these conditions, the rat's rate of lever-pressing for food or water as well as the speed with which a brightness discrimination task is performed are generally reduced. An alpha adrenergic blocker, phenoxybenzamine, increases the rate of lever-pressing for food or water and attenuates response latency in the discrimination task. Within the mesencephalic reticular system, it would thus seem that several sensory modalities are affected by the level of cholinergic or adrenergic activity. Overall, the animal's responsiveness or general level of reactivity to sensory input is enhanced by a cholinergic system and suppressed by an adrenergic one.

2. *Hypothalamus*

In a complicated experimental paradigm designed by Kalyuzhnyi (1962), a rabbit was conditioned simultaneously to procure food when a green light shone and to depress a lever to avoid foot shock when a red light switched on. Crystalline carbachol applied to the posterior hypothalamus improves the conditioned responding for food but impairs shock avoidance responding. When norepinephrine is deposited at the same locus, the opposite effect on the conditioned response is observed. This result seems to confirm an independence of the two conditioned behaviors, and it probably represents the second reported observation of a species difference in the adrenergic feeding mechanism (Chapter 7).

During the rat's performance of a Sidman shock avoidance task, the placement

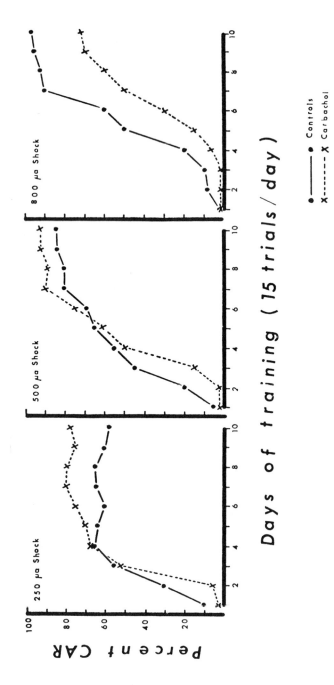

Fig. 12-11 Acquisition of conditioned avoidance responses in a double-grill apparatus. The experimental animals received 1.5 μg of carbachol 5 minutes before each 15 minute daily training session. The control animals were given sham injections. (From Grossman, 1968b)

of crystalline carbachol enhances learning if the deposit is in the lateral hypothalamus but inhibits it when implanted in the septum (Sepinwall, 1966). When implanted in the ventromedial hypothalamus, carbachol also facilitates learning, but not nearly to the degree of enhancement observed after cholinergic stimulation of that region (Sepinwall, 1969). A pharmacological antagonism is demonstrable because a deposit of atropine in the ventromedial hypothalamus has the opposite effect in that the avoidance performance is impaired. However, since sodium pentobarbital injected into the hypothalamus also has the same net effect as atropine, the specificity of an anticholinergic action is uncertain. Nevertheless, it would appear that the reinforcement pathway for avoidance learning which may pass through the lateral hypothalamus could be part of a larger cholinergic circuit.

A tranquilizer such as chlorpromazine or other phenothiazine derivative may also have a direct action on the hypothalamus of the rat (Grossman, 1968a). In some instances, the direct application of a phenothiazine raises and in others reduces the responding in a typical shock avoidance task; however, in the dose used no large effect is usually observed. Moreover, no consistent diminution of conditioned avoidance behavior is noted when the drug is implanted in the septum or amygdala. Slow-wave, high amplitude EEG wave activity may occur following the application of a chlorpromazine derivative to the rat's mesencephalon as well.

3. *Thalamus*

Repeating the experiments done on mesencephalic sites, Grossman et al. (1965) found that the rat's learning of a shock avoidance response in a shuttle box is severely retarded following the application of crystals of carbachol in various midline and other thalamic nuclei. As shown in Fig. 12-12, the asymptote performance of the rat is affected primarily by cholinergic stimulation of the reticular nucleus. In every case, the rat nevertheless does make the appropriate response to escape shock, which indicates that the animal's motor system is not incapacitated by the cholinomimetic. Cholinergic stimulation of the midline or reticular nuclei also lowers the bar-pressing rate for food and reduces exploratory behavior as well. Atropine increases locomotor activity but depresses lever-pressing for food. The impaired learning, therefore, seems to reflect neither a motivational process nor a sensorimotor disability. Rather, the cholinergic interference with this nonspecific thalamic projection system probably alters the associative processes involved in learning.

To answer the question of whether a nonspecific motivational process is involved in the disruption of avoidance learning produced by cholinergic stimulation of the rat's thalamus, an additional experiment was carried out by Grossman and Peters (1966). When crystalline atropine is applied to the reticular nucleus, the acquisition of the avoidance response as well as the asymptote in performance, shown in Fig. 12-13, is significantly disrupted. On the other hand, the rat's

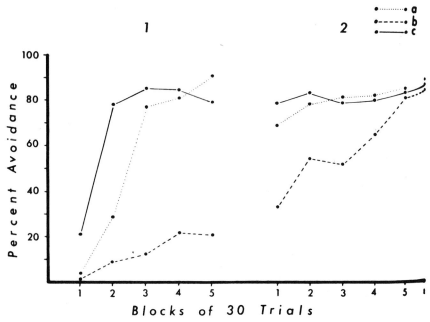

Fig. 12-12 Avoidance performance in a shuttle box (1) following cholinergic stimulation of the thalamic reticular formation and (2) after sham-stimulation. Group a. midline placements; Group b. bilateral placements in or above reticular nucleus; Group c. unoperated control Ss. (From Grossman, S. P. *et al.*, 1965. *J. Comp. Physiol. Psychol.* **59**:57–65. Copyright 1965, by the American Psychological Association. Reprinted by permission)

learning and performance, illustrated in Fig. 12-13, both improve following the cholinergic blockade of the midline thalamic nuclei by atropine. The identical results are obtained when the rat is tested under the same conditions in a black-white discrimination task. On the basis of the blockade of muscarinic receptors and other possible local effects of atropine, the midline nuclei appear to be related to the nonspecific motivational process of general arousal. On the other hand, the more lateral nuclei of the thalamus could be required for learning of a specific response and for the retention mechanism.

Using crystalline carbachol purportedly in milligram amounts that were deposited in the thalamus of the rat, Blanchard *et al.* (1972) ostensibly ruled out the possibility that the deficit in active or passive avoidance learning is due to an

Fig. 12-13 Acquisition and performance of a shuttle box avoidance response following the central application of atropine (sections 1 and 3) or sham-stimulation (section 2). (From Grossman, S. P. and R. H. Peters. 1966. *J. Comp. Physiol. Psychol.* **61**:325–332. Copyright 1966, by the American Psychological Association. Reprinted by permission)

alteration simply in the activity level of the animal. A carbachol implant failed to influence either the flinch or jump threshold of the rat to foot shock or the threshold to escape from a foot shock. Since the rat is indeed capable of learning an avoidance response at a low intensity of foot shock, the impairment produced by cholinergic stimulation is probably not due to an associative deficit. Blanchard *et al.* suggest instead that carbachol reduces the capability of the rat to react defensively to threatening stimuli.

4. *Septum*

McCleary has proposed that the result of a lesion to a structure in the limbic system such as the septum can be considered in terms of a loss of response inhibition (McCleary, 1966). Hamilton *et al.* (1968) tested this assumption by temporarily blocking the septal activity of a cat with atropine. In a passive avoidance task, 6 of 8 cats showed a deficit in passive avoidance learning after crystals of atropine were implanted bilaterally in the septum. That is, the cat approached food even though this response was punished by shock to the paws. Neither reversal learning in a discrimination task nor the acquisition of an active avoidance responses in a shuttle box was affected by the local cholinergic blockade of the septum produced by atropine. The pattern of extinction in the active

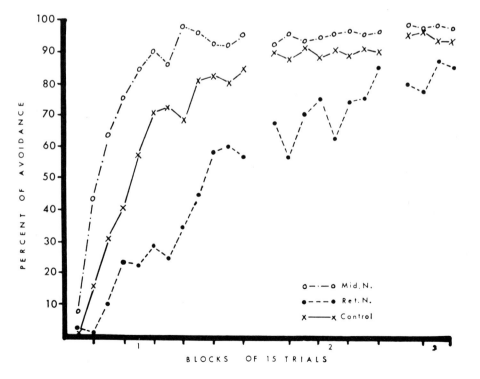

shock avoidance task, however, mimicked the effect of a lesion since the response of an atropine-treated cat extinguished at a significantly slower rate. This finding, coupled with the results in the passive avoidance task, suggests that the septal blockade evokes a perseverative deficit following the disruption of a normal inhibitory cholinergic pathway. Thus, the so-called disinhibition following a septal lesion could involve a cholinergic inhibitory circuit. Obviously, pharmacological and other controls are needed to confirm such a supposition.

As a follow-up to this, Hamilton and Grossman (1969) examined the notion that a tendency to over-respond, which impairs passive avoidance performance, follows a septal lesion which in turn prevents the inhibition of a previously learned response. First a cat was trained to jump on a shelf in order to escape shock. Then after scopolamine or atropine was applied bilaterally to the septum, the cat learned to avoid the shock on cue from a light. Scopolamine or atropine impaired this type of avoidance learning. Scopolamine, the more potent compound, even prevented each cat from reaching the same asymptote as the control. A peripheral injection of either cholinergic blocking agent in a much larger dose had the same general effect. This suggests that the site of action of the cholinolytic in many of the previous learning studies could be the septum.

A carbachol implant in the septum of the rat enhances drinking in the fasted or satiated rat while suppressing food intake in either (Chapter 7) (Grossman, 1964b). Similarly, cholinergic stimulation of the septum of a rat impairs not only the learning of a lever response for food or an avoidance response in a shuttle box, but also the performance of the avoidance task if learned earlier. Adrenergic stimulation of the septum or its blockade with Dibenzyline has no effect on ingestive behavior, but norepinephrine does improve the rat's avoidance performance. This result could reflect a reciprocal relationship between two motivational mechanisms served by cholinoceptive synapses. While the one for drinking dominates, the other for avoiding pain is suppressed. The atropine reversal of the blockade of drinking and the simultaneous facilitation of avoidance argues against this somewhat elementary interpretation, and to examine this premise, water should seemingly be made available to the rat in the shock avoidance situation.

In another test of the role of a cholinergic pathway in avoidance learning, Kelsey and Grossman (1969) found that an atropine implant in the septum of the rat facilitated the acquisition of a conditioned avoidance response in a two-way shuttle box. In addition, atropine did not alter the rat's spontaneous activity nor did it cause perseverative responding during reversal training of the avoidance behavior. Although the rat did not display a general aversion to the stimulus light, atropine may have enhanced the visual sensitivity to the conditioned stimulus. Learning was facilitated when the rat had to jump away from the lighted compartment into one which was darkened.

Although carbachol injected in a high dose into the septum of the cat also impairs two-way active avoidance performance in a shuttle box, the behavioral deficit is not as severe as that seen in the rat (Holloway, 1972). However, those cats which showed overt signs of behavioral arousal such as an orienting response to a stimulus seemed to suffer the greatest impairment. Interestingly, norepinephrine injected at homologous sites in the septum of the cat simply increased the latency of the cat's avoidance response, whereas carbachol reduced the latency scores. Thus, some sort of generalized nonspecific activation of behavior rather than an action on the learning mechanism could account for the performance decrement.

When a dose of 400 µg of procaine in an enormous volume of 20 µl is injected into the septum of the rat, a behavioral effect similar to that of an electrolytic lesion occurs (Duncan, 1971). The injection results in an impaired fear conditioning in which a conditioning tone is paired with foot shock. A normal rat's usual immobility following the presentation of the tone that signals the shock is also reduced by such an injection of the local anesthetic into the septum. Instead, the typical immobility is interspersed with bouts of running, jumping and sniffing. These results suggest that an emotional component contributes to the suspected associative deficit arising from septal dysfunction.

5. Caudate Nucleus

The application of crystals of a cholinomimetic substance to the caudate nucleus of the cat evokes contralateral circling that is accompanied by such severe postural weakness that the animal drags its hind or forelimbs behind (Stevens et al., 1961). A state of lethargy from which the cat is easily aroused can also be observed. If the animal is trained to jump a barrier in response to a buzzer in order to avoid shock delivered to the floor of the cage, an asymptote of 85% correct avoidance responses or better is easily reached by the cat. When carbachol is deposited in the caudate nucleus, the conditioned avoidance response is typically lost for a period of 4 to 24 hours. One cat did not respond for 6 hours to the conditioned stimulus or exhibit the unconditioned response to foot shock. The failure in avoidance performance of the cat could be due to either motor impairment caused by the local cholinergic excitation or simply to the inability of the animal to attend to and hear the sound of the conditioning buzzer.

An implant of scopolamine in the dorsal caudate nucleus reliably inhibits shock avoidance learning in a shuttle box situation (Neill and Grossman, 1970). On the other hand, crystals of the cholinolytic agent placed more ventrally enhance rather remarkably the acquisition of an avoidance response to foot shock. The anatomical loci of these effects are presented in Fig. 12-14. During the initial stages of habituation to the task, each rat in which scopolamine had been placed in the ventral caudate nucleus showed a somewhat higher level of spontaneous activity. Since carbachol may exert either an excitatory or inhibitory change in activity, the consideration of all behavioral inhibition in the realm of a single cholinergic system is certainly not warranted. In this connection, the cholinomimetic when deposited in the ventral striatum has the opposite effect on

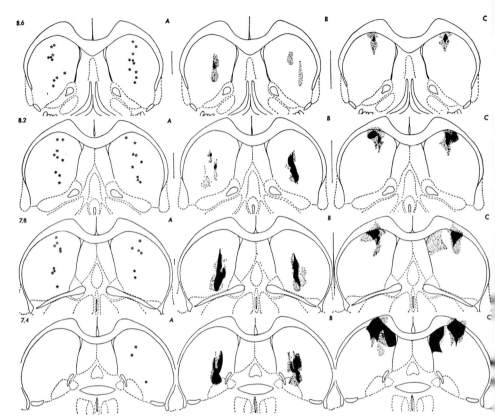

Fig. 12-14 A. All dorsal (empty stars) and ventral (filled stars) cannula placements which received scopolamine; B. ventral lesions (black area represents overlap of two or more lesions, stippled area represents extent of single lesions which did not overlap); C. dorsal lesions (same conditions as for B). Drawings after the de Groot (1959) atlas of the rat brain. (From Neill, D. B. and S. P. Grossman. 1970. *J. Comp. Physiol. Psychol.* **71**:311–317. Copyright 1970, by the American Psychological Association. Reprinted by permission)

avoidance behavior as a lesion placed in the same locus. Thus, a ventrally placed lesion may destroy a non-cholinergic system, possibly a dopaminergic pathway related to a learning mechanism.

6. *Amygdala*

In a dramatic demonstration of the long-lasting action of carbachol placed in the amygdala, a rat shows virtually no ability to learn a simple shock avoidance task as much as 3 weeks after the deposit of crystals of the cholinomimetic (Belluzzi and Grossman, 1969). A single seizure-producing dose of carbachol produces a long-lasting inhibition of learning which could be abolished entirely by scopolamine implanted at the same locus. Scopolamine applied alone to the amygdala facilitates the acquisition of the avoidance response, and the performance of a rat subjected to the cholinergic blockade is in fact superior to that of the control.

In a well-designed study, Goddard (1969) demonstrated that a very small dose of carbachol injected into the amygdala of a rat impairs its acquisition of a conditioned avoidance response to foot shock. The curves of the latency of response are plotted in Fig. 12-15. Just as impressive is the finding, shown in Fig. 12-16, that passive avoidance learning is severely impaired when the rat's training trials are distributed but not when they are massed. Goddard's important observation indicates that the cholinergic excitation of the amygdaloid nucleus interferes with a task which requires long-term retention across trials. Carbachol, however, fails to disturb learning of an active avoidance task whether or not the trials are massed or distributed; the retention of the responses is similarly preserved. Also, transfer of training from the passive avoidance to active avoidance task is not impaired by the cholinomimetic. Quite surprising is the finding that the carbachol-injected rat consumes food pellets in the active avoidance situation. In brief, the

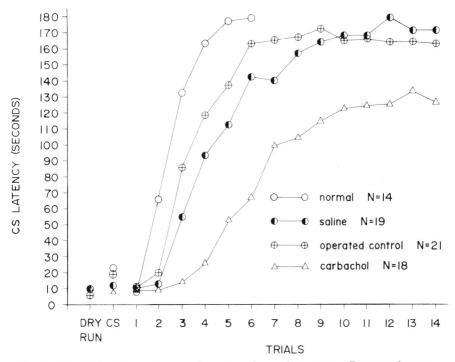

Fig. 12-15 CER: Time between CS onset and next lever press. Dry run—latency from an unsignaled point in time, no CS or US given; CS—first presentation of CS, no US given. (From Goddard, G. V. 1969. *J. Comp. Physiol. Psychol.* 68: 1–18. Copyright 1969, by the American Psychological Association. Reprinted by permission)

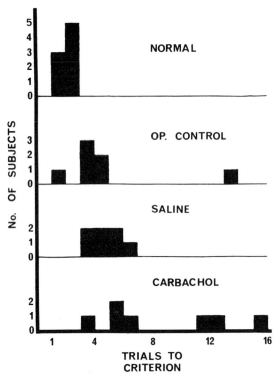

Fig. 12-16 Passive avoidance, distributed training. Frequency distribution of learning scores for all Ss. (From Goddard, G. V. 1969. *J. Comp. Physiol. Psychol.* **68**:1–18. Copyright 1969, by the American Psychological Association. Reprinted by permission)

main action of cholinergic activation of the amygdala is the loss of a fear-motivated response which is inhibited particularly when long-term retention of a problem is required.

That the action of cholinomimetic stimulation of the rat's amygdala does not produce a nonspecific deficit in learning has been shown recently. Crystalline carbachol deposited in the amygdaloid complex has no disturbing effect on the rat's acquisition of a food-motivated visual discrimination task (Belluzzi, 1972). However, cholinergic stimulation of the homologous site before the rat is given trials in a shuttle box enhances the animal's ability to learn a two-way avoidance task, but impairs the acquisition of a one-way active avoidance response. A similar implant of crystalline eserine essentially reproduces the effect of carbachol. Presumably this deficit is caused by the handling of the animal necessitated by the technique used in that the rat treated with carbachol is hyperreactive. Thus, the mechanism required for learning a new problem is not necessarily altered by carbachol, but rather the factor of emotionality is at the root of this noteworthy behavioral change.

B. Discrimination Learning

The usage of an appetitive reward to analyze the cholinergic substrate of discriminative processes has revealed several facts. For example, Khavari and Russell (1966) have shown that cholinergic stimulation of the lateral hypothalamus produces a specific change in motivated or directed behavior. After carbachol crystals are implanted in the hypothalamus of the rat, the animal runs down a runway to obtain water at the same speed as a rat deprived of water for 24 hours. When carbachol again is used to stimulate the rat's lateral hypothalamus, the animal can learn a T-maze at the same rate as a rat trained under fluid deprivation; similarly, the maze habit is retained in an identical way. Extinction curves also correspond to those of the rats that learned under cholinergic stimulation or under a condition of water deprivation. These results clearly show that the drinking response evoked by carbachol deposited in the hypothalamus has the same characteristics as that motivated by the natural thirst generated by a fluid deficit. In the appetitive situation, cholinergic stimulation of the hypothalamus can act on a basic motivational system (Chapter 8).

The application of crystals of carbachol or ACh to the mesencephalic reticular formation also reduces exploratory behavior and impairs the performance of a rat in either of two situations: a black-white discrimination problem with food as a reward or in a lever-pressing task in which pellets are given on a VR-5 schedule of reinforcement (Grossman and Grossman, 1966). This finding shows that the action of these cholinergic compounds may be opposite to those produced by a lesion and can be inhibitory even at the level of origin of the reticular activating system (Chkhartishvili, 1969).

When atropine is applied to the so-called satiety center of the rat (Chapter 7), food intake *per se* is not affected, but lever-responding for a food pellet or droplet of water is attenuated. The discrimination performance in a T-maze in which food pellets serve as the reinforcer is also much more inferior after atropine is implanted in the ventromedial hypothalamus (Grossman, 1966a). Since the presence of atropine in this structure facilitates the rat's performance in a simple shock avoidance task, one interpretation could be that the ventromedial hypothalamus mediates affective reactivity through a cholinergic system. This would account for an interference with appetitive behavior by a cholinolytic and the improvement in escaping from shock.

The injection of a single dose of norepinephrine or ethobutamoxane into the nucleus centromedian of the thalamus enhances the visual discrimination performance of the cat in a simple task in which a lever-press delivers milk reinforcement (Avery and Nance, 1970b). The improvement arises simply as a result of a reduced number of inter-trial non-reinforced responses. This result is somewhat surprising since the adrenergic blocking agent applied locally should exert an effect diametrically opposite to that of norepinephrine. Cholinergic stimulation of the same site with carbachol reduces the responding for milk whereas atropine increases the level of non-reinforced responding during the inter-trial interval. Both events, of course, would lead to a much poorer discriminative performance.

IV. HORMONES AND LEARNING

An increase in the electrical excitability of the brain of an animal or human undergoing adrenocortical therapy is a well-known phenomenon. As a result, the growing research interest in the actions of the steroid as well as peptide hormones on psychological states has focused on the question of how these substances affect the conditioning process (de Wied, 1966). The fact that ACTH and related peptides given systemically inhibit the extinction of an avoidance response even in the adrenalectomized animal signifies a direct action of the hormones on learned behavior.

A. Adrenal Mechanisms

As reviewed in Chapter 4, there is already some basis for the idea that a corticosteroid has a direct neural influence on behavioral processes and on adrenal function. Crystalline cortisol implanted in the mesencephalic reticular formation of the rat acts not only to suppress the stress-induced release of ACTH, but it also facilitates the rapid extinction of a conditioned avoidance response (Bohus, 1968). Implanted in the median eminence, cortisol also enhances the rate of extinction which correlates very closely with the rate of ACTH release. Thus, the action of the steroid in promoting the extinction process could be due to the inhibition of ACTH release from the pituitary. A direct test of this, of course, would be to place the trophic hormone in brain substance in an attempt to retard extinction.

A peripherally administered corticosteroid facilitates the extinction of a response in a conditioned avoidance task. Crystals of either dexamethasone or of corticosterone deposited in a number of areas of the thalamus or in the ventricle likewise advance the extinction process (Van Wimersma-Greidanus and de Wied, 1969). Although a lesion in the thalamus is known to interfere with the maintenance of responding in a conditioned avoidance situation, it is not certain how these two steroids act on these structures. At any rate, glucocorticoids in this case also have a local inhibitory action in the diencephalon.

In comparing the action of ACTH to a corticosteroid on the rat's avoidance behavior during response extinction, Bohus (1970a) has found that cortisone promotes extinction, as illustrated in Fig. 12 17, when it is deposited in the medial thalamic nuclei, anterior hypothalamus or rostral septum. When ACTH is administered subcutaneously, a significant inhibitory effect on the rate of extinction arises only if the rat bears a hypothalamic or septal implant of cortisone. In this case, ACTH causes the responses to perseverate during the extinction phase. Therefore, within the thalamic relay nuclei there may be a

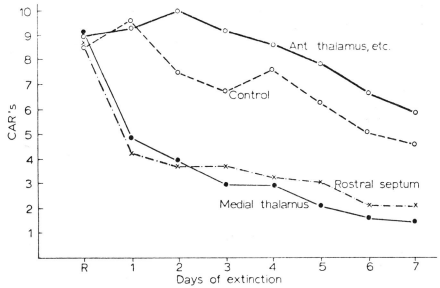

Fig. 12-17   Effect of cortisone acetate implantation on extinction of a pole-jumping avoidance response. (From Bohus, B. 1970b. *Pituitary, Adrenal, and the Brain*. D. de Wied and J. A. W. M. Weijnen (eds.) pp. 171–184. Elsevier Publishing Co., Amsterdam, The Netherlands)

neuronally competitive antagonism between ACTH and cortisone. Alternatively, ACTH may simply not interfere with the inhibition of the ascending reticular influence which is thought to be necessary for extinction to take place. Since Bohus (1970b) has also demonstrated that a cortisone implant in the amygdala of the rat has the same enhancing effect on the rate of extinction, the entire limbic system may be sensitive to an influence of the adrenal gland.

Extinction of a rat's conditioned avoidance response measured in a shuttle-box or a pole-jumping task is differentially affected by polypeptide analogues of ACTH. An implant of crystalline ACTH-(1-10) into the sites encompassing the caudal diencephalon and rostral mesencephalon inhibits the extinction of the avoidance response (Van Wimersma-Greidanus and de Wied, 1971). However, the administration of [D-phe^7]-ACTH-(1-10), another long-lasting ACTH ana-logue has the opposite effect in that the extinction of the same pole-jump response is facilitated. These observations are in general agreement with the results of a lesion to the same area, particularly the nucleus parafascicularis of the thalamus. Such an ablation interferes with the extinction of the rat's avoidance responding. These peptides demonstrate in an exceptional way the importance of structure-function relationships with respect to their opposite effect on the behavior of the rat. Although the mechanism of action is uncertain, response extinction may be modified by an alteration in the input from the reticular activating system at the level of the mesencephalon to the nonspecific thalamic nuclei.

B. Thyroid Function

Although there is a substantial amount of peripheral evidence on the role of the thyroid principle in learning (Chapter 4), there is very little information about the direct action of thyroxine on the central nervous system.

The Russian workers, Amiragova and Berlina (1970a) have utilized a straight-forward Pavlovian paradigm to show that the injection of thyroxine into the posterior hypothalamus of the dog facilitates the conditioned reflex for food. The hormone-induced reaction causes the dog to lick and turn its head toward the conditioning stimulus and to the food box in anticipation of food. Intra-hypothalamic thyroxine also causes an increase in salivation in response to either the conditioned or unconditioned stimulus.

To test whether a central adrenergic mechanism could be involved in the dog's responses, Amiragova and Berlina (1970b) then injected an adrenergic blocking agent, aminazine, just prior to the infusion of thyroxine. When both substances were infused in the antero-medial part of the thalamus, aminazine inhibited the conditioned reflex for food, and the volume of saliva usually elaborated declined significantly. Amiragova and Berlina made the assumption that the blockade of the adrenergic receptor sites in the thalamic relay nuclei serves to disconnect an ascending pathway which passes from the dog's hypothalamus to its cerebral cortex. When the adrenolytic agent temporarily severs this activating mechanism, the conditioned reflex behavior is inhibited. Although attractive, such a supposition would first require volume, pharmacological and anatomical controls.

V. MEMORY MECHANISMS

The technique of chemical stimulation offers a special advantage to the scientist whose interest is in understanding the mechanism for the memory of a given event. By the use of an appropriate substance, a temporary, reversible lesion can be produced in brain tissue before a task is acquired or at some specified interim after the learning to a criterion measure is completed.

Unfortunately, in any test of recall it is possible to determine neurochemically only when retention or retrieval is perturbed, not when it is enhanced. Furthermore, a performance measure is used to assess the extent of retention. Historically, it has been exceedingly difficult to distinguish between a deficit caused in a motor or sensory pathway from an actual deficit in the storage or retrieval of a learned response.

A. Cortical Aspect of Retention

Several investigators have altered the function of various regions of the cerebral cortex to ascertain the relationship between the neural sites serving the learning process and those involved in memory storage. For instance, focal epileptiform activity produced by alumina cream placed on the superficial cortex of the monkey retards the acquisition of all sorts of behavioral tasks. Generally, the memory for each task if learned prior to the epileptogenic lesion is not disrupted. Of special significance is the finding that the nature of the impairment in learning depends upon the region of the cortex which is required for the performance of a specific type of task (Stamm and Warren, 1961). Furthermore, focal epileptogenic discharges in certain regions such as the monkey's amygdala can interfere with the solution of a complex problem for which the utilization of previous experience is essential (Stamm and Knight, 1963). Even the transfer of training between two sets of somesthetic discrimination problems presented to a monkey can be incapacitated by focal epileptic activity induced by alumina cream placed on the parietal or temporal cortex (Stamm and Rosen, 1971).

When cobalt powder is placed on the parietal cortex or other neocortical sites of the rat to produce a focal epileptogenic disturbance, the conditioning to avoid shock by jumping onto a suspended pole is drastically attenuated (Kunz and Klingberg, 1969). Unlike the anatomical selectivity observed in the monkey, the site of the implant does not seem to matter, probably because of the widespread propagation of the convulsive electrical disturbance over the rat's cerebral cortex. What is also important is the finding that an avoidance response even if conditioned earlier is not retained after the cobalt lesion. This too does not correspond with the absence of interference to the memory storage of a monkey probably because of the disseminated epileptogenic activity.

Penicillin applied similarly to the neocortex of the rat fails to alter the rate of acquisition of a spatial discrimination in a T-maze or retard the solution of the reversal of the same maze problem (Schuman and Isaacson, 1970). Although the rat shows an increased irritability and a heightened level of activity in an open field, there is no correlation between the rat's performance and the penicillin lesion.

B. Hippocampus and Memory

Based on clinical evidence, Penfield and Milner (1958) and many others believe that the primary cerebral site for the registration of a bit of memory is contained within the hippocampus. However, the animal literature which would be taken to support this view is equivocal at the moment.

It is well known that a classically conditioned response can be blocked temporarily by neocortical spreading depression. Recently Bureš and his collaborators have begun to study the anatomical regions of the cortex that are involved in the KCl-induced decrement in performance of a response (Megirian and Bureš, 1970). Others have investigated the powerful action of spreading depression on subcortical structures implicated in memory formation.

Grossman and Mountford (1964) have used Bureš's method of localized spreading depression (e.g., 1972) to produce a reversibly dysfunctional hippocampus.

In a simple maze task in which a fasted rat is offered a food pellet for making the correct choice in a black-white discrimination, neither the acquisition score, reflected by the frequency of correct choices, nor the retention score shows any effect of local hippocampal depression produced by crystalline KCl, equivalent to a 100% solution. However, a decrement in performance is clear-cut following the bilateral application of KCl. That is, the rat responds more slowly to the opening of the start door, approaches the choice point more slowly and requires far more time to make a decision at the T-junction in the maze. Since the speed of the rat's running through the alley is relatively unaffected, it thus appears that the deficit is not due to a generalized motor disturbance. Following the hippocampal application of KCl, a rapid extinction of the maze habit occurs that is similar to that of a poorly-motivated rat. Thus, a nonspecific motivational change over and above an impairment in association is apparently related to the performance deficit.

Using a conditioned suppression technique in which a tone previously paired with shock was switched on while a thirsty rat was drinking water, Avis and Carlton (1968) did find that spreading depression blocks the retention of the rat's conditioned aversion toward licking the water spout. After a 25% KCl solution is injected bilaterally into the rat's hippocampus, the rat fails to retain the negative association signalled by the tone, and it continues to drink water. The results would suggest that the temporary interruption of hippocampal electrical activity disrupts the storage of a memory, at least that trace that pertains to a repugnant situation. If hippocampal spreading depression is not introduced for at least 24 hours after a conditioning session, then the condition of suppression is retained and the retograde amnesia does not appear. In this connection Auerbach and Carlton (1971) find that adrenal corticosteroid activation, an index of emotionality, is similarly attenuated by KCl injected into the hippocampus.

The temporal factors of retrograde amnesia following hippocampal spreading depression have been subsequently explored by Kapp and Schneider (1971) who used the same conditioned suppression technique. When crystalline KCl is applied to the hippocampus within 10 seconds after a conditioning session is completed, the retention of each rat is impaired when tested 4 to 21 days later. If on the other hand, the KCl crystals are deposited 24 hours after the training session, then significant amnesia is observed only 4 days later. Thereafter, there is a substantial recovery of the conditioned suppression to lick a water tube similar to that described by Hughes (1969). Apparently, the spreading wave of electrical negativity elicited by KCl (a) permanently disrupts the storage of a short-term memory, and (b) temporarily disrupts the retrieval of a longer term memory. These effects are reminiscent of the time-dependent recovery from amnesia in the human patient.

1. *Stimulation of Seizure Foci*

Since the hippocampus has been implicated in so many aspects of memory function in general and in the consolidation process in particular, Grossman (1969)

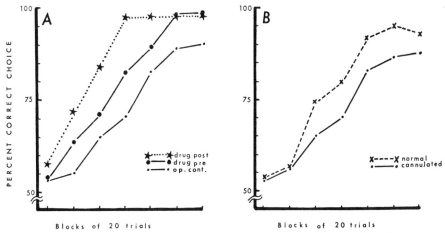

Fig. 12-18 Acquisition of a brightness discrimination in a T-maze. Panel A compares the performance of animals which received bilateral injections of 5 to 10 µg of pentylenetetrazol into the hippocampus 5 minutes before or immediately after each daily training session with that of sham-injected controls. Panel B shows the effects of the cannula implantation. (From Grossman, 1969)

has investigated the action of central nervous stimulants on this structure. A large number of experiments demonstrate unequivocally that a drug such as Metrazol, picrotoxin or strychnine given systemically immediately after each learning experience facilitates the acquisition of the behavior to be learned. When crystals of the powerful convulsant drug, Metrazol, are deposited in the hippocampus, the rat learns a simple brightness discrimination in a T-maze far more rapidly. With food pellets used as the reinforcement, the greatest improvement in learning, as illustrated in Fig. 12-18, occurs when Metrazol is implanted immediately after a daily set of six trials. All of the performance measures including the number of correct choices, the trials to criterion, and the results of a brightness reversal task, in which the previously rewarded brightness-value of the stimulus was made incorrect, revealed the same facilitating effect of intrahippocampal Metrazol. This finding supports the idea that a non-convulsive dose of a subcortical stimulant can aid the learning process and memory storage by improving the consolidation mechanism. One probable site of action is the hippocampus.

Ordinary escape from foot shock is not affected by an epileptogenic focus in the hippocampus of the rat; however, after crystalline penicillin is deposited unilaterally in this limbic structure, active avoidance learning in a two-way shuttle box is totally disrupted (Olton, 1970). As shown in Fig. 12-19, the training series had to be discontinued after a run of 250 unsuccessful trials. Either sodium sulfadiazine or penicillin applied to the septum or entorhinal region does not significantly interfere with the acquisition of the avoidance response. Thus, the abnormal seizure activity within the ipsilateral and contralateral mirror focus in

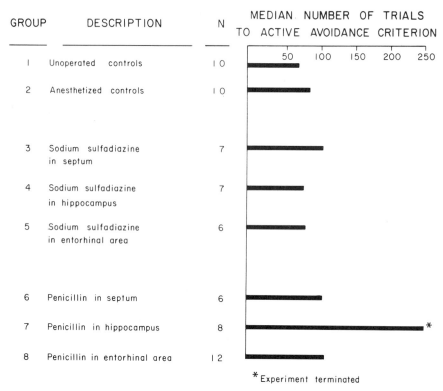

Fig. 12-19 Summary of experimental design and data from active avoidance. The bar graph indicates the number of trials to the beginning of criterion performance, 19 avoidance responses in 20 consecutive trials. (From Olton, 1970)

the hippocampus is not identical to a functional ablation, since a small lesion in this structure may facilitate avoidance learning.

In contrast to the response seen when the hippocampus is ablated bilaterally, the application of a large dose of penicillin either unilaterally or bilaterally to the hippocampus severely retards the rat's acquisition of a two-way active avoidance response to shock delivered to its cage floor (Schmaltz, 1971). Focal epileptiform or spike activity can also be recorded from the penicillin site within 10 minutes after the implantation; these abnormal discharges may persist for up to a month. Interestingly, if the rat is trained in the task before the deposition of penicillin in the hippocampus, the retention of the task is only partially attenuated. This would seem to rule out a performance deficit or motor disability as the basis for the impairment. Sodium sulfadiazine, another antibiotic which does not possess epileptogenic properties when placed even in a high dose in the hippocampus, fails to alter the rate of learning. A relationship between the perturbation in local EEG activity and the behavioral disturbance is thereby possible.

2. *Cholinergic Action*

In the mid-1950s, MacLean *et al.* (1955) began to explore the effect on conditioning of crystalline carbachol placed in the hippocampus. Not surprisingly, a cat or monkey was ordinarily unable to respond appropriately so as to avoid electric shock to the feet because of the severe psychomotor seizures produced by the cholinomimetic.

In another study a simple T-maze task was used in which water was made available for 5 seconds. Each rat was trained to alternate choices between the two goal areas. An injection of carbachol in a 1 μl volume into the hippocampus produced a doubling in the number of errors made by the rat at the same time that the running speed or the latency of choice was unaffected (Greene and Lomax, 1970). This significant impairment was not due to a motivational deficit but more probably to a perturbation of a cholinergic pathway, which disrupts the correct order in which a learned response is recalled. Thus, some interference with the storage process of a short-term memory is caused by the activation of cholinoceptive neurons.

Cholinergic stimulation of the caudate-putamen complex immediately after a passive avoidance learning trial disrupts any memory of that experience for up to 24 hours (Deadwyler *et al.*, 1972). However, when crystals of carbachol are placed in the lateral hypothalamus, there is no inhibition of the retention. Possibly a cholinergic system that passes through the caudate nucleus is involved in the phenomenon of retrograde amnesia, and the cholinomimetic mimics localized electrical stimulation. Support of this notion derives from the seizure activity in the EEG recorded from the cortex within 10 minutes after the implantation of carbachol.

Warburton and Russell (1969) have used a "go, no-go" lever-pressing task in which periods of reinforced responding are separated by intervals of no reinforcement for the emitted operant behavior. As illustrated in Fig. 12-20, a microinjection of atropine into the hippocampus increases the rat's perseverative errors in responding when no response should have been made; carbachol injected in the same region tends to suppress this kind of error and responding in general. Whether the effect of carbachol can be viewed as a mediation of an inhibitory pathway or whether the cholinomimetic evokes abnormal electrical activity such as focal seizure and thus a nonspecific functional disruption of hippocampal processes are two distinct although uncertain possibilities.

When atropine sulfate or its quaternary derivative, methyl atropine, is also injected into the hippocampus, the performance of a rat in a complex learning task is severely disrupted (Khavari and Maickel, 1967). Thus, the cholinergic suppression of the hippocampus produces a marked deficit in a well-learned pattern of behavior in that the rat is unable to withhold its responding and thus

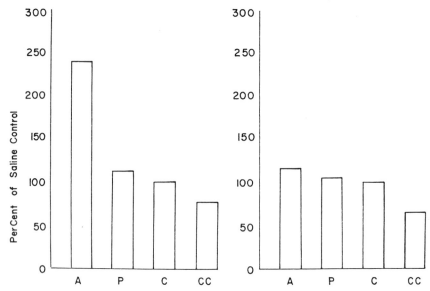

Fig. 12-20 Changes in alternation errors (left) and inter-trial interval (ITI) (right) responding following intrahippocampal injection of atropine (A), physostigmine (P), normal saline control (C), and carbachol (CC). (From Warburton, D. M. and R. W. Russel. 1969. *Life Sciences*. 8:617–627. Pergamon Press, New York)

perseverates. Given intraperitoneally, methyl atropine has no effect whereas the sulphate form of the salt which passes the blood-brain barrier produces a similar deficit.

Amphetamine is a sympathomimetic that is thought to release norepinephrine from its bound state at nerve terminals and to prevent its re-uptake. The net result would be an increase in the catecholamine concentration in the region of the receptor sites. In examining the direct central effect of this neural stimulant, Khavari (1969) trained animals on an intricate reinforcement schedule to press a level to obtain a 9% sucrose solution in response to a light-tone stimulus complex. A bilateral injection of 10 μg of *d*-amphetamine into the rat's lateral hypothalamus impairs performance in the same way as a larger dose when the compound is given either intraventricularly or intraperitoneally. Although a micro-injection of amphetamine into the hippocampus of the rat had no effect, this result would be expected because of the low endogenous concentration of catecholamines in this limbic structure. Presumably, a descending noradrenergic pathway which passes through the lateral hypothalamus is activated by amphetamine, which disrupts the rat's ongoing behavior.

It is noteworthy that the injection of atropine, scopolamine, or amphetamine into the cerebral ventricles also affects adversely a rat's learning capacity (Khavari, 1971). Perseverative errors similar to those seen in passive avoidance increase as the rat fails to press a lever when it should, and continues to lever-press when it should not. This very elegant demonstration that both a cholinolytic and sympathomimetic amine can exert the same central action would fit Carlton's (1963; 1969) formulation of a mutual antagonism between the cholinergic and adrenergic pathways.

C. Protein Synthesis and RNA

Periodically, reports appear that strongly implicate the intraneuronal synthesis of macromolecules in the formation of a long-term memory (e.g., Albert, 1966). It is well known, for instance, that drug-induced inhibition of cerebral protein synthesis in the mouse or chicken markedly impairs the retention of a learned response, but only after an interval of several hours has elapsed (e.g., Barondes, 1969; Mark and Watts, 1971; Watts and Mark, 1971). Basically, it is believed that new information arriving in the cerebrum causes the production of specific messenger RNA which is used in the formation of new protein molecules—the coded material of a permanent memory trace. Within the past few years, some exciting experiments have been undertaken to uncover the anatomical sites at which the synthesis of new protein may constitute a vital link in the establishment of a particular memory.

The destruction of cerebral RNA by ribonuclease interferes with the rat's acquisition of the simple task of pressing a lever to obtain a food pellet in a light-dark discrimination (Jaffard and Cardo, 1970). When ribonuclease was injected into the parietal or occipital cortex, the learning of these responses was impaired at the same time that the activity of the animal was unaffected. An injection given after the rat had learned either of the responses did not impair the animal's retention. Thus, there seems to be a very vital difference in terms of the effect on the acquisition and on the recall of a task. This depends on the locus in the brain at which the metabolism of nucleic acid is pharmacologically suppressed. A similar result has been obtained in the rabbit by Tushmalova and Melkova (1970) who blocked the conditioned reflex to obtain food after 300 μg of ribonuclease were infused into the animal's dorsal hippocampus.

An intriguing variation of the usual experiment paradigm with the rat has been presented by Codish (1971). Newly hatched chicks were imprinted to follow a mechanical surrogate hen which clucked and turned in a circle. After 1.2 μg of actinomycin D were injected in the region of the hippocampus in a huge 12 μl volume 30 minutes after the imprinting experience, the customary persistent response of following the surrogate disappeared completely in all of the birds. After 1 week, the imprinted response was absent in the actinomycin D group but present in saline control chicks. Thus, this special form of early memory would seem to require an intact cellular system for RNA synthesis.

A critical experiment on the effect of inhibiting protein synthesis has been completed by Daniels (1971) who examined the rat's retention of a shock-motivated, brightness discrimination in a Y-maze. The bilateral injection into the rat's hippocampus of 20 μg of acetoxycycloheximide, which is also an inhibitor of protein synthesis, has no deleterious effect on the acquisition of the task nor on its retention 3 hours later. However, the recall of the discrimination was severely impaired 6 hours, 24 hours or 7 days after the injection of acetoxycycloheximide. Daniels also found that if the drug was given just after learning or 5 hours before a test of recall, the rat's retention was unaffected. This important finding indicates that the establishment of a long-term memory in a rat is profoundly altered by the inhibition of protein synthesis whereas short-term retention is not. Further, Daniels suggests that both short- and long-term memory systems are initiated during the initial stages of acquisition and that they run parallel to one another rather than in serial succession.

That the anatomical locus of altered synthesis of ribonucleic acid is a crucial factor has been demonstrated by Nakajima (1969). When actinomycin D is injected in a relatively low dose of 1 μg into the hippocampus of the rat, the learning of a shock-motivated position discrimination in a T-maze is conspicuously disturbed. Those animals that ultimately do acquire the task also suffer difficulty in the relearning of the task. On the other hand, when the antibiotic is infused in an identical manner in the antero-dorsal neocortex of other rats, they experience no deficit in solving the discrimination problem. Similar chromatolytic lesions were noted by Nakajima in the histological sections. Further, still other rats in which the hippocampus was lesioned electrolytically do show retention of the task even though RNA synthesis could not take place in this structure. Coupled with this fact and the sudden development about 3 days later of epileptogenic discharges in the hippocampus of the actinomycin D-treated rats, it would appear that the profound deficits in learning and memory produced by the drug are the consequence of abnormal electrical activity rather than the lack of synthesis of macromolecules. Of course, it may be that these two functional events may not be mutually exclusive particularly within the cellular elements of hippocampal neurons.

Following this report, Nakajima (1972b) made the startling pronouncement that the effect of actinomycin D is actually unrelated to memory. Again the antibiotic was injected into the hippocampus of the rat at various intervals before or after the learning of the T-maze discrimination. Nakajima discovered that the rat's performance at the time of the retention test was impaired several days after actinomycin D was injected regardless of the time when the maze task had been learned. Moreover, the performance of a rat that had already learned the maze problem began to deteriorate about 3 days after the injection. This is shown in Fig. 12-21. These surprising findings do not correspond with those obtained in the goldfish (Agranoff et al., 1967) or mouse (Squire and Barondes, 1970) since retention in these two species is disturbed only when actinomycin D is given 1 hour after the original learning, but not after 3 hours.

This discrepancy in the results may be due perhaps to the actual problem asso-

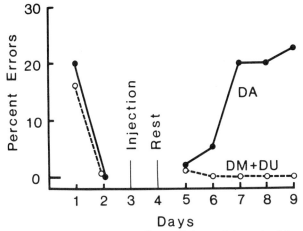

Fig. 12-21 Results of Experiment 2. Group DA was injected with actinomycin, Group DM with mannitol, and Group DU uninjected. The results of Groups DM and DU were combined because there was no essential difference between the two control groups. (From Nakajima, 1972a)

ciated with the volume of drug solution, relative to brain size, injected in the fish or mouse; however, even this does not explain the uniform temporal relationships documented in the two smaller species. Nevertheless, the phenomenon of an antibiotic-induced retrograde amnesia requires additional research before it can be viewed as a universal phenomenon related to the storage and retrieval of a memory trace within a specific anatomical locus.

VI. CONCLUDING CONSIDERATIONS

Variation in the experimental approach employed to study such a subtle transformation in behavior as learning introduces an almost insurmountable difficulty for those who wish to make a trenchant interpretation of the vast set of experiments in this field. To reiterate a segment of the Introduction, impairment in learning may really reflect an impairment in performance and have little to do with the ability of an animal to acquire a new response pattern. Similarly, a deficit in recall of a newly acquired repertoire of responses again may reflect an incapacity to perform a task and actually have little relationship to its retention.

Permeating the neurochemical experiments on the mechanisms of memory is the singularly crucial element of the temporal factor. In reality, the experimenter can prove almost any point that he wishes to make merely by selecting a decisive interval, often adventitiously, between a drug treatment prior to or after the initial training of an animal. Keeping in mind these points, there are several conclusions that can nevertheless be drawn from the foregoing investigations in this chapter.

A. Reward Mechanisms

From the research reports in which drugs are administered systemically, one would surmise that a central ACh system inhibits rewarded behavior. Such a broad generalization, however, must constitute an oversimplification because of two facts. First, a rat will emit a lever-press to self-infuse ACh to a structure in the limbic system. Second, a cholinolytic acting on muscarinic receptors in the mesencephalon attenuates hypothalamic self-stimulation in the dog. Although these findings provide a fairly sound basis for the importance of an ACh mechanism in the facilitation of the positive reward mechanism, they do not account for the blocking action of a cholinomimetic or for other contradictory observations. Therefore, the possibility cannot be disputed that there is an ACh system which facilitates the reward mechanism and a separate one which inhibits it.

How do the monoamines that are present in the limbic system, such as 5-HT, norepinephrine and dopamine function in the manifestation of a positive reward? At the present time there is abundant controversy based again on the experiments with drugs such as pCPA and αMpT; when given systemically, they deplete somewhat irregularly the cerebral stores of endogenous 5-HT and norepinephrine. From the important experiments of Margules on the injection of norepinephrine directly into the reward pathway or its terminus, it would appear that this catecholamine is involved synaptically in the mediation of reward or the inhibition of punishment. Although a definitive statement is difficult to construct, an integrated noradrenergic system may be anatomically comprised of the medial forebrain bundle together with its termination in the amygdala.

Important correlative information has come to light concerning the reward-inducing activity of the catecholamines (Arbuthnott et al., 1971). In spite of the fact that norepinephrine, epinephrine or serotonin infused into the hypothalamus counteracts the self-stimulating properties of compounds possessing excitatory effects (Olds et al., 1964), Stein and Wise (1969) have demonstrated that O-methylated metabolites of norepinephrine are released into fluid perfused through the rat's amygdala or hypothalamus by means of push-pull cannulae. The elevation in the metabolite level occurs only when the animal is self-stimulating its medial forebrain bundle with electric current, but not during the non-rewarding electrical stimulation of brain tissue. Furthermore, a high rate of electrical stimulation is reinstated in the rat by norepinephrine given intraventricularly after the lever-pressing behavior is suppressed by an enzyme inhibitor of norepinephrine synthesis (Wise and Stein, 1969). Although the evidence provided by these studies could be viewed as being indirect from a number of viewpoints, it should be recognized that this represents the beginning of some powerful support for the concept that norepinephrine release constitutes a principal neurohumoral link in the anatomical circuit containing the mechanism for positive reward.

B. Cholinergic Enhancement or Interference with Learning?

A cursory scanning of the Master Summary Table which follows reveals that the consequence of cholinergic stimulation, for the most part, is an impairment of avoidance conditioning or other form of learning. Quite significantly, this is considered independently of the locus of stimulation in the mesencephalon, hypothalamus, thalamus, amygdala, septum, caudate nucleus or hippocampus. Although experiments on the pharmacological antagonism of a cholinomimetic's deleterious effect have not been completed in as many anatomical sites, again we find a striking concordance centering on the improvement in an animal's performance in some of the discrimination and avoidance tasks studied (Warburton, 1972).

The few instances in which the local application of atropine contributes to a deficit in learning of an avoidance task or in an alternation problem also suggest a facilitating role for endogenous ACh. Equally as germane are those experiments in which carbachol, whose almost exclusive use in this particular field is regrettable, tends to improve the acquisition of an avoidance response. Within certain undesignated pathways, ACh may mediate a more efficient performance and thus improve the animal's learning. Such a speculation might be demonstrable only through the use of a small physiological dose, primarily because of the assumed sensitivity of the neuronal elements in this extremely labile system. If anything as subtle as an environmental stimulus pattern coupled with a reinforcement is sufficient to alter an animal's performance, then it is easy to imagine how a powerful drug deposited directly in the brain could be expected to affect the behavior in one direction only—downward! At the moment, the most laudable approach to a resolution of these discrepancies would seem to be the elaboration of a dose-response curve for each effect. Currently, the evidence in aggregate points to a dual cholinergic mechanism: one enhances the learning process while the other inhibits it.

The meaning of the intriguing results of an alteration in adrenal activity or thyroid function on the cerebral structures involved in the learning of a task or in the extinction of a learned response is presently unclear. What is difficult to know is whether the hormone is acting directly on a neuronal circuit or perhaps indirectly through the metabolism of another substance such as glucose. Whether changes in performance are the result of an effect on motor output or sensory input is yet another of the vital questions which require further research for clarification.

C. Neurohumoral Influence on Memory

Not unexpectedly, several impressive experiments done with judicious anatomical control point to the hippocampus as a principal locus in the neurohumoral mechanism of memory storage. The results with the localized reversible lesion of spreading depression or with convulsive and other drugs corroborate the earlier deductions based on experiments employing electrical stimulation or ablation. Again we note that a disturbance to the cholinergic synapses that are so heavily concentrated in the hippocampus can disrupt the recall of a learned task or impair an animal's performance after its training is completed.

Many questions of interminable fascination are raised by the experiments reported here. Is there a humoral code for a short-term memory? Is there a humoral code for a long-term memory? Are they encoded by the same chemical factor or complex of factors but differentiated on a morphological basis? Or are there individual chemical factors coding an engram within the same locus? How does the mechanism for retrieval operate so that a mental flash or an event, person, object or concept does not erupt spontaneously without reason?

Given that newly synthesized protein material in the cytoplasm of designated cerebral neurons does encode a memory trace or even a portion of it, a translation of the code into a synaptic reaction ultimately must take place. What is truly significant is that the decoding mechanism that raises the trace above the threshold of recall must always operate with alacrity. Why?

As this passage is read, visualize the number "7." Its entry into the conscious state is immediate. Now visualize the color of the first automobile ever owned. The latency of recall is just as short. The only difference is that the second image requires an incredibly greater number of elements to bring the more complex memory of car color above threshold. Finally, recall the most beautiful mountain vista ever witnessed as a youth—the vision of the fir trees, the greenery, the versants, the peaks, all come into cognitive focus with uncanny verisimilitude without any appreciable delay. Beginning probably within milliseconds, the recollection is just as instantaneous as the concept "7" or the color of the first-owned automobile. The object of this discussion is simply to emphasize the point that a network of neurons in the hippocampus or other structure that presumably codes such a vivid memory would have to utilize a humoral factor at each succeeding synapse that transmits impulses rapidly.

How a transformation arising from a cytoplasmic protein molecule can achieve this by way of activating the release of a substance such as ACh from its vesicles constitutes a puzzle to end all puzzlements. Whatever chemical is stored in a given configuration in nucleoprotein or in the soma must, by way of active axoplasmic transport, reach the nerve ending and trigger the release of material from the synaptic vesicles. This enables coded information to pass to the neurons which in turn enables a verbalization or other motor response to occur.

Unmistakably, we are only on the very threshold of comprehending how a chemical could possibly affect the memory trace or its cerebral acquisition. Even so, it is reassuring to know that these studies using the micro-injection technique have revealed some important first-order relationships between certain humoral systems and the processes of learning and memory.

VII. Master Summary Table
Chemicals that Exerted an Effect when Given at a Specific Site in the Brain

Chemical	Dose	Volume	Site	Species	State*	Response	Reference
Acetoxycycloheximide	20 μg	10 μl	Hippocampus	Rat	U	Impaired memory 6 hours, 24 hours, or 7 days after learning.	Daniels (1971)
Acetylcholine (ACh)	≈ .5-5 μg	crystal	Mesencephalic reticular formation	Rat	U	Impaired discrimination performance, impaired acquisition of lever-pressing, impaired exploratory behavior.	Grossman and Grossman (1966)
	≈ .1-5 μg	crystal	Mesencephalic reticular formation	Rat	U	Decreased avoidance performance.	Grossman (1966b; 1968b)
	320 μg	16 μl	Mesencephalon	Cat	U	Impaired conditioned reflexes.	Chkhartishvili (1969)
Actinomycin D	1.2 μg	12 μl	Hippocampus	Chicken	U	Eliminated imprinted behavior to surrogate hen.	Codish (1971)
	1 μg	2 μl	Hippocampus	Rat	U	Impaired learned performance on a maze task.	Nakajima (1972b)
	1 μg	2 μl	Hippocampus	Rat	U	Spike discharges, deficit in learning and retention of T-Maze discrimination.	Nakajima (1969)
Adrenocorticotrophic hormone [ACTH (1-10)]	≈ 10 μg	crystal	Mesencephalon, caudal thalamus	Rat	U	Inhibited extinction of avoidance response.	van Wimersma-Greidanus and de Wied (1971)
[D-phe[7]]-ACTH (1-10)	≈ 10 μg	crystal	Mesencephalon, caudal thalamus	Rat	U	Facilitated extinction of avoidance response.	van Wimersma-Greidanus and de Wied (1971)
Aminazine	≈ 50-100 μg/kg	?	Antero-medial thalamus	Dog	U	Inhibited conditioned reflex.	Amiragova and Berlina (1970a)

*U = unanesthetized and unrestrained; C = constrained, confined or curarized; A = anesthetized.

VII. Master Summary Table (Continued)

Chemical	Dose	Volume	Site	Species	State*	Response	Reference
d-Amphetamine	10 μg	5 μl	Hippocampus	Rat	U	Did not impair bar-pressing.	Khavari (1969)
	10 μg	1 μl	Hypothalamus	Rat	U	Impaired bar-pressing performance.	Khavari (1969)
Atropine	?	crystal	Medial hypothalamus	Rat	U	Disinhibition of punished behavior.	Margules and Stein (1966)
	≈.5–5 μg	crystal	Ventromedial hypothalamus	Rat	U	Discrimination performance; improved avoidance performance.	Grossman (1966a)
	≈.5–5 μg	crystal	Septum	Rat	U	Improved avoidance performance.	Grossman (1964b)
	≈1.5 μg	crystal	Thalamic reticular and midline nuclei	Rat	U	Increased exploratory activity.	Grossman et al. (1965)
	≈4–5 μg	crystal	Ventromedial hypothalamus	Rat	U	Reduced conflict behavior.	Sepinwall and Grodsky (1969)
	≈5 μg	crystal	Lateral hypothalamus, ventromedial hypothalamus	Rat	U	Impaired avoidance performance.	Sepinwall (1969)
	≈5–14 μg	crystal	Ventromedial hypothalamus	Rat	U	Increased passive avoidance deficit.	Margules and Stein (1969b)
	≈10–20 μg	crystal	Internal capsule	Rat	U	Acceptance of shock.	Margules (1971b)
	4 μg	.6 μl	Hippocampus	Rat	U	Increased alternation errors.	Warburton and Russell (1969)
	50 μg	5–10 μl	Hippocampus	Rat	U	Impaired performance in complex bar-pressing task.	Khavari and Maickel (1967)
	≈10–20 μg	crystal	Septum	Cat	U	Impaired passive avoidance learning.	Hamilton et al. (1968)
	≈10–20 μg	crystal	Septum	Cat	U	Impaired acquisition of active avoidance learning.	Hamilton and Grossman (1969)

Drug	Dose	Site	Species		Effect	Reference
	80 µg	Caudate nucleus	Cat	U	Inhibition of a conditioned instrumental response.	Prado-Alcalá et al. (1972)
	100 µg	Nucleus centro-median of thalamus	Cat	U	Increased non-reinforced responding.	Avery and Nance (1970b)
	≈2-5 µg	Ventromedial hypothalamus	Monkey	C	Increased punished responding; reduced food and water intake.	Miczek and Grossman (1972)
Atropine (methyl)	≈1-2 µg	Midline thalamic nucleus	Rat	U	Enhanced avoidance learning and performance.	Grossman and Peters (1966)
	≈2-7 µg	Septum	Rat	U	Facilitated shock avoidance learning.	Kelsey and Grossman (1969)
	≈1-2 µg	Reticular nucleus of thalamus	Rat	U	Impaired avoidance learning and performance.	Grossman and Peters (1966)
	50 µg	Hippocampus	Rat	U	Impaired performance in complex bar-pressing task.	Khavari and Maickel (1967)
	≈7-17 µg	Ventromedial hypothalamus	Rat	U	Produced passive avoidance deficit; increased locomotor activity.	Margules and Stein (1969a)
Carbachol	?	Medial hypothalamus	Rat	U	Restored effects of punishment.	Margules and Stein (1966)
	≈.5-1 µg	Mesencephalic reticular formation	Rat	U	Decreased avoidance performance.	Grossman (1966b; 1968b)
	≈1.5 µg	Thalamic reticular and midline nuclei	Rat	U	Impaired avoidance learning.	Grossman et al. (1965)
	≈1.7 µg	Midbrain tegmentum	Rat	U	Suppressed hypothalamic self-stimulation.	Routtenberg (1965)
	≈.5-2 µg	Amygdala	Rat	U	Convulsions; aggression; facilitated two-way shuttle box learning; impaired one-way avoidance learning.	Belluzzi (1972)
	≈.5-3 mg	Thalamus	Rat	U	Impaired active and passive avoidance.	Blanchard et al. (1972)
	≈3 µg	Dorsal mesencephalor.	Rat	U	Suppressed hypothalamic self-stimulation.	Routtenberg and Olds (1966)

VII. Master Summary Table (*Continued*)

Chemical	Dose	Volume	Site	Species	State*	Response	Reference
Carbachol	≃ .5–5 µg	crystal	Septum	Rat	U	Impaired avoidance learning and performance.	Grossman (1964b)
	≃ .5–5 µg	crystal	Mesencephalic reticular formation	Rat	U	Impaired discrimination performance; impaired acquisition of lever-pressing; impaired exploratory behavior.	Grossman and Grossman (1966)
	≃ 3–5 µg	crystal	Lateral hypothalamus	Rat	U	Motivated drinking.	Khavari and Russell (1966)
	≃ 4–5 µg	crystal	Lateral hypothalamus	Rat	U	Reduced conflict behavior.	Sepinwall and Grodsky (1969)
	≃ 4–5 µg	crystal	Ventromedial hypothalamus	Rat	U	Suppressed approach-avoidance.	Sepinwall and Grodsky (1969)
	≃ 5 µg	crystal	Lateral hypothalamus, ventromedial hypothalamus	Rat	U	Enhanced avoidance performance.	Sepinwall (1969)
	≃ 5–14 µg	crystal	Ventromedial hypothalamus	Rat	U	Reduced passive avoidance deficit.	Margules and Stein (1969b)
	≃ 5–15 µg	crystal or .5–2 µl	Septum	Rat	U	Impaired avoidance learning.	Sepinwall (1966)
	≃ 5–15 µg	crystal or .5–2 µl	Lateral hypothalamus	Rat	U	Enhanced avoidance learning.	Sepinwall (1966)
	.014–.11 µg	.003 µl	Lateral hypothalamus	Rat	U	Enhanced local self-injection.	Olds *et al.* (1964)
	.01–.25 µg	1 µl	Amygdala	Rat	U	Impaired shock avoidance learning; disrupts passive avoidance learning when retention required.	Goddard (1959)

Drug	Dose	Form	Site	Species	U/C	Effect	Reference
	.4 µg	.6 µl	Hippocampus	Rat	U	Suppression of perseverative errors.	Warburton and Russell (1971)
	2.5 µg	1 µl	Hippocampus	Rat	U	Impaired alternation learning.	Greene and Lomax (1970)
	1.1–4.3 µg	.25–1 µl	Dorsal mesencephalon	Rat	U	Suppressed hypothalamic self-stimulation.	Routtenberg and Olds (1966)
	≈10–15 µg	crystal	Posterior hypothalamus	Rabbit	U	Improved responding for food; impaired shock avoidance.	Kalyuzhnyi (1962)
	8–16 µg	2 µl	Septum	Cat	U	Impaired two-way active avoidance.	Holloway (1972)
	16 µg	2 µl	Nucleus centro-median of thalamus	Cat	U	Suppressed reinforced responding.	Avery and Nance (1970b)
	≈25–50 µg	crystal	Caudate nucleus	Cat	U	Impairment of conditioned avoidance response.	Stevens et al. (1961)
	≈.5–1 µg	crystal	Ventromedial hypothalamus	Monkey	C	Reduced punished responding; reduced food and water intake.	Miczek and Grossman (1972)
Chlorpromazine derivatives	5 µg	crystal or 1 µl	Hypothalamus	Rat	U	Changes in avoidance responding.	Grossman (1968a)
Corticosterone	≈7 µg	crystal	Nucleus parafascicularis	Rat	U	Facilitated extinction of conditioned avoidance response.	van Wimersa-Greidanus and de Wied (1969)
Cortisol	≈5 µg	crystal	Median eminence	Rat	U	Slightly facilitated extinction of conditioned avoidance response.	Bohus (1968)
	≈5 µg	crystal	Mesencephalic reticular formation	Rat	U	Facilitated extinction of conditioned avoidance response.	Bohus (1968)
Cortisone	?	crystal	Medial thalamus, anterior hypothalamus, septum	Rat	U	Rapid extinction of avoidance responding.	Bohus (1970a and b)

VII. Master Summary Table (Continued)

Chemical	Dose	Volume	Site	Species	State*	Response	Reference
Dexamethasone	≈10 µg	crystal	Thalamus (posterior, medial)	Rat	U	Facilitated extinction of conditioned avoidance response.	van Wimersa-Greidanus and de Wied (1969)
Epinephrine	.011–.016 µg	.003 µl	Lateral hypothalamus	Rat	U	Attenuated local self-injection.	Olds et al. (1964)
Ethobutamoxane	27 µg	2 µl	Nucleus centromedian of thalamus	Cat	U	Enhanced visual discrimination performance.	Avery and Nance (1970b)
Glutamate	8.82 µg	2 µl	Lateral hypothalamus	Rat	U	Facilitated self-stimulation.	Nakajima (1972a)
Glutamate	8.82 µg	2 µl	Ventral tegmentum	Rat	U	Reduced hypothalamic self-stimulation rate.	Nakajima (1972a)
γ-Aminobutyric acid (GABA)	.046–.062 µg	.003 µl	Lateral hypothalamus	Rat	U	Attenuated local self-injection.	Olds et al. (1964)
dl-4-[2-Hydroxy-3-isopropylamino-propoxy] indole (LB-46)	≈10–20 µg	crystal	Amygdala	Rat	U	Reinstated passive avoidance behavior.	Margules (1971a)
Iproniazid	1.4 µg	1.4 µl	Hypothalamus	Rat	U	Self-injection.	Olds and Olds (1958)
Isoproterenol	≈10–20 µg	crystal	Amygdala	Rat	U	Reduced acceptance of shock responses.	Margules (1971a)
Metamyzil	5–10 µg	1–2 µl	Hypothalamus	Dog	U	Inhibited self-stimulation, agitation.	Kraus and Lapina (1972)
Metrazol	≈5–10 µg	crystal	Hippocampus	Rat	U	Enhanced discrimination learning.	Grossman (1969)
Muscarine	≈5–14 µg	crystal	Ventromedial hypothalamus	Rat	U	Reduced passive avoidance deficit.	Margules and Stein (1969b)
Nembutal	25–100 µg	.5–2 µl	Lateral hypothalamus, ventromedial hypothalamus	Rat	U	Impaired avoidance performance.	Sepinwall (1969)

Drug	Dose	Form	Brain region	Animal		Effect	Reference
Neostigmine	≈7–17 µg	crystal	Ventromedial hypothalamus	Rat	U	Suppressed punished and non-punished responding.	Margules and Stein (1969a)
Norepinephrine	?	crystal	Amygdala	Rat	U	Acceptance of punished responses.	Margules (1968)
	≈.5–5 µg	crystal	Septum	Rat	U	Improved avoidance performance.	Grossman (1964b)
	≈10–20 µg	crystal	Amygdala	Rat	U	Increased acceptance of shock responses (punishment).	Margules (1971a and b)
	.075 µg	.003 µl	Lateral hypothalamus	Rat	U	Attenuated local self-injection.	Olds et al. (1964)
	≈10–15 µg	crystal	Posterior hypothalamus	Rabbit	U	Improved shock avoidance performance; inhibited food responses.	Kalyuzhnyi (1962)
	40–80 µg	2 µl	Septum	Cat	U	Increased latency of avoidance in two-way shuttle-box performance.	Holloway (1972)
	80 µg	2 µl	Nucleus centro-median of thalamus	Cat	U	Enhanced visual discrimination performance.	Avery and Nance (1970b)
Penicillin	?	crystal	Hippocampus	Rat	U	Disrupted two-way active avoidance learning.	Olton (1970)
	≈300–500 µg	crystal	Hippocampus	Rat	U	Impaired acquisition of avoidance task; focal spike discharges.	Schmaltz (1971)
Phenoxybenzamine	2–16 µg	1 µl or crystal	Mesencephalic reticular formation	Rat	U	Enhanced lever-pressing.	Grossman (1968b)
Phentolamine	≈10–20 µg	crystal	Amygdala	Rat	U	Reinstated passive avoidance behavior.	Margules (1971a)
Physostigmine	?	crystal	Medial hypothalamus	Rat	U	Restored effects of punishment.	Margules and Stein (1966)
	?	crystal	Amygdala	Rat	U	Impaired one-way avoidance learning.	Belluzzi (1972)
	≈5–14 µg	crystal	Ventromedial hypothalamus	Rat	U	Reduced passive avoidance deficit.	Margules and Stein (1969b)

VII. Master Summary Table (Continued)

Chemical	Dose	Volume	Site	Species	State*	Response	Reference
Physostigmine	≈7–17 µg	crystal	Ventromedial hypothalamus	Rat	U	Suppressed punished and non-punished responding.	Margules and Stein (1969a)
Potassium chloride (KCl)	≈1–5 µg	crystal	Hippocampus	Rat	U	Impaired brightness discrimination.	Grossman and Mountford (1964)
	≈14 µg	crystal	Hippocampus	Rat	U	Spreading depression; impaired retention.	Kapp and Schneider (1971)
	1 mg	4 µl	Hippocampus	Rat	A	Attenuated EEG, disrupted retention of CER.	Hughes (1969)
	.75–1.87 mg	3–7.5 µl	Hippocampus	Rat	U	Attenuated corticosteroid elevation during CER.	Auerbach and Carlton (1971)
	1.25–3 mg	5–12 µl	Hippocampus	Rat	U	Spreading depression; inhibited retention of a conditioned response.	Avis and Carlton (1968)
Procaine	40 µg	2 µl	Medial forebrain bundle, lateral hypothalamus	Rat	U	Suppression of electrical self-stimulation to septum, POA; lever-pressing for food pellet.	Madryga and Albert (1971)
	100 µg	2 µl	Lateral hypothalamus, ventral tegmentum	Rat	U	Reduced hypothalamic self-stimulation rate.	Nakajima (1972a)
	400 µg	20 µl	Septum	Rat	U	Impaired classical conditioning, fear, excitation.	Luncan (1971)
Ribonuclease	100 µg	2.5 µl	Occipital cortex, parietal cortex	Rat	U	Impaired acquisition of lever-pressing and visual discrimination.	Jaffard and Cardo (1970)
	300 µg	5 µl	Dorsal hippocampus	Rabbit	U	Blocked conditioned reflex to obtain food.	Tushmalova and Melkova (1970)
Scopolamine	≈2–4 µg	crystal	Amygdala	Rat	U	Reversed carbachol learning deficit.	Belluzzi and Grossman (1969)

Substance	Dose	Volume	Site	Species		Effect	Reference
	≈5–10 µg	crystal	Ventral caudate nucleus	Rat	U	Facilitated avoidance learning.	Neill and Grossman (1970)
	≈5–10 µg	crystal	Dorsal caudate nucleus	Rat	U	Impaired avoidance learning.	Neill and Grossman (1970)
	≈5–14 µg	crystal	Ventromedial hypothalamus	Rat	U	Increased passive avoidance deficit.	Margules and Stein (1969b)
	≈10–20 µg	crystal	Septum	Cat	U	Impaired acquisition of active avoidance learning.	Hamilton and Grossman (1969)
Serotonin (5-HT)	.091–.12 µg	.003 µl	Lateral hypothalamus	Rat	U	Attenuated local self-injection.	Olds et al. (1964)
NaEDTA	.033–.068 µg	.003 µl	Lateral hypothalamus	Rat	U	Enhanced local self-injection.	Olds et al. (1964)
Na phosphate	.043–.064 µg	.003 µl	Lateral hypothalamus	Rat	U	Enhanced local self-injection.	Olds et al. (1964)
Na pyrophosphate	.033–.067 µg	.003 µl	Lateral hypothalamus	Rat	U	Enhanced local self-injection.	Olds et al. (1964)
Thyroxine	≈10 µg/kg	?	Centromedial thalamus	Dog	U	Failed to alter conditioned reflex after hypothalamic thyroxine.	Amiragova and Berlina (1970a)
	≈10 µg/kg	25 µl	Posterior hypothalamus	Dog	U	Enhanced conditioning of reflex for food.	Amiragova and Berlina (1970a)

13 *Epilogue*

I. INTRODUCTION

Since this Epilogue evolved gradually as the information in each chapter was considered, Chapter 13 is not an afterthought. Whether the ideas contained here are eventually verified is inconsequential. Hopefully, they will provide some basis of reflection for the open-minded scientist, young or old, who is intellectually captivated by one or more of the extraordinary effects that can be witnessed after the brain is stimulated directly by a chemical substance.

If taken in their entirety, the findings reported in these chapters form a theoretical framework for some intriguing conjectures about the brain and the remarkable operations that this organ performs. Notwithstanding the fact that a considerable number of the experiments described in the foregoing text may lack a dose response curve, or information about pharmacological blockade, or a comprehensive anatomical mapping of the loci of effect, many of these investigations are nevertheless informative. Most all are suggestive.

A. Anatomical Uniqueness

For a start, a mere glance at each Master Summary Table emphasizes an underlying principle of anatomical specificity. That is, a given response to a chemical occurs primarily when a restricted region of brain tissue or part of a defined pathway is excited or inhibited. If morphological concepts are retained as a cornerstone of the understanding of neural function, it is almost axiomatic that the localization of action of a drug or any other chemical for that matter is now within reasonable scientific grasp. The extent of the resolution provided by the ventricular and other more traditional approaches to the issue of morphological localization wanes appreciably in contrast to an experiment having greater anatomical precision. What is so fascinating is that this general observation about morphological specificity extends across each topic of investigation de-

648

scribed in Chapters 3 through 12, whether in relation to a given structure or a circuit of structures linked together by a demarcated fiber system.

Of special importance is one discomforting fact revealed again by the perusal of the Master Summary Tables. The anatomical correlations formulated in terms of chemical sensitivity are largely fragmentary; within every corner of this field, gaps in our knowledge of immense proportion do exist today. Regrettably, the chief morphological emphasis in several disciplines has centered on only one major structure. Two such examples come to mind immediately: (1) the median eminence which occupies the spotlight for the neuroendocrine researchers; and (2) the rostral portion of the hypothalamus which has received lopsided attention by investigators whose interest lies in the mechanism of thermoregulation.

Of course, one could argue that this situation has arisen not without good reason. After all, these structures are unusually sensitive to chemical modification in terms of the respective measures taken and seem to possess unique receptors within their delimited anatomical borders. Nonetheless, it is clear that if other structures are explored with equal zeal and not dismissed offhandedly as having nothing to do with a given function, some significant new advances may burgeon forth. To be sure, neuroendocrinologists are now entertaining the possibility that a portion of the limbic system such as the hippocampus may share an important role in the action of a steroid (Chapters 4 and 5). In reality, subcortical neurons may integrate hormonal information which influences the animal's behavior rather than the physiological component of a sexual, adrenal or other response.

To make coherent sense of each reaction that is elicited chemically is by no means an easy task, particularly with respect to the anatomy of the forebrain and midbrain. For example, if the entries on the Master Summary Tables for the lateral hypothalamus or the amygdala are examined, it is readily apparent that these two structures may serve several neural masters. In fact, the functional capacity of each is exceptionally diverse.

By chemically stimulating the lateral hypothalamus, one can influence an animal's gastric secretion, its heart rate, blood pressure, hormonal activity, respiration, body temperature, feeding behavior, fluid intake, motivational level, sleep-wakefulness cycle, EEG pattern, emotionality, motor response, stereotypic behavior, killing propensity, or the animal's performance in a learning task.

Chemical stimulation of the amygdala can act to excite or inhibit the animal's general autonomic activity, emotionality, sleep, conditioning of a behavioral response, aggression, epileptic seizures, vocalization, attention, catatonia, tremor, twitching, drinking, feeding, sexual behavior, lactation, ACTH release, vomiting and salivation. The same sort of astounding catalogue of effects is seen for a surprising proportion of individual structures that have been tested using the approach of chemical stimulation.

B. Basis of Anatomical Diversity

What does this complex state of anatomical affairs signify?

First, in considering a reaction mediated by a structure, it is mandatory to know which chemical alters which response under what circumstance. At once, the myriad of reactions exemplified above can be classified according to the category of the compound that is used for stimulating the structure. Otherwise, such information about the lateral hypothalamus or amygdala is wantonly misleading.

Second, a concept that has been considered for about 10 years or more (cf. Wayner, 1964) becomes even clearer: a circumscribed region of the brain does not necessarily constitute a center for a given function. Although a subcortical structure may perform a major function and as such comprise a vital morphological link in a given system (Millhouse, 1969), almost every structure or subpart of it may be able to serve several functions. Hence, the traditional idea expressed so often that a specific "center" controls a given functional process necessarily falls by the wayside. More properly, it might be well to replace the word center with a term such as "primary monitoring zone": *primary* because there are obviously secondary regions which take over a portion of a function, after some days or weeks, when the primary neurons are lesioned; *monitoring* since the confluence of input to sensors or detectors including steroid, CO_2, osmo-, gluco-, or thermoreceptors, has determined historically the features of a so-called center; and *zone* because this word can denote a region set off from adjoining structures yet can retain the intrinsic meaning of a broad circuit of neurons that is characterized by a uniform function.

Third, a part of the variety of physiological reactions capable of being produced by chemical excitation could be attributed to a lack of precise anatomical localization. It would be delusive at this time to gainsay the possibility that some of the reported responses may be due to a partial spillover of the chemical from the site of its application to a contiguous structure.

Fourth, an observer on the lookout only for a change in one type of physiological or behavioral process may overlook a causal relationship. For example, an animal that gulps down a large volume of water will in turn experience a sharp fall in body temperature, which may then alter respiratory rate. The point here is that to monitor the intake of water but not body temperature, or to record focal EEG activity but not the level of arousal, or to measure a stereotyped movement but not tremor, will yield only a partial answer. To chronicle only one type of isolated response could lead to a misinterpretation of fact and conceivably to some sort of discrepancy.

Fifth, to accept or reject a hypothesis about an integrated function on the basis of one species alone is anatomically foolhardy. Speculation about an individual chemical mechanism in the brain of the rat, sometimes with total disregard of a pertinent finding in another species such as the cat or monkey, is an all-too-common practice among some scientists. Since the morphology of each species is founded on a comparative basis, it is logical to conceive of the neurohumoral properties of an anatomical substrate in a similar way.

II. ARE FUNCTIONS OF THE FOREBRAIN AND MIDBRAIN CHEMICALLY CODED?

Ever since the word "coding" was used popularly to document a chemical configuration that determines the patterning of genes, this term has been employed widely in the neurosciences to describe a particular systematization of physiological signals or messages in the vertebrate or invertebrate nervous system.

Within the present context, a chemical coding extant within brain tissue would be defined as the neurohumoral systematization at the level of the synaptic membrane of a specific response, whether behavioral or physiological. This means that a synaptic element involved in a given function and located in a very restricted part of the brain could be activated by the presence or release of one substance but suppressed by the presence or release of a second substance. Presumably, a physiological imbalance sensed locally or signalled remotely by the afferent input for that function would serve as the trigger to release one or the other opposing substance.

One who adopts the view of a chemical code does so usually after stepping back from an experiment in which two chemicals applied to brain tissue have evoked startlingly opposite effects. Immediately, the pivotal question arises: "How could these responses occur?"

A. Concept of a Neurochemical Code

In its simplest form, the concept of neurochemical coding could account for the phenomenon of the excitation of a set of neurons by one substance and their inhibition by another substance (Miller, 1965; Myers and Sharpe, 1968b). The response of these neurons could activate a designated pathway and thereby evoke a chain of specific behavioral or physiological reactions. Therefore, as a starting premise, one must acknowledge that the transmission of a nerve impulse is initiated by a chemical event.

Although the concept is theoretically attractive on the surface because of its relative simplicity and capacity to explain many results, whether each coding system in all of its infinite complexity can be entirely deciphered is presently uncertain. The principal reason for this is that the nerve terminal is an exceedingly complicated structure as is revealed by every kind of cytochemical analysis, iontophoretic study or determination of the chemical constituents of the particulate matter at the nerve ending. Moreover, the evolutionary aspects of the coding mechanism and the associated anatomical circuitry across the animal kingdom are so intricate that they almost reach beyond human comprehension.

Certainly at this stage in our progress, no one person possesses sufficient information to pass judgment on the acceptability of the concept of a neuro-humoral code. Therefore, some pertinent evidence will now be considered towards an evaluation of this intriguing concept.

B. Dualism in Neurohumoral Coding

Cutting across different fields of investigation are a number of observations which reflect a neurochemical dualism in the expression of a hypothesized coding mechanism. For many an endogenous substance that is found to excite a given region and stimulate a specific response, an alternative neurohumoral substance is known to counter that response.

A few illustrations of this dualism are presented here in terms of two humoral factors applied at an identical anatomical locus. (1) Serotonin given in the rostral part of the hypothalamus increases local blood flow, whereas norepinephrine reduces blood flow when applied similarly (Chapter 3). (2) Progesterone deposited in the ventromedial hypothalamus suppresses the synthesis of progestin, but estrogen application at the same locus facilitates its synthesis (Chapter 5). (3) Serotonin elevates body temperature when infused into the anterior hypothalamus whereas norepinephrine produces hypothermia (Chapter 6). (4) Norepinephrine injected in the rostral hypothalamus evokes feeding whereas angiotensin reduces eating behavior (Chapter 7). (5) Epinephrine deposited in the amygdala suppresses drinking, whereas cholinergic stimulation of this structure enhances the intake of water (Chapter 8). (6) Dopamine injected into the caudate nucleus antagonizes the intense tremor evoked by acetylcholine applied at the same locus (Chapter 10). (7) ACh injected into the hypothalamus evokes the killing of a prey, whereas norepinephrine at the same site suppresses it (Chapter 11). (8) ACh impairs the performance of a learned avoidance response whereas norepinephrine improves this performance when they are injected into the septum (Chapter 12).

A note of caution must be sounded with regard to a mechanistic interpretation of the palpable "on-off" nature of two functionally opposing substances. The dualism is undoubtedly an oversimplification that is derived originally from the conceptual dichotomy of cholinergic versus adrenergic receptors in the sympathetic nervous system. Actually, there is reasonable evidence that three or more substances within a circumscribed region may well be involved simultaneously in the efferent activity that controls a set of responses. For instance, Na^+, angiotensin, ACh and a monoamine are already implicated in the diencephalic mechanisms underlying the drinking of fluids (Chapter 8). Similarly, serotonin, norepinephrine, ACh, a prostaglandin, Na^+, and Ca^{2+} are believed to play a critical part in the hypothalamic control of body temperature (Chapter 7).

A remarkable corollary of the coding process is the anatomical selectivity in the activation of a class of receptors. Within a given species, a single substance may exert quite antagonistic actions, illustrated as follows: (1) ACh inhibits or facilitates colonic motility depending upon how laterally the ACh implant is positioned in the rostral hypothalamus (Chapter 3). (2) Serotonin may cause either an elevation or decrease in plasma 17-hydroxycorticosteroids as a result of a slight alteration in the horizontal plane in the hippocampus at which the amine is deposited (Chapter 4). (3) Estrogen applied in the median eminence of the female impairs gonadal development but in the anterior hypothalamus acts to advance the time of vaginal opening (Chapter 5). (4) Although stimulation of nicotinic receptors in the hypothalamus evokes a change in body temperature, a hyper- or hypothermia is contingent on the site of an injection of nicotine in the rostral-caudal axis (Chapter 6). (5) Norepinephrine enhances or suppresses the drinking of water depending on the locus of its deposition in the hypothalamus (Chapter 8). (6) Sleep, arousal or rage is reported to occur after ACh is placed in different parts of the cat's hypothalamus (Chapters 9 and 11). (7) Contralateral movement including circling is determined by whether the right or left corpus striatum is stimulated by ACh (Chapter 10). (8) Glutamate either raises or lowers the rate of hypothalamic self-stimulation with electric current depending upon whether the amino acid is injected into the hypothalamus or midbrain, respectively (Chapter 12).

Although a compound may either excite or depress a local group of neurons, the possibility cannot be excluded that a response may occur as a result of the blockade of an inhibitory system. In this case, the chemical substance would only appear to possess an excitatory property. For example, the feeding evoked by norepinephrine injected into the hypothalamus (Chapter 7) may ensue because the catecholamine actually suppresses a satiety circuit; in turn, the normal inhibition of feeding is not prevented. Research that raises this possibility is still in a very early stage.

The concordance of a pharmacological manipulation with that of chemical stimulation is vital to the supposition that a centrally occurring substance has a localized physiological role (Chapter 1). When taken as a whole, the specific blockade of a class of receptors, the elevation of the content of a substance, and the prevention of its degradation contribute toward a convincing case for the functional significance of that compound.

Going hand in hand with the criterion of identical actions (Werman, 1972), evidence of equal consequence is provided by the lability of the endogenous substance as reflected by its release into the extracellular space. Even so, it is not enough that a given substance effuses spontaneously from cerebral tissue and passes into a cerebral ventricle or into the cisterna magna. It is also not enough that electrical stimulation of adjacent brain tissue can cause the interstitial extravasation of the substance. As in the case of the false transmitter, which selectively accumulates and displaces an amine in the nerve ending (Kopin, 1971), such a release may be unrelated to the reason for its presence.

C. Local Release of a Humoral Factor

The crux of the whole issue of the functional specificity of a given substance is whether its *in vivo* release can be differentially enhanced or suppressed.

To demonstrate this is not an elementary matter. The reasons for this are as follows: (1) the change in the level of release of the substance from a resting base line must be evoked by a quantifiable physiological stimulus; (2) the change in the output of the substance must occur in a specified direction, i.e., either increased or decreased; (3) the augmentation or reduction in the release of the substance must correlate with one or more aspects of the functional state of the animal which was altered in the first place; (4) the pattern of localized release from neural tissue should coincide temporally with the pharmacological action of that same substance when it is applied or micro-injected at the homologous site; (5) the activation or prevention of the release of the substance should be altered by an appropriate pharmacological agent known to exert such enhancing or attenuating effects when acting on the nerve cell.

1. Brain Transfusion Studies

One direct way of determining whether a physiologically active factor is released from the brain is to collect it from the brain of one animal and then transfer it to the brain of a second animal (e.g., Myers, 1967a). The earliest work using this paradigm was done in Pieron's laboratory in the early part of this century (Chapter 9). When CSF was collected from a sleep-deprived dog and was re-injected into the cisterna magna of a normal dog, the recipient became somnolent. As a result, the exciting prospect arose of a "hypnogenic factor" which is responsible for the induction of the sleeping state. Promising research in different laboratories such as those of Pappenheimer and Monnier (Chapter 9) has been devoted similarly to the examination of the CSF of the sleep-deprived animal. Fascinating attempts to determine the chemical nature of a sleep-promoting substance are now in progress. In fact, Monnier and his group have succeeded in purifying and isolating a factor which is collected by the extracorporeal dialysis of plasma that is recirculated in a sleeping rabbit (Monnier *et al.*, 1972; Schoenenberger *et al.*, 1972).

Evidence has also been obtained for the presence of a thermogenic factor in the cerebrospinal fluid of the monkey (Myers, 1967b). When CSF is taken from a monkey exposed to cold air and transfused directly to the third ventricle of a normothermic monkey, the recipient begins to shiver and to develop a fever. Other isolated experiments have suggested that a humoral factor is present in the CSF of a hungry or satiated animal. For example, CSF which is collected from a food-deprived donor monkey causes a second monkey to eat food biscuits when this CSF is perfused through the recipient's lateral hypothalamus (Myers, 1969b). The effect of this CSF on ingestive behavior is a potent one, since the latency of onset is very short and the duration is up to an hour.

To try to identify the specific sites at which these temperature and feeding factors are released, Myers and Sharpe (1968c) collected perfusate from push-pull cannulae implanted in the thermosensitive zone of the monkey's hypothalamus—the anterior region (Chapter 6). When this perfusate is transfused directly to the homologous site of a recipient, the body temperature of the second monkey does not change. However, if the donor monkey's body is cooled and the transfusion procedure repeated, the recipient shivers and its temperature rises. Conversely, if the donor's body is warmed, the temperature of the recipient monkey declines during the transfusion of the perfusate. In both cases, the hypothalamus of the recipient responds to the factor in a compensatory manner, as if the temperature of its own periphery had been lowered or raised.

These potent, but unknown factors exert different actions when the position of the push-pull cannulae is located in a different part of the recipient monkey's hypothalamus. For example, when push-pull perfusate is collected from the anterior hypothalamus of a warmed monkey, and is then transfused directly to the lateral rather than anterior hypothalamus of an entirely normal monkey, the recipient suddenly drinks water instead of losing heat (Myers and Sharpe, 1968b). This response could mean that the factor activating the cells of the anterior hypothalamus along the heat-loss pathway may simultaneously stimulate neurons involved in water balance. Homeostatically, the ingestion of fluid is a very effective means of losing heat as well as of replenishing the water that is depleted during evaporative heat loss. The specificity of the anatomical locus could account for the independence of these two responses under the common circumstance in which a change in temperature may occur without drinking.

Another result has been reported by Drucker-Colín et al. (1970) who used the push-pull cannula system to perfuse the midbrain reticular formation of a donor cat in slow and/or fast wave sleep (Chapter 9). After this mesencephalic effluent obtained from the sleeping animal is transfused to the homologous region in the mesencephalon of an alert recipient cat, fast wave sleep alternating with slow wave sleep is recorded on the EEG. Since perfusate collected in the same way from identical sites in an awake cat never produces any signs of sleep in a recipient cat, it would appear that Drucker-Colín et al. may have been able to extract a hypnogenic factor from the neurons of the cat's mesencephalon. Anatomical and other controls will help to clarify this interesting possibility.

What could be termed a hunger factor is released into the perfusate collected from the perifornical region of a fasted monkey. On transfusion to an homologous site of a food-satiated monkey, the perfusate causes a fully satiated recipient monkey to eat biscuits (Chapter 7). Similarly, when a donor monkey is satiated prior to the cross-perfusion between the ventromedial nuclei of the two animals, the fasted recipient fails to eat (Yaksh and Myers, 1972a). Thus, factors that appear to be functionally specific are released at anatomically circumscribed sites. Furthermore, their physiological potency depends on the animal's level of hunger or satiety.

Although the strategy of these experiments is obvious, their significance is not always abundantly clear. Basically, they provide the first *in vivo* clue that distinct humoral factors exist which may be: (a) present within a restricted area of the brain; (b) released by a specific physiological stimulus; (c) pharmacologically specific in relation to the response that is elicited; and (d) anatomically circumscribed in terms of their release from a donor and subsequent action on neurons in the forebrain of a recipient.

Considering these points, the stage is now set to ask three vital questions: What is the identity of the substances constituting each of the factors? What is the nature of their morphological distribution? What is the functional condition under which the evoked release occurs?

2. *Estimation of Substances in Cortical or Ventricular Perfusates*

That the release of humoral factors occurs locally within the extracellular space of the brain or more diffusely into the ventricular cavity is unquestionable. To demonstrate the functional specificity of such a release has not been so easy, principally because most experiments have been performed of necessity under anesthesia, which is frequently a complicating biological recourse. Yet, a very large number of investigators have shown quite convincingly that both identifiable and unknown substances are spontaneously liberated into a physiological salt solution when it is perfused through the cerebral ventricles, passed over the cerebral cortex, or restricted parts of each. A few examples illustrate the diversity of these notable observations.

As reviewed comprehensively by Pepeu (1972), ACh has been detected in effluent collected from the cerebral cortex (e.g., Mitchell, 1963; Szerb, 1964; Phillis and York, 1968) as well as from the anterior horn of the ventricle adjacent to the caudate nucleus (Beleslin *et al.*, 1964). While morphine, chlorpromazine, ethyl alcohol and other drugs can suppress the cortical release of ACh (Beleslin and Polak, 1965; Phillis and Jhamandas, 1971), atropine and other substances often enhance the output of ACh (Armitage *et al.*, 1969; Bartolini and Pepeu, 1967; Collier and Mitchell, 1966; Elie and Panisset, 1970; MacIntosh and Perry, 1950; Szerb, 1964).

Serotonin is released into the third ventricle (Feldberg and Myers, 1966) or into the anterior horn (Holman and Vogt, 1972), and there is evidence from radioactive tracer and other studies that serotonin output into the perfused ventricles can be enhanced by different drugs (Goodrich, 1969; Tilson and Sparber, 1972). Similarly, the resting release of norepinephrine and dopamine into the ventricular cavity has been determined. In some cases, the output of these monoamines is increased by the electrical stimulation of a subcortical structure, or by the systemic administration of amphetamine and other agents, or as a result of behavioral activation (Portig *et al.*, 1968; Carr and Moore, 1969; Portig and Vogt, 1969; Moir *et al.*, 1970; Philippu, 1970; Philippu *et al.*, 1970; Sweet and Reis, 1971; Sparber and Tilson, 1972). An unknown prostaglandin-like factor has also been detected in the ventricular perfusate (Feldberg and Myers, 1966; Beleslin and Myers, 1971; Beleslin *et al.*, 1971).

How the ventricular release or the increased output of a given substance relates to an anatomically specific system cannot be precisely ascertained. The walls of each cerebral ventricle including the third ventricle are comprised of many superficial nuclei, each delegated to a distinct set of functions. Undoubtedly, the nerve endings from a number of convergent fiber systems contribute to the overall output of factors that are liberated into the CSF "sink" (Löfgren, 1959).

3. *Activity of Perfusate Collected by Push-Pull Cannulae*

Recent technical developments with the push-pull cannula system (Chapter 2) have tended to overcome this limitation of a ventricular perfusion to some degree. The morphological advantage afforded by the technique of localized perfusion is sufficiently impressive that the disadvantage of the small local damage that arises with its usage is outweighed.

In the early 1960s, the development of the double cannula system for analyzing the exchange of electrolytes and ACh in the brain of a rhesus monkey was pioneered by Delgado. Ordinarily, an experiment with a push-pull perfusion system is performed in one of two ways: either (a) the effluent is assayed on a highly sensitive organ preparation such as a segment of smooth muscle from the intestine, or (b) the brain is first labelled with a radioactive compound that is taken up in nerve tissue and the radioactivity of successive samples of perfusate is determined.

ACh is released spontaneously from different parts of the caudate nucleus, and an unidentified inhibitory factor also appears which reduces the contractility of the guinea pig ileum assay (Delgado and Rubinstein, 1964). Electrical stimulation with low frequency pulses of the thalamus of the cat also enhances the resting release of ACh in the caudate nucleus (McLennan, 1964).

In both the hypothalamus and thalamus of the rhesus monkey, four types of ACh and serotonin releasing sites have been delineated (Myers and Beleslin, 1970); i.e., those that: release ACh; release only serotonin; release both ACh and serotonin; or do not release either of the amines. Although the sites that liberate ACh and serotonin in the push-pull perfusate are scattered widely throughout the diencephalon, there are anatomical distinctions. A greater number of serotonin sites are found within the anterior and posterior parts of the hypothalamus, whereas a greater proportion of sites in the thalamus release ACh than in the hypothalamus. ACh and serotonin have also been detected in the solution perfused within the superior colliculi of the rhesus monkey (Beleslin and Myers, 1970). Moreover, an unknown contractile substance similar to a prostaglandin is also released into the push-pull perfusate at sites distributed throughout the limbic system of the cat and monkey (Beleslin and Myers, 1971). In the cat, 5-HT is present in hypothalamic perfusate (Randić and Padjen, 1968) and ACh is found in a push-pull solution perfused through discrete sites of the thalamus (Phillis *et al.*, 1968).

Since dopamine contained in the caudate nucleus may in this instance be a functional end product of monoamine synthesis rather than act solely as a metabolic precursor of norepinephrine, the dynamics of dopamine release have also been examined. Dopamine is found in the push-pull perfusate of the caudate nucleus and its resting output can be augmented by electrical stimulation of the medial thalamus of the cat (McLennan, 1964). However, McKenzie and Szerb (1968) did not detect an appreciable quantity of dopamine in the effluent collected from the cat's caudate nucleus unless a drug such as d-amphetamine was included in the perfusion medium that was passed through the push-pull cannulae.

Within the caudate nucleus, hypothalamus or amygdala of the monkey, both dopamine and norepinephrine are newly synthesized locally. This synthesis is reflected in their release into a push-pull perfusion solution that contains two of their precursors, tyrosine or DOPA (Roth et al., 1969). The bulk of these results has been confirmed in the cat by Riddell and Szerb (1971). Furthermore, the addition of several drugs including d-amphetamine to the perfusion medium as well as electrical stimulation of the medial forebrain bundle or substantia nigra causes a striking elevation in dopamine output from the caudate nucleus (Riddell and Szerb, 1971). The release of dopamine from the putamen and its subsequent elevation by electrical stimulation of the nigro-striatal fiber system has also been established (McLennan, 1965).

In a series of experiments, Sulser and co-workers have demonstrated that radio-labelled norepinephrine injected in the rat's ventricle can be detected in a solution perfused through the anterior hypothalamus (Sulser and Dingell, 1968). Further, the radioactivity in the perfusate attributed to the monoamine and certain of its metabolites is increased or otherwise modified by the systemic administration of reserpine, desmethylimipramine, p-chloroamphetamine and pargyline (Sulser et al., 1969; Strada and Sulser, 1971; 1972). These results verify lucidly the fact that the dynamics of catecholamine activity in the diencephalon can be altered directly by one of several drugs that are presumed to exert an action on the central stores of the amine.

4. *Localized Release of Substances Evoked by a Physiological or Behavioral Stimulus*

Within an identified locus, the correlated release of a substance with a physiological or behavioral change has obvious implications that are as far-reaching as any other observation at the present time.

In an initial effort to relate an animal's respiratory activity to the level of ACh in the medulla, Metz (1966; 1971) perfused the medulla of the anesthetized dog with a solution containing an anticholinesterase before, during and after the animal inhaled 12% CO_2. During hypercapnia, the output of ACh increased sharply within the local area at which an earlier micro-injection of bicarbonate solution had evoked hyperpnea (Chapter 3). Interestingly, Metz also showed that the enhanced EEG activity of the perfused region was correlated positively with the augmented release of ACh, although a change in ACh liberation did occur without any EEG activation following hypoxia. What is important is that an *in vivo* correlation is demonstrated between the medullary regulation of respiration and the magnitude of ACh output in this self-same structure.

When the brain of an anesthetized rat is labelled with either tritiated norepinephrine or serotonin, a stream of air containing odorants such as pyridine or almond extract blown over the animal's nostrils produces a three- to tenfold rise in the efflux of tritium in the perfusate collected from the olfactory bulb (Chase and Kopin, 1968). Although a noise or stimulation of the forepaw fails to alter this efflux, the odorants do evoke a concomitant release of ^{14}C inulin, which after injection remains in the extracellular space. This perplexing finding has never been adequately explained nor followed-up with the improved controls to which Chase and Kopin allude. Parenthetically, two points are germane: (1) the external diameter of the pull cannula was about 2 mm which encroaches upon the entire olfactory apparatus of the diminutive bulb of the rat and (2) the rate of perfusion was 200 μl/minute.

A simple intraperitoneal injection also elevates the radioactivity of a push-pull perfusate collected from the amygdala but not from the hypothalamus (Winson and Gerlach, 1971). In this case, the radioactivity of both ^{3}H-norepinephrine and ^{14}C urea, again injected into the cerebral ventricles before the perfusion, increases just in the samples collected after the injection. This result could be interpreted as being due to stress. Although the flow rate of 170 μl/minute, the size of the two cannulae, and the use of a potentially damaging method of gravity flow (Myers, 1972) could contribute to the efflux of extracellular urea, it is not clear which technical problem would account for the absence of any change in the radioactivity in the hypothalamic perfusate.

A set of behavioral experiments has also demonstrated a functionally induced increase in norepinephrine release. In a memorable paper, Stein and Wise (1969) showed that electrical self-stimulation of rewarding sites in the medial forebrain bundle elicited a marked increase in radioactivity in the push-pull perfusate. The brain of the rat had been labelled earlier with ^{3}H-norepinephrine given intraventricularly, and the loci of perfusion were the hypothalamus and amygdala. Non-rewarding control stimulation with electric current of other sites did not alter the tritium efflux. During the rewarding stimulation, 88% of the radioactivity in the effluent was accounted for by the O-methylated metabolites of norepinephrine. This important observation was taken by Stein *et al.* (1972) to support the notion (Chapter 12) that the release of the catecholamine from nerve terminals in the medial forebrain bundle contributes to the mechanism of positive reinforcement. This idea has been extended further to the etiology of schizophrenia as stemming from progressive damage to the noradrenergic reward system (Stein and Wise, 1972).

A remarkable concordance of the identical action of a group of compounds with their collectability (Werman, 1972) has been established thus far for only one function—thermoregulation. Corresponding to the shivering and rise in temperature of a monkey after serotonin is injected into the anterior hypothalamus (Chapter 6) is the 2- to 24-fold increase in serotonin output from homologus sites, which is evoked when the trunk of the monkey is cooled externally (Myers *et al.*, 1969). The functional specificity of the indoleamine release during the period of heat production has also been demonstrated in that warming of the monkey's body fails to alter serotonin output in the push-pull perfusate collected from the same hypothalamic region (Myers and Beleslin, 1971).

In the cat, an identical sort of evocation of ^{3}H- or ^{14}C-norepinephrine from the anterior hypothalamus occurs during an interval when the body of the animal is warmed externally but not when cooled (Myers and Chinn, 1973). The locus of release corresponds to a site at which the micro-injection of norepinephrine activates a heat-loss response and a consequent fall in the cat's body temperature (Chapter 6). Finally, ACh is released at a large proportion of sites all along an efferent heat production pathway when the monkey is cooled peripherally. This cholinergic system extends from the very rostral part of the hypothalamus to the most caudal aspect of the mesencephalon (Myers and Waller, 1973). Again, the sites of ACh release correspond precisely to those at which a micro-injection of ACh evokes a rise in temperature (Chapter 6).

Overall, the functional pattern of the release of serotonin, norepinephrine and ACh conforms with the influence on the animal's body temperature that each of these amines exerts when it is applied to the brain-stem. By this physiological consonance, the viewpoint that these humoral substances do play an underlying role in the hypothalamic mechanism for thermoregulation (Chapter 6) is greatly strengthened. Point by point, the endogenous presence of each amine, their mimicry of action as revealed by chemical stimulation, and the specificity of their evoked release within the same morphological boundaries illustrate a meaningful physiological congruency. In line with Werman's concepts, can we now conclude that these substances fulfill the requirements of a transmitter and can be so designated?

III. NEUROTRANSMITTER: CONCEPT REVISITED

Recently, there has been a somewhat incautious tendency among many neuroscientists to paste the label of transmitter on almost any endogenous compound that produces some sort of response when it is applied by a cannula or micropipette to nerve tissue (e.g., Valzelli, 1972; Motta and Martini, 1972). Clearly, not to query this uncritical labeling would be a prevarication, particularly in view of three questions which come to mind immediately: What should a transmitter do? Is there a reason for the existence of more than one transmitter substance? Can the primary postsynaptic action of a transmitter in the mammalian brain be altered by the release of another substance from vesicles in a secondary neuron?

In recapitulating Chapters 3 through 12, we find that within the mammalian diencephalon alone a total of 21 endogenous substances are implicated already in one or more functions: 5 biogenic amines, 10 peptides, 3 amino acids, 2 cations and 1 fatty acid.   Also postulated to exist in the hypothalamus are three types of cholinergic receptor, four types of monoamine receptor, and several other classes of receptor protein. From a physiological standpoint, how can we make any kind of neurological sense out of this veritable morass of substances and presumed receptors?

First of all, it is admittedly difficult to know which chemical substance of all those identified in brain extracts might be classified as a neurotransmitter. In fact, it is entirely conceivable that ACh is still the only likely neuro- transmitter within the mammalian forebrain and midbrain (Burgen, 1964); parenthetically, the cerebellum may represent an exception with respect to amino acids. If this is so, then other endogenous substances would have to be designated in different categories according to the characteristics of their action.

In Chapter 1, the main principles were reviewed upon which the stringent criteria for a transmitter are based. In being liberated from an axon terminal, a transmitter would act instantaneously on the substance-specific receptor con- tained on the postsynaptic membrane of a second neuron. This would serve to alter the established equilibrium potential of the second neuron. At the junction at which the net effect is the propagation of an impulse, the synapse itself is not necessarily defined by the category of receptor alone but rather by the ultra- structural elements of the presynaptic membrane (Bloom *et al.*, 1971). Ap- parently, chemical recognition in the form of receptor sensitivity is distributed rather widely on the surface of the nerve cell.

A. Supplementary Criteria for a Neurotransmitter

With respect to the main issues, three supplemental criteria (Chapter 1) are hypothesized here to be essential to the process of synaptic transmission in the mammal, at least in the fore- and midbrain.

1. *Temporal Requirement*

The temporal characteristic of rapidity is proposed to be indispensable for the chemically triggered passage of an impulse in terms of the rise and decay times of the membrane depolarization as well as for the mechanism of synaptic inac- tivation of the substance.

Viewed from a broad functional perspective, a cortical process ostensibly requires a mechanism that would operate in the millisecond range. That is, the recall of an image or a memory, a vocalization such as a verbal expression, the volitional initiation of a muscle contraction, the execution of a particular motor pattern such as a jump or eyeblink, the visual scanning of the printed word as these lines are read—all require a reflexive-like, millisecond responsiveness in the entire pathway of the specific neurons involved. These processes would not seem to require any sort of secondary chemical code, in the hormonal or regulatory sense, other than that which would switch the neuron circuit on or off with alacrity.

At the very opposite extreme, a preponderance of vital functions operate temporally on a second, minute or hourly basis, or on an even longer time span. To illustrate, a shift in the nutritional level brought about by food deprivation will lead ultimately to the act of feeding. The monitoring activity and the signals that specify the nutritional state are relatively long-term in nature. They do not require a sequence of instantaneous responses until the actual ingestive processes including mastication and swallowing occur. That is, the factor of speed in the synaptic transmission of feeding behavior is essential on a millisecond basis only for the efferent pathways underlying the act of eating.

A water deficit typifies another condition that is monitored again over a relatively long interval, perhaps on a minute by minute basis. On the other hand, the more critical but related state of hypovolemia could be monitored on a somewhat shorter scale, perhaps on a second by second basis. Both of these conditions may lead to the act of drinking water, which would require again the millisecond transmission of motor impulses for the ingestion of fluid. Other survival or vegetative systems including those serving sleep, body temperature, sexual, and other endocrine activity which are regulated in large measure by subcortical structures also do not require a response that operates in the millisecond range.

Taking another step of comparison, it is reasonable to contrast the temporal differences between the liberation of a hypothalamic releasing factor such as TRF with the output of ACh. For example, the ACh activity in the precentral gyrus that could evoke a staccato-like flicking of the hind-paw as a cat scratches a flea on its ear does not in any way resemble the action of TRF on the elaboration of thyroxine. Clearly, the time dimension of each is separated on the basis of functional celerity versus sluggishness. Other neurohumoral substances can be categorized equally well on a temporal continuum between these extremes.

2. *Ubiquitary Distribution*

Anatomical ubiquity of a substance used as a transmitter is proposed here as a requisite with respect to equal availability within all parts of the brain. Teleologically, one would expect that a substance that transmits an impulse from one neuron to the next would be present in all parts of the brain.

Although varying in concentration, ACh is certainly distributed widely and in high concentration throughout the prosencephalon and mesencephalon. However, other biogenic amines and the polypeptides do not share this attribute of morphological ubiquity. The hypophyseal releasing factors are concentrated in the very ventral portion of the diencephalon (Chapter 4 and 5). The monoamines are also differentiated anatomically in the rat and other species in uniquely restricted pathways which follow specified routes. Moreover, the projections of the neurons containing the monoamines touch upon certain nuclei in the brain but not others (Chapter 1). Norepinephrine and serotonin neurons are scattered sparsely or are virtually absent in many areas of the telencephalon but are particularly dense, often interdigitated and well-defined in the brain-stem. In addition, neurons in certain structures such as the caudate nucleus or substantia nigra may metabolize an amine such as dopamine in a special way so that the monoamine is an end product in itself (Woodruff, 1971). Again in respect to the proportionality of regional concentration, dopamine is not ubiquitous.

Curiously enough, the fiber systems containing serotonin and norepinephrine are intensely conjoined both functionally and anatomically (e.g., Bieger et al., 1972) to the diencephalic and mesencephalic systems that integrate and control the vegetative processes. Within these regions each substance has been implicated in a relatively long-term monitoring, feedback, state-signaling or other homeostatic process.

3. *Specialization of the Nerve Ending*

For a pulsed and quantal release of a transmitter substance as well as its subsequent degradation, it is hypothesized here that the general morphology and the metabolic nature of the pre- and postsynaptic component elements of the transmitter mechanism should be uniform.

The diversity in specialization of the nerve ending in the mammalian CNS at the ultrastructural and metabolic levels is so well known that further elaboration is not necessary. What is vital is the probability that this diversity in itself may reflect a unique specialization insofar as the function of the substance that is released.

ACh is hydrolyzed directly at the postsynaptic membrane by acetylcholinesterase, but serotonin depends primarily on extracellular monoamine oxidase for its degradation. Even more curious is the fact that norepinephrine is inactivated in large part by its own re-uptake in the terminal bouton rather than through metabolic degradation by monoamine oxidase. In the case of these two monoamines, it is not unlikely that the termination of the depolarizing event is a less direct chemical mechanism than that which destroys a quantum of liberated ACh. If each served the self-same function to transmit a nerve impulse across a synaptic cleft, it is difficult to concoct a reason why all three substances should rely on such vastly different mechanisms of inactivation.

The peptidergic releasing hormones are even more dissimilar. Unlike amines, they are apparently synthesized within the cell body of the neuron and are then carried to neurosecretory storage granules by way of axoplasmic transport. Whether or not the peptides are partially inactivated within the synaptic cleft following their secretion is presently uncertain. If each of the endogenous substances were a transmitter, it is indeed puzzling why a parsimonious and identical pattern is not followed for the manufacture, exocytotic release and terminal inactivation.

B. Classification of Substances

A recondite sort of vocabulary has unfolded to describe the influence of an endogenous chemical substance on synaptic transmission or the propagation of a nerve impulse.   In various scientific sectors, such terms as mediator, carrier, modulator, trigger, communicator, modifier, moderator, interactor, messenger or transmitter are commonplace.   These words are often modified by an adjective such as possible, putative, promising, candidate, presumed, likely, probable or the!   The idea must be reiterated, however, that the capacity of a hodge-podge of chemical compounds to alter the activity of neurons does not in any way signify that one or another is a transmitter in the classical sense or has any bearing on the transmission process.

Several of these terms will be redefined further in order to explain and clarify hypothetically those properties of an endogenous substance that can be correlated with a given function.

1. *Transmitter.* An endogenous substance that is found at the axon terminus. It can depolarize a neuron, is readily synthesized, instantaneously degraded, and is ubiquitous anatomically.   Not only does ACh meet these requirements, but it is the only substance known that is extremely difficult to identify in an *in vivo* preparation unless its enzymatic destruction is prevented by an anticholinesterase.   As we have seen in Chapters 3 through 12, ACh has been implicated in virtually every response that has been studied by the method of chemical stimulation.

Not surprisingly, ACh or a cholinomimetic analogue possesses excitatory and inhibitory properties which would be expected of a substance that could alter the polarization characteristics of an adjacent neuron.

2. *Modulator.* An endogenous substance that is identifiable in nerve cells but is not a transmitter as defined here.   It functions in a homeostatic way to change, adjust or regulate the rate of depolarization or hyperpolarization of a neuron.   On release, a modulator may exert its influence either at the synapse or the axonal membrane.   The release of a modulator may be triggered directly by afferent impulses or by a change in the concentration of an electrolyte, nutrient, hormone, toxin or a foreign protein in the circulating plasma.   The modulators would include the monoamines that have been localized in discrete pathways or regions.

Neuronal transmission could be modulated in at least one of several ways including: (1) a shift of the membrane's threshold of depolarization induced by ACh; (2) the alteration in the trans-membrane flux of the cations; (3) competition for receptor sites or other effect on the postsynaptic membrane; (4) a counter effect by virtue of another amine's action on the nerve cell; or (5) the metabolic disturbance to a cellular enzyme such as ATPase or adenyl cyclase. Some cogent evidence for these ideas can be found in the accounts of Aprison (1962), Bianchi (1968), Shore (1972) and Smythies (1972).

A modulator may be unifunctional in that its release maintains or alters the steady-state firing of a neuron population. Or it may be released in harmony with another modulator, the balance in both of which would sustain the firing pattern of a designated pathway. In this case, the cessation in the release of one modulator would let the other modulator dominate the pattern of neuronal discharge. More and more evidence is accumulating that amines such as norepinephrine and serotonin influence the metabolism, uptake and storage of each other (e.g., Jester and Horst, 1972).

3. *Mediator.* A blood-borne endogenous substance that is not synthesized in nerve cells. A mediator would facilitate either the rate of synaptic transmission of an impulse or its axonal conduction. Or a mediator may act to release a transmitter or alter the action of a modulator. A circulating polypeptide such as angiotensin could serve as a mediator within specific regions of the brain.

4. *Moderator.* Also a blood-borne endogenous substance that is not synthesized in nerve cells. A moderator would slow down or attenuate the rate of synaptic transmission or modify the axonal conductance of an impulse. A moderator may also suppress the release of a transmitter or affect the action of a modulator. Plasma glucose may serve in certain cases as a moderator of a certain set of central neurons; conceivably one substance could mediate or moderate depending upon the local concentration reaching the neurons.

5. *Modifier.* Any exogenous drug or chemical that alters uniformly the function of neurons in a nucleus, in a fiber bundle or the entire nervous system. A modifier serves to enhance or suppress the process of impulse transmission by altering such mechanisms as the depolarization of the cells, the degradation of ACh, or the intracellular metabolism of essential factors. Typical modifiers would be a barbiturate anesthetic and an anticholinesterase such as eserine which affects endogenous ACh.

C. How Does a Neurohumoral Code Function?

Considering a collection of neurons within a circumscribed region, there are several ways in which their collective firing pattern could be influenced by the liberation of a modulator found in a nerve terminal, the release of which may not by itself initiate a depolarization. First, a modulator could govern the overall proportion of neurons that are fired in the sense of recruitment. Second, the rate of impulse propagation could be regulated through the release of the modulator on the axonal membrane. Third, the collective membrane equilibrium potentials of a group of neurons could be shifted for a relatively prolonged interval by the direct or feedback action of a modulator on Na^+ transport (Duncan, 1967), cyclic AMP (Siggins *et al.*, 1970) or an enzyme such as Ca^{2+} ATPase or $Na^+ - K^+$ activated ATPase (Shore, 1972). Fourth, a modulator may alter the rate of combination with the receptor of a transmitter substance, another modulator, or a mediator such as a prostaglandin (Smythies, 1972).

If we assume a specificity of neuron sensitivity to a given chemical, a local physical stimulus, or input from the periphery via an afferent pathway, then a structure could be coded neurohumorally in one of two general ways. First, the balance in the release of two modulators from neurons within the structure may be determined by afferent signals to that structure which in turn trigger an efferent response. Second, the local excitation of specialized neurons termed detectors or sensors caused by a change in the constituent in the blood coursing through the microvasculature (i.e., a mediator or moderator) would likewise trigger an efferent pathway. What then is the function of ACh?

1. The Role of ACh

On the basis of the experiments reported in this book and other information (e.g., Pepeu, 1972), it is logical to conclude that ACh transmits impulses along afferent as well as efferent fiber systems within the brain. On the basis of the direct application of cholinomimetics or cholinergic blocking agents, it is clear that there are numerous cholinergic pathways which are either excitatory or inhibitory. Most impressive is the singular fact that ACh is the only substance that can influence every physiological or behavioral response thus far examined, independent of species and circumstance. For this reason, it is proposed that ACh represents the final common neurochemical substance responsible for the transmission of all efferent signals.

In this sense, ACh may not always act as a principal initiator of a response in the forebrain or midbrain, but rather secondarily in the overall chain of events. That is, ACh could convey synaptically the output of a hypothalamic structure, for example, which is coded either by a (a) modulator or (b) mediator-moderator system as described above. Thus, the membrane of a cholinergic neuron, so called because it liberates ACh from its terminal vesicles, could be mono-aminoceptive. Similarly, the membrane of a serotonin or norepinephrine containing neuron could in turn be sensitive to a mediator or moderator.

From all of the studies utilizing the micro-injection and application of ACh, this choline ester is implicated in the overall efferent signalling of responses concerned with heart rate, respiration, adrenal corticosteroid activity, lordosis, prolactin elaboration, body temperature, feeding, drinking, sleep, seizures, pain, tremor, specific motor patterning, EEG synchronization, emotional reactivity, motivated behavior, and even the learning of a task. Immediately, one might question whether ACh applied locally could evoke every sort of excitatory response. The answer is probably that it can. As yet, the proper experiment has probably not been satisfactorily completed in some disciplines,[1] primarily because of the morphological difficulties still inherent in the procedure of chemically dissecting, so to speak, a fiber pathway or similar network of neurons.

In actual practice, the magnitude of ACh release in a given nucleus or pathway could be dictated in the first instance by the neuronal release of serotonin, norepinephrine or dopamine or by an extrinsic mediator or moderator in plasma or cerebral tissue. The latter would include an electrolyte, glucose, bacteria, a prostaglandin, steroid, angiotensin or other substance. It is now possible to examine some specific examples of the relationships between a modulator and transmitter as well as between a mediator, moderator and a transmitter. Table 13-1 presents a provisional conceptualization of the effect of a specific input to a structure, the resultant action on a modulator and the subsequent effect of ACh release on the corresponding response. As shown in the table, a mediator or moderator may serve as a chemical input to the structure or may modify the release of a modulator. Quite remarkably, there is both direct and indirect evidence from *in vivo* and *in vitro* experiments that serotonin or norepinephrine do have the capacity to alter the levels of acetylcholinesterase, choline acetylase and the release of ACh (e.g., Aprison, 1962; Singer *et al.*, 1971; Ho and Loh, 1972; Myers, 1973).

One of the many facts that is presently unclear is whether there is an intervening mediator in the link between the osmotic and volemic stimuli to drink and the activity of ACh. Furthermore, the role of ACh in the final expression of feeding behavior has also not been reconciled. In general, however, these principles may be applied to many of the reported findings. With respect to a modulatory action, some of the dilatory characteristics of the latency of the reaction to an endogenous compound are now explicable.

An excellent illustrative comparison of the actions of a mediator, a modulator and a transmitter is provided by the hyperthermic response produced by leucocytes, serotonin and ACh (Chapter 6). Acting directly on the cells of the hypothalamus, leucocyte pyrogen (mediator) produces a prolonged fever after a relatively long latency with a slope that often requires two hours to reach an asymptote. On the other hand, serotonin (modulator) acts with a much shorter latency, has a similar slope and magnitude but has a somewhat shorter duration. Still more different is the almost immediate, spike-like rise in temperature evoked by ACh (transmitter) of very short duration but striking intensity. Although the net effect on the hypothalamic mechanism for temperature of a mediator, modulator and transmitter is identical, i.e., hyperthermia, the salient

---

[1] To illustrate, ACh injected into sites in the diencephalon of a cat has never elicited feeding or drinking (Chapters 7 and 8). The reason for this may simply be that the appropriate structure has not been stimulated, or a suitable dose has not been used, or a sufficiently circumscribed population of neurons has not been stimulated.

TABLE 13-1   Summary of Evidence for Modulator Control of ACh Release to Evoke a Given Response
Note that the input may be comprised of a direct anatomical coupling or the influence of a
blood-borne constituent impinging upon the structure.

Function	Input	Structure	Modulator	Transmitter	Response
Temperature	Ascending pathway; local temperature (?); pyrogen (?)	hypothalamus	serotonin / norepinephrine } balance	ACh	Thermogenesis
Sleep	Blood-borne peptide?	mesencephalon	serotonin / norepinephrine } balance	ACh (?)	Cortical EEG synchronization
Water balance	Na$^+$; angiotensin; ADH	hypothalamus	catecholamine (?)	ACh	Drinking
Motor movement	Descending cortical pathway	caudate nucleus	dopamine	ACh	Tremor
Emotion	Afferent pathway	hypothalamus	norepinephrine	ACh	Rage
Hunger	Glucose serum factors (?)	hypothalamus	norepinephrine	ACh (?)	Feeding

point here is that each endogenous substance exerts its effect in a very different way.

Of tangential importance is the finding alluded to earlier that the elevation in the level of serotonin or norepinephrine in the anterior hypothalamus of a monkey provokes a marked change in the subsequent release of ACh from sites located more caudally. This observation that a monoamine can act on nervous tissue to liberate ACh is the antithesis of the Burn-Rand concept which proposes that ACh may evoke the synaptic release of a catecholamine in the autonomic nervous system. Nevertheless, there is also evidence of a cholinergic to adrenergic coupling in the brain of the rabbit (e.g., Glisson *et al.*, 1972).

In conclusion, several important facts must be taken into account to uncover the purpose of a given chemical substance. These include: (1) whether the substance is widely distributed or confined to the structure under study; (2) the difference in latency, magnitude, duration and direction of action when the substance is applied locally in graded doses; (3) the capacity of a related compound to attenuate or potentiate one or more of the actions of the substance; (4) its dependence on other intact and chemically defined pathways; and (5) the point-by-point comparison of the effect of the substance with another that possesses the same pharmacological attributes. In the final analysis the classification of any endogenous compound according to its function in a given specific anatomical system will rest on an analysis of the totality of its action.

IV. THE BLACK BOX IS GRAY

Nearly 20 years ago, a famous American behaviorist commented informally to the author about the intricacies of the so-called black box, the brain's functional essence. His view was that a substantial understanding about the mammalian central nervous system based on a substantive body of knowledge could not possibly come to pass until the year 2000 or well beyond. Following on from this is the belief that one's scientific effort in this field should be expended to define carefully the features of the environmental input to the black box as well as to describe most explicitly the entire nature of the organism's response. As valid as the notion may still be, this casual prediction at the three-quarter mark of our century does not seem to have materialized.

In all quarters, great strides are being taken continually by neurophysiologists, biochemists, electron microscopists, neuropharmacologists, and many others who are successfully sorting out the contents of this dark box. To be sure, the ultrastructure, the interconnections and the chemical dynamics persist in being bewilderingly complex. But immense gains in factual knowledge make it safe to conclude that the hue of the box can no longer be considered as black. Instead its overall color, in my opinion, has taken on a conceptual cast of gray.

Only through the tremendous out-pouring of research from laboratories, large and small throughout the world, has the lightening of this box been achieved.

As each one makes a distinguishing impact in one way or another, the tight lid of this now gray box is already wedged open, and by a formidable wedge at that. In this last fourth of the twentieth century, the breach will open ever wider as the coadunation of each biological discipline, dedicated to a comprehension of the gray box, continues toward the common goal. Indeed, the elements of understanding do not lie beyond us on the horizon of the coming millennium. They are here with us now, today.

References

van Abeelen, J., L. Gilissen, Th. Hanssen and A. Lenders. 1972. Effects of intrahippocampal injections with methylscopolamine and neostigmine upon exploratory behaviour in two inbred mouse strains. *Psychopharmacologia.* **24**: 470–475.

Abrahams, V. C. and M. Pickford. 1956. The effect of anticholinesterases injected into the supraoptic nuclei of chloralosed dogs on the release of the oxytocic factor of the posterior pituitary. *J. Physiol.* **133**: 330–333.

Abrahams, V. C., S. M. Hilton and J. L. Malcolm. 1962. Sensory connexions to the hypothalamus and midbrain, and their role in the reflex activation of the defence reaction. *J. Physiol.* **164**: 1–16.

Adams, D. B. 1968. The activity of single cells in the midbrain and hypothalamus of the cat during affective defense behavior. *Arch. Ital. Biol.* **106**: 243–269.

Agranoff, B. W., R. E. Davis, L. Casola and R. Lim. 1967. Actinomycin D blocks formation of memory of shock-avoidance in goldfish. *Science.* **158**: 1600–1601.

Aida, S. 1956. Experimental research on the function of the amygdaloid nuclei in psychomotor epilepsy. *Folia Psychiat. Neurol.* **10**: 181–207.

Ajmone-Marsan, C. 1969. Acute effects of topical epileptogenic agents, pp. 299–319. *In* H. H. Jasper, A. A. Ward and A. Pope (eds.) *Basic Mechanisms of the Epilepsies.* Little, Brown & Co., Boston.

Albert, D. J. 1966. Memory in mammals: evidence for a system involving nuclear ribonucleic acid. *Neuropsychologia.* **4**: 79–92.

Albert, D. J., L. H. Storlien, D. J. Wood and G. K. Ehman. 1970. Further evidence for a complex system controlling feeding behavior. *Physiol. Behav.* **5**: 1075–1082.

Alexander, R. S. 1946. Tonic and reflex functions of medullary sympathetic cardiovascular centers. *J. Neurophysiol.* **9**: 205–217.

Allikmets, L. H. 1972. Influence of dopamin-, adren- and serotoninergic substances on cholinergic emotional reactions of hypothalamic origin. *J. High. Nerv. Act.* **22**: 597–602.

Allikmets, L. and J. M. R. Delgado. 1968. Injection of antidepressants in the amygdala of awake monkeys. *Arch. Int. Pharmacodyn. Ther.* **175**: 170–178.

Allikmets, L., J. M. R. Delgado and S. A. Richards. 1968. Intra-mesencephalic injection of imipramine, promazine and chlorprothixene in awake monkeys. *Int. J. Neuropharmacol.* **7**: 185–193.

Allikmets, L. H., V. A. Vahing and I. P. Lapin. 1969. Dissimilar influences of imipramine, benactyzine and promazine on effects of micro-injections of noradrenaline, acetylcholine and serotonin into the amygdala in the cat. *Psychopharmacologia.* **15**: 392–403.

Altaffer, F. B., F. De Balbian Verster, S. Hall, C. J. Long and P. D'Encarnacao. 1970. A simple and inexpensive cannula technique for chemical stimulation of the brain. *Physiol. Behav.* **5**: 119–121.

671

Amiragova, M. G. and M. A. Berlina. 1970a. Effect of thyroid hormones injected in the posterior hypothalamic nucleus on conditioned reflex activity. *Doklady Akad. Nauk SSSR.* **191:** 720–722.

Amiragova, M. G. and M. A. Berlina. 1970b. Mechanisms of hormonal-effect transmission from posterior hypothalamus to cerebral cortex. *Doklady Akad. Nauk SSSR.* **191:** 1186–1188.

Amiragova, M. G. and R. I. Svirskaia. 1968. Effect of thyroid hormone injected into the posterior hypothalamus on the summed electrical activity of the cortex. *Doklady Akad. Nauk SSSR.* **179:** 1246–1248.

Anand, B. K. and J. R. Brobeck. 1951. Hypothalamic control of food intake in rats and cats. *Yale J. Biol. Med.* **24:** 123–140.

Anand, B. K., S. Dua and B. Singh. 1961a. Electrical activity of the hypothalamic 'feeding centres' under the effect of changes in blood chemistry. *EEG Clin. Neurophysiol.* **13:** 54–59.

Anand, B. K., U. Subberwal, S. K. Manchanda and B. Singh. 1961b. Glucoreceptor mechanism in the hypothalamic feeding centres. *Ind. J. Med. Res.* **49:** 717–724.

Anand, B. K., G. S. Chhina, K. N. Sharma, S. Dua and B. Singh. 1964. Activity of single neurons in the hypothalamic feeding centers: effect of glucose. *Amer. J. Physiol.* **207:** 1146–1154.

Andén, N.-E., S. G. Butcher and K. Fuxe. 1970. Protection of the neostriatal dopamine stores against reserpine by local treatment with metatyramine. *Acta Pharmacol. Toxicol.* **28:** 39–48.

Andersson, B. 1952. Polydipsia caused by intrahypothalamic injections of hypertonic NaCl-solutions. *Experientia.* **8:** 157–159.

Andersson, B. 1953. The effect of injections of hypertonic NaCl-solutions into different parts of the hypothalamus of goats. *Acta Physiol. Scand.* **28:** 188–201.

Andersson, B. 1971a. Receptors subserving hunger and thirst, pp. 187–216. *In* E. Neil (ed.) *Handbook of Sensory Physiology,* Vol. III. Springer-Verlag, Berlin.

Andersson, B. 1971b. Thirst- and brain control of water balance. *Amer. Sci.* **59:** 408–415.

Andersson, B. and S. M. McCann. 1955. A further study of polydipsia evoked by hypothalamic stimulation in the goat. *Acta Physiol. Scand.* **33:** 333–346.

Andersson, B. and O. Westbye. 1970. Synergistic action of sodium and angiotensin on brain mechanisms controlling fluid balance. *Life Sci.* **9:** 601–608.

Andersson, B., L. Eriksson and O. Fernández. 1971. Reinforcement by Na^+ of centrally mediated hypertensive response to angiotensin II. *Life Sci.* **10:** 633–638.

Andersson, B., L. Eriksson and R. Oltner. 1970. Further evidence for angiotensin-sodium interaction in central control of fluid balance. *Life Sci.* **9:** 1091–1096.

Andersson, B., R. Grant and S. Larsson. 1956. Central control of heat loss mechanisms in the goat. *Acta Physiol. Scand.* **37:** 261–280.

Andersson, B., L. Eriksson, O. Fernández, C.-G. Kolmodin and R. Oltner. 1972. Centrally mediated effects of sodium and angiotensin II on arterial blood pressure and fluid balance. *Acta Physiol. Scand.* **85:** 398–407.

Andreas, K. and W. Oelssner. 1969. Die Hemmung der "tail-flick"-Reaktion durch Arekolin und Oxotremorin an dezerebrierten und medullotomierten Ratten. *Acta Biol. Med. Ger.* **23:** 669–678.

Andreas, K. and A. H. Staib. 1971. Die Hemmung der "tail-flick"-Reaktion durch gezielte Oxotremorininjektionen in verschiedene Hirnareale der Ratte. *Acta Biol. Med. Ger.* **26:** 1071–1075.

Ankier, S. I. and M. B. Tyers. 1969. A technique for the continuous micro-infusion of chemicals into discrete parts of the brain in unrestrained rats. *Brit. J. Pharmacol.* **37:** 548P.

Antelman, S. M., A. K. Johnson and A. E. Fisher. 1972. Survival of cholinergic drinking following nephrectomy. *Physiol. Behav.* **8:** 1169–1170.

Antunes-Rodrigues, J. and M. R. Covian. 1971. Water and sodium chloride intake following microinjection of carbachol into the septal area of the rat brain. *Experientia.* 27: 784–785.

Aprison, M. H. 1962. On a proposed theory for the mechanism of action of serotonin in brain, pp. 133–146. *In* J. Wortis (ed.) *Recent Advances in Biological Psychiatry*, Vol. IV. Plenum Press, New York.

Arai, Y. and R. A. Gorski. 1968. Inhibition of ovarian compensatory hypertrophy by hypothalamic implantation of gonadotrophin in androgen-sterilized rats: evidence for "internal" feedback. *Endocrinology.* 82: 871–873.

Arbuthnott, G., K. Fuxe and U. Ungerstedt. 1971. Central catecholamine turnover and self-stimulation behavior. *Brain Res.* 27: 406–413.

Armitage, A. K., G. H. Hall and C. M. Sellers. 1969. Effects of nicotine on electrocortical activity and acetylcholine release from the cat cerebral cortex. *Brit. J. Pharmacol.* 35: 152–160.

Armitage, A. K., G. H. Hall, A. S. Milton and C. F. Morrison. 1967. Effects of nicotine injected into and perfused through the cerebral ventricles of the cat. *Ann. N. Y. Acad. Sci.* 142: 27–39.

Arnold, M. G. (ed.) 1970. *Feelings and Emotions.* Academic Press, New York. pp. 1–339.

Auerbach, P. and P. L. Carlton. 1971. Retention deficit correlated with a deficit in the corticoid response to stress. *Science.* 173: 1148–1149.

Averill, R. L. W. 1970. Disappearance of ^{131}I-labeled thyroxine (^{131}I-T$_4$) from agar pellets implanted in the hypothalamus of rats. *Endocrinology.* 87: 176–178.

Avery, D. D. 1970. Hyperthermia induced by direct injections of carbachol in the anterior hypothalamus. *Neuropharmacology.* 9: 175–178.

Avery, D. D. 1971. Intrahypothalamic adrenergic and cholinergic injection effects on temperature and ingestive behavior in the rat. *Neuropharmacology.* 10: 753–763.

Avery, D. D. 1972. Thermoregulatory effects of intrahypothalamic injections of adrenergic and cholinergic substances at different environmental temperatures. *J. Physiol.* 220: 257–266.

Avery, D. D. and D. M. Nance. 1970a. Behavioral correlates of chemical stimulation in the cat thalamus. *Psychon. Sci.* 19: 7–8.

Avery, D. D. and D. M. Nance. 1970b. Injections of neurohumors in the cat thalamus and visual discrimination performance. *Psychon. Sci.* 21: 143–144.

Avis, H. H. 1972. Hippocampal injections of KCl and shock-induced bradycardia in the rat. *Psychon. Sci.* 27: 283–284.

Avis, H. H. and P. L. Carlton. 1968. Retrograde amnesia produced by hippocampal spreading depression. *Science.* 161: 73–75.

Babb, T. L., Babb, M., Mahnke, J. H. and Verzeano, M. 1971. The action of cholinergic agents on the electrical activity of the non-specific nuclei of the thalamus. *Int. J. Neurol.* 8: 198–210.

Babichev, V. N. and G. Telegdy. 1968. The effect of hypothalamic lesion and oestrogen implantation on progestin secretion in the rat. *Acta Physiol. Acad. Sci. Hung.* 33: 447–454.

Baile, C. A. and J. Mayer. 1968. Effects of insulin-induced hypoglycemia and hypoace-toemia on eating behavior in goats. *J. Dairy Sci.* 51: 1495–1499.

Baillie, P. and S. D. Morrison. 1963. The nature of the suppression of food intake by lateral hypothalamic lesions in rats. *J. Physiol.* 165: 227–245.

Bainbridge, J. G. and A. P. Labhsetwar. 1971. The role of oestrogens in spontaneous ovulation: location of site of action of positive feedback of oestrogen by intracranial implantation of the anti-oestrogen I.C.I. 46474. *J. Endocrinol.* 50: 321–327.

Baker, A. B., H. A. Matzke and J. R. Brown. 1950. Poliomyelitis III. Bulbar poliomyelitis; a study of medullary function. *AMA Arch. Neurol. Psychiat.* 63: 257–281.

Baker, W. W. 1965. Tremorine suppression of hippocampal strychnine foci. *Arch. Int. Pharmacodyn. Ther.* 155: 273–281.

Baker, W. W. 1972. Excitatory responses following intracaudate injection of N-methyl-*dl*-aspartic acid. *Arch. Int. Pharmacodyn. Ther.* **196:** 226-234.

Baker, W. W. and F. Benedict. 1967. Local electrographic responses to intrahippocampal *d*-tubocurarine and related neuromuscular blocking agents. *Proc. Soc. Exptl. Biol. Med.* **124:** 607-611.

Baker, W. W. and F. Benedict. 1968a. Differential responses of hippocampal repetitive discharges to scopolamine and pentobarbital. *Exptl. Neurol.* **21:** 187-200.

Baker, W. W. and F. Benedict. 1968b. Analysis of local discharges induced by intrahippocampal microinjection of carbachol or diisopropylfluorophosphate (DFP). *Int. J. Neuropharmacol.* **7:** 135-147.

Baker, W. W. and F. Benedict. 1970. Influence of increased local cholinergic activity on discharge patterns of hippocampal foci. *EEG Clin. Neurophysiol.* **28:** 499-509.

Baker, W. W. and M. Kratky. 1967. Acute effects of chlorpromazine and imipramine on hippocampal foci. *Arch. Int. Pharmacodyn. Ther.* **165:** 265-275.

Baker, W. W. and M. Kratky. 1968. Differential suppression of spontaneous and evoked hippocampal electrical activities by local tetracaine. *Arch. Int. Pharmacodyn. Ther.* **173:** 395-410.

Baker, W. W. and M. Kratky. 1971. Suppression of hippocampal DFP discharges by chlorpromazine, imipramine and desipramine. *Arch. Int. Pharmacodyn. Ther.* **189:** 109-122.

Baker, W. W., M. Kratky and F. Benedict. 1965. Electrographic responses to intrahippocampal injections of convulsant drugs. *Exptl. Neurol.* **12:** 136-145.

Bakke, J. L., N. Lawrence and S. Robinson. 1972. Late effects of thyroxine injected into the hypothalamus of the neonatal rat. *Neuroendocrinology.* **10:** 183-195.

Balagura, S. 1971. Neurochemical regulation of food intake, pp. 181-193. *In* L. Martini (ed.) *The Hypothalamus.* Academic Press, New York.

Balagura, S. and M. Kanner. 1971. Hypothalamic sensitivity to 2-deoxy-*D*-glucose and glucose: effects on feeding behavior. *Physiol. Behav.* **7:** 251-255.

Baldwin, B. A. and D. L. Ingram. 1966. Effects of cooling the hypothalamus in the pig. *J. Physiol.* **186:** 72-73P.

Bandler, R. J. 1969. Facilitation of aggressive behaviour in rat by direct cholinergic stimulation of the hypothalamus. *Nature.* **224:** 1035-1036.

Bandler, R. J. 1970. Cholinergic synapses in the lateral hypothalamus for the control of predatory aggression in the rat. *Brain Res.* **20:** 409-424.

Bandler, R. J. 1971a. Direct chemical stimulation of the thalamus: effects on aggressive behavior in the rat. *Brain Res.* **26:** 81-93.

Bandler, R. J. 1971b. Chemical stimulation of the rat midbrain and aggressive behaviour. *Nature New Biol.* **229:** 222-223.

Bandler, R. J., C. C. Chi and J. P. Flynn. 1972. Biting attack elicited by stimulation of the ventral midbrain tegmentum of cats. *Science.* **177:** 364-366.

Banerjee, U., W. Feldberg and V. P. Georgiev. 1970a. Microinjections of tubocurarine, leptazol, strychnine and picrotoxin into the cerebral cortex of anaesthetized cats. *Brit. J. Pharmacol.* **40:** 6-22.

Banerjee, U., T. F. Burks, W. Feldberg and C. A. Goodrich. 1970b. Temperature responses and other effects of 5-hydroxytryptophan and 5-hydroxytryptamine when acting from the liquor space in unanaesthetized rabbits. *Brit. J. Pharmacol.* **38:** 688-701.

Barbour, H. G. 1912. Die Wirkung unmittelbarer Erwärmung und Abkühlung der Wärmezentra auf die Körpertemperatur. *Arch. Exper. Pathol. Pharmakol.* **70:** 1-26.

Barbour, H. G. 1921. The heat-regulating mechanism of the body. *Physiol. Rev.* **1:** 295-326.

Bard, P. 1960. Anatomical organization of the central nervous system in relation to control of the heart and blood vessels. *Physiol. Rev.* **40:** 3-26.

Barfield, R. J. 1969. Activation of copulatory behavior by androgen implanted into the preoptic area of the male fowl. *Horm. Behav.* **1**: 37–52.

Bargmann, W. 1960. The neurosecretory system of the diencephalon. *Endeavour.* **19**: 125–133.

Barofsky, I. and A. Feldstein. 1970. Serotonin and its metabolites; their respective roles in the production of hypothermia in the mouse. *Experientia.* **26**: 990–991.

Barondes, S. H. 1969. The mirror focus and long-term memory storage, pp. 371–374. *In* H. H. Jasper, A. A. Ward and A. P. Pope (eds.) *Basic Mechanisms of the Epilepsies.* Little, Brown & Co., Boston.

Bartolini, A. and G. Pepeu. 1967. Investigations into the acetylcholine output from the cerebral cortex of the cat in the presence of hyoscine. *Brit. J. Pharmac. Chemother.* **31**: 66–73.

Basu-Ray, B. N., S. N. Dutta and S. N. Pradhan. 1972a. Effects of microinjections of ouabain into certain medullary areas in cats. *J. Pharmacol. Exptl. Ther.* **181**: 357–361.

Basu-Ray, B. N., W. M. Booker, S. N. Dutta and S. N. Pradhan. 1972b. Effects of microinjection of ouabain into the hypothalamus in cats. *Brit. J. Pharmacol.* **45**: 197–206.

Baxter, B. L. 1967. Comparison of the behavioral effects of electrical or chemical stimulation applied at the same brain loci. *Exptl. Neurol.* **19**: 412–432.

Baxter, B. L. 1968. Elicitation of emotional behavior by electrical or chemical stimulation applied at the same loci in cat mesencephalon. *Exptl. Neurol.* **21**: 1–10.

Baxter, B. L. 1969. Induction of both emotional behavior and a novel form of REM sleep by chemical stimulation applied to cat mesencephalon. *Exptl. Neurol.* **23**: 220–229.

Beckman, A. L. 1970. Effect of intrahypothalamic norepinephrine on thermoregulatory responses in the rat. *Amer. J. Physiol.* **218**: 1596–1604.

Beckman, A. L. and H. J. Carlisle. 1969. Effect of intrahypothalamic infusion of acetylcholine on behavioural and physiological thermoregulation in the rat. *Nature.* **221**: 561–562.

Beckman, A. L. and E. Satinoff. 1972. Arousal from hibernation by intrahypothalamic injections of biogenic amines in ground squirrels. *Amer. J. Physiol.* **222**: 875–879.

Beideman, L. R. and R. Goldstein. 1970. Specificity of carbachol in the elicitation of drinking. *Psychon. Sci.* **20**: 261–262.

Beleslin, D. B. and R. D. Myers. 1970. The release of acetylcholine and 5-hydroxytryptamine from the mesencephalon of the unanesthetized rhesus monkey. *Brain Res.* **23**: 437–442.

Beleslin, D. B. and R. D. Myers. 1971. Release of an unknown substance from brain structures of unanesthetized monkeys and cats. *Neuropharmacology.* **10**: 121–124.

Beleslin, D. and R. L. Polak. 1965. Depression by morphine and chloralose of acetylcholine release from the cat's brain. *J. Physiol.* **177**: 411–419.

Beleslin, D., E. A. Carmichael and W. Feldberg. 1964. The origin of acetylcholine appearing in the effluent of perfused cerebral ventricles of the cat. *J. Physiol.* **173**: 368–376.

Beleslin, D. B., B. Ž. Radmanović and M. M. Rakić. 1971. Release during convulsions of an unknown substance into the cerebral ventricles of the cats. *Brain Res.* **35**: 625–627.

Belluzzi, J. D. 1972. Long-lasting effects of cholinergic stimulation of the amygdaloid complex in the rat. *J. Comp. Physiol. Psychol.* **80**: 269–282.

Belluzzi, J. D. and S. P. Grossman. 1969. Avoidance learning: long-lasting deficits after temporal lobe seizure. *Science.* **166**: 1435–1437.

Benedetti, W. L., R. Lozdziejsky, M. A. Sala, J. M. Monti and E. Griño. 1969. Blockade of ovulation after atropine implants in the lateral hypothalamus of the rat. *Experientia.* **25**: 1158–1159.

Benkert, O. and B. Köhler. 1972. Intrahypothalamic and intrastriatal dopamine and norepinephrine injections in relation to motor hyperactivity in rats. *Psychopharmacologia.* **24**: 318–325.

Bennett, I. L., R. G. Petersdorf and W. R. Keene. 1957. Pathogenesis of fever: evidence for direct cerebral action of bacterial endotoxins. *Assoc. Amer. Phys. Trans.* **70**: 64–73.

Benzinger, T. H. 1969. Heat regulation: homeostasis of central temperature in man. *Physiol. Rev.* **49**: 671–759.

Berger, B. D., C. D. Wise and L. Stein. 1971. Norepinephrine: reversal of anorexia in rats with lateral hypothalamic damage. *Science.* **172**: 281–284.

Bergmann, F., A. Zerachia and Y. Gutman. 1968a. The antidipsic effect of sulphonamides implanted in the hypothalamus of rats. *Experientia.* **24**: 375–376.

Bergmann, F., A. Zerachia and Y. Gutman. 1968d. The influence of drugs, implanted into the hypothalamus, on hypovolemic thirst. *Physiol. Behav.* **3**: 693–694.

Bergmann, F., A. Zerachia and Y. Gutman. 1970a. Aphagia, produced by deposition of drugs into the hypothalamus of rats. *Physiol. Behav.* **5**: 417–420.

Bergmann, F., M. Chaimovitz, Y. Gutman and A. Zerachia. 1968c. Effect of mercury derivatives, implanted into the hypothalamus, on the water intake of albino rats. *Brit. J. Pharmacol. Chemother.* **32**: 483–492.

Bergmann, F., A. Costin, M. Chaimovitz and A. Zerachia. 1970b. Seizure activity evoked by implantation of ouabain and related drugs into cortical and subcortical regions of the rabbit brain. *Neuropharmacology.* **9**: 441–449.

Bergmann, F., A. Zerachia, M. Chaimovitz and Y. Gutman. 1968b. Influence of drugs, implanted into the hypothalamus, on the water consumption of rats. *J. Pharmacol. Exptl. Ther.* **159**: 222–228.

Bergmann, F., M. Chaimovitz, A. Costin, Y. Gutman and Y. Ginath. 1967. Water intake of rats after implantation of ouabain into the hypothalamus. *Amer. J. Physiol.* **213**: 328–332.

Bern, H. A. and F. G. W. Knowles. 1966. Neurosecretion, pp. 139–186. *In* L. Martini and W. F. Ganong (eds.) *Neuroendocrinology*, Vol. I. Academic Press, New York.

Beyer, C., G. Moralí and M. L. Cruz. 1971. Effect of 5-α-dihydrotestosterone on gonadotropin secretion and estrous behavior in the female wistar rat. *Endocrinology.* **89**: 1158–1161.

Bianchi, C. P. 1968. *Cell Calcium.* Butterworth and Co., Ltd., London. pp. 1–131.

Bieger, D., L. Larochelle and O. Hornykiewicz. 1971. A model for the quantitative study of central dopaminergic and serotoninergic activity. *Europ. J. Pharmacol.* **18**: 128–136.

Black, P. 1970. *Physiological Correlates of Emotion.* Academic Press, New York. pp. 1–309.

Black, R. G., J. Abraham and A. A. Ward, Jr. 1967. The preparation of tungstic acid gel and its use in the production of experimental epilepsy. *Epilepsia.* **8**: 58–63.

Blanchard, R. J. and D. C. Blanchard. 1966. Home cage behavior following chemical stimulation of the lateral hypothalamus. *Psychon. Sci.* **5**: 1–2.

Blanchard, R. J., K. Fukunaga and D. C. Blanchard. 1972. Alterations of defensive reactions in the rat after cholinergic stimulation of midline thalamic nuclei. *Physiol. Behav.* **8**: 817–822.

Blass, E. M. 1968. Separation of cellular from extracellular controls of drinking in rats by frontal brain damage. *Science.* **162**: 1501–1503.

Blass, E. M. and H. W. Chapman. 1971. An evaluation of the contribution of cholinergic mechanisms to thirst. *Physiol. Behav.* **7**: 679–686.

Blass, E. M. and A. N. Epstein. 1971. A lateral preoptic osmosensitive zone for thirst in the rat. *J. Comp. Physiol. Psychol.* **76**: 378–394.

Bligh, J. 1966. Effects on temperature of monoamines injected into the lateral ventricles of sheep. *J. Physiol.* **185**: 46–47P.

Bligh, J. 1972. Neuronal models of mammalian temperature regulation, pp. 105–120. *In* J. Bligh and R. E. Moore (eds.) *Essays on Temperature Regulation.* North-Holland, London.

Bligh, J., W. H. Cottle and M. Maskrey. 1971. Influence of ambient temperature on the thermoregulatory responses to 5-hydroxytryptamine, noradrenaline and acetylcholine injected into the lateral cerebral ventricles of sheep, goats and rabbits. *J. Physiol.* **212:** 377–392.

Bloch, G. J. and J. M. Davidson. 1967. Antiandrogen implanted in brain stimulates male reproductive system. *Science.* **155:** 593–595.

Bloch, G. J. and J. M. Davidson. 1971. Behavioral and somatic responses to antiandrogen cyproterone. *Horm. Behav.* **2:** 11–25.

Block, M. L. and A. E. Fisher. 1970. Anticholinergic central blockade of salt-aroused and deprivation-induced drinking. *Physiol. Behav.* **5:** 525–527.

Bloom, F. E., B. J. Hoffer and G. R. Siggins. 1971. Studies on norepinephrine-containing afferents to purkinje cells of rat cerebellum. I. Localization of the fibers and their synapses. *Brain Res.* **25:** 501–521.

Blum, B. and E. Liban. 1960. Experimental bastemporal epilepsy in the cat. *Neurology.* **10:** 546–554.

Blum, B. and E. Liban. 1963. The cold tungstic acid gel method for production of experimental epilepsy. *Bull. Res. Coun. Israel.* **10E:** 146–148.

Blundell, J. E. and L. J. Herberg. 1970. Adrenergic stimulation of the rat diencephalon and its effect on food intake and hoarding activity. *Quart. J. Exp. Psychol.* **22:** 125–132.

van Bogaert, A. 1936a. Hypothalamus et réactions cardio-vasculaires d'origine centrale. *Arch. Int. Pharmacodyn. Ther.* **53:** 137–176.

van Bogaert, A. 1936b. Régulation hypothalamo-hypophysaire de l'appareil circulatoire. *Arch. Maladies Coeur.* **29:** 15–38.

Bogdanove, E. M. 1957. Selectivity of the effects of hypothalamic lesions on pituitary trophic hormone secretion in the rat. *Endocrinology.* **60:** 689–697.

Bogdanove, E. M. 1963a. Secretion and release of LH and FSH: Discussion, pp. 236–237. *In* A. V. Nalbandov (ed.) *Advances in Neuroendocrinology.* University of Illinois Press, Urbana.

Bogdanove, E. M. 1963b. Direct gonad-pituitary feedback: an analysis of effects of intracranial estrogenic depots on gonadotrophin secretion. *Endocrinology.* **73:** 696–712.

Bogdanove, E. M. and E. V. Crabill. 1961. Thyroid-pituitary feedback: direct or indirect? A comparison of the effects of intrahypothalamic and intrapituitary thyroid autotransplants on pituitary thyroidectomy reactions in the rat. *Endocrinology.* **69:** 581–595.

Bohus, B. 1968. Pituitary ACTH release and avoidance behavior of rats with cortisol implants in mesencephalic reticular formation and median eminence. *Neuroendocrinology.* **3:** 355–365.

Bohus, B. 1970a. The medial thalamus and the opposite effect of corticosteroids and adrenocorticotrophic hormone on avoidance extinction in the rat. *Acta Physiol. Acad. Sci. Hung.* **38:** 217–223.

Bohus, B. 1970b. Central nervous structures and the effect of ACTH and corticosteroids on avoidance behaviour: A study with intracerebral implantation of corticosteriods in the rat, pp. 171–184. *In* D. de Wied and J. A. W. M. Weijnen (eds.) *Pituitary, Adrenal, and the Brain.* Elsevier, Amsterdam.

Bohus, B. and E. Endröczi. 1964. Effect of intracerebral implantation of hydrocortisone on adrenocortical secretion and adrenal weight after unilateral adrenalectomy. *Acta Physiol. Acad. Sci. Hung.* **25:** 11–19.

Bohus, B. and K. Lissák. 1967. The sites of feedback action of corticosteriod at extrahypothalamic level. *Gener. Comp. Endocrinol.* **9:** 434–435.

Bohus, B. and D. Strashimirov. 1970. Localization and specificity of corticosteroid "feedback receptors" at the hypothalamo-hypophyseal level; comparative effects of various steroids implanted in the median eminence or the anterior pituitary of the rat. *Neuroendocrinology.* **6:** 197–209.

Bohus, B., K. Lissák and B. Mezei. 1965. The effect of thyroxine implantation in the hypothalamus and the anterior pituitary on pituitary-adrenal function in rats. *Neuroendocrinology.* **1:** 15–22.

Bohus, B., Cs. Nyakas and K. Lissák. 1968. Involvement of suprahypothalamic structures in the hormonal feedback action of corticosteroids. *Acta Physiol. Acad. Sci. Hung.* **34:** 1–8.

Bøler, J., F. Enzmann, K. Folkers, C. Y. Bowers and A. V. Schally. 1969. The identity of chemical and hormonal properties of the thyrotropin releasing hormone and pyroglutamyl-histidyl-proline amide. *Biochem. Biophys. Res. Commun.* **37:** 705–710.

Bondareff, W., A. Routtenberg, R. Narotzky and D. G. McLone. 1970. Intrastriatal spreading of biogenic amines. *Exptl. Neurol.* **28:** 213–229.

Bonvallet, M. and V. Bloch. 1961. Bulbar control of cortical arousal. *Science.* **133:** 1133–1134.

Boom, R., G. Chávez-Ibarra, J. J. Del Villar and R. Hernández-Peón. 1965. Changes of colonic motility induced by electrical and chemical stimulation of the forebrain and hypothalamus in cats. *Int. J. Neuropharmacol.* **4:** 169–175.

Booth, D. A. 1967. Localization of the adrenergic feeding system in the rat diencephalon. *Science.* **158:** 515–517.

Booth, D. A. 1968a. Amphetamine anorexia by direct action on the adrenergic feeding system of rat hypothalamus. *Nature.* **217:** 869–870.

Booth, D. A. 1968b. Effects of intrahypothalamic glucose injection on eating and drinking elicited by insulin. *J. Comp. Physiol. Psychol.* **65:** 13–16.

Booth, D. A. 1968c. Mechanism of action of norepinephrine in eliciting an eating response on injection into the rat hypothalamus. *J. Pharmacol. Exptl. Ther.* **160:** 336–348.

Booth, D. A. 1972. Unlearned and learned effects of intrahypothalamic cyclic AMP injection on feeding. *Nature New Biol.* **237:** 222–224.

Booth, D. A. and N. E. Miller. 1969. Lateral hypothalamus mediated effects of a food signal on blood glucose concentration. *Physiol. Behav.* **4:** 1003–1009.

Booth, D. A. and D. Quartermain. 1965. Taste sensitivity of eating elicited by chemical stimulation of the rat hypothalamus. *Psychon. Sci.* **3:** 525–526.

Borison, H. L., P. S. R. K. Haranath and L. E. McCarthy. 1972. Respiratory responses to chemical pulses in the cerebrospinal fluid of cats. *Brit. J. Pharmacol.* **44:** 605–616.

Boros-Farkas, M. and A. Illei-Donhoffer. 1969. The effect of hypothalamic injections of noradrenaline, serotonin, pyrogen, γ-amino-n-butyric acid, triiodothyronine, triiodothyroacetic acid, DL-phenylalanine, DL-alanine and DL-γ-amino-β-hydroxybutyric acid on body temperature and oxygen consumption in the rat. *Acta. Physiol. Acad. Sci. Hung.* **36:** 105–116.

Bossy, J. 1970. *Atlas of Neuroanatomy and Special Sense Organs.* W. B. Saunders Company, Philadelphia, pp. 1–348.

Breckenridge, B. M. and R. D. Lisk. 1969. Cyclic adenylate and hypothalamic regulatory functions. *Proc. Soc. Exptl. Biol. Med.* **131:** 934–935.

Bremer, F. 1935. Cerveau «isolé» et physiologie du sommeil. *C. R. Soc. Biol. (Paris).* **118:** 1235–1241.

Brezenoff, H. E. 1972. Cardiovascular responses to intrahypothalamic injections of carbachol and certain cholinesterase inhibitors. *Neuropharmacology.* **11:** 637–644.

Brezenoff, H. E. and D. J. Jenden. 1969. Modification of arterial blood pressure in rats following microinjection of drugs into the posterior hypothalamus. *Int. J. Neuropharmacol.* **8:** 593–600.

Brezenoff, H. E. and D. J. Jenden. 1970. Changes in arterial blood pressure after microinjections of carbachol into the medulla and IVth ventricle of the rat brain. *Neuropharmacology.* **9:** 341–348.

Brezenoff, H. E. and P. Lomax. 1970. Temperature changes following microinjections of histamine into the thermoregulatory centers of the rat. *Experientia.* **26:** 51–52.

Brezenoff, H. E. and T. S. Wirecki. 1970. The pharmacological specificity of muscarinic receptors in the posterior hypothalamus of the rat. *Life Sci.* 9: 99–109.

Brobeck, J. R., J. Tepperman and C. N. H. Long. 1943. Experimental hypothalamic hyperphagia in the albino rat. *Yale J. Biol. Med.* 15: 831–853.

Brody, J. F., P. A. DeFeudis and F. V. DeFeudis. 1969. Effects of microinjections of L-glutamate into the hypothalamus on attack and flight behaviours in cats. *Nature.* 224: 1330.

Broekkamp, C. and J. M. van Rossum. 1972. Clonidine induced intrahypothalamic stimulation of eating in rats. *Psychopharmacologia.* 25: 162–168.

Bronzino, J. D., P. J. Morgane and W. C. Stern. 1972b. EEG synchronization following application of serotonin to area postrema. *Amer. J. Physiol.* 223: 376–383.

Bronzino, J. D., P. J. Morgane, W. C. Stern and S. Bottaro. 1972a. A new design for an exploring chemode. *EEG Clin. Neurophysiol.* 32: 195–198.

Brookhart, J. M., F. L. Dey and S. W. Ranson. 1941. The abolition of mating behavior by hypothalamic lesions in guinea pigs. *Endocrinology.* 28: 561–565.

Brooks, G. F., A. Koch and J. Wong. 1970. Kinetics of sodium transfer from blood to brain of the dog. *Amer. J. Physiol.* 218: 693–702.

Bunge, R. P. 1970. Structure and function of neuroglia: some recent observations, pp. 782–797. *In* F. O. Schmitt (ed.) *The Neurosciences, Second Study Program.* The Rockefeller University Press, New York.

Bureš, J. and O. Burešová. 1972. Inducing cortical spreading depression, pp. 319–343. *In* R. D. Myers (ed.) *Methods in Psychobiology*, Vol. 2. Academic Press, London.

Bureš, J., G. Hartmann and L. D. Lukyanova. 1967. Blockade of thalamocortical and pyramidal pathways by striatal spreading depression in rats. *Exptl. Neurol.* 18: 404–415.

Bureš, J., I. B. Kozlovskaya and E. Fifková. 1964. Excitability changes in non-specific thalamic nuclei during striatal depression in the rat. *Arch. Int. Physiol. Biochim.* 72: 776–786.

Bureš, J., O. Burešová, E. Fifková and G. Rabending. 1965. Reversible deafferentation of cerebral cortex by thalamic spreading depression. *Exptl. Neurol.* 12: 55–67.

Burešová, O., E. Fifková and J. Bureš. 1966. Pupillary paralysis evoked by thalamic spreading depression in rats. *Exp. Brain Res.* 2: 168–175.

Burešová, O., I. Shima, J. Bureš and E. Fifková. 1963. Unit activity in regions affected by the spreading depression. *Physiol. Bohemoslov.* 12: 488–494.

Burgen, A. S. V. 1964. Book review: The Physiology of Synapses. *Nature.* 204: 412.

Burgen, A. S. V. and L. M. Chipman. 1951. Cholinesterase and succinic dehydrogenase in the central nervous system of the dog. *J. Physiol.* 114: 296–305.

Butcher, L. L. and S. S. Fox. 1968. Motor effects of copper in the caudate nucleus: reversible lesions with ion-exchange resin beads. *Science.* 160: 1237–1238.

Cabanac, M. and J. D. Hardy. 1969. Réponses unitaires et thermorégulatrices lors de réchauffements et refroidissements localisés de la région préoptique et du mésencéphale chez le lapin. *J. Physiol. (Paris).* 61: 331–347.

Canal, N. and A. Ornesi. 1961. Serotonina encefalica e ipertermia da vaccino. *Atti Accad. Med. Lombarda.* 16: 69–73.

Carlton, P. L. 1963. Cholinergic mechanisms in the control of behavior by the brain. *Psychol. Rev.* 70: 19–39.

Carlton, P. L. 1969. Brain-acetylcholine and inhibition, pp. 286–327. *In* J. T. Tapp (ed.) *Reinforcement and Behavior.* Academic Press, New York.

Carmichael, E. A., W. Feldberg and K. Fleischhauer. 1964. Methods for perfusing different parts of the cat's cerebral ventricles with drugs. *J. Physiol.* 173: 354–367.

Carr, L. A. and K. E. Moore. 1969. Norepinephrine: release from brain by d-amphetamine *in vivo. Science.* 164: 322–323.

Carr, L. A. and K. E. Moore. 1970. Effects of amphetamine on the contents of norepinephrine and its metabolites in the effluent of perfused cerebral ventricles of the cat. *Biochem. Pharmacol.* **19:** 2361–2374.

Cesa-Bianchi, M. G., M. Mancia and R. Mutani. 1967. Experimental epilepsy induced by cobalt powder in lower brain-stem and thalamic structures. *EEG Clin. Neurophysiol.* **22:** 525–536.

Chai, C. Y., C. L. Chen and T. H. Yin. 1971. Central sites of action and effects of acetyl-strophanthidin on body temperature in monkeys. *Exptl. Neurol.* **33:** 618–628.

Chambers, W. F. and R. J. Sobel. 1971. Effect of thyroxine-agar tube application to the rat hypothalamus. *Neuroendocrinology.* **7:** 37–45.

Chase, T. N. and I. J. Kopin. 1968. Stimulus-induced release of substances from olfactory bulb using the push-pull cannula. *Nature.* **217:** 466–467.

Chen, C. L., J. L. Voogt and J. Meites. 1968. Effect of median eminence implants of FSH, LH or prolactin on luteal function in the rat. *Endocrinology.* **83:** 1273–1277.

Chi, C. C. 1970. Afferent connections to the ventromedial nucleus of the hypothalamus in the rat. *Brain Res.* **17:** 439–445.

Chi, C. C. and J. P. Flynn. 1968. The effects of hypothalamic and reticular stimulation on evoked responses in the visual system of the cat. *EEG Clin. Neurophysiol.* **24:** 343–356.

Chiaraviglio, E. and S. Taleisnik. 1969. Water and salt intake induced by hypothalamic implants of cholinergic and adrenergic agents. *Amer. J. Physiol.* **216:** 1418–1422.

Chisholm, B., and G. Singer. 1970. A new type of cannula for central administration of drugs in rats. *Physiol. Behav.* **5:** 1069–1070.

Chkhartishvili, B. V. 1969. EEG and behavioral changes following injection of acetylcholine in different parts of the midbrain reticular formation of cats. *Bull. Acad. Sci. Georgian SSR.* **54:** 196–200.

Chowers, I. and S. M. McCann. 1963. The effects on ACTH and gonadotrophin secretion of implants of gonadal steroids in the hypothalamo-hypophysial region. *Israel Med. J.* **22:** 420–432.

Chowers, I. and S. M. McCann. 1967. Comparison of the effect of hypothalamic and pituitary implants of estrogen and testosterone on reproductive system and adrenal of female rats. *Proc. Soc. Exptl. Biol. Med.* **124:** 260–266.

Chowers, I., N. Conforti and S. Feldman. 1967. Effects of corticosteroids on hypothalamic corticotropin releasing factor and pituitary ACTH content. *Neuroendocrinology.* **2:** 193–199.

Chowers, I., N. Conforti and S. Feldman. 1968. Local effect of cortisol in the preoptic area on temperature regulation. *Amer. J. Physiol.* **214:** 538–542.

Chowers, I., S. Feldman and J. M. Davidson. 1963. Effects of intrahypothalamic crystalline steroids on acute ACTH secretion. *Amer. J. Physiol.* **205:** 671–673.

Chowers, I., H. T. Hammel, S. B. Stromme and S. M. McCann. 1964. Comparison of effect of environmental and preoptic cooling on plasma cortisol levels. *Amer. J. Physiol.* **207:** 577–582.

Chusid, J. G. and L. M. Kopeloff. 1962. Epileptogenic effects of pure metals implanted in motor cortex of monkeys. *J. Appl. Physiol.* **17:** 697–700.

Chusid, J. G. and L. M. Kopeloff. 1967. Epileptogenic effects of metal powder implants in motor cortex of monkeys. *Int. J. Neuropsychiat.* **3:** 24–28.

Chusid, J. G., L. M. Kopeloff and N. Kopeloff. 1955. Motor epilepsy of parietal lobe origin in the monkey. *Neurology.* **5:** 108–112.

Cicero, T. J. and R. D. Myers. 1969. Preference-aversion functions for alcohol after cholinergic stimulation of the brain and fluid deprivation. *Physiol. Behav.* **4:** 559–562.

Clemens, J. A. and J. Meites. 1968. Inhibition by hypothalamic prolactin implants of prolactin secretion, mammary growth and luteal function. *Endocrinology.* **82:** 878–881.

Clöetta, M. and H. Fischer. 1930. Über die Wirkung der Kationen Ca, Mg, Sr, Ba, K and Na bei intrazerebraler Injektion. *Arch. Exper. Pathol. Pharmakol.* **158:** 254–281.

Code, C. F. 1967. Control of food and water intake, pp. 1–459. *In: Handbook of Physiology. Section 6: Alimentary Canal.* American Physiological Society, Washington, D.C.

Codish, S. D. 1971. Actinomycin D injected into the hippocampus of chicks: effects upon imprinting. *Physiol. Behav.* **6**: 95–96.

Cohen, D. L. and J. R. Sladek. 1972. Evidence for the limited spread of intracerebrally applied serotonin. *Brain Res.* **45**: 630–634.

Colin-Jones, D. G. and R. L. Himsworth. 1970. The location of the chemoreceptor controlling gastric acid secretion during hypoglycaemia. *J. Physiol.* **206**: 397–409.

Collier, B. and J. F. Mitchell. 1966. The central release of acetylcholine during stimulation of the visual pathway. *J. Physiol.* **184**: 239–254.

Collier, H. O. J. 1969. A pharmacological analysis of aspirin, pp. 333–405. *In* S. Garattini, A. Goldin, F. Hawking and I. J. Kopin (eds.) *Advances in Pharmacology and Chemotherapy* Vol. 7. Academic Press, New York, London.

Colvin, G. B. and C. H. Sawyer. 1969. Induction of running activity by intracerebral implants of estrogen in ovariectomized rats. *Neuroendocrinology.* **4**: 309–320.

Comroe, J. H. 1943. The effects of direct chemical and electric stimulation of the respiratory center in the cat. *Amer. J. Physiol.* **139**: 490–498.

Connor, J. D., G. V. Rossi and W. W. Baker. 1966a. Analysis of the tremor induced by injection of cholinergic agents into the caudate nucleus. *Int. J. Neuropharmacol.* **5**: 207–216.

Connor, J. D., G. V. Rossi and W. W. Baker. 1966b. Characteristics of tremor in cats following injections of carbachol into the caudate nucleus. *Exptl. Neurol.* **14**: 371–382.

Connor, J. D., G. V. Rossi and W. W. Baker. 1967. Antagonism of intracaudate tremor by local injections of catecholamines. *J. Pharmacol. Exptl. Ther.* **155**: 545–551.

Cools, A. R. 1972. Athetoid and choreiform hyperkinesias produced by caudate application of dopamine in cats. *Psychopharmacologia.* **25**: 229–237.

Cools, A. R. and J. M. van Rossum. 1970. Caudal dopamine and stereotype behavior of cats. *Arch. Int. Pharmacodyn. Ther.* **187**: 163–173.

Coons, E. E. and D. Quartermain. 1970. Motivational depression associated with norepinephrine-induced eating from the hypothalamus: resemblance to the ventromedial hyperphagic syndrome. *Physiol. Behav.* **5**: 687–692.

Cooper, I. S. 1954. Intracerebral injection of procaine into the globus pallidus in hyperkinetic disorders. *Science.* **119**: 417–418.

Cooper, K. E. 1972a. Central mechanisms for the control of body temperature in health and febrile states, pp. 33–54. *In* C. B. B. Downman (ed.) *Modern Trends in Physiology.* Butterworths, London.

Cooper, K. E. 1972b. The body temperature "set-point" in fever, pp. 149–162. *In* J. Bligh and R. E. Moore (eds.) *Essays on Temperature Regulation.* North-Holland, London.

Cooper, K. E., W. I. Cranston and A. J. Honour. 1965. Effects of intraventricular and intrahypothalamic injection of noradrenaline and 5-HT on body temperature in conscious rabbits. *J. Physiol.* **181**: 852–864.

Cooper, K. E., W. I. Cranston and A. J. Honour. 1967. Observations on the site and mode of action of pyrogens in the rabbit brain. *J. Physiol.* **191**: 325–337.

Corbin, A. 1966. Pituitary and plasma LH of ovariectomized rats with median eminence implants of LH. *Endocrinology.* **78**: 893–896.

Corbin, A. and A. I. Cohen. 1966. Effect of median eminence implants of LH on pituitary LH of female rats. *Endocrinology.* **78**: 41–46.

Corbin, A. and J. C. Story. 1967. "Internal" feedback mechanism: response of pituitary FSH and of stalk-median eminence follicle stimulating hormone-releasing factor to median eminence implants of FSH. *Endocrinology.* **80**: 1006–1012.

Corbin, A., G. Mangili, M. Motta and L. Martini. 1965. Effect of hypothalamic and mesencephalic steroid implantations on ACTH feedback mechanisms. *Endocrinology.* **76**: 811–818.

Corbit, J. D. 1969. Behavioral regulation of hypothalamic temperature. *Science.* **166:** 256–257.

Cordeau, J. P., A. Moreau, A. Beaulnes and C. Laurin. 1963. EEG and behavioral changes following microinjections of acetylcholine and adrenaline in the brain stem of cats. *Arch. Ital. Biol.* **101:** 30–47.

Cornog, Jr., J. L., N. K. Gonatas and J. R. Feierman. 1967. Effects of intracerebral injection of ouabain on the fine structure of rat cerebral cortex. *Amer. J. Pathol.* **51:** 573–590.

Costall, B. and R. J. Naylor. 1972a. Modification of amphetamine effects by intracerebrally administered anticholinergic agents. *Life Sci.* **11:** 239–253.

Costall, B. and R. J. Naylor. 1972b. Possible involvement of a noradrenergic area of the amygdala with stereotyped behaviour. *Life Sci.* **11:** 1135–1146.

Costall, B., R. J. Naylor and J. E. Olley. 1972a. On the involvement of the caudate-putamen, globus pallidus and substantia nigra with neuroleptic and cholinergic modification of locomotor activity. *Neuropharmacology.* **11:** 317–330.

Costall, B., R. J. Naylor and J. E. Olley. 1972b. Stereotypic and anticataleptic activities of amphetamine after intracerebral injections. *Europ. J. Pharmacol.* **18:** 83–94.

Courville, J., J. Walsh and J. P. Cordeau. 1962. Functional organization of the brain stem reticular formation and sensory input. *Science.* **138:** 973–975.

Coury, J. N. 1967. Neural correlates of food and water intake in the rat. *Science.* **156:** 1763–1765.

Covian, M. R., C. G. Gentil and J. Antunes-Rodrigues. 1972. Water and sodium chloride intake following microinjections of angiotensin II into the septal area of the rat brain. *Physiol. Behav.* **9:** 373–390.

Cox, B. and D. Potkonjak. 1969. An investigation of the tremorgenic effects of oxotremorine and tremorine after stereotaxic injection into rat brain. *Int. J. Neuropharmacol.* **8:** 291–297.

Cranston, W. I. and M. D. Rawlins. 1972. Effects of intracerebral micro-injection of sodium salicylate on temperature regulation in the rabbit. *J. Physiol.* **222:** 257–266.

Cranston, W. I. and C. Rosendorff. 1971. Local blood flow, cerebrovascular autoregulation and CO_2 responsiveness in the rabbit hypothalamus. *J. Physiol.* **215:** 577–590.

Craven, R. P. and P. G. McDonald. 1971. The effect of intrahypothalamic infusions of dopamine and noradrenaline on ovulation in the adult rat. *Life Sci.* **10:** 1409–1415.

Crawshaw, L. I. 1972. Effects of intracerebral 5-hydroxytryptamine injection on thermoregulation in rat. *Physiol. Behav.* **9:** 133–140.

Cremer, J. E. and J. Bligh. 1969. Body-temperature and response to drugs. *Brit. Med. Bull.* **25:** 299–306.

Curtis, D. R. and J. M. Crawford. 1969. Central synaptic transmission-microelectrophoretic studies. *Ann. Rev. Pharmacol.* **9:** 209–240.

Cushing, H. 1930. Neurohypophysial mechanisms from a clinical standpoint. *The Lancet.* **219:** 175–184.

Dallman, M. F. and F. E. Yates. 1968. Anatomical and functional mapping of central neural input and feedback pathways of the adreno-cortical system. *Mem. Soc. Endocrinol. (London).* **17:** 39–72.

D'Angelo, S. A., J. Snyder and J. M. Grodin. 1964. Electrical stimulation of the hypothalamus: simultaneous effects on the pituitary-adrenal and thyroid systems of the rat. *Endocrinology.* **75:** 417–427.

Daniels, D. 1971. Acquisition, storage, and recall of memory for brightness discrimination by rats following intracerebral infusion of acetoxycycloheximide. *J. Comp. Physiol. Psychol.* **76:** 110–118.

Daniels-Severs, A., E. Ogden and J. Vernikos-Danellis. 1971. Centrally mediated effects of angiotensin II in the unanesthetized rat. *Physiol. Behav.* **7:** 785–787.

David, M. A., F. Fraschini and L. Martini. 1966. Control of LH secretion: role of a "short" feedback mechanism. *Endocrinology.* **78:** 55–60.

Davidson, J. M. 1966a. Control of gonadotropin secretion in the male, pp. 565-611. *In* L. Martini and W. F. Ganong (eds.) *Neuroendocrinology*, Vol. I. Academic Press, New York.

Davidson, J. M. 1966b. Activation of the male rat's sexual behavior by intracerebral implantation of androgen. *Endocrinology.* 79: 783-794.

Davidson, J. M. 1969. Feedback control of gonadotropin secretion, pp. 343-388. *In* W. F. Ganong and L. Martini (eds.) *Frontiers in Neuroendocrinology*. Oxford University Press, New York.

Davidson, J. M. and G. J. Bloch. 1969. Neuroendocrine aspects of male reproduction. *Biol. Reprod.* 1: 67-92.

Davidson, J. M. and S. Feldman. 1962. Andrenocorticotropin secretion inhibited by implantation of hydrocortisone in the hypothalamus. *Science.* 137: 125-126.

Davidson, J. M. and S. Feldman. 1963. Cerebral involvement in the inhibition of ACTH secretion by hydrocortisone. *Endocrinology.* 72: 936-946.

Davidson, J. M. and S. Feldman. 1967. Effects of extrahypothalamic dexamethasone implants on the pituitary-adrenal system. *Acta Endocrinol.* 55: 240-246.

Davidson, J. M. and S. Levine. 1972. Endocrine regulation of behavior. *Ann. Rev. Physiol.* 34: 375-408.

Davidson, J. M. and C. H. Sawyer. 1961a. Effects of localized intracerebral implantation of oestrogen on reproductive function in the female rabbit. *Acta Endocrinol.* 37: 385-393.

Davidson, J. M. and C. H. Sawyer. 1961b. Evidence for an hypothalamic focus of inhibition of gonadotropin by androgen in the male. *Proc. Soc. Exptl. Biol. Med.* 107: 4-7.

Davidson, J. M. and E. R. Smith. 1966. Testosterone feedback in the control of somatic and behavioral aspects of male reproduction. *Excp. Med. Int. Cong.* 132: 805-813.

Davidson, J. M., L. E. Jones and S. Levine. 1968. Feedback regulation of adrenocorticotropin secretion in "basal" and "stress" conditions: acute and chronic effects of intrahypothalamic corticoid implantation. *Endocrinology.* 82: 655-663.

Davidson, J. M., S. Feldman, L. E. Jones and S. Levine. 1967. The central nervous system and pituitary-adrenocortical feedback mechanisms. *Rassegna Di Neurologia Vegetativa.* 27: 9-27.

Davidson, J. M., P. Johnston, G. J. Bloch, E. R. Smith and R. F. Weick. 1970. Comparative responses to androgen of anatomic, behavioral and other parameters. *Excp. Med. Int. Cong.* 219: 727-730.

Davis, J. R. and R. E. Keesey. 1971. Norepinephrine-induced eating: its hypothalamic locus and an alternate interpretation of action. *J. Comp. Physiol. Psychol.* 77: 394-402.

Davis, J. D., R. L. Gallagher and R. Ladove. 1967a. Food intake controlled by a blood factor. *Science.* 156: 1247-1248.

Davis, M., A. Nonneman and S. E. Glickman. 1967b. Chemical stimulation of the midbrain reticular system. *Phychol. Rep.* 20: 507-509.

Dawson, G. D. and O. Holmes. 1966. Cobalt applied to the sensorimotor area of the cortex cerebri of the rat. *J. Physiol.* 185: 455-470.

Deadwyler, S. A., D. Montgomery and E. J. Wyers. 1972. Passive avoidance and carbachol excitation of the caudate nucleus. *Physiol. Behav.* 8: 631-635.

Debons, A. F., I. Krimsky and A. From. 1970. A direct action of insulin on the hypothalamic satiety center. *Amer. J. Physiol.* 219: 938-943.

Decima, E. and R. George. 1964. A simple cannula for intracerebral injections in chronic animals. *EEG Clin. Neurophysiol.* 17: 438-439.

Decsi, L. and M. K. Várszegi. 1969. Fear and escape reaction evoked by the intrahypothalamic injection of *d*-tubocurarine in unrestrained cats. *Acta Physiol. Acad. Sci. Hung.* 36: 95-104.

Decsi, L. and M. K. Várszegi. 1971. Effect of tranquilizers on the emotional-behavioral reactions evoked by direct chemical stimulation of the hypothalamus. *Societas Pharma-*

cologica Hungarica: V. Conferentia Hungarica Pro Therapia et Investigatione in Pharmacologia, Budapest, pp. 171–176.

Decsi, L., M. K. Vászegi and J. Méhes. 1969. Direct chemical stimulation of various subcortical brain areas in unrestrained cats, pp. 182–211. *In* K. Lissák (ed.) *Recent Developments of Neurobiology in Hungary*, Vol. II. Akadémiai Kiadó, Budapest.

DeHaven, K. E. and F. G. Carpenter. 1964. Interaction between CO_2 and citrate ions in the medullary reticular formation. *Amer. J. Physiol.* 207: 298–302.

Delezenne, C. 1900. Serums nervrotoxiques. *Ann. l'Institut. Pasteur.* 14: 686–704.

van Delft, A. M. L. and J. I. Kitay. 1972. Effect of ACTH on single unit activity in the diencephalon of intact and hypophysectomized rats. *Neuroendocrinology.* 9: 188–196.

Delgado, J. M. R. 1962. Pharmacological modifications of social behavior, pp. 265–292. *In* W. D. M. Paton (ed.) *Pharmacological Analysis of Central Nervous Action.* Pergamon Press, Oxford.

Delgado, J. M. R. 1966. Intracerebral perfusion in awake monkeys. *Arch. Int. Pharmacodyn. Ther.* 161: 442–462.

Delgado, J. M. R. and B. K. Anand. 1953. Increase of food intake induced by electrical stimulation of the lateral hypothalamus. *Amer. J. Physiol.* 172: 162–168.

Delgado, J. M. R. and F. V. DeFeudis. 1969. Effects of lithium injections into the amygdala and hippocampus of awake monkeys. *Exptl. Neurol.* 25: 255–267.

Delgado, J. M. R. and L. M. Kitahata. 1967. Reversible depression of hippocampus by local injections of anesthetics in monkeys. *EEG.Clin. Neurophysiol.* 22: 453–464.

Delgado, J. M. R. and L. Rubinstein. 1964. Intracerebral release of neurohumors in unanesthetized monkeys. *Arch. Int. Pharmacodyn. Ther.* 150: 530–546.

Delgado, J. M. R., F. V. DeFeudis and I. Bellido. 1971b. Injections of GABA and glutamate into the amygdalae of awake monkeys. *Commun. Behav. Biol.* 5: 347–357.

Delgado, J. M. R., M. C. Lico, H. Bracchitta and D. R. Snyder. 1971a. Brain excitability and behavioral reactivity in monkeys under meprobamate. *Arch. Int. Pharmacodyn. Ther.* 194: 5–17.

Delgado, J. M. R., F. V. DeFeudis, R. H. Roth, D. K. Ryugo and B. M. Mitruka. 1972. Dialytrode for long term intracerebral perfusion in awake monkeys. *Arch. Int. Pharmacodyn. Ther.* 198: 9–21.

Dement, W. C. 1972. Sleep deprivation and the organization of the behavioral states, pp. 321–361. *In* C. D. Clemente, D. Purpura and F. E. Mayer (eds.) *Sleep and the Maturing Nervous System.* Academic Press, New York.

Demole, V. 1927. Pharmakologisch-anatomische Untersuchungen zum Problem des Schlafes. *Arch. Exper. Pathol. Pharmakol.* 120: 229–258.

Denenberg, V. H. and R. D. Myers. 1958. Learning and hormone activity: I. Effects of thyroid levels upon the acquisition and extinction of an operant response. *J. Comp. Physiol. Psychol.* 51: 213–219.

Desiraju, T., M. G. Banerjee and B. K. Anand. 1968. Activity of single neurons in the hypothalamic feeding centers: effect of 2-deoxy-*D*-glucose. *Physiol. Behav.* 3: 757–760.

Deter, R. L. and R. A. Liebelt. 1964. Goldthioglucose as an experimental tool. *Texas Rep. Biol. Med.* 22: 229–243.

Deuben, R. R. and J. P. Buckley. 1970. Identification of a central site of action of angiotensin II. *J. Pharmacol. Exptl. Ther.* 175: 139–146.

Dey, F. L., C. Fisher, C. M. Berry and S. W. Ranson. 1940. Disturbances in reproductive functions caused by hypothalamic lesions in female guinea pigs. *Amer. J. Physiol.* 129: 39–46.

Dichter, M. and W. A. Spencer. 1969a. Penicillin-induced interictal discharges from the cat hippocampus. I. Characteristics and topographical features. *J. Neurophysiol.* 32: 649–662.

Dichter, M. and W. A. Spencer. 1969b. Penicillin-induced interictal discharges from the cat hippocampus. II. Mechanisms underlying origin and restriction. *J. Neurophysiol.* **32**: 663–687.

Dikshit, B. B. 1935. Action of acetylcholine on the "sleep centre." *J. Physiol.* **83**: 42P.

Dill, R. E., H. L. Dorman and W. M. Nickey. 1968a. A simple method for recording tremors in small animals. *J. Appl. Physiol.* **24**: 598–599.

Dill, R. E., W. M. Nickey and M. D. Little. 1968b. Dyskinesias in rats following chemical stimulation of the neostriatum. *Texas Rep. Biol. Med.* **26**: 101–106.

DiStefano, J. H., III. 1972. Precision microbicannulation device for neuroendocrine or neurophysiologic applications. *J. Appl. Physiol.* **33**: 159–163.

Döcke, F. and G. Dörner. 1969. A possible mechanism by which progesterone facilitates ovulation in the rat. *Neuroendocrinology.* **4**: 139–149.

Döcke, F., G. Dörner and K.-H. Voigt. 1968. A possible mechanism of the ovulation-inhibiting effect of chlormadinone acetate in the rat. *J. Endocrinol.* **41**: 353–362.

Dörner, G., F. Döcke and S. Moustafa. 1968a. Differential localization of a male and a female hypothalamic mating centre. *J. Reprod. Fert.* **17**: 583–586.

Dörner, G., F. Döcke and S. Moustafa. 1968b. Homosexuality in female rats following testosterone implantation in the anterior hypothalamus. *J. Reprod. Fert.* **17**: 173–175.

Douglas, W. W. 1970. Polypeptides–angiotensin, plasma kinins, and other vasoactive agents; prostaglandins, pp. 663–676. *In* L. S. Goodman and A. Gilman (eds.) *The Pharmacological Basis of Therapeutics, Fourth Edition.* Macmillan Company, New York.

Dow, R. S., A. Fernández-Guardiola and E. Manni. 1962. The production of cobalt experimental epilepsy in the rat. *EEG Clin. Neurophysiol.* **14**: 399–407.

Drucker-Colín, R., J. Rojas-Ramírez, J. Vera-Trueba, G. Monroy-Ayala and R. Hernández-Peón. 1970. Effect of crossed-perfusion of the midbrain reticular formation upon sleep. *Brain Res.* **23**: 269–273.

Dudar, J. D. and J. C. Szerb. 1970. A. The push-pull cannula (PPC). B. Bioassay of acetylcholine on leech muscle suspended in a microbath. *Exp. Physiol. Biochem.* **3**: 341–350.

Duke, H. N., M. Pickford and J. A. Watt. 1950. The immediate and delayed effects of diisopropylfluorphosphate injected into the supraoptic nuclei of dogs. *J. Physiol.* **111**: 81–88.

Duncan, C. J. 1967. *The Molecular Properties and Evolution of Excitable Cells.* Pergamon Press, London, pp. 1–253.

Duncan, P. M. 1971. Effect of temporary septal dysfunction on conditioning and performance of fear responses in rats. *J. Comp. Physiol. Psychol.* **74**: 340–348.

Dunér, H. 1953. The effect of local injections of glucose into the hypothalamus on the secretion of adrenaline and noradrenaline from the suprarenal. *Acta Physiol. Scand.* Suppl. 102, **28**: 54–77.

Dutta, S. N., D. A. Davis, W. M. Booker and S. N. Pradhan. 1971. Responses to microinjections of angiotensin into the hypothalamus of cats. *Neuropharmacology.* **10**: 231–236.

Echavarria-Mage, M-T., B. Senault and J. Delacour. 1972. Effets de microinjections de 6-hydroxydopamine dans le système nigro-strié sur un apprentissage chez le Rat blanc. *C. R. Acad. Sci. (Paris)* **275**: 1155–1158.

Ehrenpreis, S., J. H. Fleisch and T. W. Mittag. 1969. Approaches to the molecular nature of pharmacological receptors. *Pharmacol. Rev.* **21**: 131–181.

Eichelman, B. S., N. B. Thoa and K. Y. Ng. 1972. Facilitated aggression in the rat following 6-hydroxydopamine administration. *Physiol. Behav.* **8**: 1–3.

Elie, R. and J.-C. Panisset. 1970. Effect of angiotensin and atropine on the spontaneous release of acetylcholine from cat cerebral cortex. *Brain Res.* **17**: 297–305.

Endröczi, E., G. Hartmann and K. Lissák. 1963b. Effect of intracerebrally administered cholinergic and adrenergic drugs on neocortical and archicortical electrical activity. *Acta Physiol. Acad. Sci. Hung.* **24**: 199–209.

Endröczi, E., K. Lissák and M. Tekeres. 1961. Hormonal "feedback" regulation of pituitary-adrenocortical activity. *Acta Physiol. Acad. Sci. Hung.* **18**: 291–299.

Endröczi, E., G. Schreiberg and K. Lissák. 1963a. The role of central nervous activating and inhibitory structures in the control of pituitary-adreno-cortical function. Effects of intracerebral cholinergic and adrenergic stimulation. *Acta Physiol. Acad. Sci. Hung.* **24**: 211–221.

Epstein, A. N. 1960. Reciprocal changes in feeding behavior produced by intrahypothalamic chemical injections. *Amer. J. Physiol.* **199**: 969–974.

Epstein, A. N., J. T. Fitzsimons and B. J. Rolls. 1970. Drinking induced by injection of angiotensin into the brain of the rat. *J. Physiol.* **210**: 457–474.

Ernst, A. M. 1969. The role of biogenic amines in the extra-pyramidal system. *Acta Physiol. Pharmacol. Neerl.* **15**: 141–154.

Ernst, A. M. 1972. Relationship of the central effect of dopamine on gnawing compulsion syndrome in rats and the release of serotonin. *Arch. Int. Pharmacodyn. Ther.* **199**: 219–225.

Ernst, A. M. and P. G. Smelik. 1966. Site of action of dopamine and apomorphine on compulsive gnawing behavior in rats. *Experientia.* **22**: 837–839.

Essman, W. B. 1970. Some neurochemical correlates of altered memory consolidation. *N.Y. Acad. Sci.* **32**: 948–973.

von Euler, C. 1950. Slow "temperature potentials" in the hypothalamus. *J. Cell. Comp. Physiol.* **36**: 333–350.

von Euler, C. 1961. Physiology and pharmacology of temperature regulation. *Pharmacol. Rev.* **13**: 361–398.

von Euler, C. and B. Holmgren. 1956. The thyroxine 'receptor' of the thyroid-pituitary system. *J. Physiol.* **131**: 125–136.

Evetts, K. D., J. T. Fitzsimons and P. E. Setler. 1972. Eating caused by 6-hydroxy-dopamine-induced release of noradrenaline in the diencephalon of the rat. *J. Physiol.* **223**: 35–47.

Faeth, W. H. and A. E. Walker. 1957. Studies on effect of the injection of alumina (aluminum oxide) cream into the basal ganglia. *AMA Arch. Neurol. Psychiat.* **78**: 562–567.

Faeth, W. H., A. E. Walker and W. A. Warner. 1955. The electroencephalographic concomitants of experimental subcortical epilepsy. *Acta Neurol. Latinoamer.* **1**: 239–255.

Faeth, W. H., A. E. Walker and W. A. Warner. 1956. Experimental subcortical epilepsy. *AMA Arch. Neurol. Psychiat.* **75**: 548–562.

Faure, J. M. A. 1968. États de veille et de sommeil dans la régulation neuro-endocrinienne. *Actualites Neurophysiol.* **8**: 251–292.

Feider, A. 1967. Feedback control of carbachol-induced drinking. *J. Comp. Physiol. Psychol.* **64**: 336–338.

Feldberg, W. 1963. *A Pharmacological Approach to the Brain from its Inner and Outer Surface.* Edward Arnold Ltd., London, pp. 1–128.

Feldberg, W. 1968. The monoamines of the hypothalamus as mediators of temperature responses, pp. 349–397. *In* J. M. Robson and R. S. Stacey (eds.) *Recent Advances in Pharmacology.* Churchill, London.

Feldberg, W. and K. Fleischhauer. 1967. Site of origin of the abnormal discharge in the electrocorticogram produced by tubocurarine perfused through the anterior horn of a lateral ventricle. *J. Physiol.* **191**: 487–500.

Feldberg, W. and V. J. Lotti. 1970. Direct and indirect activation of the hippocampus by tubocurarine. *J. Physiol.* **210**: 697–716.

Feldberg, W. and R. D. Myers. 1964a. Effects on temperature of amines injected into the cerebral ventricles. A new concept of temperature regulation. *J. Physiol.* 173: 226-237.

Feldberg, W. and R. D. Myers. 1964b. Temperature changes produced by amines injected into the cerebral ventricles during anaesthesia. *J. Physiol.* 175: 464-478.

Feldberg, W. and R. D. Myers. 1965a. Changes in temperature produced by microinjections of amines into the anterior hypothalamus of cats. *J. Physiol.* 177: 239-245.

Feldberg, W. and R. D. Myers. 1965b. Hypothermia produced by chloralose acting on the hypothalamus. *J. Physiol.* 179: 509-517.

Feldberg, W. and R. D. Myers. 1966. Appearance of 5-hydroxytryptamine and an unidentified pharmacologically active lipid acid in effluent from perfused cerebral ventricles. *J. Physiol.* 184: 837-855.

Feldberg, W. and P. N. Saxena. 1970. Mechanism of action of pyrogen. *J. Physiol.* 211: 245-261.

Feldberg, W. and P. N. Saxena. 1971. Further studies on prostaglandin E_1 fever in cats. *J. Physiol.* 219: 739-745.

Feldman, S. 1971. Electrical activity of the brain following cerebral microinfusion of cortisol. *Epilepsia.* 12: 249-262.

Feldman, S., N. Conforti and J. M. Davidson. 1966. Adrenocortical responses in rats with corticosteroid and reserpine implants. *Neuroendocrinology.* 1: 228-239.

Feldman, S., N. Conforti and J. M. Davidson. 1967. Long-term effects of intracerebral corticoid implants. *Acta Endocrinol.* 55: 440-450.

Feldman, S., N. Conforti, I. Chowers and J. M. Davidson. 1969. Differential responses to various ACTH-releasing stimuli in rats with hypothalamic implants of corticosteroids. *Neuroendocrinology.* 5: 290-302.

Fencl, V., T. B. Miller and J. R. Pappenheimer. 1966. The respiratory responses to disturbances of acid-base balance, with deductions concerning the ionic composition of cerebral interstitial fluid, pp. 414-430. *In* W. F. Caveness and A. E. Walker (eds.) *Head Injury.* Lippincott Co., Philadelphia.

Fendler, K. and E. Endröczi. 1966. Effects of hypothalamic steroid implants on compensatory ovarian hypertrophy of rats. *Neuroendocrinology.* 1: 129-137.

Ferrari, W., G. L. Gessa, L. Vargiu, F. Crabai and M. Pisano. 1966. Localizzazione della zona cerebrale responsabile della sintomatologia da iniezione endoliquorale di peptidi con attivita ACTH ed MSH simili. *Boll. Soc. Ital. Biol. Sper.* 42: 1154-1157.

Fifková, E. 1964. Spreading EEG depression in the neo-, paleo- and archicortical structures of the brain of the rat. *Physiol. Bohemoslov.* 13: 1-15.

Fifková, E. 1966. Spreading depression in subcortical structures in rabbit. *Brain Res.* 2: 61-70.

Fifková, E. and J. Bureš. 1964. Spreading depression in the mammalian striatum. *Arch. Int. Physiol. Biochim.* 72: 171-179.

Fifková, E. and J. Syka. 1964. Relationships between cortical and striatal spreading depression in rat. *Exptl. Neurol.* 9: 355-366.

Fischer, J., J. Holubář and V. Malík. 1967. A new method of producing chronic epileptogenic cortical foci in rats. *Physiol. Bohemoslov.* 16: 272-277.

Fischer, J., J. Holubář and V. Malík. 1968. Neurohistological study of the development of experimental epileptogenic cortical cobalt-gelatine foci in rats and their correlation with the onset of epileptic electrical activity. *Acta Neuropath.* 11: 45-54.

Fisher, A. E. 1956. Maternal and sexual behavior induced by intracranial chemical stimulation. *Science.* 124: 228-229.

Fisher, A. E. 1966. Control of sexual behavior by gonadal steroids. III. Chemical and electrical stimulation of the brain in the male rat, pp. 117-130. *In* R. A. Gorski and R. E. Whalen (eds.) *Brain and Behavior*, Vol. III. University of California Press, Los Angeles.

Fisher, A. E. and J. N. Coury. 1962. Cholinergic tracing of a central neural circuit underlying the thirst drive. *Science.* **138**: 691-693.

Fisher, A. E. and J. N. Coury. 1964. Chemical tracing of neural pathways mediating the thirst drive, pp. 515-531. *In* M. J. Wayner (ed.) *Thirst.* Pergamon Press, New York.

Fisher, A. E. and R. A. Levitt. 1967. Drinking induced by carbachol: thirst circuit or ventricular modification? *Science.* **157**: 839-841.

Fisher, C., W. R. Ingram and S. W. Ranson. 1938. *Diabetes Insipidus and the Neurohormonal Control of Water Balance: A Contribution to the Structure and Function of the Hypothalamico-Hypophyseal System.* Edwards Brothers, Inc., Ann Arbor, pp. 1-212.

Fisher, C., H. W. Magoun and S. W. Ranson. 1938. Dystocia in Diabetes Insipidus. The relation of pituitary oxytocin to parturition. *Amer. J. Obstet. Gynecol.* **36**: 1-9.

Fitzsimons, J. T. 1971a. The hormonal control of water and sodium intake, pp. 103-128. *In* L. Martini and W. F. Ganong (eds.) *Frontiers in Neuroendocrinology.* Oxford University Press, Oxford.

Fitzsimons, J. T. 1971b. The effect on drinking of peptide precursors and of shorter chain peptide fragments of angiotensin II injected into the rat's diencephalon. *J. Physiol.* **214**: 295-303.

Fitzsimons, J. T. 1972. Thirst. *Physiol. Rev.* **52**: 468-561.

Flerkó, B. 1966. Control of gonadotropin secretion in the female, pp. 613-668. *In* L. Martini and W. F. Ganong (eds.) *Neuroendocrinology*, Vol. 1. Academic Press, New York.

Flerkó, B. and J. Szentágothai. 1957. Oestrogen sensitive nervous structure in the hypothalamus. *Acta Endocrinol.* **26**: 121-127.

Fletcher, A. and S. N. Pradhan. 1969. Responses to microinjections of *d*-tubocurarine into the hypothalamus of cats. *Int. J. Neuropharmacol.* **8**: 373-377.

Florey, E. 1960. Physiological evidence for naturally occurring inhibitory substances, pp. 72-84. *In* E. Roberts, C. F. Baxter, A. V. Harreveld, C. A. G. Wiersma, W. R. Adey and K. F. Killam (eds.) *Inhibition in the Nervous System and Gamma-Aminobutyric Acid.* Pergamon Press, New York.

Fog, R. L. and H. Pakkenberg. 1971. Behavioral effects of dopamine and *p*-hydroxyamphetamine injected into corpus striatum of rats. *Exptl. Neurol.* **31**: 75-86.

Fog, R. L., A. Randrup and H. Pakkenberg. 1967. Aminergic mechanisms in corpus striatum and amphetamine-induced stereotyped behaviour. *Psychopharmacologia.* **11**: 179-183.

Fog, R. L., A. Randrup and H. Pakkenberg. 1968. Neuroleptic action of quaternary chlorpromazine and related drugs injected into various brain areas in rats. *Psychopharmacologia.* **12**: 428-432.

Fog, R. L., A. Randrup and H. Pakkenberg. 1969. Chlorpromazine and related neuroleptic drugs in relation to the corpus striatum in rats. *Excp. Med. Int. Cong. Ser.* **180**: 278-280.

Fog, R. L., A. Randrup and H. Pakkenberg. 1970. Lesions in corpus striatum and cortex of rat brains and the effect of pharmacologically induced stereotyped, aggressive and cataleptic behaviour. *Psychopharmacologia.* **18**: 346-356.

Fog, R. L., A. Randrup and H. Pakkenberg. 1971. Intrastriatal injection of quaternary butyrophenones and oxypertine: neuroleptic effect in rats. *Psychopharmacologia.* **19**: 224-230.

Folkman, J., V. H. Mark, F. Ervin, K. Suematsu and R. Hagiwara. 1968. Intracerebral gas anesthesia by diffusion through silicone rubber. *Anesthesiology.* **29**: 419-425.

Forssberg, A. and S. Larsson. 1954. Studies of isotope distribution and chemical composition in the hypothalamic region of hungry and fed rats. *Acta Physiol. Scand.* **32**: 41-63.

Foster, R. S., D. J. Jenden and P. Lomax. 1967. A comparison of the pharmacologic effects or morphine and N-methyl-morphine. *J. Pharmacol. Exptl. Ther.* **157**: 185-195.

Foulkes, J. A. and N. Robinson. 1968. [^{14}C] leucine incorporation and axoplasmic flow in the rat brain stem reticular formation. *Brain Res.* **11**: 638-647.

Franklin, K. B. J. and D. Quartermain. 1970. Comparison of the motivational properties of deprivation-induced drinking with drinking elicited by central carbachol stimulation. *J. Comp. Physiol. Psychol.* **71**: 390–395.

Fraschini, F. 1968. The pineal gland and the control of LH and FSH secretion. *Excp. Med. Int. Cong.* **184**: 637–644.

Fraschini, F., R. Collu and L. Martini. 1970. Effects of pineal indoles on the hypothalamic-pituitary-gonadal axis. *Excp. Med. Int. Cong.* **219**: 830–838.

Fraschini, F., B. Mess and L. Martini. 1968b. Pineal gland, melatonin and the control of luteinizing hormonal secretion. *Endocrinology.* **82**: 919–924.

Fraschini, F., B. Mess, F. Piva and L. Martini. 1968a. Brain receptors sensitive to indole compounds: function in control of luteinizing hormone secretion. *Science.* **159**: 1104–1105.

Freeman, W. J. and D. D. Davis. 1959. Effects on cats of conductive hypothalamic cooling. *Amer. J. Physiol.* **197**: 145–148.

Freund, H. 1911. Üher das Kochsalzfieber. *Arch. Exper. Pathol. Pharmakol.* **65**: 225–238.

Friedman, M. J. and A. Wikler. 1970. The effect of intrahypothalamic microinjection of hemicholinium (HC-3) on the hippocampal theta rhythm of cats. *Psychopharmacologia.* **17**: 345–353.

Frigyesi, T., A. Ige, A. Iulo and R. Schwartz. 1971. Denigration and sensorimotor disability induced by ventral tegmental injection of 6-hydroxy-dopamine in the cat. *Exptl. Neurol.* **33**: 78–87.

Fuxe, K. 1965. Evidence for the existence of monoamine neurons in the central nervous system. IV. The distribution of monoamine nerve terminals in the central nervous system. *Acta Physiol. Scand.* Suppl. 247, **64**: 37–85.

Fuxe, K. and U. Ungerstedt. 1970. Histochemical, biochemical and functional studies on central monoamine neurons after acute and chronic amphetamine administration, pp. 257–288. *In* E. Costa and S. Garattini (eds.) *Amphetamines and Related Compounds.* Raven Press, New York.

Fuxe, K., A. Dahlström and N.-A. Hillarp. 1966. Central monoamine neurons and monoamine neuro-transmission. *Excp. Med. Int. Cong.* **87**: 419–434.

Fuxe, K., B. Hamberger and T. Hökfelt. 1968. Distribution of noradrenaline nerve terminals in cortical areas of the rat. *Brain Res.* **8**: 125–131.

Fuxe, K., T. Hökfelt and U. Ungerstedt. 1970. Morpholotical and functional aspects of central monoamine neurons. *Int. Rev. Neurobiol.* **13**: 93–126.

Gala, R. R., P. B. Markarian and M. R. O'Neill. 1970. The influence of neural blocking agents implanted into the hypothalamus of the rat on induced deciduomata formation. *Life Sci.* **9**: 1055–1064.

Gandelman, R., J. Panksepp and J. Trowill. 1968. Preference behavior and differences between water deprivation-induced and carbachol-induced drinkers. *Commun. Behav. Biol.* **1**: 341–346.

Ganong, W. F. 1966. Neuroendocrine integrating mechanisms, pp. 1–13. *In* L. Martini and W. F. Ganong (eds.) *Neuroendocrinology*, Vol. 1. Academic Press, New York.

Gardner, J. E. and A. E. Fisher. 1968. Induction of mating in male chicks following preoptic implantation of androgen. *Physiol. Behav.* **3**: 709–712.

Gastaut, H., R. Naquet and R. Vigouroux. 1953. Un cas d'épilepsie amygdalienne expérimentale chez le chat. *EEG Clin. Neurophysiol.* **5**: 291–294.

Gastaut, H., R. Vigouroux and R. Naquet. 1952. Lésions épileptogènes amygdalo-hippocampiques provoquées chez le chat par injection de "crème d'alumine." *Revue Neurol.* **87**: 607–609.

Gastaut, H., R. Naquet., A. Meyer, J. B. Cavanagh and E. Beck. 1959. Experimental psychomotor epilepsy in the cat electro-clinical and anatomo-pathological correlations. *J. Neuropath. Exp. Neurol.* **18:** 270–293.

Geller, I. and J. Seifter. 1960. The effects of meprobamate, barbiturates, *d*-amphetamine and promazine on experimentally induced conflict in the rat. *Psychopharmacologia.* **1:** 482–492.

Gellhorn, E. and E. S. Redgate. 1955. Hypotensive drugs (Acetylcholine, mecholyl, histamine) as indicators of the hypothalamic excitability of the intact organism. *Arch. Int. Pharmacodyn. Ther.* **102:** 162–178.

George, R., W. L. Haslett and D. J. Jenden. 1964. A cholinergic mechanism in the brainstem reticular formation: induction of paradoxical sleep. *Int. J. Neuropharmacol.* **3:** 541–552.

George, R., W. L. Haslett and D. J. Jenden. 1966. The production of tremor by cholinergic drugs: central sites of action. *Int. J. Neuropharmacol.* **5:** 27–34.

Gerhard, L. 1968. *Atlas of the Mes- and Diencephalon of the Rabbit.* Springer-Verlag, Heidelberg, pp. 1–183.

Gesell, R. 1940. A neurophysiological interpretation of the respiratory act. *Ergebn. Physiol.* **43:** 477–639.

Gessa, G. L., G. Krishna, J. Forn, A. Tagliamonte and B. B. Brodie. 1970. Behavioral and vegetative effects produced by dibutyryl cyclic AMP injected into different areas of the brain, pp. 371–381. *In* P. Greengard and E. Costa (eds.) *Advances in Biochemical Psychopharmacology*, Vol. 3. Raven Press, New York.

Gessa, G. L., M. Pisano, L. Vargiu, F. Crabai and W. Ferrari. 1967. Stretching and yawning movements after intracerebral injection of ACTH. *Rev. Can. Biol.* **26:** 229–236.

Giardina, A. R. and A. E. Fisher. 1971. Effect of atropine on drinking induced by carbachol, angiotensin and isoproterenol. *Physiol. Behav.* **7:** 653–655.

Gildenberg, P. L. 1957. Studies in stereoencephalotomy. VIII: Comparison of the variability of subcortical lesions produced by various procedures. *Confinia Neurol.* **17:** 299–309.

Glaser, G. H. 1972. Experimental derangements of extracellular ionic environment, pp. 317–345. *In* D. P. Purpura, J. K. Penry, D. B. Tower, D. M. Woodbury and R. D. Walter (eds.) *Experimental Models of Epilepsy.* Raven Press, New York.

Glassman, E. 1969. The biochemistry of learning: an evaluation of the role of RNA and and protein. *Ann. Rev. Biochem.* **38:** 605–646.

Glick, S. M. 1969. The regulation of growth hormone secretion, pp. 141–182. *In* W. F. Ganong and L. Martini (eds.) *Frontiers in Neuroendocrinology.* Oxford University Press, New York.

Gliddon, J. B. 1970. Effects of glucose, glucose-6-phosphate, and fructose-6-phosphate on the electrical activity in the ventromedial hypothalamus in rats. *Brain Res.* **22:** 429–433.

Glisson, S. N., A. G. Karczmar and L. Barnes. 1972. Cholinergic effects on adrenergic neurotransmitters in rabbit brain parts. *Neuropharmacology.* **11:** 465–477.

Gloor, P. 1969. Epileptogenic action of penicillin. *Ann. N.Y. Acad. Sci.* **166:** 350–360.

Gloor, P., G. Hall and F. Coceani. 1966. Differential sensitivity of various brain structures to the epileptogenic action of penicillin. *Exptl. Neurol.* **16:** 333–348.

Goddard, G. V. 1969. Analysis of avoidance conditioning following cholinergic stimulation of amygdala in rats. *J. Comp. Physiol. Psychol.* **68:** 1–18.

Gogan, F. 1968. Sensibilité hypothalamique à la testostérone chez le canard. *Gen. Comp. Endocrinol.* **11:** 316–327.

Goldberg, A. M., J. J. Pollock, E. R. Hartman and C. R. Craig. 1972. Alterations in cholinergic enzymes during the development of cobalt-induced epilepsy in the rat. *Neuropharmacology.* **11:** 253–259.

Goldblatt, H. 1948. *The Renal Origin of Hypertension.* Charles C Thomas, Springfield. pp. 1–126.

Goldman, H. W., D. Lahr and E. Friedman. 1971. Antagonistic effects of alpha and beta-adrenergically coded hypothalamic neurones on consummatory behaviour in the rat. *Nature*. **231**: 453–455.

Goodrich, C. A. 1969. Effect of monoamineoxidase inhibitors on 5-hydroxytryptamine output from perfused cerebral ventricles of anaesthetized cats. *Brit. J. Pharmacol*. **37**: 87–93.

Gordon, J. H., J. Bollinger and S. Reichlin. 1972. Plasma thyrotropin responses to thyrotropin-releasing hormone after injection into the third ventricle, systemic circulation, median eminence and anterior pituitary. *Endocrinology*. **91**: 696–701.

Gorski, R. A. 1966. Localization and sexual differentiation of the nervous structures which regulate ovulation. *J. Reprod. Fert*. Suppl. 1, 67–88.

Gorski, R. A. 1971. Gonadal hormones and the perinatal development of neuroendocrine function, pp. 237–290. *In* L. Martini and W. F. Ganong (eds.) *Frontiers in Neuroendocrinology*. Oxford University Press, New York.

Gorski, R. A. and C. A. Barraclough. 1962. Studies on hypothalamic regulation of FSH secretion in the androgen-sterilized female rat. *Proc. Soc. Exptl. Biol. Med*. **110**: 298–300.

Gorski, R. A. and J. W. Wagner. 1965. Gonadal activity and sexual differentiation of the hypothalamus. *Endocrinology*. **76**: 226–239.

Grafe, E. and E. Grünthal. 1929. Über isolierte Beeinflussung des Gesamtstoffwechsels vom Zwischenhirn aus. *Klin. Wschr*. **8**: 1013–1016.

Grant, L. D. and L. E. Jarrard. 1968. Functional dissociation within hippocampus. *Brain Res*. **10**: 392–401.

Grant, R. 1950. Emotional hypothermia in rabbits. *Amer. J. Physiol*. **160**: 285–290.

Green, J. D. and W. R. Adey. 1956. Electrophysiological studies of hippocampal connections and excitability. *EEG Clin. Neurophysiol*. **8**: 245–262.

Green, J. D., C. D. Clemente and J. deGroot. 1957. Rhinencephalic lesions and behavior in cats; an analysis of the Klüver-Bucy syndrome with particular reference to normal and abnormal sexual behavior. *J. Comp. Neurol*. **108**: 505–545.

Greene, E. G. 1968. Cholinergic stimulation of medial septum. *Psychon. Sci*. **10**: 157–158.

Greene, E. G. and P. Lomax. 1970. Impairment of alternation learning in rats following microinjection of carbachol into the hippocampus. *Brain Res*. **18**: 355–359.

Greep, R. O. 1963. Synthesis and summary, pp. 511–517. *In* A. V. Nalbandov (ed.) *Advances in Neuroendocrinology*. University of Illinois Press, Urbana.

Greer, M. A. 1957. Studies on the influence of the central nervous system on anterior pituitary function. *Rec. Prog. Hormone Res*. **13**: 67–104.

Greer, M. A., J. W. Kendall, Jr. and C. Duyck. 1963. Failure of heterotopic rat pituitary transplants to maintain andrenocortical secretion. *Endocrinology*. **72**: 499–501.

Grimm, R. J., J. G. Frazee, T. Kawasaki and M. Savić. 1970a. Cobalt epilepsy in the squirrel monkey. *EEG Clin. Neurophysiol*. **29**: 525–528.

Grimm, R. J., J. G. Frazee, C. C. Bell, T. Kawasaki and R. S. Dow. 1970b. Quantitative studies in cobalt model epilepsy: the effect of cerebellar stimulation. *Int. J. Neurol*. **7**: 126–140.

Grimm, Y. and J. W. Kendall. 1968. A study of feedback suppression of ACTH secretion utilizing glucocorticoid implants in the hypothalamus: the comparative effects of cortisol, corticosterone, and their 21-acetates. *Neuroendocrinology*. **3**: 55–63.

de Groot, J. 1959. The rat hypothalamus in stereotaxic coordinates. *J. Comp. Neurol*. **113**: 389–400.

Grossman, S. P. 1960. Eating or drinking elicited by direct adrenergic or cholinergic stimulation of hypothalamus. *Science*. **132**: 301–302.

Grossman, S. P. 1962a. Direct adrenergic and cholinergic stimulation of hypothalamic mechanisms. *Amer. J. Physiol*. **202**: 872–882.

Grossman, S. P. 1962b. Effects of adrenergic and cholinergic blocking agents on hypothalamic mechanisms. *Amer. J. Physiol.* **202:** 1230–1236.

Grossman, S. P. 1963. Chemically induced epileptiform seizures in the cat. *Science.* **142:** 409–411.

Grossman, S. P. 1964a. Behavioral effects of chemical stimulation of the ventral amygdala. *J. Comp. Physiol. Psychol.* **57:** 29–36.

Grossman, S. P. 1964b. Effect of chemical stimulation of the septal area on motivation. *J. Comp. Physiol. Psychol.* **58:** 194–200.

Grossman, S. P. 1964c. Behavioural effects of direct chemical stimulation of central nervous system structures. *Int. J. Neuropharmacol.* **3:** 45–58.

Grossman, S. P. 1966a. The VMH: a center for affective reactions, satiety, or both? *Physiol. Behav.* **1:** 1–10.

Grossman, S. P. 1966b. Acquisition and performance of avoidance responses during chemical stimulation of the midbrain reticular formation. *J. Comp. Physiol. Psychol.* **61:** 42–49.

Grossman, S. P. 1968a. Behavioral and electrophysiological effects of intracranial microjections of phenothiazines. *Commun. Behav. Biol.* **1:** 9–17.

Grossman, S. P. 1968b. Behavioral and electroencephalographic effects of micro-injections of neurohumors into the midbrain reticular formation. *Physiol. Behav.* **3:** 777–786.

Grossman, S. P. 1968c. Hypothalamic and limbic influences on food intake. *Fed. Proc.* **27:** 1349–1359.

Grossman, S. P. 1969. Facilitation of learning following intracranial injections of pentylenetetrazol. *Physiol. Behav.* **4:** 625–628.

Grossman, S. P. 1972. Neurophysiologic aspects: extrahypothalamic factors in the regulation of food intake. *Adv. Psychosom. Med.* **7:** 49–72.

Grossman, S. P. and L. Grossman. 1966. Effects of chemical stimulation of the midbrain reticular formation on appetitive behavior. *J. Comp. Physiol. Psychol.* **61:** 333–338.

Grossman, S. P. and H. Mountford. 1964. Learning and extinction during chemically induced disturbance of hippocampal functions. *Amer. J. Physiol.* **207:** 1387–1393.

Grossman, S. P. and R. H. Peters. 1966. Acquisition of appetitive and avoidance habits following atropine-induced blocking of the thalamic reticular formation. *J. Comp. Physiol. Psychol.* **61:** 325–332.

Grossman, S. P. and W. E. Stumpf. 1969. Intracranial drug implants: an autoradiographic analysis of diffusion. *Science.* **166:** 1410–1412.

Grossman, S. P., R. H. Peters, P. E. Freedman and H. I. Willer. 1965. Behavioral effects of cholinergic stimulation of the thalamic reticular formation. *J. Comp. Physiol. Psychol.* **59:** 57–65.

Grunden, L. R. 1969. Action of intracerebroventricular epinephrine on gross behavior, locomotor activity and hexobarbital sleeping times in rats. *Int. J. Neuropharmacol.* **8:** 573–586.

Grunden, L. R. and G. E. Linburn. 1969. Permanent cannula-injection system for intracerebral injections in small animals. *J. Pharm. Sci.* **58:** 1147–1148.

Guerrero-Figueroa, E., R. Guerrero-Figueroa, and R. G. Heath. 1966a. Trigeminal evoked responses during chemical stimulation of cortical and some subcortical structures. *The Bulletin of the Tulane University Medical Faculty,* Vol. 25, pp. 323–335.

Guerrero-Figueroa, R. and D. M. Gallant. 1967. Effects of pinoxepin and imipramine on the mesencephalic reticular formation and amygdaloid complex in the cat: Neurophysiological and clinical correlations in human subjects. *Curr. Ther. Res.* **9:** 387–403.

Guerrero-Figueroa, R., A. Barros and F. De Balbian Verster. 1963b. Some inhibitory effects of attentive factors on experimental epilepsy. *Epilepsia.* **4:** 225–240.

Guerrero-Figueroa, R., F. De Balbian Verster and R. G. Heath. 1962. Mirror focus in specific subcortical nuclei. *Trans. Am. Neurol. Assoc.* **87:** 207–209.

Guerrero-Figueroa, R., B. Lester and R. G. Heath. 1965. Changes of hippocampal epileptiform activity during wakefulness and sleep. *Acta Neurol. Latinoamer.* **11**: 330–349.

Guerrero-Figueroa, R., M. M. Rye and D. M. Gallant. 1967. Effects of diazepam on three per second spike and wave discharges. *Curr. Ther. Res.* **9**: 522–535.

Guerrero-Figueroa, R., M. M. Rye and C. Guerrero-Figueroa. 1968. Effects of diazepam on secondary subcortical epileptogenic tissues. *Curr. Ther. Res.* **10**: 150–166.

Guerrero-Figueroa, R., M. M. Rye and R. G. Heath. 1969a. Effects of two benzodiazepine derivates on cortical and subcortical epileptogenic tissues in the cat and monkey. I. Limbic system structures. II. Cortical and centrencephalic structures. *Curr. Ther. Res.* **11**: 27–50.

Guerrero-Figueroa, R., A. Barros, R. G. Heath and G. Gonzaléz. 1964a. Experimental subcortical epileptiform focus. *Epilepsia.* **5**: 112–139.

Guerrero-Figueroa, R., A. Barros, B. Lester and R. G. Heath. 1966b. Electrophysiological studies of hippocampal epileptiform discharges during emotional stages. *Acta Neurol. Latinoamer.* **12**: 6–28.

Guerrero-Figueroa, R., A. Barros, F. De Balbian Verster and R. G. Heath. 1963a. Experimental "petit mal" in kittens. *Arch. Neurol.* **9**: 297–306.

Guerrero-Figueroa, R., F. De Balbian Verster, A. Barros and R. G. Heath. 1964b. Cholinergic mechanism in subcortical mirror focus and effects of topical application of γ-aminobutyric acid and acetylcholine. *Epilepsia.* **5**: 140–155.

Guerrero-Figueroa, R., D. M. Gallant, C. Guerrero-Figueroa and J. Gallant. 1973. Electrophysiological analysis of the action of four benzodiazepine derivatives on the central nervous system, pp. 489–510. *In* S. Garattini and L. O. Randall (eds.) *The Benzodiazepines*, Raven Press, New York.

Guerrero-Figueroa, R., M. M. Rye, D. M. Gallant and C. L. Morse. 1969b. Effects of a new butyrophenone compound (AL-1021) on subcortical and cortical nervous system structures in the cat. *Curr. Ther. Res.* **11**: 121–133.

Gutman, Y. and M. Chaimovitz. 1966. Effect of chlorothiazide on water consumption in the rat. *Nature.* **209**: 410–411.

Gutman, Y., F. Bergmann and A. Zerachia. 1971a. Influence of hypothalamic deposits of antidipsic drugs on renal excretion. *Europ. J. Pharmacol.* **13**: 326–329.

Gutman, Y., M. Chaimovitz, A. Zerachia and F. Bergmann. 1970. Effect of hypothalamic implantation of ouabain on urine production in the rat. *Physiol. Behav.* **5**: 497–501.

Gutman, Y., M. Chaimovitz, F. Bergmann and A. Zerachia. 1971b. Hypothalamic implantation of ouabain and electrolyte excretion: evidence for central effect on sodium balance. *Physiol. Behav.* **6**: 399–401.

Hadžović, S. 1971. Hypothalamus and central effects of 5-hydroxytryptamine. *Jugoslav. Physiol. Pharmacol. Acta.* **7**: 109–113.

Hadžović, S. and A. M. Ernst. 1969. The effect of 5-hydroxytryptamine and 5-hydroxytryptophan on extra-pyramidal function. *Europ. J. Pharmacol.* **6**: 90–95.

Hafemann, D. R., A. Costin and T. J. Tarby. 1969. Neurophysiological effects of tetrodotoxin in lateral geniculate body and dorsal hippocampus. *Brain Res.* **12**: 363–373.

Hafemann, D. R., A. Costin and T. J. Tarby. 1970. Electrophysiological effects of enzymes introduced into the lateral geniculate body of the cat. *Exptl. Neurol.* **27**: 238–247.

Hagino, N. 1967. Site of positive feedback on ovarian hormones in immature female rats. *Jap. J. Physiol.* **17**: 190–199.

Hagino, N., M. Watanabe and J. Goldzieher. 1969. Inhibition by adrenocorticotrophin of gonadotrophin-induced ovulation in i nature female rats. *Endocrinology.* **84**: 308–314.

Haley, T. J. 1957. Intracerebral injection of psychotomimetic and psychotherapeutic drugs into conscious mice. *Acta Pharmacol. Toxicol.* **13**: 107–112.

Hall, G. H. and R. D. Myers. 1972. Temperature changes produced by nicotine injected into the hypothalamus of the conscious monkey. *Brain Res.* 37: 241-251.

Hamilton, C. L. and P. J. Ciaccia. 1971. Hypothalamus, temperature regulation and feeding in the rat. *Amer. J. Physiol.* 221: 800-809.

Hamilton, L. W. and S. P. Grossman. 1969. Behavioral changes following disruption of central cholinergic pathways. *J. Comp. Physiol. Psychol.* 69: 76-82.

Hamilton, L. W., R. A. McCleary and S. P. Grossman. 1968. Behavioral effects of cholinergic septal blockade in the cat. *J. Comp. Physiol. Psychol.* 66: 563-568.

Hammel, H. T. 1965. Neurons and temperature regulation, pp. 71-97. *In* W. S. Yamamoto and J. R. Brobeck (eds.) *Physiological Controls and Regulations.* W. B. Saunders Company, Philadelphia.

Hammel, H. T. 1968. Regulation of internal body temperature. *Ann. Rev. Physiol.* 30: 641-710.

Hardy, J. D. 1961. Physiology of temperature regulation. *Physiol. Rev.* 41: 521-606.

Hardy, J. D. 1965. The "set-point" concept in physiological temperature regulation, pp. 98-116. *In* W. S. Yamamoto and J. R. Brobeck (eds.) *Physiological Controls and Regulations.* W. B. Saunders Company, Philadelphia.

Hardy, J. D. 1972a. Models of temperature regulation—a review, pp. 163-186. *In* J. Bligh and R. E. Moore (eds.) *Essays on Temperature Regulation.* North-Holland, London.

Hardy, J. D. 1972b. Peripheral inputs to the central regulator for body temperature, pp. 3-21. *In* S. Ito, K. Ogata and H. Yoshimura (eds.) *Advances in Climatic Physiology.* Igaku Shoin, Ltd., Tokyo.

Hardy, J. D., R. F. Hellon and K. Sutherland. 1964. Temperature-sensitive neurones in the dog's hypothalamus. *J. Physiol.* 175: 242-253.

Harris, G. W. 1963. Secretion and release of TSH: Discussion, pp. 205-210. *In* A. V. Nalbandov (ed.) *Advances in Neuroendocrinology.* University of Illinois Press, Urbana.

Harris, G. W. 1964. The central nervous system and the endocrine glands. *Triangle.* 6: 242-251.

Harris, G. W. and R. P. Michael. 1958. Hypothalamic mechanisms and the control of sexual behavior in the female cat. *J. Physiol.* 142: 26P.

Harris, G. W. and R. P. Michael. 1964. The activation of sexual behavior by hypothalamic implants of oestrogen. *J. Physiol.* 171: 275-301.

Harris, G. W., R. P. Michael and P. P. Scott. 1958. Neurological site of action of stilboestrol in eliciting sexual behavior, pp. 236-254. *In* G. E. W. Wolstenholme and C. M. O'Connor (eds.) *CIBA Foundation Symposium on the Neurological Basis of Behavior.* J & A Churchill, London.

Harrison, T. S. 1961. Some factors influencing thyrotropin release in the rabbit. *Endocrinology.* 68: 466-478.

Hartmann, G., E. Endröczi and K. Lissák. 1966. The effect of hypothalamic implantation of 17 β-oestradiol and systemic administration of prolactin (LTH) on sexual behaviour in male rabbits. *Acta Physiol. Acad. Sci. Hung.* 30: 53-59.

Harvey, J. A., A. Heller and R. Y. Moore. 1963. The effect of unilateral and bilateral medial forebrain bundle lesions of brain serotonin. *J. Pharmacol.* 140: 103-110.

Hasama, B. 1930. Pharmakologische und physiologische Studien über die Schweisszentren. *Arch. Exper. Pathol. Pharmakol.* 153: 291-308.

Hashimoto, M. 1915a. Fieberstudien. I. Mitteilung: Über die spezifische Überempfindlichkeit des Wärmezentrums an sensibilisierten tieren. *Arch. Exper. Pathol. Pharmakol.* 70: 370-393.

Hashimoto, M. 1915b. Fieberstudien. II. Mitteilung: Über den Einfluss unmittelbarer Erwärmung und Abkühlung des Wärmezentrums auf die Temperaturwirkungen von verschiedenen pyrogenen und antipyretischen Substanzen. *Arch. Exper. Pathol. Pharmakol.* **70**: 394-425.

Hayward, J. N. and M. A. Baker. 1968. Diuretic and thermoregulatory responses to preoptic cooling in the monkey. *Amer. J. Physiol.* **214**: 843-850.

Heath, R. G. 1964. Pleasure response of human subjects to direct stimulation of the brain: physiologic and psychodynamic considerations, pp. 219-243. *In* R. G. Heath (ed.) *The Role of Pleasure in Behavior.* Harper & Row, New York.

Heath, R. G. 1972. Pleasure and brain activity in man. Deep and surface electroencephalograms during orgasm. *J. Nerv. Ment. Dis.* **154**: 3-18.

Heath, R. G. and F. De Balbian Verster. 1961. Effects of chemical stimulation to discrete brain areas. *Amer. J. Psychiat.* **117**: 980-990.

Heath, R. G. and W. L. Founds. 1960. A perfusion cannula for intracerebral microinjections. *EEG Clin. Neurophysiol.* **12**: 930-932.

Heath, R. G. and R. Guerrero-Figueroa. 1965. Psychotic behavior with evoked septal dysrhythmia: effects of intracerebral acetylcholine and gamma aminobutyric acid. *Amer. J. Psychiat.* **121**: 1080-1086.

Hebb, C. 1970. CNS at the cellular level: identity of transmitter agents. *Ann. Rev. Physiol.* **32**: 165-192.

Hedge, G. A. 1971. ACTH secretion due to hypothalamo-pituitary effects of adenosine-3', 5'-monophosphate and related substances. *Endocrinology.* **89**: 500-506.

Hedge, G. A. 1972. The effects of prostaglandins on ACTH secretion. *Endocrinology.* **91**: 925-933.

Hedge, G. A. and P. G. Smelik. 1968. Corticotropin release: inhibition by intrahypothalamic implantation of atropine. *Science.* **159**: 891-892.

Hedge, G. A., M. B. Yates, R. Marcus and F. E. Yates. 1966. Site of action of vasopressin in causing corticotropin release. *Endocrinology.* **79**: 328-340.

Hellon, R. F. 1967. Thermal stimulation of hypothalamic neurones in unanaesthetized rabbits. *J. Physiol.* **193**: 381-395.

Hellon, R. F. 1969. Environmental temperature and firing rate of hypothalamic neurones. *Experientia.* **25**: 610.

Hellon, R. F. 1972. Central transmitters and thermoregulation, pp. 71-85. *In* J. Bligh and R. E. Moore (eds.) *Essays on Temperature Regulation.* North-Holland, London.

Hemingway, A. 1963. Shivering. *Physiol. Rev.* **43**: 397-422.

Hemingway, A., P. Forgrave and L. Birzis. 1954. Shivering suppression by hypothalamic stimulation. *J. Neurophysiol.* **17**: 375-386.

Henderson, W. R. and W. C. Wilson. 1936. Intraventricular injection of acetylcholine and eserine in man. *Quart. J. Exp. Physiol.* **26**: 83-95.

Hendler, N. H. and W. D. Blake. 1969. Hypothalamic implants of angiotensin II, carbachol, and norepinephrine on water and NaCl solution intake in rats. *Commun. Behav. Biol.* **4**: 41-48.

Henjyoji, E. Y. and R. S. Dow. 1965. Cobalt-induced seizures in the cat. *EEG Clin. Neurophysiol.* **19**: 152-161.

Herberg, L. J. and K. B. J. Franklin. 1972. Adrenergic feeding: its blockade or reversal by posterior VMH lesions; and a new hypothesis. *Physiol. Behav.* **8**: 1029-1034.

Hernández-Peón, R. 1962. Sleep induced by localized electrical or chemical stimulation of the forebrain. *EEG Clin. Neurophysiol.* **14**: 423-424.

Hernández-Peón, R. 1965. Central neuro-humoral transmission in sleep and wakefulness, pp. 96-116. *In* K. Akert, C. Bally and J. P. Schade (eds.) *Progress in Brain Research*, Vol. 18. Elsevier, Amsterdam.

Hernández-Peón, R. and G. Chávez-Ibarra. 1963. Sleep induced by electrical or chemical stimulation of the forebrain. *EEG Clin. Neurophysiol.* **24**: 188-198.

Hernández-Peón, R., G. Chávez-Ibarra, P. J. Morgane and C. Timo-Iaria. 1962. Cholinergic pathways for sleep, alertness and rage in the limbic midbrain circuit. *Acta Neurol. Latinoamer.* 8: 93–96.

Hernández-Peón, R., G. Chávez-Ibarra, P. J. Morgane and C. Timo-Iaria. 1963. Limbic cholinergic pathways involved in sleep and emotional behavior. *Exptl. Neurol.* 8: 93–111.

Hervey, G. R. 1959. The effects of lesions in the hypothalamus in parabiotic rats. *J. Physiol.* 145: 336–352.

Herz, A. and J. Metyš. 1968. Inhibition of nociceptive responses by substances acting on central cholinoceptive systems, pp. 321–334. *In* A. Soulairac, J. Cahn and J. Charpentier (eds.) *Pain, Proceedings of the International Symposium on Pain, Paris, 1967.* Academic Press, London.

Herz, A. and H. J. Teschemacher. 1971. Activities and sites of antinociceptive action of morphine-like analgesics and kinetics of distribution following intravenous, intracerebral and intraventricular application. *Adv. Drug Res.* 6: 79–119.

Herz, A., W. Zieglgänsberger and Hj. Von Freytag-Loringhoven. 1970b. Development of fields of focal potentials in the caudate nucleus following micro-electrophoretic application of glutamic acid and GABA. *EEG Clin. Neurophysiol.* 28: 247–258.

Herz, A., K. Albus, J. Metyš, P. Schubert and H. J. Teschemacher. 1970a. On the central sites for the antinociceptive action of morphine and fentanyl. *Neuropharmacology.* 9: 539–551.

Hetherington, A. W. and S. W. Ranson. 1939. Experimental hypothalamico-hypophyseal obesity in the rat. *Proc. Soc. Exptl. Biol. Med.* 41: 465–466.

Hess, W. R. 1954. *Diencephalon. Autonomic and Extrapyramidal Functions.* Grune & Stratton, Inc., New York, pp. 1–79.

Hess, W. R. 1957. *The Functional Organization of the Diencephalon.* J. R. Hughes (ed.), Grune & Stratton, Inc., New York, pp. 1–180.

Hilton, S. M. and A. W. Zbrożyna. 1963. Amygdaloid region for defence reactions and its efferent pathway to the brain stem. *J. Physiol.* 165: 160–173.

Himsworth, R. L. 1970. Hypothalamic control of adrenaline secretion in response to insufficient glucose. *J. Physiol.* 206: 411–417.

Himsworth, R. L., P. W. Carmel and A. G. Frantz. 1972. The location of the chemoreceptor controlling growth hormone secretion during hypoglycemia in primates. *Endocrinology.* 91: 217–226.

Hiroi, M., S. Sugita and M. Suzuki. 1965. Ovulation induced by implantation of cupric sulfate into the brain of the rabbit. *Endocrinology.* 77: 963–967.

Hirono, M., M. Igarashi and S. Matsumoto. 1970. Short- and auto-feedback control of pituitary FSH secretion. *Neuroendocrinology.* 6: 274–282.

Hiroshige, T., H. Kunita, C. Ogura and S. Itoh. 1968. Effect on ACTH release of intrapituitary injections of posterior pituitary hormones and several amines in the hypothalamus. *Jap. J. Physiol.* 18: 609–619.

Ho, A. K. S. and H. H. Loh. 1972. Evidence of adrenergic-cholinergic interaction in the central nervous system. II. Dopamine and its analogues. *Europ. J. Pharmacol.* 19: 145–150.

Hoebel, B. G. 1964. Electrode-cannulas for electrical or chemical treatment of multiple brain sites. *EEG Clin. Neurophysiol.* 16: 399–402.

Hoebel, B. G. 1971. Feeding: neural control of intake. *Ann. Rev. Physiol.* 33: 533–568.

Hoebel, B. G. and P. Teitelbaum. 1962. Hypothalamic control of feeding and self-stimulation. *Science.* 135: 375–377.

von Hohlweg, W. and E. Daume. 1959. Über die Wirkung intrazerebral verabreichten Dienoestroldiacetats bei Ratten. *Endokrinologie.* 38: 46–51.

von Hohlweg, W. and K. Junkmann. 1932. Die hormonal-nervöse Regulierung der Funktion des Hypophysenvorderlappens. *Klin. Wschr.* 11: 321–323.

Holloway, F. A. 1972. Effects of septal chemical injections on asymptotic avoidance performance in cats. *Physiol. Behav.* **8**: 463–469.

Holman, R. B. and M. Vogt. 1972. Release of 5-hydroxytryptamine from caudate nucleus and septum. *J. Physiol.* **223**: 243–254.

Holmes, J. H. and L. J. Cizek. 1951. Observations on sodium chloride depletion in the dog. *Amer. J. Physiol.* **164**: 407–414.

Holmes, J. H. and M. I. Gregersen. 1950. Observation on drinking induced by hypertonic solutions. *Amer. J. Physiol.* **162**: 326–337.

Holubář, J. and J. Fischer. 1967. Electrophysiological properties of the epileptogenic cortical foci produced by a new cobalt-gelatine method in rats. An attempt to correlate the electrophysiological, histological and histochemical data. *Physiol. Bohemoslov.* **16**: 278–284.

Hornykiewicz, O. 1966. Dopamine (3-hydroxytyramine) and brain function. *Pharmacol. Rev.* **18**: 925–964.

Horovitz, Z. P. 1966. The amygdala and depression. *Excp. Med. Int. Cong. Ser.* **122**: 121–129.

Houpt, K. A. and A. N. Epstein. 1971. The complete dependence of beta-adrenergic drinking on the renal dipsogen. *Physiol. Behav.* **7**: 897–902.

Hughes, R. A. 1969. Retrograde amnesia in rats produced by hippocampal injections of potassium chloride: gradient of effect and recovery. *J. Comp. Physiol. Psychol.* **68**: 637–644.

Hull, C. D., N. A. Buchwald and G. Ling. 1967. Effects of direct cholinergic stimulation of forebrain structures. *Brain Res.* **6**: 22–35.

Hulst, S. G. T. 1972. Intracerebral implantation of carbachol in the rat: its effect on water intake and body temperature. *Physiol. Behav.* **8**: 865–872.

Hulst, S. G. T. and D. deWied. 1967. Changes in body temperature and water intake following intracerebral implantation of carbachol in rats. *Physiol. Behav.* **2**: 367–371.

Huston, J. P. and J. Bureš. 1970. Drinking and eating elicited by cortical spreading depression. *Science.* **169**: 702–704.

Hutchinson, R. R. and J. W. Renfrew. 1967. Modification of eating and drinking: interactions between chemical agent, deprivation state, and site of stimulation. *J. Comp. Physiol. Psychol.* **63**: 408–416.

Hutchison, J. B. 1967. Initiation of courtship by hypothalamic implants of testosterone propionate in castrated doves (*Streptopelia risoria*). *Nature.* **216**: 591–592.

Hutchison, J. B. 1969. Changes in hypothalamic responsiveness to testosterone in male Barbary doves (*Streptopelia risoria*). *Nature.* **222**: 176–177.

Hutchison, J. B. 1971. Effects of hypothalamic implants of gonadal steroids on courtship behaviour in Barbary doves (*Streptopelia risoria*). *J. Endocrinol.* **50**: 97–113.

Igić, R., P. Stern and E. Basagić. 1970. Changes in emotional behaviour after application of cholinesterase inhibitor in the septal and amygdala region. *Neuropharmacology.* **9**: 73–75.

Ilyutchenok, R. Y. 1969. Action of drugs on memory and learning, pp. 55–78. *Proceedings of the 4th International Congress on Pharmacology, Basel, Switzerland.* Schwabe & Co., Basel.

Ingenito, A. J., J. P. Barrett and L. Procita. 1972. Direct central and reflexly mediated effects of nicotine on the peripheral circulation. *Europ. J. Pharmacol.* **17**: 375–385.

Inutsuka, T. 1969. Electroencephalographic and behavioral changes following penicillin injection into the thalamus and the modification by drugs. *Fukuoka Igaku Zasshi.* **60**: 16–33.

Isenschmid, R. and L. Krehl. 1912. Über den Einfluss des Gehirns auf die Wärmeregulation. *Arch. Exper. Pathol. Pharmakol.* **70**: 109–134.

698 REFERENCES

Ivaldi, G., G. L. Avanzino and I. Macri. 1964. A bipolar electrode needle for the introduction of crystals into the brain. *EEG Clin. Neurophysiol.* **17**: 330-332.

Iversen, L. L. 1970. Neurotransmitters, neurohormones, and other small molecules in neurons, pp. 768-782. *In* F. O. Schmitt (ed.) *The Neurosciences. Second Study Program.* The Rockefeller University Press, New York.

Izquierdo, I., A. G. Nasello and E. S. Marichich. 1970. Effects of potassium on rat hippocampus: the dependence of hippocampal evoked and seizure activity on extracellular potassium levels. *Arch. Int. Pharmacodyn. Ther.* **187**: 318-328.

Jackson, D. L. 1967. A hypothalamic region responsive to localized injection of pyrogens. *J. Neurophysiol.* **30**: 586-602.

Jackson, H. M. and D. W. Robinson. 1971. Evidence for hypothalamic α and β adrenergic receptors involved in the control of food intake of the pig. *Brit. Vet. J.* **127**: li-liii.

Jacob, J., J. M. Girault and R. Peindaries. 1972. Actions of 5-hydroxytryptamine and 5-hydroxytryptophan injected by various routes on the rectal temperature of the rabbit. *Neuropharmacology.* **11**: 1-16.

Jacobson, S. 1972. Taste, olfaction, and the emotional brain, pp. 425-436. *In* B. A. Curtis, S. Jacobson and E. M. Marcus (eds.) *An Introduction to the Neurosciences.* W. B. Saunders Company, Philadelphia.

Jaffard, R. and B. Cardo. 1970. Influence of intracortical injections of ribonuclease on the acquisition and retention of operant behavior and visual discrimination. *Physiol. Behav.* **5**: 1303-1308.

Jancsó-Gábor, A., J. Szolcsányi and N. Jancsó. 1970. Stimulation and desensitization of the hypothalamic heat-sensitive structures by capsaicin in rats. *J. Physiol.* **208**: 449-459.

Janowitz, H. D. and A. C. Ivy. 1949. Role of blood sugar levels in spontaneous and insulin-induced hunger in man. *J. Appl. Physiol.* **1**: 643-645.

Javoy, F., M. Hamon and J. Glowinski. 1970. Disposition of newly synthesized amines in cell bodies and terminals of central catechol aminergic neurons. (1) Effect of amphetamine and thioproperazine on the metabolism of CA in the caudate nucleus, the substantia nigra and the ventromedial nucleus of the hypothalamus. *Europ. J. Pharmacol.* **10**: 178-188.

Jell, R. M. and P. Gloor. 1971. Distribution of thermosensitive and nonthermosensitive preoptic and anterior hypothalamic neurons in unanesthetized cats, and effects of some anesthetics. *Canad. J. Physiol. Pharmacol.* **50**: 890-901.

Jester, J. and W. D. Horst. 1972. Influence of serotonin on adrenergic mechanisms. *Biochem. Pharmacol.* **21**: 333-338.

Jewell, P. A. and E. B. Verney. 1957. An experimental attempt to determine the site of the neurohypophysial osmoreceptors in the dog. *Phil. Trans. Roy. Soc. (London). B.* **240**: 197-324.

Jiménez-Díaz, C., J. M. Linazasoro and A. Merchante. 1959. Further study of the part played by the kidneys in the regulation of thirst. *Bull. Inst. Med. Res.* **12**: 60-67.

Johnston, P. and J. M. Davidson. 1972. Intracerebral androgens and sexual behavior in the male rat. *Horm. Behav.* **3**: 345-357.

Jouvet, M. 1967. Neurophysiology of the states of sleep. *Physiol. Rev.* **47**: 117-177.

Jouvet, M. 1969. Biogenic amines and the states of sleep. *Science.* **163**: 32-41.

Jouvet, M. 1972. The role of monoamines and acetylcholine-containing neurons in the regulation of the sleep-waking cycle, pp. 166-307. *In: Ergebnisse der Physiologie.* Springer-Verlag, Heidelberg.

Joynt, R. J. 1964. Functional significance of osmosensitive units in the anterior hypothalamus. *Neurology.* **14**: 584-590.

Jung, R. and R. Hassler. 1960. The extrapyramidal motor system, pp. 863-927. *In* J. Field, H. W. Magoun and V. E. Hall (eds.) *Handbook of Physiology*, Vol. II. Waverly Press, Inc., Baltimore.

Kabat, H., B. J. Anson, H. W. Magoun and S. W. Ranson. 1935. Stimulation of the hypothalamus with special reference to its effect on gastro-intestinal motility. *Amer. J. Physiol.* 112: 214–226.

Kajihara, A. and J. W. Kendall, 1969. Studies on the hypothalamic control of TSH secretion. *Neuroendocrinology.* 5: 53–63.

Kalyuzhnyi, L. B. 1962. Food and defensive conditioned reflexes in rabbits after injection of norepinephrine and carbacholine into hypothalamus. Zh. Vysshei Nervnoi *Deyatel'nosti im. I. P. Pavlova.* 12: 318–322.

Kamberi, I. A. and S. M. McCann. 1972. Effects of implants of testosterone in the median eminence and pituitary on FSH secretion. *Neuroendocrinology.* 9: 20–29.

Kanematsu, S. and C. H. Sawyer. 1963a. Effects of hypothalamic estrogen implants on pituitary LH and prolactin in rabbits. *Amer. J. Physiol.* 205: 1073–1076.

Kanematsu, S. and C. H. Sawyer. 1963b. Effects of intrahypothalamic implants of reserpine on lactation and pituitary prolactin content in the rabbit. *Proc. Soc. Exptl. Biol. Med.* 113: 967–969.

Kanematsu, S. and C. H. Sawyer. 1964. Effects of hypothalamic and hypophysial estrogen implants on pituitary and plasma LH in ovariectomized rabbits. *Endocrinology.* 75: 579–585.

Kanematsu, S. and C. H. Sawyer. 1965. Blockade of ovulation in rabbits by hypothalamic implants of norethindrone. *Endocrinology.* 76: 691–699.

Kaplanski, J. and P. G. Smelik. 1973. Analysis of the inhibition of the ACTH release by hypothalamic implants of atropine. *Acta Endocrinol.* 73: 651–659.

Kapp, B. S. and A. M. Schneider. 1971. Selective recovery from retrograde amnesia produced by hippocampal spreading depression. *Science.* 173: 1149–1151.

Karasszon, D. 1968. Somnolence in rhesus monkey following intracerebral inoculation. *Acta Vet. Acad. Sci. Hung.* 18: 257–263.

Karplus, J. P. and A. Kreidl, 1927. Gehirn und Sympathicus. VII. Mitteilung. Über Beziehungen der Hypothalamuszentren zu Blutdruck und innerer Sekretion. *Pflügers Arch. Physiol.* 215: 667–670.

Kato, J. and C. A. Villee. 1967. Preferential uptake of estradiol by the anterior hypothalamus of the rat. *Endocrinology.* 80: 567–575.

Katz, S. H., M. Molitch and S. M. McCann. 1967. Feedback of hypothalamic growth hormone (GH) implants upon the anterior pituitary (AP), p. 86. *Proceedings of the Forty-ninth Meeting of the Endocrine Society.*

Katz, S. H., M. Molitch and S. M. McCann. 1969. Effect of hypothalamic implants of GH on anterior pituitary weight and GH concentration. *Endocrinology.* 85: 725–734.

Kawakami, M., T. Koshino and Y. Hattori. 1966. Changes in the EEG of the hypothalamus and limbic system after administration of ACTH, SU-4885 and ACH in rabbits with special reference to neurohumoral feedback regulation of pituitary-adrenal system. *Jap. J. Physiol.* 16: 551–569.

Kawakami, M., H. Negoro and E. Terasawa. 1965. Influence of immobilization stress upon the paradoxical sleep (EEG afterreaction) in the rabbit. *Jap. J. Physiol.* 15: 1–16.

Kawakami, M., K. Seto and K. Yoshida. 1968. Influence of corticosterone implantation in limbic structure upon biosynthesis of adrenocortical steroid. *Neuroendocrinology.* 3: 349–354.

Kawakami, M., K. Seto, K. Yoshida and T. Miyamoto. 1969. Biosynthesis of ovarian steroids in the rabbit: influence of progesterone or estradiol implantation into the hypothalamus and limbic structures. *Neuroendocrinology.* 5: 303–321.

Kelsey, J. E. and S. P. Grossman. 1969. Cholinergic blockade and lesions in the ventro-medial septum of the rat. *Physiol. Behav.* 4: 837–845.

Kendall, J. W., Y. Grimm and G. Shimshak. 1969. Relation of cerebrospinal fluid circulation to the ACTH-suppressing effects of corticosteroid implants in the rat brain. *Endocrinology.* 85: 200–208.

Kennedy, G. C. 1953. The effect of lesions in the hypothalamus on appetite. *Proc. Nutr. Soc. (Lon.)* **12**: 160–165.

Kent, E. W. 1972. Behavior of CNS single units in the vicinity of topically applied crystalline neurohumors. *Physiol. Behav.* **8**: 987–991.

Khavari, K. A. 1969. Effects of central versus intraperitoneal D-amphetamine administration on learned behavior. *J. Comp. Physiol. Psychol.* **68**: 226–234.

Khavari, K. A. 1971. Adrenergic-cholinergic involvement in modulation of learned behavior. *J. Comp. Physiol. Psychol.* **74**: 284–291.

Khavari, K. A. and R. P. Maickel. 1967. Atropine and atropine methyl bromide effects on behavior of rats. *Int. J. Neuropharmacol.* **6**: 301–306.

Khavari, K. A. and R. W. Russell. 1966. Acquisition, retention and extinction under conditions of water deprivation and of central cholinergic stimulation. *J. Comp. Physiol. Psychol.* **61**: 339–345.

Khavari, K. A., P. Heebink and J. Traupman. 1968. Effects of intraventricular carbachol and eserine on drinking. *Psychon. Sci.* **11**: 93–94.

Khavari, K. A., A. J. Feider, D. M. Warburton and R. A. Martin. 1967. Bilateral cannulae for central administration of drugs in rats. *Life Sci.* **6**: 235–240.

Kim, J. K. and F. G. Carpenter. 1961. Excitation of medullary neurons by chemical agents. *Amer. J. Physiol.* **201**: 1187–1191.

Kirkpatrick, W. E. and P. Lomax. 1967. The effect of atropine on the body temperature of the rat following systemic and intracerebral injection. *Life Sci.* **6**: 2273–2278.

Kirkpatrick, W. E. and P. Lomax. 1970. Temperature changes following iontophoretic injection of acetylcholine into the rostral hypothalamus of the rat. *Neuropharmacology.* **9**: 195–202.

Kirkpatrick, W. E. and P. Lomax. 1971. Temperature changes induced by chlorpromazine and N-methyl chlorpromazine in the rat. *Neuropharmacology.* **10**: 61–66.

Kirkpatrick, W. E., D. J. Jenden and P. Lomax. 1967. The effect of N-(4-diethylamino-2-butynyl)-succinimide (DKJ 21) on oxotremorine induced hypothermia in the rat. *Int. J. Neuropharmacol.* **6**: 273–277.

Klingberg, F., I. Kästner and M. Müller. 1969. Wechselwirkungen zwischen neokortikalen Kobaltherden, verschiedenen Reizeffekten und dem Verhalten der Ratte. *Acta Biol. Med. Germ.* **23**: 397–412.

Knaape, H. H. and P. Wiechert. 1970. Krampfaktivität nach intracerebraler injektion von *L*-glutamat. *J. Neurochem.* **17**: 1171–1175.

Knigge, K. M. 1962. Gonadotropic activity of neonatal pituitary glands implanted in the rat brain. *Amer. J. Physiol.* **202**: 387–391.

Knigge, K. M. and S. A. Joseph. 1971. Neural regulation of TSH secretion: sites of thyroxin feedback. *Neuroendocrinology.* **8**: 273–288.

Knizley, H. 1972. The hippocampus and septal area as primary target sites for corticosterone. *J. Neurochem.* **19**: 2737–2745.

Knox, G. V. and P. Lomax. 1972. The effect of nicotine on thermosensitive units in the rostral hypothalamus. *Proc. West. Pharmacol. Soc.* **15**: 179–183.

Koella, W. P. and J. Czicman. 1966. Mechanisms of the EEG-synchronizing action of serotonin. *Amer. J. Physiol.* **211**: 926–934.

Koelle, G. B. 1965. Neurohumoral transmission and the autonomic nervous system, pp. 399–440. *In* L. S. Goodman and A. Gilman (eds.) *The Pharmacological Basis of Therapeutics, Third Edition.* The Macmillan Company, New York.

Kollros, J. J. 1943. Experimental studies of the development of the corneal reflex in amphibia. II. Localized maturation of the reflex mechanism effected by thyroxin-agar implants into the hindbrain. *Physiol. Zoöl.* **16**: 269–279.

Komisaruk, B. R. 1966. Localization in brain of reproductive behavior responses to progesterone in ring doves. (Unpublished thesis, Rutgers University.)

Komisaruk, B. R. 1967. Effects of local brain implants of progesterone on reproductive behavior in doves. *J. Comp. Physiol. Psychol.* **64**: 219–224.

König, J. F. R. and R. A. Klippel. 1963. *The Rat Brain: A Stereotaxic Atlas of the Forebrain and Lower Parts of the Brain Stem.* Williams and Wilkins, Baltimore, pp. 1–162.

Kopeloff, L. M. 1960. Experimental epilepsy in the mouse. *Proc. Soc. Exptl. Biol. Med.* **104**: 500–504.

Kopeloff, L. M., S. E. Barrera and N. Kopeloff. 1942. Recurrent convulsive seizures in animals produced by immunologic and chemical means. *Amer. J. Psychiat.* **98**: 881–902.

Kopeloff, N., J. R. Whittier, B. L. Pacella and L. M. Kopeloff. 1950. The epileptogenic effect of subcortical alumina cream in the rhesus monkey. *EEG Clin. Neurophysiol.* **2**: 163–168.

Kopin, I. J. 1971. Unnatural amino acids as precursors of false transmitters. *Fed. Proc.* **30**: 904–907.

Kordon, C. 1971. Blockade of ovulation in the immature rat by local microinjection of α-methyl-dopa into the arcuate region of the hypothalamus. *Neuroendocrinology.* **7**: 202–209.

Kordon, C. and J. Glowinski. 1970. Role of brain catecholamines in the control of anterior pituitary functions, pp. 85–100. *In* L. Martini and J. Meites (eds.) *Neurochemical Aspects of Hypothalamic Function.* Academic Press, New York.

Kordon, C. and F. Gogan. 1964. Localisation par une technique de microimplantation de structures hypothalamiques responsables du feed-back par la testostérone chez la canard. *Compt. Rend. Soc. Biol.* **158**: 1795–1798.

Kosaka, M., E. Simon, R. Thauer and O.-E. Walther. 1969. Effect of thermal stimulation of spinal cord on respiratory and cortical activity. *Amer. J. Physiol.* **217**: 858–864.

Kostowski, W. 1971. Effects of some cholinergic and anticholinergic drugs injected intra-cerebrally to the midline pontine area. *Neuropharmacology.* **10**: 595–605.

Kottler, P. D. and R. E. Bowman. 1968. A simple intracranial needle guide for preventing backflow of injectant. *J. Exp. Anal. Behav.* **11**: 536.

Kovács, S. and M. Vértes. 1961. Wirkung der intracerebralen Thyroxin-Implantation auf die Funktion des Hypophysen-Schilddrüsen-Systems. *Endokrinologie.* **40**: 159–164.

Koval, L. A. 1969. The influence of adrenaline, acetylcholine and pituitrine injections into the hypothalamus on the motility of gastrointestinal tract and the reflectory interrelations between its different parts. *Problemy Fiziologii Gipotalamusa.* **3**: 29–38.

Krasne, F. B. 1962. General disruption resulting from electrical stimulation of ventro-medial hypothalamus. *Science.* **138**: 822–823.

Kraus, V. A. and I. A. Lapina. 1972. Effect of direct electrical and chemical stimulation on the excitability of the hypothalamic nuclei and the self-stimulation reaction in dogs. *Zh Vyssh Nerv Deiat.* **22**: 1226–1233.

Krebs, H. and D. Bindra. 1971. Noradrenaline and "chemical coding" of hypothalamic neurones. *Nature New Biol.* **229**: 178–180.

Krieger, D. T. and H. P. Krieger. 1964. The effects of intrahypothalamic injection of drugs on ACTH release in the cat. *Excp. Med. Int. Cong.* **83**: 640–645.

Krieger, D. T. and H. P. Krieger. 1970a. Effect of dexamethasone on pituitary-adrenal activation following intrahypothalamic implantation of "neurotransmitters." *Endocrinology.* **87**: 179–182.

Krieger, H. P. and D. T. Krieger. 1970b. Chemical stimulation of the brain: effect on adrenal corticoid release. *Amer. J. Physiol.* **218**: 1632–1641.

Krieger, H. P. and D. T. Krieger. 1971. Pituitary-adrenal activation by implanted neuro-transmitters and ineffectiveness of dexamethasone in blocking this activation, pp. 98–106. *In: Influence of Hormones on the Nervous System.* Karger, Basel.

Krikstone, B. J. and R. A. Levitt. 1970. Interactions between water deprivation and chemical brain stimulation. *J. Comp. Physiol. Psychol.* **71**: 334–340.

Kulkarni, A. S. 1967. A hypothermic effect of serotonin injected into the lateral cerebral ventricle of the cat. *Int. J. Neuropharmacol.* **6**: 333–335.

Kumagai, H., F. Sakai and Y. Otsuka. 1962a. EEG response to subcortical microinjection of *d*-tubocurarine chloride and other drugs in cats. *Arch. Int. Pharmacodyn. Ther.* **139**: 588–595.

Kumagai, H., F. Sakai and Y. Otsuka. 1962b. Analysis of central effect of *d*-tubocurarine chloride in the cat. *Int. J. Neuropharmacol.* **1**: 157–159.

Kunz, F. and F. Klingberg. 1969. Der Einfluss neokortikaler Kobaltherde auf die Ausarbeitung bedingter Fluchtreflexe bei Ratten. *Acta Biol. Med. Germ.* **23**: 443–456.

Kurochkin, I. G. and Y. V. Burov. 1971. Effect of psychotropic substances on the behaviour of cats conditioned by introduction of acetylcholine into the hypothalamus. *Farmakol. Toksikol.* **34**: 21–25.

Kym, O. 1934. Die Beeinflussung des durch verschiedene fiebererzeugende Stoffe erregten Temperaturzentrums durch lokale Applikation von Ca, K und Na. *Arch. Exper. Pathol. Pharmakol.* **176**: 408–424.

Labhsetwar, A. P. and J. G. Bainbridge. 1971. Inhibition of ovulation by intracranial implantation of progesterone in the 4-day cyclic rat. *J. Reprod. Fert.* **27**: 445–449.

Lajtha, A. 1969. *Handbook of Neurochemistry*. Plenum Press, New York.

Lalley, P. M., G. V. Rossi and W. W. Baker. 1970. Analysis of local cholinergic tremor mechanisms following selective neurochemical lesions. *Exptl. Neurol.* **27**: 258–275.

Lalley, P. M., G. V. Rossi and W. W. Baker. 1971. Alterations in tremor regulation after intracaudate injections of calcium ions or disodium edetate. *Neuropharmacology.* **10**: 613–619.

Langlois, J. M. and Y. Poussart. 1969. Electrocortical activity following cholinergic stimulation of the caudate nucleus in the cat. *Brain Res.* **15**: 581–583.

Lavy, S. and S. Stern. 1970. Bradycardic effect of propranolol administered into the central nervous system. *Arch. Int. Pharmacodyn. Ther.* **184**: 257–266.

Lazaris, Ya. A., I. A. Serebrovskaya, L. Z. Tel' and Z. E. Bavel'skii. 1967. Edema of the lungs in albino rats and rabbits after injection of aconitine into the hypothalamus. *Bull. Exp. Biol. Med.* **63**: 19–22.

Leaf, R. C., L. Lerner and Z. P. Horovitz. 1969. The role of the amygdala in the pharmacological and endocrinological manipulation of aggression, pp. 120–131. *In* S. Garattina and E. Sigg (eds.) *Aggressive Behavior*. Wiley, New York.

Leão, A. A. P. 1972. Spreading depression, pp. 173–196. *In* D. P. Purpura, J. K. Penry, D. B. Tower, D. M. Woodbury and R. D. Walter (eds.) *Experimental Models of Epilepsy*. Raven Press, New York.

Leaton, R. N. and R. H. Rech. 1972. Locomotor activity increases produced by intra-hippocampal and intraseptal atropine in rats. *Physiol. Behav.* **8**: 539–541.

Ledebur, I. X. and R. Tissot. 1966. Modification de l'activité électrique cérébrale du lapin sous l'effet de micro-injections de précurseurs des monoamines dans les structures somnogènes bulbaires et pontiques. *EEG Clin. Neurophysiol.* **20**: 370–381.

Legendre, R. and H. Piéron. 1910. Des résultats histophysiologiques de l'injection intra-occipito-atlantoïdienne de liquides insomniques. *C. R. Soc. Biol. (Paris).* **1**: 1108–1109.

Legendre, R. and H. Piéron. 1912. Recherches sur le besoin de sommeil consécutif à une veille prolongée; *Zeitschrift für Allgemeine Physiologie.* **14**: 235–262.

Lehr, D., J. Mallow and M. Krukowski. 1967. Copious drinking and simultaneous inhibition of urine flow elicited by Beta-adrenergic stimulation and contrary effect of alpha-adrenergic stimulation. *J. Pharmacol. Exptl. Ther.* **158**: 150–163.

Leibowitz, S. F. 1970a. Hypothalamic β-adrenergic "satiety" system antagonizes an α-adrenergic "hunger" system in the rat. *Nature.* **226**: 963–964.

Leibowitz, S. F. 1970b. Reciprocal hunger-regulating circuits involving alpha- and beta-adrenergic receptors located, respectively, in the ventromedial and lateral hypothalamus. *Proc. Nat. Acad. Sci.* **67**: 1063–1070.

Leibowitz, S. F. 1971. Hypothalamic alpha- and beta-adrenergic systems regulate both thirst and hunger in the rat. *Proc. Nat. Acad. Sci.* 68: 332–334.

Leibowitz, S. F. 1972. Central adrenergic receptors and the regulation of hunger and thirst. *Neurotransmitters.* 50: 327–358.

Leibowitz, S. F. and N. E. Miller. 1969. Unexpected adrenergic effect of chlorpromazine: eating elicited by injection into rat hypothalamus. *Science.* 165: 609–611.

Leighton, K. M. and L. C. Jenkins. 1970. Experimental studies of the central nervous system related to anaesthesia: IV. Effects of pentobarbital placement in caudate nucleus. *Canad. Anaesth. Soc. J.* 17: 112–118.

Leusen, I. 1972. Regulation of cerebrospinal fluid composition with reference to breathing. *Physiol. Rev.* 52: 1–56.

Levitt, R. A. 1968. Anticholinergic brain stimulation and thirst induced by 23 hour water deprivation. *Psychon. Sci.* 12: 21–22.

Levitt, R. A. 1969. Biochemical blockade of cholinergic thirst. *Psychon. Sci.* 15: 274–276.

Levitt, R. A. 1970. Temporal decay of the blockade of carbachol drinking by atropine. *Physiol. Behav.* 5: 627–628.

Levitt, R. A. 1971. Cholinergic substrate for drinking in the rat. *Psychol. Rep.* 29: 431–448.

Levitt, R. A. and R. P. Boley. 1970. Drinking elicited by injection of eserine or carbachol into rat brain. *Physiol. Behav.* 5: 693–695.

Levitt, R. A. and P. B. Buerger. 1970. Interactions between cholinergic mechanisms and the salt arousal of drinking. *Learn. Motiv.* 1: 297–303.

Levitt, R. A. and A. E. Fisher. 1966. Anticholinergic blockade of centrally induced thirst. *Science.* 154: 520–522.

Levitt, R. A. and A. E. Fisher. 1967. Failure of central anticholinergic brain stimulation to block natural thirst. *Physiol. Behav.* 2: 425–428.

Levitt, R. A. and B. J. Krikstone. 1968. Cortical spreading depression and thirst. *Physiol. Behav.* 3: 421–423.

Levitt, R. A. and J. Y. O'Hearn. 1972. Drinking elicited by cholinergic stimulation of CNS fibers. *Physiol. Behav.* 8: 641–644.

Levitt, R. A., C. S. White and D. M. Sander. 1970. Dose-response analysis of carbachol-elicited drinking in the rat limbic system. *J. Comp. Physiol. Psychol.* 72: 345–350.

Lewis, P. R. and C. C. D. Shute. 1967. The cholinergic limbic system: projections to hippocampal formation, medial cortex, nuclei of the ascending cholinergic reticular system, and the subfornical organ and supra-optic crest. *Brain.* 90: 521–540.

Lichtensteiger, W. 1970. Effects of endocrine manipulations on the metabolism of hypothalamic monoamines, pp. 101–133. *In* L. Martini and J. Meites (eds.) *Neurochemical Aspects of Hypothalamic Function.* Academic Press, New York.

von Liebermeister, C. 1860. Physiologische Untersuchungen über die quantitativen Veränderungen der Wärmeproduction. *Arch. Anat. Physiol. Wissenschaft. Med.* 520–541; 589–623.

Light, R. U. and S. M. Bysshe. 1933. The administration of drugs into the cerebral ventricles of monkeys: pituitrin, certain pituitary fractions, pitressin, pitocin, histamine, acetyl choline, and pilocarpine. *J. Pharmacol. Exptl. Ther.* 47: 17–36.

Liljestrand, A. 1953. Respiratory reactions elicited from medulla oblongata of the cat. *Acta Physiol. Scand.* 29: 321–393.

Lilly, J. C. 1958. Electrode and cannulae implantation in the brain by a simple percutaneous method. *Science.* 127: 1181–1182.

Linazasoro, J. M., C. J. Díaz and H. C. Mendoza. 1954. The kidney and thirst regulation. *Bull. Inst. Med. Res. (Madrid).* 7: 53–61.

Lippert, T. H. and N. G. Waton. 1969. The origin of histamine in the pituitary gland. *Med. Exp.* 19: 119–123.

Lisk, R. D. 1960. Estrogen-sensitive centers in the hypothalamus of the rat. *J. Exptl. Zool.* **145:** 197–207.

Lisk, R. D. 1962a. Testosterone-sensitive centers in the hypothalamus of the rat. *Acta Endocrinol.* **41:** 195–204.

Lisk, R. D. 1962b. Diencephalic placement of estradiol and sexual receptivity in the female rat. *Amer. J. Physiol.* **203:** 493–496.

Lisk, R. D. 1963. Maintenance of normal pituitary weight and cytology in the spayed rat following estradiol implants in the arcuate nucleus. *Anat. Rec.* **146:** 281–286.

Lisk, R. D. 1965a. Neurosecretion in the rat: changes occurring following neural implant of estrogen. *Neuroendocrinology.* **1:** 83–92.

Lisk, R. D. 1965b. Reproductive capacity and behavioural oestrus in the rat bearing hypothalamic implants of sex steroids. *Acta Endocrinol.* **48:** 209–219.

Lisk, R. D. 1966a. Control of sexual behavior by gonadal steroids. II. Hormonal implants in the central nervous system and behavioral receptivity in the female rat, pp. 98–117. *In* R. A. Gorski and R. E. Whalen (eds.) *Brain and Behavior*, Vol. III. University of California Press, Los Angeles.

Lisk, R. D. 1966b. The hypothalamus and hormone sensing systems. *Excp. Med. Int. Cong.* **132:** 952–957.

Lisk, R. D. 1967a. Neural control of gonad size by hormone feedback in the desert iguana *Dipsosaurus dorsalis dorsalis. Gen. Comp. Endocrinol.* **8:** 258–266.

Lisk, R. D. 1967b. Neural localization for androgen activity of copulatory behavior in the male rat. *Endocrinology.* **80:** 754–761.

Lisk, R. D. 1968. Brain investigation techniques in the study of reproduction and sex behavior, pp. 287–302. *In* M. Diamond (ed.) *Perspectives in Reproduction and Sexual Behavior.* Indiana University Press, Bloomington.

Lisk, R. D. 1969a. Estrogen: direct effects on hypothalamus or pituitary in relation to pituitary weight changes. *Neuroendocrinology.* **4:** 368–373.

Lisk, R. D. 1969b. Progesterone: biphasic effects on the lordosis response in adult or neonatally gonadectomized rats. *Neuroendocrinology.* **5:** 149–160.

Lisk, R. D. 1970. Mechanisms regulating sexual activity in mammals. *J. Sex. Res.* **6:** 220–228.

Lisk, R. D. and M. Newlon. 1963. Estradiol: evidence for its direct effect on hypothalamic neurons. *Science.* **139:** 223–224.

Lisk, R. D. and A. J. Suydam. 1967. Sexual behavior patterns in the prepubertally castrate rat. *Anat. Rec.* **157:** 181–189.

Little, M. D. and R. E. Dill. 1969. Mescaline and other O-methylated β-phenylethylamines: intrastriatal induction of tremor in rats. *Brain Res.* **13:** 360–366.

Livingston, R. B. 1967. Brain circuitry relating to complex behavior, pp. 499–515. *In* G. C. Quarton, T. Melnechuk and F. O. Schmitt (eds.) *The Neurosciences. A Study Program.* The Rockefeller University Press, New York.

Loeschcke, H. H., H. P. Koepchen and K. H. Gertz. 1958. Über den Einfluss von Wasserstoffionenkonzentration und CO_2-Druck im Liquor cerebrospinalis auf die Atmung. *Pflügers Arch.* **266:** 569–585.

Löfgren, F. 1959. New aspects of the hypothalamic control of the adenohypophysis. *Acta Morphol. Neerlando. Scand.* **2:** 220–229.

Löfgren, F. 1960. On the transport-mechanism between the hypothalamus and the anterior pituitary. *Kungl. Fysiografiska Sallskrapets I Lund Forhandlingar* **30:** 115–121.

Lomax, P. 1966a. The distribution of morphine following intracerebral microinjection. *Experientia.* **22:** 249–250.

Lomax, P. 1966b. The hypothermic effect of pentobarbital in the rat: sites and mechanisms of action. *Brain Res.* **1:** 296–302.

Lomax, P. 1967. Investigations on the central effects of morphine on body temperature. *Arch. Biol. Med. Exp.* **4:** 119–124.

Lomax, P. 1970. Drugs and body temperature. *Int. Rev. Neurobiol.* **12**: 1–43.

Lomax, P. and R. S. Foster. 1969. Temperature changes induced by imidazoline sympathomimetics in the rat. *J. Pharmacol. Exptl. Ther.* **167**: 159–165.

Lomax, P. and D. J. Jenden. 1966. Hypothermia following systematic and intracerebral injection of oxotremorine in the rat. *Int. J. Neuropharmacol.* **5**: 353–359.

Lomax, P., R. S. Foster and W. E. Kirkpatrick. 1969. Cholinergic and adrenergic interactions in the thermoregulatory centers of the rat. *Brain Res.* **15**: 431–438.

Lomax, P., N. Kokka and R. George. 1970. Thyroid activity following intracerebral injection of morphine in the rat. *Neuroendocrinology.* **6**: 146–152.

Lotti, V. J., N. Kokka and R. George. 1969. Pituitary-adrenal activation following intrahypothalamic microinjection of morphine. *Neuroendocrinology.* **4**: 326–332.

Lotti, V. J., P. Lomax and R. George. 1965a. Temperature responses in the rat following intracerebral microinjection of morphine. *J. Pharmacol. Exptl. Ther.* **150**: 135–139.

Lotti, V. J., P. Lomax and R. George. 1965b. N-allylnormorphine antagonism of the hypothermic effect of morphine in the rat following intracerebral and systemic administration. *J. Pharmacol. Exptl. Ther.* **150**: 420–425.

Lotti, V. J., P. Lomax and R. George. 1966a. Acute tolerance to morphine following systemic and intracerebral injection in the rat. *Int. J. Neuropharmacol.* **5**: 35–42.

Lotti, V. J., P. Lomax and R. George. 1966b. Heat production and heat loss in the rat following intracerebral and systemic administration of morphine. *Int. J. Neuropharmacol.* **5**: 75–83.

Lovett, D. and G. Singer. 1971. Ventricular modification of drinking and eating behavior. *Physiol. Behav.* **6**: 23–26.

McCann, S. M. and V. D. Ramírez. 1964. The neuroendocrine regulation of hypophyseal luteinizing hormone secretion. *Rec. Prog. Hormone Res.* **20**: 131–181.

McCarthy, L. E. and H. L. Borison. 1972. Separation of central effects of CO_2 and nicotine on ventilation and blood pressure. *Respir. Physiol.* **15**: 321–330.

McCleary, R. A. 1966. Response-modulating functions of the limbic system: initiation and suppression, pp. 209–266. *In: Progress in Physiological Psychology*, Vol. 1. Academic Press, New York.

McEwen, B. S., J. M. Weiss and L. S. Schwartz. 1969. Uptake of corticosterone by rat brain and its concentration by certain limbic structures. *Brain Res.* **16**: 227–241.

McEwen, B. S., J. M. Weiss and L. S. Schwartz. 1970. Retention of corticosterone by cell nuclei from brain regions of adrenalectomized rats. *Brain Res.* **17**: 471–482.

McEwen, B. S., R. E. Zigmond and J. L. Gerlach. 1972. Sites of steroid binding and action in the brain, pp. 205–291. *In* G. H. Bourne (ed.) *The Structure and Function of Nervous Tissue.* Academic Press, New York.

McFarland, D. J. and B. Rolls. 1972. Suppression of feeding by intracranial injections of angiotensin. *Nature.* **236**: 172–173.

McGuire, J. L. and R. D. Lisk. 1968. Estrogen receptors in the intact rat. *Proc. Nat. Acad. Sci.* **61**: 497–503.

McGuire, J. L. and R. D. Lisk. 1969. Localization of estrogen receptors in the rat hypothalamus. *Neuroendocrinology.* **4**: 289–295.

McKenzie, G. M. and J. C. Szerb. 1968. The effect of dihydroxyphenylalanine, pheniprazine and dextroamphetamine on the *in vivo* release of dopamine from the caudate nucleus. *J. Pharmacol. Exptl. Ther.* **162**: 302–308.

McLennan, H. 1963. *Synaptic Transmission.* W. B. Saunders Company, Philadelphia. pp. 1–134.

McLennan, H. 1964. The release of acetylcholine and of 3-hydroxytyramine from the caudate nucleus. *J. Physiol.* **174**: 152–161.

McLennan, H. 1965. The release of dopamine from the putamen. *Experientia.* **21**: 725–726.

van Maanen, J. H. and P. G. Smelik. 1968. Induction of pseudopregnancy in rats following local depletion of monoamines in the median eminence of the hypothalamus. *Neuroendocrinology.* **3:** 177–186.

MacDonnell, M. F. and J. P. Flynn. 1964. Attack elicited by stimulation of the thalamus of cats. *Science.* **144:** 1249–1250.

MacIntosh, F. C. and W. L. M. Perry. 1950. Biological estimation of acetylcholine, pp. 78–92. *In* R. W. Gerard (ed.) *Methods in Medical Research*, Vol. 3. Year Book Publishers, Chicago.

MacLean, P. D. 1954. The limbic system and its hippocampal formation. *J. Neurosurg.* **11:** 29–44.

MacLean, P. D. 1957a. Chemical and electrical stimulation of hippocampus in unrestrained animals. I. Methods and electroencephalographic findings. *AMA Arch. Neurol. Psychiat.* **78:** 113–127.

MacLean, P. D. 1957b. Chemical and electrical stimulation of hippocampus in unrestrained animals. II. Behavioral findings. *AMA Arch. Neurol. Psychiat.* **78:** 128–142.

MacLean, P. D. 1958. The limbic system with respect to self-preservation and preservation of the species. *J. Nerv. Ment. Dis.* **127:** 1–11.

MacLean, P. D. 1962. New findings relevant to the evolution of psychosexual functions of the brain. *J. Nerv. Ment. Dis.* **135:** 289–301.

MacLean, P. D. 1970a. The triune brain, emotion, and scientific bias, pp. 336–349. *In* F. O. Schmitt (ed.) *The Neurosciences, Second Study Program.* The Rockefeller University Press, New York.

MacLean, P. D. 1970b. The limbic brain in relation to the psychoses, pp. 129–146. *In* P. Black (ed.) *Physiological Correlates of Emotion.* Academic Press, New York.

MacLean, P. D. and J. M. R. Delgado. 1953. Electrical and chemical stimulation of frontotemporal portion of limbic system in the waking animal. *EEG Clin. Neurophysiol.* **5:** 91–100.

MacLean, P. D., S. Flanigan, J. P. Flynn, C. Kim and J. R. Stevens. 1955. Hippocampal function: tentative correlations of conditioning, EEG, drug and radioautographic studies. *Yale J. Biol. Med.* **23:** 380–395.

Macphail, E. M. 1968. Effects of intracranial cholinergic stimulation in rats on drinking, EEG, and heart rate. *J. Comp. Physiol. Psychol.* **65:** 42–49.

Macphail, E. M. 1969. Cholinergic stimulation of dove diencephalon: a comparative study. *Physiol. Behav.* **4:** 655–657.

Macphail, E. M. and N. E. Miller. 1968. Cholinergic brain stimulation in cats: failure to obtain sleep. *J. Comp. Physiol. Psychol.* **65:** 499–503.

Madryga, F. J. and D. J. Albert. 1971. Procaine injections into MFB-LHA during septal and preoptic self-stimulation. *Physiol. Behav.* **6:** 695–701.

Magoun, H. W., F. Harrison, J. R. Brobeck and S. W. Ranson. 1938. Activation of heat loss mechanisms by local heating of the brain. *J. Neurophysiol.* **1:** 101–114.

Makino, T., V. S. Fang, K. Yoshinaga and R. O. Greep. 1972. Effect of implantation of anti-LH serum into median eminence on rat pituitary and serum LH. *Proc. Soc. Exptl. Biol. Med.* **140:** 703–706.

Mancia, M. and R. Lucioni. 1966. EEG and behavioural changes induced by subcortical introduction of cobalt powder in chronic cats. *Epilepsia.* **7:** 308–317.

Mandl, F. 1951. Chemical lobotomy (infiltration therapy of the frontal lobe). *Acta Med. Orient.* **10:** 1–4

Mangili, G., M. Motta and L. Martini. 1966. Control of adrenocorticotropic hormone secretion, pp. 297–370. *In* L. Martini and W. F. Ganong (eds.) *Neuroendocrinology*, Vol. 1. Academic Press, New York.

Manning, J. W. 1965. Intracranial representation of cardiac innervation, pp. 16–33. *In* W. C. Randall (ed.) *Nervous Control of the Heart.* The Williams and Wilkins Company, Baltimore.

Mantegazzini, P., K. Poeck and G. Santibañez-H. 1959. The action of adrenaline and noradrenaline on the cortical electrical activity of the "encéphale isolé" cat. *Arch. Ital. Biol.* 97: 222–242.

Marczynski, T. J., N. Yamaguchi, G. M. Ling and L. Grodzinska. 1964. Sleep induced by the administration of melatonin (5-methoxy-N-acetyltryptamine) to the hypothalamus in unrestrained cats. *Experientia.* 20: 435–437.

Margules, D. L. 1968. Noradrenergic basis of inhibition between reward and punishment in amygdala. *J. Comp. Physiol. Psychol.* 66: 329–334.

Margules, D. L. 1969a. Noradrenergic rather than serotonergic basis of reward in the dorsal tegmentum. *J. Comp. Physiol. Psychol.* 67: 32–35.

Margules, D. L. 1969b. Noradrenergic synapses for the suppression of feeding behavior. *Life Sci.* 8: 693–704.

Margules, D. L. 1970a. Alpha-adrenergic receptors in hypothalamus for the suppression of feeding behavior by satiety. *J. Comp. Physiol. Psychol.* 73: 1–12.

Margules, D. L. 1970b. Beta-adrenergic receptors in the hypothalamus for learned and unlearned taste aversions. *J. Comp. Physiol. Psychol.* 73: 13–21.

Margules, D. L. 1971a. Alpha and beta adrenergic receptors in amygdala: reciprocal inhibitors and facilitators of punished operant behavior. *Europ. J. Pharmacol.* 16: 21–26.

Margules, D. L. 1971b. Localization of anti-punishment actions of norepinephrine and atropine in amygdala and entopeduncular nucleus of rats. *Brain Res.* 35: 177–184.

Margules, D. L. and L. Stein. 1966. Neuroleptics vs. tranquilizers: evidence from animal behavior studies of mode and site of action. *Excp. Med. Int. Cong.* 129: 108–120.

Margules, D. L. and L. Stein. 1969a. Cholinergic synapses in the ventromedial hypothalamus for the suppression of operant behavior by punishment and satiety. *J. Comp. Physiol. Psychol.* 67: 327–335.

Margules, D. L. and L. Stein. 1969b. Cholinergic synapses of a periventricular punishment system in the medial hypothalamus. *Amer. J. Physiol.* 217: 475–480.

Margules, D. L., M. J. Lewis, J. A. Dragovich and A. S. Margules. 1972. Hypothalamic norepinephrine: circadian rhythms and the control of feeding behavior. *Science.* 178: 640–643.

Marinesco, G., O. Sager and A. Kreindler. 1929. Experimentelle Untersuchungen zum Problem des Schlafmechanismus. *Z. Ges. Neurol. Psychiat.* 119: 277–306.

Mark, R. F. and Watts, M. E. 1971. Drug inhibition of memory formation in chickens. I. Long-term memory. *Proc. R. Soc. Lond.* 178: 439–454.

Marley, E. and G. Nistico. 1972. Effects of catecholamines and adenosine derivatives given into the brain of fowls. *Brit. J. Pharmacol.* 46: 619–636.

Marley, E. and T. J. Seller. 1972. Effects of muscarine given into the brain of fowls. *Brit. J. Pharmacol.* 44: 413–434.

Marley, E. and J. D. Stephenson. 1968. Intracerebral micro-infusion of drugs under controlled conditions in young chickens. *J. Physiol.* 196: 97–99P.

Marley, E. and J. D. Stephenson. 1970. Effects of catecholamines infused into the brain of young chickens. *Brit. J. Pharmacol.* 40: 639–658.

Martini, L. and J. Meites. 1970. *Neurochemical Aspects of Hypothalamic Function.* Academic Press, New York, pp. 1–159.

Maskrey, M. and J. Bligh. 1971. Interactions between the thermoregulatory responses to injections into a lateral cerebral ventricle of the Welsh mountain sheep of putative neurotransmitter substances, and of local changes in anterior hypothalamic temperature. *Int. J. Biometeor.* 15: 129–133.

Mason, J. W. 1958. The central nervous system regulation of ACTH secretion, pp. 645–670. *In* H. H. Jasper, L. D. Procton, R. S. Knighton, W. C. Noshay and R. T. Costello (eds.) *Reticular Formation of the Brain.* Little, Brown & Co., Boston.

Masserman, J. H. 1937. Effects of sodium amytal and other drugs on the reactivity of the hypothalamus of the cat. *AMA Arch. Neurol. Psychiat.* 37: 617–628.

Masserman, J. H. 1938a. Destruction of the hypothalamus in cats. Effect on activity of the cerebral nervous system and its reaction to sodium amytal. *AMA Arch. Neurol. Psychiat.* 39: 1250–1271.

Masserman, J. H. 1938b. The effect of strychnine sulphate on the emotional mimetic functions of the hypothalamus of the cat. *J. Pharmacol. Exptl. Ther.* 64: 335–354.

Masserman, J. H. 1939. Action of metrazol (pentamethylenetetrazol) on the hypothalamus of the cat. *AMA Arch. Neurol. Psychiat.* 41: 504–510.

Masserman, J. H. 1940a. Effects of analeptic drugs on the hypothalamus of the cat. *Proc. Assoc. Res. Nerv. Ment. Dis.* 20: 624–634.

Masserman, J. H. 1940b. Stimulant effects of ethyl alcohol in cortico-hypothalamic functions. *J. Pharmacol. Exptl. Ther.* 70: 450–453.

Masserman, J. H. 1941. Is the hypothalamus a center of emotion? *Psychosom. Med.* 3: 3–25.

Masserman, J. H. and L. Jacobson. 1940. Effects of ethyl alcohol on the cerebral cortex and the hypothalamus of the cat. *AMA Arch. Neurol. Psychiat.* 43: 334–340.

Matsumoto, K., T. Ohmoto, S. Namba and T. Miyamoto. 1971. Influence of GABOB and GABA solutions on the cortical evoked potentials after thalamic stimulations of cats and human. *Brain Nerve (Tokyo)* 23: 357–363.

Matsuura, T. and J. Bureš. 1971. The minimum volume of depolarized neural tissue required for triggering cortical spreading depression in rat. *Exp. Brain Res.* 12: 238–249.

Mayer, J. 1953. Genetic, traumatic and environmental factors in the etiology of obesity. *Physiol. Rev.* 33: 472–508.

Mayer, J. and N. B. Marshall. 1956. Specificity of gold thioglucose for ventromedial hypothalamic lesions and hyperphagia. *Nature.* 178: 1399–1400.

Medawar, P. B. 1972. *The Hope of Progress.* Methuen & Co., Ltd., London, pp. 1–133.

Megirian, D. and J. Bureš. 1970. Unilateral cortical spreading depression and conditioned eyeblink responses in the rabbit. *Exptl. Neurol.* 27: 34–45.

Metyš, J., N. Wagner, J. Metyšová and A. Herz. 1969a. Studies on the central antinociceptive action of cholinomimetic agents. *Int. J. Neuropharmacol.* 8: 413–425.

Metyš, J., J. Metyšová, N. Wagner, N. Schöndorf and A. Herz. 1969b. Hemmung nociceptiver Reaktionen durch Cholinomimetica und durch Morphin nach intraventrikulärer und intracerebraler Injektion. *Arzneimittel-forsch.* 19: 432–433.

Metz, B. 1961. The brain ACh-AChE-ChA system in respiratory control. *Neurology.* 11: 37–45.

Metz, B. 1966. Hypercapnia and acetylcholine release from the cerebral cortex and medulla. *J. Physiol.* 186: 321–332.

Metz, B. 1971. Correlation between the electrical activity and acetylcholine release from the cerebral cortex and medulla during hypercapnia. *Canad. J. Physiol. Pharmacol.* 49: 331–337.

Meyer, C. C. 1972. Inhibition of precocial copulation in the domestic chick by progesterone brain implants. *J. Comp. Physiol. Psychol.* 79: 8–12.

Meyer, C. C. and T. M. Ruby. 1970. A stereotaxic attachment for implanting crystalline steroids in the brain. *Physiol. Behav.* 5: 1181–1182.

Meyer, H. H. 1913. Theorie des Fiebers und seiner Behandlung. *Verhandl. Deut. Bes. Inner. Med.* 30: 15–25.

Michael, R. P. 1961. An investigation of the sensitivity of circumscribed neurological areas to hormonal stimulation by means of the application of oestrogens directly to the brain of the cat, pp. 465–480. In S. S. Kety and J. Elkes (eds.) *Regional Neurochemistry.* Pergamon Press, Oxford.

Michael, R. P. 1965. Oestrogens in the central nervous system. *Brit. Med. Bull.* 21: 87–90.

Michael, R. P. 1966. Control of sexual behavior by gonadal steroids. I. Action of hormones on the cat brain, pp. 81–98. *In* R. A. Gorski and R. E. Whalen (eds.) *Brain and Behavior*, Vol. III. University of California Press, Los Angeles.

Michael, R. P. 1968. Neural and non-neural mechanisms in the reproductive behaviour of primates. *Excp. Med. Int. Cong.* **184**: 302–309.

Miczek, K. A. and S. P. Grossman. 1972. Punished and unpunished operant behavior after atropine administration to the VMH of squirrel monkeys. *J. Comp. Physiol. Psychol.* **81**: 318–330.

Mihailović, Lj. T. and D. Čupić. 1971. Epileptiform activity evoked by intracerebral injection of anti-brain antibodies. *Brain Res.* **32**: 97–124.

Mihailović, Lj. T. and B. D. Janković. 1961. Effects of intraventricularly injected anti-N. caudatus antibody on the electrical activity of the cat brain. *Nature.* **192**: 665–666.

Militello, L., G. Amato and A. Rizzo. 1970. Effecti della stimolazione chimica del nucleo caudato sull'activita' spontanea ed evocata della corteccia cerebrale, nel gatto. *Boll. Della Soc. Ital. Biol. Sper.* **46**: 957–961.

Miller, F. R. 1937. The local action of eserine on the central nervous system. *J. Physiol.* **91**: 212–221.

Miller, F. R. 1943. Direct stimulation of the hypoglossal nucleus by acetylcholine in extreme dilutions. *Proc. Soc. Exptl. Biol. Med.* **54**: 285–287.

Miller, F. P., R. H. Cox, Jr. and R. P. Maickel. 1968. Intrastrain differences in serotonin and norepinephrine in discrete areas of rat brain. *Science.* **162**: 463–464.

Miller, N. E. 1965. Chemical coding of behavior in the brain. *Science.* **148**: 328–338.

Miller, N. E. and C. W. Chien. 1968. Drinking elicited by injecting eserine into preoptic area of rat brain. *Commun. Behav. Biol.* **1**: 61–63.

Miller, N. E., C. J. Bailey and J. A. F. Stevenson. 1950. Decreased "hunger" but increased food intake resulting from hypothalamic lesions. *Science.* **112**: 256–259.

Miller, N. E., K. S. Gottesman and N. Emery. 1964. Dose response to carbachol and norepinephrine in rat hypothalamus. *Amer. J. Physiol.* **206**: 1384–1388.

Millhouse, O. E. 1969. A golgi study of the descending medial forebrain bundle. *Brain Res.* **15**: 341–363.

Milner, J. S., D. M. Nance and D. E. Sheer. 1971. Effects of hypothalamic and amygdaloid chemical stimulation on appetitive behavior in the cat. *Psychon. Sci.* **23**: 25–26.

Milton, A. S. and S. Wendlandt. 1970. A possible role for prostaglandin E_1 as a modulator for temperature regulation in the central nervous system of the cat. *J. Physiol.* **207**: 76–77P.

Milton, A. S. and S. Wendlandt. 1971. Effects on body temperature of prostaglandins of the A, E, and F series on injection into the third ventricle of unanaesthetized cats and rabbits. *J. Physiol.* **218**: 325–336.

Mims, C. A. 1960. Intracerebral injections and the growth of viruses in the mouse brain. *Brit. J. Exper. Pathol.* **41**: 52–59.

Mishkinsky, J., K. Khazen and F. G. Sulman. 1969. Mammotropic effect of fluphenazine enanthate in the rat. *Neuroendocrinology.* **4**: 321–325.

Mishkinsky, J., Z. K. Lajtos and F. G. Sulman. 1968. Initiation of lactation by hypothalamic implantation of perphenazine. *Endocrinology.* **78**: 919–922.

Mitchell, D., J. W. Snellen and A. R. Atkins. 1970. Thermoregulation during fever: change of set-point or change of gain. *Pflügers Arch.* **321**: 293–302.

Mitchell, J. F. 1963. The spontaneous and evoked release of acetylcholine from the cerebral cortex. *J. Physiol.* **165**: 98–116.

Mitchell, R. A., H. H. Loeschcke, W. H. Massion and J. W. Severinghaus. 1963. Respiratory responses mediated through superficial chemosensitive areas on the medulla. *J. Appl. Physiol.* **18**: 523–533.

Moir, A. T. B., G. W. Ashcroft, T. B. Crawford, D. Eccleston and H. C. Guldberg. 1970.

Cerebral metabolites in cerebrospinal fluid as a biochemical approach to the brain. *Brain.* **93**: 357–368.

Monnier, M. M. 1938. Physiologie des formations réticulées. II. Respiration. Effets de l'excitation faradique du bulbe chez le chat. *Rev. Neurol.* **69**: 517–523.

Monnier, M. and A. M. Hatt. 1971. Humoral transmission of sleep. V. New evidence from production of pure sleep hemodialysate. *Pflügers Arch.* **329**: 231–243.

Monnier, M. and L. Hösli. 1965. Humoral transmission of sleep and wakefulness. II. Hemodialysis of a sleep inducing humor during stimulation of the thalamic somnogenic area. *Pflügers Arch.* **282**: 60–75.

Monnier, M. and G. A. Schoenenberger. 1972. Some physical-chemical properties of the rabbit's "sleep hemodialysate". *Experientia.* **28**: 32–33.

Monnier, M., A. M. Hatt, L. B. Cueni and G. A. Schoenenberger. 1972. Humoral transmission of sleep. VI. Purification and assessment of a hypnogenic fraction of "sleep dialysate" (factor delta). *Pflügers Arch.* **331**: 257–265.

Montgomery, R. B. and J. S. M. Armstrong. 1973. Cafeteria behaviour in rat after hypothalamic cholinergic and adrenergic stimulation. *Reports from the Psychological Laboratories*, Vol. I, Latrobe University, Australia.

Montgomery, R. B. and G. Singer. 1969a. Histochemical fluorescence as an index of spread of centrally applied neurochemicals. *Science.* **165**: 1031–1032.

Montgomery, R. B. and G. Singer. 1969b. Lack of effect on drinking of stimulation of the ventral amygdala of rat with GABA. *J. Comp. Physiol. Psychol.* **69**: 623–627.

Montgomery, R. B., G. Singer, A. T. Purcell, J. Narbeth and A. G. Bolt. 1969. Central control of hunger in the rat. *Nature.* **223**: 1278–1279.

Montgomery, R. B., G. Singer, A. T. Purcell, J. Narbeth and A. G. Bolt. 1971. The effects of intrahypothalamic injections of desmethylimipramine on food and water intake of the rat. *Psychopharmacologia.* **19**: 81–86.

Moore, C. R. and D. Price. 1932. Gonad hormone functions, and the reciprocal influence between gonads and hypophysis with its bearing on the problem of sex hormone antagonism. *Amer. J. Anatomy.* **50**: 13–67.

Morelli, L. 1968. Effetti elettrocorticografici di microiniezioni di benzoato di estradiolo nell'ipotalamo. *Arch. Sci. Biol.* **52**: 325–335.

Morgane, P. J. 1961a. Alterations in feeding and drinking behavior of rats with lesions in globi pallidi. *Amer. J. Physiol.* **201**: 420–428.

Morgane, P. J. 1961b. Evidence of a 'hunger motivational' system in the lateral hypothalamus of the rat. *Nature.* **191**: 672–674.

Morgane, P. J. 1962. Reinforcing effects of self-injected cholinergic agents into hypothalamic 'drinking' areas in rats. *Fed. Proc.* **21**: 352.

Morgane, P. J. 1972. Maturation of neurobiochemical systems related to the ontogeny of sleep behavior, pp. 141–162. *In* C. D. Clemente, D. P. Purpura and F. E. Mayer (eds.) *Sleep and the Maturing Nervous System.* Academic Press, New York.

Morgane, P. J. and H. L. Jacobs. 1969. Hunger and satiety. *World Rev. Nutr. Diet.* **10**: 100–213.

Morgane, P. J. and W. C. Stern. 1972. Relationship of sleep to neuroanatomical circuits, biochemistry, and behavior. *Ann. N.Y. Acad. Sci.* **193**: 95–111.

Morgane, P. J., J. D. Bronzino and W. C. Stern. 1972. An exploring chemitrode device for direct chemical stimulation of the brain. *J. Appl. Physiol.* **32**: 138–142.

Morris, H., R. Walker and D. L. Margules. 1970. A cannula of variable depth for chemical stimulation of the brain. *EEG Clin. Neurophysiol.* **29**: 521–523.

Morselli, P. L., S. Garattini, E. Marcucci, E. Mussini, W. Rewersky, L. Valzelli and R. A. Peters. 1968. The effect of injections of fluorocitrate into the brains of rats. *Biochem. Pharmacol.* **17**: 195–202.

Moruzzi, G. 1972. The sleep-waking cycle, pp. 1–165. *In: Ergebnisse der Physiologie.* Springer-Verlag, Heidelberg.

Moruzzi, G. and H. W. Magoun. 1949. Brain stem reticular formation and activation of the EEG. *EEG Clin. Neurophysiol.* **1**: 455–473.

Motta, M. 1969. The brain and the physiological interplay of long and short feedback systems. *Proceedings of the 3rd International Congress on Endocrinology*, pp. 523–531.

Motta, M. and L. Martini. 1972. Hypothalamic releasing factors: a new class of "neurotransmitters." *Arch. Int. Pharmacodyn. Ther.* **196**: 191–204.

Motta, M., F. Fraschini and L. Martini. 1969. "Short" feedback mechanisms in the control of anterior pituitary function, pp. 211–253. *In* W. F. Ganong and L. Martini (eds.) *Frontiers in Neuroendocrinology.* Oxford University Press, New York.

Motta, M., G. Mangili and L. Martini. 1965. A "short" feedback loop in the control of ACTH secretion. *Endocrinology.* **77**: 392–395.

Motta, M., F. Fraschini, G. Giuliani and L. Martini. 1968. The central nervous system, estrogen and puberty. *Endocrinology.* **83**: 1101–1107.

Mountford, D. 1969. Drinking following carbachol stimulation of hippocampal formation or lateral ventricles. *Psychon. Sci.* **16**: 124–125.

Müller, E. E., T. Saito, A. Arimura and A. V. Schally. 1967. Hypoglycemia, stress and growth hormone release: blockade of growth hormone release by drugs acting on the central nervous system. *Endocrinology.* **80**: 109–117.

Murphey, D. L. and R. E. Dill. 1972. Chemical stimulation of discrete brain loci as a method of producing dyskinesia models in primates. *Exptl. Neurol.* **34**: 244–254.

Mutani, R. 1967a. Cobalt experimental amygdaloid epilepsy in the cat. *Epilepsia.* **8**: 73–92.

Mutani, R. 1967b. Cobalt experimental hippocampal epilepsy in the cat. *Epilepsia.* **8**: 223–240.

Mutani, R. 1967c. Epilessia sperimentale rinecefalica de cobalto: registrazioni in profondita. *Boll. Soc. Ital. Biol. Sper.* **43**: 1175–1178.

Mutani, R., T. Doriguzzi, R. Fariello and P. M. Furlan. 1969. Studio dell'azione di alcuni farmaci antiepilettici. I. Effetti sul focus epilettogeno sperimentale indotto dalla introduzione di cobalto nell'ippocampo del gatto. *Sistema Nervoso.* **21**: 160–171.

Myers, J. M., F. E. Nulsen, H. Dillon, C. S. Drayer, M. M. Pearson, F. C. Grant and L. H. Smith. 1953. An obsessive-compulsive reaction treated with prefrontal procaine injection. *J. Amer. Med. Assoc.* **153**: 1015–1016.

Myers, R. D. 1961. Behavioral changes after intradiencephalic chemical stimulation of cats with chronically implanted cannulae. *Proc. East. Psychol. Assoc., 32nd Ann. Meeting.*

Myers, R. D. 1963. An intracranial chemical stimulation system for chronic or self-infusion. *J. Appl. Physiol.* **18**: 221–223.

Myers, R. D. 1964a. Emotional and autonomic responses following hypothalamic chemical stimulation. *Canad. J. Psychol.* **18**: 6–14.

Myers, R. D. 1964b. Modification of drinking patterns by chronic intracranial chemical infusion, pp. 533–549. *In* M. J. Wayner (ed.) *Thirst.* Pergamon Press, New York.

Myers, R. D. 1966. Injection of solutions into cerebral tissue: relation between volume and diffusion. *Physiol. Behav.* **1**: 171–174.

Myers, R. D. 1967a. Transfusion of cerebrospinal fluid and tissue bound chemical factors between the brains of conscious monkeys: a new neurobiological assay. *Physiol. Behav.* **2**: 373–377.

Myers, R. D. 1967b. Release of chemical factors from the diencephalic region of the unanaesthetized monkey during changes in body temperature. *J. Physiol.* **188**: 50–51P.

Myers, R. D. 1968. Discussion of serotonin, norepinephrine, and fever. *Adv. Pharmacol.* **6**: 318–321.

Myers, R. D. 1969a. Thermoregulation and norepinephrine. *Science.* **165**: 1030–1031.

Myers, R. D. 1969b. Chemical mechanisms in the hypothalamus mediating eating and drinking in the monkey. *Ann. N.Y. Acad. Sci.* **157**: 918–933.

Myers, R. D. 1969c. Temperature regulation: neurochemical systems in the hypothalamus, pp. 506–523. *In* W. Nauta, W. Haymaker and E. Anderson (eds.) *The Hypothalamus.* Charles Thomas, Springfield.

Myers, R. D. 1970a. An improved push-pull cannula system for perfusing an isolated region of the brain. *Physiol. Behav.* **5**: 243–246.

Myers, R. D. 1970b. The role of hypothalamic transmitter factors in the control of body temperature, pp. 648–666. *In* J. D. Hardy (ed.) *Physiological and Behavioral Temperature Regulation.* Charles Thomas, Springfield.

Myers, R. D. 1971a. Methods for chemical stimulation of the brain, pp. 247–280. *In* R. D. Myers (ed.) *Methods in Psychobiology.* Academic Press, London.

Myers, R. D. 1971b. Hypothalamic mechanisms of pyrogen action in the cat and monkey, pp. 131–153. *In* G. E. B. Wolstenholme and J. Birch (eds.) *Ciba Foundation Symposium on Pyrogen and Fever.* Churchill, London.

Myers, R. D. 1971c. Primates, pp. 283–326. *In* C. C. Whittow (ed.) *Comparative Physiology of Thermoregulation*, Vol. 2. Academic Press, New York.

Myers, R. D. 1972. Methods for perfusing different structures of the brain, pp. 169–211. *In* R. D. Myers (ed.) *Methods in Psychobiology*, Vol. 2. Academic Press, New York.

Myers, R. D. 1973. The role of hypothalamic serotonin in thermoregulation, pp. 293–302. *In* J. Barchas and E. Usdin (eds.) *Serotonin and Behavior.* Academic Press, New York.

Myers, R. D. and D. B. Beleslin. 1970. The spontaneous release of 5-hydroxytryptamine and acetylcholine within the diencephalon of the unanaesthetized rhesus monkey. *Exp. Brain Res.* **11**: 539–552.

Myers, R. D. and D. B. Beleslin. 1971. Changes in serotonin release in hypothalamus during cooling or warming of the monkey. *Amer. J. Physiol.* **220**: 1746–1754.

Myers, R. D. and P. D. Brophy. 1972. Temperature changes in the rat produced by altering the sodium-calcium ratio in the cerebral ventricles. *Neuropharmacology.* **11**: 351–361.

Myers, R. D. and J. E. Buckman. 1972. Deep hypothermia induced in the golden hamster by altering cerebral calcium levels. *Amer. J. Physiol.* **223**: 1313–1318.

Myers, R. D. and C. Chinn. 1973. Evoked release of hypothalamic norepinephrine during thermoregulation in the cat. *Amer. J. Physiol.* **224**: 230–236.

Myers, R. D. and T. J. Cicero. 1968. Are the cerebral ventricles involved in thirst produced by a cholinergic substance? *Psychon. Sci.* **10**: 93–94.

Myers, R. D. and J. DeStefano. 1969. Ingestive behavior mediated centrally by adrenergic and cholinergic systems. *Purdue Neuropsychology Series Report No. 2A.*

Myers, R. D. and G. E. Martin. 1973. 6-OHDA lesions of the hypothalamus: interaction of aphagia, food palatability, set-point for weight regulation, and recovery of feeding. *Pharmacol. Biochem. Behav.* **1**: 329–345.

Myers, R. D. and L. G. Sharpe. 1968a. Intracerebral injections and perfusions in the conscious monkey, pp. 449–465. *In* H. Vagtborg (ed.) *Use of Non-Human Primates in Drug Evaluation.* Austin University, Texas.

Myers, R. D. and L. G. Sharpe. 1968b. Chemical activation of ingestive and other hypothalamic regulatory mechanisms. *Physiol. Behav.* **3**: 987–995.

Myers, R. D. and L. G. Sharpe. 1968c. Temperature in the monkey: transmitter factors released from the brain during thermoregulation. *Science.* **161**: 572–573.

Myers, R. D. and M. Tytell. 1972. Fever: reciprocal shift in brain sodium to calcium ratio as the set-point temperature rises. *Science.* **178**: 765–767.

Myers, R. D. and W. L. Veale. 1970. Body temperature: possible ionic mechanism in the hypothalamus controlling the set point. *Science.* **170**: 95–97.

Myers, R. D. and W. L. Veale. 1971a. The role of sodium and calcium ions in the hypothalamus in the control of body temperature of the unanaesthetized cat. *J. Physiol.* **212**: 411–430.

Myers, R. D. and W. L. Veale. 1971b. Spontaneous feeding in the satiated cat evoked by sodium or calcium ions perfused within the hypothalamus. *Physiol. Behav.* **6**: 507–512.

Myers, R. D. and M. B. Waller. 1973. Differential release of acetylcholine from the hypothalamus and mesencephalon of the monkey during thermoregulation. *J. Physiol.* **230**: 273–293.

Myers, R. D. and T. L. Yaksh. 1968. Feeding and temperature responses in the unrestrained rat after injections of cholinergic and aminergic substances into the cerebral ventricles. *Physiol. Behav.* .3: 917–928.

Myers, R. D. and T. L. Yaksh. 1969. Control of body temperature in the unanaesthetized monkey by cholinergic and aminergic systems in the hypothalamus. *J. Physiol.* **202**: 483–500.

Myers, R. D. and T. L. Yaksh. 1971. Thermoregulation around a new 'set-point' established in the monkey by altering the ratio of sodium to calcium ions within the hypothalamus. *J. Physiol.* **218**: 609–633.

Myers, R. D. and T. L. Yaksh. 1972. The role of hypothalamic monoamines in hibernation and hypothermia, pp. 551–575. *In* F. E. South, J. P. Hannon, J. R. Willis, E. T. Pengelley and N. R. Alpert (eds.) *Hibernation-Hypothermia. Perspectives and Challenges.* Elsevier, Amsterdam.

Myers, R. D., G. Casaday and R. B. Holman. 1967. A simplified intracranial cannula for chemical stimulation or long-term infusion of the brain. *Physiol. Behav.* **2**: 87–88.

Myers, R. D., G. H. Hall and T. A. Rudy. 1973. Drinking in the monkey evoked by nicotine or angiotensin II microinjected in hypothalamic and mesencephalic sites. *Pharmacol. Biochem. Behav.* **1**: 15–22.

Myers, R. D., A. Kawa and D. B. Beleslin. 1969. Evoked release of 5-HT and NEFA from the hypothalamus of the conscious monkey during thermoregulation. *Experientia.* **25**: 705–706.

Myers, R. D., T. A. Rudy and T. L. Yaksh. 1971a. Fever in the monkey produced by the direct action of pyrogen on the hypothalamus. *Experientia.* **27**: 160–161.

Myers, R. D., T. A. Rudy and T. L. Yaksh. 1971b. Effect in the rhesus monkey of salicylate on centrally-induced endotoxin fevers. *Neuropharmacology.* **10**: 775–778.

Myers, R. D., W. L. Veale and T. L. Yaksh. 1971c. Changes in body temperature of the unanaesthetized monkey produced by sodium and calcium ions perfused through the cerebral ventricles. *J. Physiol.* **217**: 381–392.

Myers, R. D., S. A. Bender, M. Krstić and P. D. Brophy. 1972. Feeding produced in the satiated rat by elevating the concentration of calcium in the brain. *Science.* **176**: 1124–1125.

Myers, R. D., M. Tytell, A. Kawa and T. Rudy. 1971d. Micro-injection of ^{3}H-acetylcholine, ^{14}C-serotonin and ^{3}H-norepinephrine into the hypothalamus of the rat: diffusion into tissue and ventricles. *Physiol. Behav.* **7**: 743–751.

Nachmansohn, D. 1971. Chemical events in conducting and synaptic membranes during electrical activity. *Proc. Nat. Acad. Sci.* **68**: 3170–3174.

Nadler, R. D. 1965. A simplified cannula system for implanting and injecting chemicals into the brains of small animals. *EEG Clin. Neurophysiol.* **19**: 312–313.

Nadler, R. D. 1968. Masculinization of female rats by intracranial implantation of androgen in infancy. *J. Comp. Physiol. Psychol.* **66**: 157–167.

Nadler, R. D. 1972a. Intrahypothalamic locus for induction of androgen sterilization in neonatal female rats. *Neuroendocrinology.* **9**: 349–357.

Nadler, R. D. 1972b. Intrahypothalamic exploration of androgen-sensitive brain loci in neonatal female rats. *N. Y. Acad. Sci.* **34**: 572–581.

Nakajima, S. 1964. Effects of chemical injection into the reticular formation of rats. *J. Comp. Physiol. Psychol.* **58:** 10–15.

Nakajima, S. 1969. Interference with relearning in the rat after hippocampal injection of actinomycin D. *J. Comp. Physiol. Psychol.* **67:** 457–461.

Nakajima, S. 1972a. Effects of intracranial chemical injections upon self-stimulation in in the rat. *Physiol. Behav.* **8:** 741–746.

Nakajima, S. 1972b. Proactive effect of actinomycin D on maze performance in the rat. *Physiol. Behav.* **8:** 1063–1067.

Nakayama, T., J. Eisenman and J. D. Hardy. 1961. Single unit activity of anterior hypothalamus during local heating. *Science.* **134:** 560–561.

Nakayama, T., H. T. Hammel, J. D. Hardy and J. S. Eisenman. 1963. Thermal stimulation of electrical activity of single units of the preoptic region. *Amer. J. Physiol.* **204:** 1122–1126.

Nance, D. M., J. S. Milner and D. E. Sheer. 1971. Hypothalamic anticholinergic inhibition of eating and drinking in the cat. *Psychon. Sci.* **23:** 26–28.

Narabayashi, H., T. Okuma and S. Shikiba. 1956. Procaine oil blocking of the globus pallidus. *AMA Arch. Neurol. Psychiat.* **75:** 36–48.

Nashold, B. S. 1959. Cholinergic stimulation of globus pallidus in man. *Proc. Soc. Exptl. Biol. Med.* **101:** 68–69.

Nashold, B. S. 1961. Analysis of physiologic changes after chemical and mechanical lesions of the globus pallidus and/or thalamus in persons with extrapyramidal disorders. *Rev. Canad. Biol.* **20:** 381–389.

Nashold, B. S. and J. P. Gills. 1960. Chemical stimulation of telencephalon, diencephalon and mesencephalon in unrestrained animals. *J. Neuropath. Exp. Neurol.* **19:** 580–590.

Nashold, B. S., J. R. Urbaniak and M. A. Hatcher. 1965. Chemical stimulation of red nucleus, substantia nigra, and basis pedunculi in alert cats. *Neurology.* **15:** 604–612.

Naumenko, E. V. 1967. Role of adrenergic and cholinergic structures in the control of the pituitary-adrenal system. *Endocrinology.* **80:** 69–76.

Naumenko, E. V. 1968. Hypothalamic chemoreactive structures and the regulation of pituitary-adrenal function. Effects of local injections of norepinephrine, carbachol and serotonin into the brain of guinea pigs with intact brains and after mesencephalic transection. *Brain Res.* **11:** 1–10.

Naumenko, E. V. 1969. Effect of local injection of 5-hydroxytryptamine into rhinencephalic and mesencephalic structures on pituitary-adrenal function in guinea-pigs. *Neuroendocrinology.* **5:** 81–88.

Naumenko, E. V. and R. Yu. Ilyutchenok. 1967. Central action of serotonin on the pituitary-adrenal cortex system. *Bull. Exp. Biol. Med. (USSR).* **64:** 63–65.

Nauta, W. J. H. 1958. Hippocampal projections and related neural pathways to the midbrain in the cat. *Brain.* **81:** 319–340.

Nauta, W. J. H. 1960. Limbic system and hypothalamus: anatomical aspects. *Physiol. Rev.* **40:** 102–104.

Nauta, W. J. H. 1963. Central nervous organization and the endocrine motor system, pp. 5–28. *In* A. V. Nalbandov (ed.) *Advances in Neuroendocrinology.* University of Illinois Press, Urbana.

Nauta, W. J. H. and H. J. Karten. 1970. A general profile of the vertebrate brain with sidelights on the ancestry of cerebral cortex, pp. 7–26. *In* F. O. Schmitt (ed.) *The Neurosciences. Second Study Program.* The Rockefeller University Press, New York.

Neill, D. G. and S. P. Grossman. 1970. Behavioral effects of lesions or cholinergic blockade of the dorsal and ventral caudate of rats. *J. Comp. Physiol. Psychol.* **71:** 311–317.

Nicoll, R. A. and J. L. Barker. 1971. Excitation of supraoptic neurosecretory cells by angiotensin II. *Nature New Biol.* **233:** 172–174.

Ôba, T., K. Ôta and A. Yokoyama. 1971. Inhibition of milk-ejection reflex in lactating rats by systemic administration and intracerebral implantation of atropine. *Neuroendocrinology.* **7:** 116–126.

Obrador, S. 1957. A simplified neurosurgical technique for approaching and damaging the region of the globus pallidus in Parkinson's disease. *J. Neurol. Neurosurg. Psychiat.* **20:** 47–49.

Ojeda, S. R. and V. D. Ramírez. 1969. Automatic control of LH and FSH secretion by short feedback circuits in immature rats. *Endocrinology.* **84:** 786–797.

Ojeda, S. R. and V. D. Ramírez. 1970. Failure of estrogen to block compensatory ovarian hypertrophy in prepuberal rats bearing medial basal hypothalamic FSH implants. *Endocrinology.* **86:** 50–56.

Ojeda, S. R. and V. D. Ramírez. 1972. Different pituitary-gonadal response to hemicastration in female and in male rats bearing intrahypothalamic FSH implants. *Neuroendocrinology.* **10:** 161–174.

Olds, J. and P. Milner. 1954. Positive reinforcement produced by electrical stimulation of septal area and other regions of rat brain. *J. Comp. Physiol. Psychol.* **47:** 419–427.

Olds, J. and M. E. Olds. 1958. Positive reinforcement produced by stimulating hypothalamus with iproniazid and other compounds. *Science.* **127:** 1175–1176.

Olds, J., W. S. Allan and E. Briese. 1971. Differentiation of hypothalamic drive and reward centers. *Amer. J. Physiol.* **221:** 368–375.

Olds, J., A. Yuwiler, M. E. Olds and C. Yun. 1964. Neurohumors in hypothalamic substrates of reward. *Amer. J. Physiol.* **207:** 242–254.

Olds, M. E. and E. F. Domino. 1969. Comparison of muscarinic and nicotinic cholinergic agonists on self-stimulation behavior. *J. Pharmacol. Exptl. Ther.* **166:** 189–204.

Olney, J. W. and L. G. Sharpe. 1969. Brain lesions in an infant rhesus monkey treated with monosodium glutamate. *Science.* **166:** 386–388.

Olton, D. S. 1970. Specific deficits in active avoidance behavior following penicillin injection into hippocampus. *Physiol. Behav.* **5:** 957–963.

Oomura, Y., T. Ono, H. Ooyama and M. J. Wayner. 1969. Glucose and osmosensitive neurones of the rat hypothalamus. *Nature.* **222:** 282–284.

Osterholm, J. L., J. Bell, R. Meyer and J. Pyenson. 1969. Experimental effects of free serotonin on the brain and its relation to brain injury. *J. Neurosurg.* **31:** 408–421.

Palka, Y. S. and C. H. Sawyer. 1966a. The effects of hypothalamic implants of ovarian steroids on oestrous behaviour in rabbits. *J. Physiol.* **185:** 251–269.

Palka, Y. S. and C. H. Sawyer. 1966b. Induction of estrous behavior in rabbits by hypothalamic implants of testosterone. *Amer. J. Physiol.* **211:** 225–228.

Palka, Y. S., V. D. Ramírez and C. H. Sawyer. 1966. Distribution and biological effects of tritiated estradiol implanted in the hypothalamo-hypophysial region of female rats. *Endocrinology.* **78:** 487–499.

Panksepp, J. and D. A. Booth. 1971. Decreased feeding after injections of amino-acids into the hypothalamus. *Nature.* **233:** 341–342.

Panksepp, J. and D. M. Nance. 1972. Insulin, glucose and hypothalamic regulation of feeding. *Physiol. Behav.* **9:** 447–451.

Paolino, R. M. and B. R. Bernard. 1968. Environmental temperature effects on the thermoregulatory response to systemic and hypothalamic administration of morphine. *Life Sci.* **7:** 857–863.

Papez, J. W. 1937. A proposed mechanism of emotion. *AMA Arch. Neurol. Psychiat.* **38:** 725–743.

Pappenheimer, J. R. 1967. The ionic composition of cerebral extracellular fluid and its relation to control of breathing. *Harvey Lectures Ser.* **61:** 71–94.

Pappenheimer, J. R., T. B. Miller and C. A. Goodrich. 1967. Sleep-promoting effects of cerebrospinal fluid from sleep-deprived goats. *Proc. Nat. Acad. Sci.* **58:** 513–517.

Pappenheimer, J. R., V. Fencl, S. R. Heisey and D. Held. 1965. Role of cerebral fluids in control of respiration as studied in unanesthetized goats. *Amer. J. Physiol.* **208**: 436–450.

Parks, R. E., G. W. Stein and R. A. Levitt. 1971. The effects of lateral hypothalamic or septal lesions on cholinergically elicited drinking. *Psychon. Sci.* **24**: 25–26.

Patton, H. D. and V. E. Amassian. 1960. The pyramidal tract: its excitation and functions, pp. 837–861. *In* J. Field, II. W. Magoun and V. E. Hall (eds.) *Handbook of Physiology*, Vol. II. Waverly Press, Baltimore.

Payan, H. M. 1967. Cerebral lesions produced in rats by various implants: epileptogenic effect of cobalt. *J. Neurosurg.* **27**: 146–152.

Payan, H., S. Levine and R. Strebel. 1966. Inhibition of experimental epilepsy by chemical stimulation of cerebellum. *Neurology.* **16**: 573–576.

Pecile, A. and E. E. Müller. 1966. Control of growth hormone secretion, pp. 537–564. *In* L. Martini and W. F. Ganong (eds.) *Neuroendocrinology*, Vol. I. Academic Press, New York.

Peck, J. W. and D. Novin. 1971. Evidence that osmoreceptors mediating drinking in rabbits are in the lateral preoptic area. *J. Comp. Physiol. Psychol.* **74**: 134–147.

Peindaries, R. and J. Jacob. 1971. Interactions between 5-hydroxytryptamine and a purified bacterial pyrogen when injected into the lateral cerebral ventricle of the wake rabbit. *Europ. J. Pharmacol.* **13**: 347–355.

Peiss, C. N. 1965. Concepts of cardiovascular regulation: past, present and future, pp. 154–197. *In* W. C. Randall (ed.) *Nervous Control of the Heart.* The Williams and Wilkins Company, Baltimore.

Peñaloza-Rojas, J. H. and J. Zeidenweber. 1965. Local and EEG effects of adrenaline and acetylcholine application within the olfactory bulb. *EEG Clin. Neurophysiol.* **19**: 88–90.

Penfield, W. and B. Milner. 1958. Memory deficit produced by bilateral lesions in the hippocampal zone. *AMA Arch. Neurol. Psychiat.* **79**: 475–497.

Pepeu, G. 1972. Cholinergic neurotransmission in the central nervous system. *Arch. Int. Pharmacodyn. Ther.* Suppl. 196, 229–243.

Philippu, A. 1970. Release of catecholamines from the hypothalamus by drugs and electrical stimulation. *Bayer-Symposium II*, 258–267.

Philippu, A., G. Heyd and A. Burger. 1970. Release of noradrenaline from the hypothalamus *in vivo. Europ. J. Pharmacol.* **9**: 52–58.

Philippu, A., H. Przuntek, G. Heyd and A. Burger. 1971. Central effects of sympathomimetic amines on the blood pressure. *Europ. J. Pharmacol.* **15**: 200–208.

Phillis, J. W. and K. Jhamandas. 1971. The effects of chlorpromazine and ethanol on *in vivo* release of acetylcholine from the cerebral cortex. *Comp. Gen. Pharmacol.* **2**: 306–310.

Phillis, J. W. and D. H. York. 1968. Pharmacological studies on a cholinergic inhibition in the cerebral cortex. *Brain Res.* **10**: 297–306.

Phillis, J. W., A. K. Tebēcis and D. H. York. 1968. Acetylcholine release from the feline thalamus. *J. Pharm. Pharmac.* **20**: 476–478.

Pickford, M. 1947. The action of acetylcholine in the supraoptic nucleus of the chloralosed dog. *J. Physiol.* **106**: 264–270.

Pitts, R. F., H. W. Magoun and S. W. Ranson. 1939. Localization of the medullary respiratory centers in the cat. *Amer. J. Physiol.* **126**: 673–688.

Plekss, O. J. and S. Margolin. 1968. Further evidence for an unique neurohumoral agent released from brain by morphine given intracerebrally. *Proc. Soc. Exptl. Biol. Med.* **128**: 317–321.

Poirier, L. J., P. Langelier, A. Roberge, R. Boucher and A. Kitsikis. 1972. Non-specific histopathological changes induced by the intracerebral injection of 6-hydroxy-dopamine (6-OH-DA). *J. Neurol. Sci.* **16**: 401–416.

Pomerat, C. M., W. J. Hendelman, C. W. Raiborn, Jr. and J. F. Massey. 1967. Dynamic activities of nervous tissue *in vitro*, pp. 119-178. *In* H. Hydén (ed.) *The Neuron.* Elsevier Publishing Company, Amsterdam.

Popova, N. K., L. N. Maslova and E. V. Naumenko. 1972. Serotonin and the regulation of the pituitary-adrenal system after deafferentation of the hypothalamus. *Brain Res.* **47:** 61-67.

Portig, P. J. and M. Vogt. 1969. Release into the cerebral ventricles of substances with possible transmitter function in the caudate nucleus. *J. Physiol.* **204:** 687-715.

Portig, P. J., D. F. Sharman and M. Vogt. 1968. Release by tubocurarine of dopamine and homovanillic acid from the superfused caudate nucleus. *J. Physiol.* **194:** 565-572.

Powers, J. B. 1972. Facilitation of lordosis in ovariectomized rats by intracerebral progesterone implants. *Brain Res.* **48:** 311-325.

Powley, T. L. and R. E. Keesey. 1970. Relationship of body weight to the lateral hypothalamic feeding syndrome. *J. Comp. Physiol. Psychol.* **70:** 25-36.

Prado-Alcalá, R. A., J. Grinberg-Zylberbaun, J. Alvarez-Leefmans, A. Gómez, S. Singer, and H. Brust-Carmona. 1972. A possible caudate-cholinergic mechanism in two instrumental conditioned responses. *Psychopharmacologia.* **25:** 339-346.

Price, H. L., M. L. Price and H. T. Morse. 1965. Effects of cyclopropane, halothane, and procaine on the vasomotor "center" of the dog. *Anesthesiology.* **26:** 55-60.

Przuntek, H., S. Guimarães and A. Philippu. 1971. Importance of adrenergic neurons of the brain for the rise of blood pressure evoked by hypothalamic stimulation. *Naunyn-Schmied. Arch. Pharmakol.* **271:** 311-319.

Quadagno, D. M., J. Shryne and R. A. Gorski. 1971. The inhibition of steroid-induced sexual behavior by intrahypothalamic actinomycin-D[1]. *Horm. Behav.* **2:** 1-10.

Quartermain, D. and N. E. Miller. 1966. Sensory feedback in time-response of drinking elicited by carbachol in preoptic area of rat. *J. Comp. Physiol. Psychol.* **62:** 350-353.

Rabin, B. M. 1972. Ventromedial hypothalamic control of food intake and satiety: a reappraisal. *Brain Res.* **43:** 317-342.

Rakić, L., N. A. Buchwald and E. J. Wyers. 1962. Induction of seizures by stimulation of the caudate nucleus. *EEG Clin. Neurophysiol.* **14:** 809-823.

Ralph, C. L. and R. M. Fraps. 1959. Effect of hypothalamic lesions on progesterone-induced ovulation in the hen. *Endocrinology.* **65:** 819-824.

Ralph, C. L. and R. M. Fraps. 1960. Induction of ovulation in the hen by injection of progesterone into the brain. *Endocrinology.* **66:** 269-272.

Ralston, B. L. and C. Ajmone-Marsan. 1956. Thalamic control of certain normal and abnormal cortical rhythms. *EEG Clin. Neurophysiol.* **8:** 559-582.

Ralston, B. L. and H. Langer. 1965. Experimental epilepsy of brain-stem origin. *EEG Clin. Neurophysiol.* **18:** 325-333.

Ramírez, V. D. and S. M. McCann. 1963. Comparison of the regulation of luteinizing hormone (LH) secretion in immature and adult rats. *Endocrinology.* **72:** 452-464.

Ramírez, V. D. and S. M. McCann. 1964. Induction of prolactin secretion by implants of estrogen into the hypothalamo-hypophysial region of female rats. *Endocrinology.* **75:** 206-214.

Ramírez, V. D., R. M. Abrams and S. M. McCann. 1964. Effect of estradiol implants in the hypothalamo-hypophysial region of the rat on the secretion of luteinizing hormone. *Endocrinology.* **75:** 243-248.

Randić, M. and A. Padjen. 1968. The release of 5-hydroxytryptamine in the brain by mid-brain stimulation. *Jugoslav. Physiol. Pharmacol. Acta* 4, Suppl. 1, 215-220.

Randrup, A. and I. Munkvad. 1968. Behavioural stereotypies induced by pharmacological agents. *Pharmakopsychiatrie-Neuro-Psychopharmakologie.* **1:** 18-26.

Randrup, A. and I. Munkvad. 1970. Biochemical, anatomical and psychological investigations of stereotyped behavior induced by amphetamines, pp. 695-713. *In* E. Costa and S. Garattini (eds.) *Amphetamines and Related Compounds.* Raven Press, New York.

Ranson, S. W. 1916. New evidence in favor of a chief vasoconstrictor center in the brain. *Amer. J. Physiol.* **42**: 1–8.

Ranson, S. W. 1940. Regulation of body temperature, pp. 342–399. *In: The Hypothalamus and Central Levels of Autonomic Function.* Williams and Wilkins Co., Baltimore.

Ranson, S. W. and P. R. Billingsley. 1916. Vasomotor reactions from stimulation of the floor of the fourth ventricle. *Amer. J. Physiol.* **41**: 85–90.

Ranson, S. W. and H. W. Magoun. 1939. The hypothalamus. *Ergeb. Physiol. Biol. Chem. Exp. Pharmakol.* **41**: 56–163.

Rech, R. H. and E. F. Domino. 1959. Observations on injections of drugs into the brain substance. *Arch. Int. Pharmacodyn. Ther.* **121**: 429–442.

Redgate, E. S. and E. Gellhorn. 1956a. The tonic effects of the posterior hypothalamus on blood pressure and pulse rate as disclosed by the action of intrahypothalamically injected drugs. *Arch. Int. Pharmacodyn. Ther.* **105**: 193–198.

Redgate, E. S. and E. Gellhorn. 1956b. The alteration of anterior hypothalamic excitability through intrahypothalamic injections of drugs and its significance for the measurement of parasympathetic hypothalamic excitability in the intact organism. *Arch. Int. Pharmacodyn. Ther.* **105**: 199–208.

Reichlin, S. 1966. Control of thyrotropic hormone secretion, pp. 445–536. *In* L. Martini and W. F. Ganong (eds.) *Neuroendocrinology,* Vol. 1. Academic Press, New York.

Reichlin, S., E. M. Volpert and S. C. Werner. 1966. Hypothalamic influence on thyroxine monodeiodination by rat anterior pituitary gland. *Endocrinology.* **78**: 302–306.

Reigle, T. G. and H. H. Wolf. 1971. The effects of centrally administered chlorpromazine on temperature regulation in the hamster. *Life Sci.* **10**: 121–132.

Reis, D. J. and K. Fuxe. 1969. Brain norepinephrine: evidence that neuronal release is essential for sham rage behavior following brainstem transection in cat. *Proc. Natl. Acad. Sci.* **64**: 108–112.

Reis, D. J., D. T. Moorhead II and N. Merlino. 1970. Dopa-induced excitement in the cat. *Arch. Neurol.* **22**: 31–39.

Reiter, R. J. and F. Fraschini. 1969. Endocrine aspects of the mammalian pineal gland: a review. *Neuroendocrinology.* **5**: 219–255.

Repin, I. S. and I. L. Kratskin. 1967. Hypothalamic mechanisms of fever. *Fiziol. Zh. SSSR.* **53**: 1206–1211.

Rewerski, W. J. and W. Gumulka. 1969. The effect of α-MT on hyperthermia induced by chlorpromazine. *Int. J. Neuropharmacol.* **8**: 389–391.

Rewerski, W. J. and A. Jori. 1968a. Microinjection of chlorpromazine in different parts of rat brain. *Int. J. Neuropharmacol.* **7**: 359–364.

Rewerski, W. J. and A. Jori. 1968b. Effect of desipramine injected intracerebrally in normal or reserpinized rats. *J. Pharm. Pharmac.* **20**: 293–296.

Reynolds, R. W. and C. W. Simpson. 1969a. Pulmonary edema induced by intracranial carbachol infusion in rabbits and rats. *Physiol. Behav.* **4**: 635–639.

Reynolds, R. W. and C. W. Simpson. 1969b. Chronic infusion studies on the hypothalamic regulation of food intake. *Ann. N. Y. Acad. Sci.* **157**: 755–757.

Richard, R. 1966. Estrogen effects on pituitary-adrenal function via the hypothalamus and hypophysis. *Neuroendocrinology.* **1**: 322–332.

Richter, C. P. 1935. The primacy of polyuria in diabetes insipidus. *Amer. J. Physiol.* **112**: 481–487.

Richter, D. 1964. *Comparative Neurochemistry.* Pergamon Press, Oxford, pp. 1–491.

Riddell, D. and J. C. Szerb. 1971. The release *in vivo* of dopamine synthesized from labelled precursors in the caudate nucleus of the cat. *J. Neurochem.* **18**: 989–1006.

Rindi, G., G. Sciorelli, M. Poloni and F. Acanfora. 1972. Induction of ingestive responses by cAMP applied into the rat hypothalamus. *Experientia.* **28**: 1047–1049.

Ringle, D. A. and B. L. Herndon. 1969. Effects on rats of CSF from sleep-deprived rabbits. *Pflügers Arch.* **306**: 320–328.

Robinson, B. W. 1964. Forebrain alimentary responses: some organizational principles, pp. 411–427. *In* M. J. Wayner (ed.) *Thirst.* Pergamon Press, Oxford.

Robinson, B. W. and M. Mishkin. 1968. Alimentary responses to forebrain stimulation in monkeys. *Exp. Brain Res.* 4: 330–366.

Rodgers, C. H. and O. T. Law. 1968. Effects of chemical stimulation of the "limbic system" on lordosis in female rats. *Physiol. Behav.* 3: 241–246.

Rogozea, R., J. Ungher and V. Florea-Ciocoiu. 1969. The influence of intrahippocampal gamma-amino-butyric acid on the orienting reflex. *EEG Clin. Neurophysiol.* 27: 162–168.

Rogozea, R., J. Ungher and V. Florea-Ciocoiu. 1971. The effect of intrahippocampal acetylcholine on the orienting reflex. *Revue Roumaine Neurol.* 8: 237–253.

Rolls, B. J. and B. P. Jones. 1972. Cessation of drinking following intracranial injections of angiotensin in the rat. *J. Comp. Physiol. Psychol.* 80: 26–29.

Rolls, B. J., B. P. Jones and D. J. Fallows. 1972. A comparison of the motivational properties of thirst induced by intracranial angiotensin and by water deprivation. *Physiol. Behav.* 9: 777–782.

Rose, S. P. R. 1969. Neurochemical correlates of learning and environmental change. *Febs. Letters.* 5: 305–312.

Rose, S. and J. F. Nelson. 1957. The direct effect of oestradiol on the pars distalis. *Austral. J. Exp. Biol.* 35: 605–610.

Rose, S., J. Nelson and T. R. Bradley. 1960. Regulation of TSH release. *Ann. N. Y. Acad. Sci.* 86: 647–666.

Rosendorff, C. and W. I. Cranston. 1971. Effects of intrahypothalamic and intraventricular norepinephrine and 5-hydroxytryptamine on hypothalamic blood flow in the conscious rabbit. *Circ. Res.* 28: 492–502.

Rosendorff, C. and J. J. Mooney. 1971. Central nervous system sites of action of a purified leucocyte pyrogen. *Amer. J. Physiol.* 220: 597–603.

Rosendorff, C., R. D. Lowe, H. Lavery and W. I. Cranston. 1970. Cardiovascular effects of angiotensin mediated by the central nervous system of the rabbit. *Cardiov. Res.* 4: 36–43.

Rosenthal, F. E. 1941. Cooling drugs and cooling centres. *J. Pharmacol. Exptl. Ther.* 71: 305–314.

Ross, J., C. Claybaugh, L. G. Clemens and R. A. Gorski. 1971. Short latency induction of estrous behavior with intracerebral gonadal hormones in ovariectomized rats. *Endocrinology.* 89: 32–38.

Roth, L. J. and C. F. Barlow. 1961. Drugs in the brain—autoradiography and radioassay techniques permit analysis of penetration by labeled drugs. *Science.* 134: 22–31.

Roth, R. H., L. Allikmets and J. M. R. Delgado. 1969. Synthesis and release of noradrenaline and dopamine from discrete regions of monkey brain. *Arch. Int. Pharmacodyn. Ther.* 181: 273–282.

Routtenberg, A. 1965. The effects of chemical stimulation in dorsal midbrain tegmentum on self-stimulation in hypothalamus and septal area. *Psychon. Sci.* 3: 41–42.

Routtenberg, A. 1967. Drinking induced by carbachol: thirst circuit or ventricular modification? *Science.* 157: 838–839.

Routtenberg, A. 1972. Intracranial chemical injection and behavior: a critical review. *Behav. Biol.* 7: 601–641.

Routtenberg, A. and J. Olds. 1966. Stimulation of dorsal midbrain during septal and hypothalamic self-stimulation. *J. Comp. Physiol. Psychol.* 62: 250–255.

Routtenberg, A. and J. B. Simpson. 1971. Carbachol-induced drinking at ventricular and subfornical organ sites of application. *Life Sci.* 10: 481–490.

Routtenberg, A., J. Sladek and W. Bondareff. 1968. Histochemical fluorescence after application of neurochemicals to caudate nucleus and septal area *in vivo. Science.* 161: 272–274.

Roux, E. and A. Borrel. 1898. Tétanos cérébral et immunité contrele tétanos. *Ann. l'Inst. Pasteur.* 12: 225–239.

Rozear, M., R. DeGroof and G. Somjen. 1971. Effects of micro-iontophoretic administration of divalent metal ions on neurons of the central nervous system of cats. *J. Pharmacol. Exptl. Ther.* **176**: 109–118.

Rudy, T. A. and H. H. Wolf. 1971. The effect of intrahypothalamically injected sympathomimetic amines on temperature regulation in the cat. *J. Pharmacol. Exptl. Ther.* **179**: 218–235.

Rudy, T. A. and H. H. Wolf. 1972. Effect of intracerebral injections of carbamylcholine and acetylcholine on temperature regulation in the cat. *Brain Res.* **38**: 117–130.

Ruf, K. and F. A. Steiner. 1967. Steroid-sensitive single neurons in rat hypothalamus and midbrain: identification by microelectrophoresis. *Science.* **156**: 667–669.

Russek, M. and S. Piña. 1962. Conditioning of adrenalin anorexia. *Nature.* **193**: 1296–1297.

Russek, M., G. J. Mogenson and J. A. F. Stevenson. 1967. Calorigenic, hyperglycemic and anorexigenic effects of adrenaline and noradrenaline. *Physiol. Behav.* **2**: 429–433.

Russel, M. J., M. S. Godsey and K. W. Lydell. 1972. Omnitrode: a simple cannula for chemical and bipolar electrical stimulation. *Physiol. Behav.* **8**: 773–775.

Russell, R. W., G. Singer, F. Flanagan, M. Stone and J. W. Russell. 1968. Quantitative relations in amygdaloid modulation of drinking. *Physiol. Behav.* **3**: 871–875.

Russell, S. M., A. P. S. Dhariwal, S. M. McCann and F. E. Yates. 1969. Inhibition by dexamethasone of the *in vivo* pituitary response to corticotropin-releasing factor (CRF). *Endocrinology.* **85**: 512–521.

Sahlgren, E. 1934. Experimentelle Untersuchungen über den Angriffsupnkt des Luminals im Gehirn bei Kaninchen. *Acta Psychiat. Neurol. Scand.* **9**: 129–147.

Sala, M. A., J. T. Otegui, W. L. Benedetti, J. M. Monti and E. Griñó. 1971. Blockade of ovarian compensatory hypertrophy and ovulation in the rat by hypothalamic implants of an anticholinergic drug. *J. Neuro-Visceral Relat.* **32**: 241–248.

Salama, S. and S. Wright. 1950. Action of *d*-tubocurarine chloride on the central nervous system of the cat. *Brit. J. Pharmacol.* **5**: 49–61.

Satinoff, E. 1967. Disruption of hibernation caused by hypothalamic lesions. *Science.* **155**: 1031–1033.

Sawyer, C. H. 1959. Nervous control of ovulation, pp. 1–20. *In* C. W. Lloyd (ed.) *Recent Progress in the Endocrinology of Reproduction.* Academic Press, New York.

Sawyer, C. H. and J. Hilliard. 1971. Sites of feedback action of estrogen and progesterone. *Excp. Med. Int. Cong.* **219**: 716–721.

Scapagnini, U., G. R. Van Loon, G. P. Moberg and W. F. Ganong. 1970. Effect of α-methyl-p-tyrosine on the circadian variation of plasma corticosterone in rats. *Europ. J. Pharmacol.* **11**: 266–268.

Scaramuzzi, O. E., C. A. Baile and J. Mayer. 1971. Prostaglandins and food intake of rats. *Experientia.* **27**: 256–257.

Schain, R. J. 1960. Neurohumors and other pharmacologically active substances in cerebrospinal fluid: a review of the literature. *Yale J. Biol. Med.* **33**: 15–36.

Schally, A. V., A. Arimura, C. Y. Bowers, A. B. Kastin, S. Sawano and T. W. Redding. 1968. Hypothalamic neurohormones regulating anterior pituitary function. *Rec. Prog. Hormone Res.* **24**: 497–588.

Scharrer, E. 1965. The final common path in neuroendocrine integration. *Arch. Anat. Microscop.* **54**: 359–370.

Scherp, H. W. and C. F. Church. 1937. Neurotoxic action of aluminum salts. *Proc. Soc. Exptl. Biol. Med.* **36**: 851–853.

Schmaltz, L. W. 1971. Deficit in active avoidance learning in rats following penicillin injection into hippocampus. *Physiol. Behav.* **6**: 667–674.

Schneider, H. P. G. and S. M. McCann. 1970. Dopaminergic pathways and gonadotropin releasing factors, pp. 177–191. *In* W. Bargmann and B. Scharrer (eds.) *Aspects of Neuroendocrinology.* Springer-Verlag, Heidelberg.

Schoenenberger, G. A., L. B. Cueni, M. Monnier and A. M. Hatt. 1972. Humoral transmission of sleep. VII. Isolation and physical-chemical characterization of the "sleep inducing factor delta." *Pflügers Arch.* **338:** 1–17.

Schreiner, L. and A. Kling. 1953. Behavioral changes following rhinencephalic injury in cat. *J. Neurophysiol.* **16:** 643–659.

Schubert, P., H. Teschemacher, G. W. Kreutzberg and A. Herz. 1970. Intracerebral distribution pattern of radioactive morphine and morphine-like drugs after intraventricular and intrathecal injection. *Histochemie.* **22:** 277–288.

Schuman, M. and R. L. Isaacson. 1970. Penicillin-induced epileptogenic foci in the rat cortex. *Psychon. Sci.* **18:** 185–186.

Schütz, J. 1916. Zur Kenntnis der Wirkung des Magnesiums auf die Körpertemperatur. *Arch. Exper. Pathol. Pharmakol.* **79:** 285–290.

Sciorelli, G., M. Poloni and G. Rindi. 1972. Evidence of cholinergic mediation of ingestive responses elicited by dibutyryl-adenosine-3', 5'-monophosphate in rat hypothalamus. *Brain Res.* **48:** 427–431.

Scotti de Carolis, A., H. Ziegler, P. Del Basso and V. G. Longo. 1971. Central effects of 6-hydroxydopamine. *Physiol. Behav.* **7:** 705–708.

Seager, L. D. and C. D. Wood. 1962. Aconitine induced pulmonary edema. *Proc. Soc. Exptl. Biol. Med.* **111:** 120–121.

Segura, E. T., A. O. R. De Juan, J. A. Colombo and A. Kacelnik. 1971. The sexual clasp as a reticularly controlled behavior in the toad, *Bufo arenarum* Hensel. *Physiol. Behav.* **7:** 157–160.

Selye, H. 1956. *The Stress of Life.* McGraw-Hill Book Company, Inc., New York, pp. 1–324.

Sepinwall, J. 1966. Cholinergic stimulation of the brain and avoidance behavior. *Psychon. Sci.* **5:** 93–94.

Sepinwall, J. 1969. Enhancement and impairment of avoidance behavior by chemical stimulation of the hypothalamus. *J. Comp. Physiol. Psychol.* **68:** 393–399.

Sepinwall, J. and F. S. Grodsky. 1969. Effects of cholinergic stimulation or blockade of the rat hypothalamus on discrete-trial conflict behavior. *Life Sci.* **8:** 45–52.

Severs, W. B., A. E. Daniels, H. H. Smookler, W. J. Kinnard and J. P. Buckley. 1966. Interrelationship between angiotensin II and the sympathetic nervous system. *J. Pharmacol. Exptl. Ther.* **153:** 530–537.

Shani, J., G. S. Knaggs and J. S. Tindal. 1971. The effect of noradrenaline, dopamine, 5-hydroxytryptamine and melatonin on milk yield and composition in the rabbit. *J. Endocrinol.* **50:** 543–544.

Share, L. and J. R. Claybaugh. 1972. Regulation of body fluids. *Ann. Rev. Physiol.* **34:** 235–260.

Sharpe, L. G. and R. D. Myers. 1969. Feeding and drinking following stimulation of the diencephalon of the monkey with amines and other substances. *Exp. Brain Res.* **8:** 295–310.

Sheth, U. K. and H. L. Borison. 1960. Central pyrogenic action of *Salmonella typhosa* lipopolysaccharide injected into the lateral cerebral ventricle in cats. *J. Pharmacol. Exptl. Ther.* **130:** 411–417.

Shirao, T. 1969. Effects of alumina cream lesions in the substantia nigra or on the cortex of cats. *Acta Med. Univ. Kagoshima.* **11:** 79–96.

Shore, P. A. 1972. Transport and storage of biogenic amines. *Ann. Rev. Pharmacol.* **12:** 209–226.

Shute, C. C. D. and P. R. Lewis. 1967. The ascending cholinergic reticular system: neocortical, olfactory and subcortical projections. *Brain.* **90:** 497–520.

Siggins, G. R., B. J. Hoffer and F. E. Bloom. 1970. Studies on norepinephrine-containing afferents to purkinje cells of rat cerebellum. III. Evidence for mediation of norepinephrine effects by cyclic 3',5'-adenosine monophosphate. *Brain Res.* **25:** 535–553.

Simpson, J. B. and A. Routtenberg. 1972. The subfornical organ and carbachol-induced drinking. *Brain Res.* **45:** 135–152.

Singer, G. and J. Kelly. 1972. Cholinergic and adrenergic interaction in the hypothalamic control of drinking and eating behavior. *Physiol. Behav.* **8:** 885–890.

Singer, G. and R. B. Montgomery. 1968. Neurohumoral interaction in the rat amygdala after central chemical stimulation. *Science.* **160:** 1017–1018.

Singer, G. and R. B. Montgomery. 1969. Functional relationship of lateral hypothalamus and amygdala in control of drinking. *Physiol. Behav.* **4:** 505–507.

Singer, G. and R. B. Montgomery. 1970. Functional relationships of brain circuits in control of drinking behavior. *Life Sci.* **9:** 91–97.

Singer, G., A. Ho and S. Gershon. 1971. Changes in activity of choline acetylase in central nervous system of rat after intraventricular administration of noradrenaline. *Nature New Biol.* **230:** 152–153.

Singer, G., I. Sanghvi and S. Gershon. 1972. Exploration of certain behavioral patterns induced by psychoactive agents in the rat. *Commun. Behav. Biol.* **6:** 307–314.

Slangen, J. L. and N. E. Miller. 1969. Pharmacological tests for the function of hypothalamic norepinephrine in eating behavior. *Physiol. Behav.* **4:** 543–552.

Slusher, M. A. 1966. Effects of cortisol implants in the brainstem and ventral hippocampus on diurnal corticosteroid levels. *Exp. Brain Res.* **1:** 184–194.

Slusher, M. A., J. E. Hyde and M. Laufer. 1966. Effect of intracerebral hydrocortisone on unit activity of diencephalon and midbrain in cats. *J. Neurophysiol.* **29:** 157–169.

Smelik, P. G. 1967. ACTH secretion after depletion of hypothalamic monoamines by reserpine implants. *Neuroendocrinology.* **2:** 247–254.

Smelik, P. G. 1969. The effect of a CRF preparation on ACTH release in rats bearing hypothalamic dexamethasone implants: a study on the "implantation paradox." *Neuroendocrinology.* **5:** 193–204.

Smelik, P. G. and A. M. Ernst. 1966. Role of nigro-neostriatal dopaminergic fibers in compulsive gnawing behavior in rats. *Life Sci.* **5:** 1485–1488.

Smelik, P. G. and C. H. Sawyer. 1962. Effects of implantation of cortisol into the brain stem or pituitary gland on the adrenal response to stress in the rabbit. *Acta Endocrinol.* **41:** 561–570.

Smith, C. J. V. 1972. Hypothalamic glucoreceptors—the influence of gold thioglucose implants in the ventromedial and lateral hypothalamic areas of normal and diabetic rats. *Physiol. Behav.* **9:** 391–396.

Smith, C. J. V. and D. L. Britt. 1971. Obesity in the rat induced by hypothalamic implants of gold thioglucose. *Physiol. Behav.* **7:** 7–10.

Smith, D. E., M. B. King and B. G. Hoebel. 1970. Lateral hypothalamic control of killing: evidence for a cholinoceptive mechanism. *Science.* **167:** 900–901.

Smith, E. R. and J. M. Davidson. 1967. Differential responses to hypothalamic testosterone in relation to male puberty. *Amer. J. Physiol.* **212:** 1385–1390.

Smith, E. R. and J. M. Davidson. 1968. Role of estrogen in the cerebral control of puberty in female rats. *Endocrinology.* **82:** 100–108.

Smith, E. R., R. F. Weick and J. M. Davidson. 1969. Influence of intracerebral progesterone on the reproductive system of female rats. *Endocrinology.* **85:** 1129–1136.

Smith, E. R., J. Johnson, R. F. Weick, S. Levine and J. M. Davidson. 1971. Inhibition of the reproductive system in immature rats by intracerebral implantation of cortisol. *Neuroendocrinology.* **8:** 94–106.

Smith, G. P., A. J. Strohmayer and D. J. Reis. 1972. Effect of lateral hypothalamic injections of 6-hydroxydopamine on food and water intake in rats. *Nature New Biol.* **235:** 27–29.

Smith, O. A. 1956. Stimulation of lateral and medial hypothalamus and food intake in tne rat. *Anat. Rec.* **124:** 363–364.

Smith, O. A. 1965. Cardiovascular integration by the central nervous system, pp. 684–689. *In* T. C. Ruch and H. D. Patton (eds.) *Physiology and Biophysics.* W. H. Saunders, Philadelphia.

Smythies, J. R. 1972. The adenylcyclase complex: a model of its mechanism of action in relation to the α- and β-adrenergic receptors. *Europ. J. Pharmacol.* **19:** 18–24.

Snider, R. S. and W. T. Niemer. 1961. *A Stereotaxic Atlas of the Cat Brain.* U. of Chicago Press, Chicago.

Sommer, S. R., D. Novin and M. LeVine. 1967. Food and water intake after intrahypothalamic injections of carbachol in the rabbit. *Science.* **156:** 983–984.

Soulairac, A. 1958. Les régulations psycho-physiologiques de la faim. *J. Physiol. (Paris).* **50:** 663–783.

Sparber, S. B. and H. A. Tilson. 1972. Schedule controlled and drug induced release of norepinephrine-7-^{3}H into the lateral ventricle of rats. *Neuropharmacology.* **11:** 453–464.

Spector, N. H., J. R. Brobeck and C. L. Hamilton. 1968. Feeding and core temperature in albino rats: changes induced by preoptic heating and cooling. *Science.* **161:** 286–288.

Spencer, J. and F. A. Holloway. 1972. Differentiation between carbachol and eserine during deprivation-induced drinking in the rat. *Psychon. Sci.* **28:** 16–18.

Spiegel, E. A. and E. G. Szekely. 1961. Prolonged stimulation of the head of the caudate nucleus. *Arch. Neurol.* **4:** 55–65.

Spiegel, E. A., E. G. Szekely and D. Zivanovic. 1968. Striatal bradykinesia alleviated by intracaudate injection of L-dopa. *Experientia.* **24:** 39–40.

Spiegel, E. A., H. T. Wycis, E. G. Szekely, A. Constantinovici, J. J. Egyed, P. Gildenberg, R. Lehman and M. Werthan. 1965. Role of the caudate nucleus in Parkinsonian bradykinesia. *Confin. Neurol.* **26:** 336–341.

Squire, L. R. and S. H. Barondes. 1970. Actinomycin-D: effects on memory at different times after training. *Nature.* **225:** 649–650.

Staib, A. H. and K. Andreas. 1970. Untersuchungen zur Lokalisation cholinerger Rezeptoren mit thermoregulatorishen Aktivität in Rattenhirn. *Acta Biol. Med. Germ.* **25:** 605–611.

Stamm, J. S. and M. Knight. 1963. Learning of visual tasks by monkeys with epileptogenic implants in temporal cortex. *J. Comp. Physiol. Psychol.* **56:** 254–260.

Stamm, J. S. and S. C. Rosen. 1971. Learning on somesthetic discrimination and reversal tasks by monkeys with epileptogenic implants in anteromedial temporal cortex. *Neuropsychologia.* **9:** 185–194.

Stamm, J. S. and A. Warren. 1961. Learning and retention by monkeys with epileptogenic implants in posterior parietal cortex. *Epilepsia.* **2:** 229–242.

Stark, P., J. A. Turk and C. W. Totty. 1971. Reciprocal adrenergic and cholinergic control of hypothalamic elicited eating and satiety. *Amer. J. Physiol.* **220:** 1516–1521.

Stark, P., C. W. Totty, J. A. Turk and J. K. Henderson. 1968. A possible role of a cholinergic system affecting hypothalamic-elicited eating. *Amer. J. Physiol.* **214:** 463–468.

Stein, G. W. and R. A. Levitt. 1971. Lesion effects on cholinergically elicited drinking in the rat. *Physiol. Behav.* **7:** 517–522.

Stein, L. 1964. Reciprocal action of reward and punishment mechanisms, pp. 113–139. *In* R. G. Heath (ed.) *The Role of Pleasure in Behavior.* Harper & Row, New York.

Stein, L. 1968. Chemistry of reward and punishment, pp. 105–123. *In* D. H. Efron (ed.) *Psychopharmacology: A Review of Progress 1957–1967.* U.S. Govt. Printing Office, Washington, D.C.

Stein, L. and J. Seifter. 1962. Muscarinic synapses in the hypothalamus. *Amer. J. Physiol.* **202:** 751–756.

Stein, L. and C. D. Wise. 1969. Release of norepinephrine from hypothalamus and amygdala by rewarding medial forebrain bundle stimulation and amphetamine. *J. Comp. Physiol. Psychol.* **67**: 189–198.

Stein, L. and C. D. Wise. 1972. Possible etiology of schizophrenia: progressive damage to the noradrenergic reward system by endogenous 6-hydroxydopamine. *Neurotransmitters.* **50**: 298–314.

Stein, L., C. D. Wise and B. D. Berger. 1972. Noradrenergic reward mechanisms, recovery of function, and schizophrenia, pp. 81–103. *In* J. L. McGaugh (ed.) *The Chemistry of Mood, Motivation, and Memory.* Plenum Press, New York.

Steiner, F. A., K. Ruf and K. Akert. 1969. Steroid-sensitive neurones in rat brain: anatomical localization and responses to neurohumors and ACTH. *Brain Res.* **12**: 74–85.

Sterman, M. B. and C. D. Clemente. 1962. Forebrain inhibitory mechanisms: cortical synchronization induced by basal forebrain stimulation. *Exptl. Neurol.* **6**: 91–102.

Sternbach, R. A. 1968. *Pain: A Psychophysiological Analysis.* Academic Press, New York, pp. 1–185.

Stetson, M. H. 1972. Feedback regulation of testicular function in Japanese quail: testosterone implants in the hypothalamus and adenohypophysis. *Gen. Comp. Endocrinol.* **19**: 37–47.

Stevens, J. J., C. Kim and P. D. MacLean. 1961. Stimulation of caudate nucleus. *Arch. Neurol. (Chicago).* **4**: 47–54.

Stevenson, J. A. F. 1969. Neural control of food and water intake, pp. 524–621. *In* W. Haymaker, E. Anderson and W. J. H. Nauta (eds.) *The Hypothalamus.* Charles C Thomas, Springfield.

Strada, S. J. and F. Sulser. 1971. Comparative effects of *p*-chloroamphetamine and amphetamine on metabolism and *in vivo* release of ^{3}H-norepinphrine in the hypothalamus. *Europ. J. Pharmacol.* **15**: 45–51.

Strada, S. J. and F. Sulser. 1972. Effect of monoamine oxidase inhibitors on metabolism and *in vivo* release of H^3-norepinphrine from the hypothalamus. *Europ. J. Pharmacol.* **18**: 303–308.

Strashimirov, D. 1971. Thyroid function after implantation of thyroxine in the hypothalamus and anterior pituitary of rats. *Agressologie.* **12**: 45–50.

Strashimirov, D., B. Bohus and S. Kovács. 1969. Pituitary-thyroid function of the rat after suppression of ACTH release by dexamethasone implants in the median eminence. *Acta Physiol. Acad. Sci. Hung.* **35**: 335–344.

Stricker, E. M. and N. E. Miller. 1968. Saline preference and body fluid analyses in rats after intrahypothalamic injections of carbachol. *Physiol. Behav.* **3**: 471–475.

Ström, G. 1950. Influence of local thermal stimulation of the hypothalamus of the cat on cutaneous blood flow and respiratory rate. *Acta Physiol. Scand.* Suppl. 70, **20**:47–76.

Ström, G. 1960. Central nervous regulation of body temperature, pp. 1173–1196. *In* J. Field, H. W. Magoun and V. E. Hall (eds.) *Handbook of Physiology.* Vol. II. *Neurophysiology.* Williams and Wilkins, Baltimore.

Strongman, K. T. 1973. *The Psychology of Emotion.* John Wiley & Sons, London, pp. 1–235.

Struyker Boudier, H. A. J. and J. M. van Rossum. 1972. Clonidine-induced cardiovascular effects after stereotaxic application in the hypothalamus of rats. *J. Pharm. Pharmac.* **24**: 410–411.

Stunkard, A. J., B. Van Itallie and B. B. Reis. 1955. The mechanism of satiety: effect of glucagon on gastric hunger contractions in man. *Proc. Soc. Exptl. Biol. Med.* **89**: 258–261.

Suh, T. H., C. H. Wang and R. K. S. Lim. 1936. The effect of intracisternal applications of acetylcholine and the localization of the pressor centre and tract. *Chin. J. Physiol.* **10**: 61–78.

Sulser, F. and J. V. Dingell. 1968. Adrenergic mechanisms in the central action of tricyclic antidepressants and substituted phenothiazines. *Aggressologie.* **9**: 281–287.

Sulser, F., M. L. Owens, S. J. Strada and J. V. Dingell. 1969. Modification by desipramine (DMI) of the availability of norepinephrine released by reserpine in the hypothalamus of the rat *in vivo. J. Pharmacol. Exptl. Ther.* **168**: 272–282.

Sutin, J. 1966. The periventricular stratum of the hypothalamus, pp. 263–300. *In* C. C. Pfeiffer and J. R. Smythies (eds.) *International Review of Neurobiology,* Vol. 9. Academic Press, New York.

Sutin, J., L. Van Orden and T. Tsubokawa. 1963. Effect of catecholamines and brain stem stimulation upon the hypothalamic ventromedial nucleus, pp. 244–271. *In* G. H. Glaser (ed.) *EEG and Behavior.* Basic Books, New York.

Suzuki, M., M. Hiroi and S. Sugita. 1965. Ovulation in rabbits following intravenous and intracerebral administration of copper sulphate. *Acta Endocrinol.* **50**: 512–516.

Swanson, H. E. and J. J. van der Werff ten Bosch. 1964. The early-androgen syndrome; differences in response to pre-natal and post-natal administration of various doses of testosterone propionate in female and male rats. *Acta Endocrinol.* **47**: 37–50.

Swanson, L. W., V. J. Perez and L. G. Sharpe. 1972. Accurate and reliable intracerebral delivery of minute volumes of drug solutions. *J. Appl. Physiol.* **33**: 247–251.

Sweet, R. D. and D. J. Reis. 1971. Collection of [^{3}H] norepinephrine in ventriculo-cisternal perfusate during hypothalamic stimulation in cat. *Brain Res.* **33**: 584–588.

Sypert, G. W. and A. A. Ward. 1967. The hyperexcitable neuron: microelectrode studies of the chronic epileptic focus in the intact, awake monkey. *Exptl. Neurol.* **19**: 104–114.

Szekely, E. G. and E. A. Spiegel. 1963. Vertical nystagmus induced by injection of stimulating substances into the striatum, third, or lateral ventricle. *Neurology.* **13**: 306–314.

Szerb, J. C. 1964. The effect of tertiary and quaternary atropine on cortical acetylcholine output and on the electroencephalogram in cats. *Canad. J. Physiol. Pharmacol.* **42**: 303–314.

Szolcsányi, J., F. Joó and A. Jancsó-Gábor. 1971. Mitochondrial changes in preoptic neurones after capsiacin desensitization of the hypothalamic thermodetectors in rats. *Nature.* **229**: 116–117.

Tallian, F., Cs. Nyakas and E. Endröczi. 1972. Influence of intrahypothalamic estradiol and hydrocortisone implantation on the pituitary-adrenal and pituitary-ovary functions in the rat. *Endokrinologie.* **60**: 279–284.

Teitelbaum, P. and A. N. Epstein. 1962. The lateral hypothalamic syndrome: recovery of feeding and drinking after lateral hypothalamic lesions. *Psychol. Rev.* **69**: 74–90.

Telegdy, G., G. Schreiberg and E. Endröczi. 1964. Effects of oestrogens implanted into the hypothalamus on the activity of the pituitary-adrenocortical system. *Acta Physiol. Acad. Sci. Hung.* **25**: 229–234.

Terpstra, G. K. and J. L. Slangen. 1972a. Central blockade of (methyl-) atropine on carbachol drinking: a dose-response study. *Physiol. Behav.* **8**: 715–719.

Terpstra, G. K. and J. L. Slangen. 1972b. The role of the tractus diagonalis in drinking behaviour induced by central chemical stimulation, water deprivation and salt injection. *Neuropharmacology.* **11**: 807–817.

Thomalske, G. and S. Lyagoubi. 1969. Nouveau modèle d'un foyer épileptique amygdalien d'apparition très rapide et restant très focalisé. *Neurochirurgia.* **12**: 115–122.

Tilson, H. A. and S. B. Sparber. 1972. Studies on the concurrent behavioral and neurochemical effects of psychoactive drugs using the push-pull cannula. *J. Pharmacol. Exptl. Ther.* **181**: 387–398.

Tindal, J. S. and G. S. Knaggs. 1966. Lactogenesis in the pseudopregnant rabbit after the local placement of oestrogen in the brain. *J. Endocrinol.* **34**: ii–iii.

Tindal, J. S., G. S. Knaggs and A. Turvey. 1967. Central nervous control of prolactin secretion in the rabbit: effect of local oestrogen implants in the amygdaloid complex. *J. Endocrinol.* **37:** 279–287.

Toivola, P. and C. C. Gale. 1970. Effect on temperature of biogenic amine infusion into hypothalamus of baboon. *Neuroendocrinology.* **6:** 210–219.

Toivola, P. T. K. and C. C. Gale. 1972a. Stimulation of growth hormone release by microinjection of norepinephrine into hypothalamus of baboons. *Endocrinology.* **90:** 895–902.

Toivola, P. T. K. and C. C. Gale. 1972b. Central adrenergic regulation of growth hormone secretion in baboons. *Int. J. Neurosci.* **4:** 53–63.

Toivola, P. T. K., C. C. Gale, C. J. Goodner and J. H. Werrbach. 1972. Central α-adrenergic regulation of growth hormone and insulin. *Hormones.* **3:** 193–213.

Torda, C. 1968. Effect of changes of brain norepinephrine content on sleep cycle in rat. *Brain Res.* **10:** 200–207.

Trabka, J. 1967. Contribution to the formation of theta rhythm in cat hippocampus. *Acta Physiol. Polonica.* **18:** 699–706.

Trachtenberg, M. C., C. D. Hull and N. A. Buchwald. 1970. Electrophysiological concomitants of spreading depression in caudate and thalamic nuclei of the cat. *Brain Res.* **20:** 219–231.

Trzebski, A. 1960. The action of adrenaline, noradrenaline and monoamine oxidase inhibitors injected directly into the reticular formation of the brain stem. *Bull. Acad. Pol. Sci. Cl.* **8:** 525–528.

Tsou, K. and C. S. Jang. 1964. Studies on the site of analgesic action of morphine by intracerebral micro-injection. *Sci. Sinica.* **13:** 1099–1109.

Tushmalova, N. A. and I. V. Melkova. 1970. Food-procuring conditioned reflexes of rabbits after injection of ribonuclease into different regions of the hippocampal dorsal area. *Zh. Vyssh. Nerv. Deiat.* **20:** 519–523.

Tuttle, W. W. and H. W. Elliott. 1969. Electrographic and behavioral study of convulsants in the cat. *Anesthesiology.* **30:** 48–64.

Ungerstedt, U. 1968. 6-Hydroxy-dopamine induced degeneration of central monoamine neurons. *Europ. J. Pharmacol.* **5:** 107–110.

Ungerstedt, U. 1971a. Adipsia and aphagia after 6-hydroxydopamine induced degeneration of the nigro-striatal dopamine system. *Acta Physiol. Scand.* Suppl. 367, 95–122.

Ungerstedt, U. 1971b. Histochemical studies on the effect of intracerebral and intraventricular injections of 6-hydroxydopamine on monoamine neurons in the rat brain, pp. 101–127. *In* T. Malmfors and H. Thoenen (eds.) *6-Hydroxydopamine and Catecholamine Neurons.* North-Holland Publishing Company, Amsterdam.

Ungerstedt, U. and G. W. Arbuthnott. 1970. Quantitative recording of rotational behavior in rats after 6-hydroxy-dopamine lesions of the nigrostriatal dopamine system. *Brain Res.* **24:** 485–493.

Ungerstedt, U., L. L. Butcher, S. G. Butcher, N. E. Andén and K. Fuxe. 1969. Direct chemical stimulation of dopaminergic mechanisms in the neostriatum of the rat. *Brain Res.* **14:** 461–471.

Vahing, V. A. and L. H. Allikmets. 1970. Behavioral and visceral reactions elicited by chemical stimulation of the hypothalamus and septum in cats. *Sechenov Physiol. J. USSR.* **56:** 38–47.

Vahing, V. A., L. H. Allikmets and I. P. Lapin. 1968. Onset of vomiting after microinjections of serotonin into the hypothalamus, septum and amygdala of cats receiving imimpramine. *Bull. Exp. Biol. Med. USSR.* **66:** 48–51.

Vahing, V. A., L. H. Allikmets and L. S. Mehilane. 1972. The influence of antidepressants and neuroleptics on emotional reaction provoked by cholinergic stimulation of the hypothalamus and mesencephalon. *Farmacol. Toxicol.* **35:** 398–401.

Vahing, V. A., L. S. Mehilane and L. H. Allikmets. 1971. Neurochemical analysis of hypothalamic and midbrain effector centres regulating emotional behavior. *J. High. Nerv. Act.* **21**: 551–558.

Valenstein, E. S., V. C. Cox and J. W. Kakolewski. 1970. Reexamination of the role of the hypothalamus in motivation. *Psychol. Rev.* **77**: 16–31.

Valzelli, L. 1964. A simple method to inject drugs intracerebrally. *Med. Exp.* **11**: 23–26.

Valzelli, L. 1972. Psychoactive drugs and brain neurochemical transmitters. *Arch. Int. Pharmacodyn. Ther.* **196**: 221–228.

Vane, J. R. 1971. Inhibition of prostaglandin synthesis as a mechanism of action for aspirin-like drugs. *Nature New Biol.* **231**: 232–235.

Várszegi, M. K. and L. Decsi. 1967. Some characteristics of the rage reaction evoked by chemical stimulation of the hypothalamus. *Acta Physiol. Acad. Sci Hung.* **32**: 61–68.

Veale, W. L. 1972. A stereotaxic method for the push-pull perfusion of discrete regions of brain tissue of the unanesthetized rabbit. *Brain Res.* **42**: 479–481.

Veale, W. L. and R. D. Myers. 1971. Emotional behavior, arousal and sleep produced by sodium and calcium ions perfused within the hypothalamus of the cat. *Physiol. Behav.* **7**: 601–607.

Velluti, R. and R. Hernández-Peón. 1963. Atropine blockade within a cholinergic hypnogenic circuit. *Exptl. Neurol.* **8**: 20–29.

Vermes, I. and G. Telegdy. 1972. Effect of intraventricular injection and intrahypothalamic implantation of serotonin on the hypothalamo-hypophyseal-adrenal system in the rat. *Acta Physiol. Acad. Sci. Hung.* **42**: 49–59.

Verney, E. B. 1947. The antidiuretic hormone and the factors which determine its release. *Proc. Roy. Soc. (London). B.* **135**: 25–106.

Vernikos-Danellis, J. 1964. Estimation of corticotropin-releasing activity of rat hypothalamus and neurohypophysis before and after stress. *Endocrinology.* **75**: 514–520.

Villablanca, J. 1962. Electroencephalogram in the permanently isolated forebrain of the cat. *Science.* **138**: 44–46.

Villablanca, J. and R. D. Myers. 1964. Fever production by endotoxin injections in the cat. *Arch. Biol. Med. Exp.* **1**: 102.

Villablanca, J. and R. D. Myers. 1965. Fever produced by microinjection of typhoid vaccine into hypothalamus of cats. *Amer. J. Physiol.* **208**: 703–707.

Vincent, J. D. and J. N. Hayward. 1970. Activity of single cells in the osmoreceptor-supraoptic nuclear complex in the hypothalamus of the waking rhesus monkey. *Brain Res.* **23**: 105–108.

Vincent, J. D., E. Arnauld and B. Bioulac. 1972. Activity of osmosensitive single cells in the hypothalamus of the behaving monkey during drinking. *Brain Res.* **44**: 371–384.

Voiculescu, V. and I. Voinescu. 1968. Experimental seizures of thalamic origin. *Revue Roumaine de Neurol.* **5**: 313–318.

Voogt, J. L., J. A. Clemens and J. Meites. 1969. Stimulation of pituitary FSH release in immature female rats by prolactin implant in median eminence. *Neuroendocrinology.* **4**: 157–163.

de Vries, R. A. C. 1972. Abolition of the effect of pinealectomy on hypothalamic magnocellular neurosecretory activity in male rats by hypothalamic pineal implants. *Neuroendocrinology.* **9**: 358–364.

Wade, G. N. 1972. Gonadal hormones and behavioral regulation of body weight. *Physiol. Behav.* **8**: 523–534.

Wade, G. N. and I. Zucker. 1970. Modulation of food intake and locomotor activity in female rats by diencephalic hormone implants. *J. Comp. Physiol. Psychol.* **72**: 328–336.

Van Wagenen, W. P. and C. T. Liu. 1952. Procaine block of frontal lobe white fibers as a means of predicting the effect of prefrontal lobotomy. II. Clinical evaluation. *J. Neurosurg.* **9**: 30–51.

Wagner, J. W. and J. de Groot. 1963a. Multipurpose cannula for acute and chronic intra-cerebral chemical and electrophysiological studies. *EEG Clin. Neurophysiol.* **15:** 125–126.

Wagner, J. W. and J. de Groot. 1963b. Changes in feeding behavior after intracerebral injections in the rat. *Amer. J. Physiol.* **204:** 483–487.

Wagner, J. W., W. Erwin and W. Critchlow. 1966. Androgen sterilization produced by intracerebral implants of testosterone in neonatal female rats. *Endocrinology.* **79:** 1135–1142.

Walker, A. E. and G. B. Udvarhelyi. 1965. Dissemination of acute focal seizures in the monkey. *Arch. Neurol.* **12:** 357–380.

Walter, R. D., C. L. Yeager and J. Adams. 1954. Electroencephalographic changes in procainization of the frontal lobe. *EEG Clin. Neurophysiol.* **6:** 299–302.

Warburton, D. M. 1972. The cholinergic control of internal inhibition, pp. 431–460. *In* R. Boakes and M. S. Halliday (eds.) *Inhibition and Learning.* Academic Press, London.

Warburton, D. M. and R. W. Russell. 1969. Some behavioral effects of cholinergic stimulation in the hippocampus. *Life Sci.* **8:** 617–627.

Watts, M. E. and R. F. Mark. 1971. Drug inhibition of memory formation in chickens. II. Short-term memory. *Proc. R. Soc. Lond.* **178:** 455–464.

Wayner, M. J. 1964. *Thirst.* Pergamon Press, London, pp. 1–570.

Weick, R. F. and J. M. Davidson. 1970. Localization of the stimulatory feedback effect of estrogen on ovulation in the rat. *Endocrinology.* **87:** 693–700.

Weiner, R. I., R. A. Gorski and C. H. Sawyer. 1972. Hypothalamic catecholamines and pituitary gonadotropic function, pp. 236–244. *In: Brain-Endocrine Interaction. Median Eminence: Structure and Function: Int. Symp. Munich, 1971.* Karger, Basel.

Weiner, R. I., C. A. Blake, L. Rubinstein and C. H. Sawyer. 1971. Electrical activity of the hypothalamus: effects of intraventricular catecholamines. *Science.* **171:** 411–412.

Weiss, P. A. 1970. Neuronal dynamics and neuroplasmic flow, pp. 840–850. *In* F. O. Schmitt (ed.) *The Neurosciences. Second Study Program.* The Rockefeller University Press, New York.

Weiss, T. and E. Fifková. 1963. The effect of neocortical and caudatal spreading depression on "circling movements" induced from the caudate nucleus. *Physiol. Bohemoslov.* **12:** 332–338.

Welsch, C. W., M. Sar, J. A. Clemens and J. Meites. 1968. Effects of estrogen on pituitary prolactin levels of female rats bearing median eminence implants of prolactin. *Proc. Soc. Exptl. Biol. Med.* **129:** 817–820.

Werman, R. 1966. A review-criteria for identification of a central nervous system transmitter. *Comp. Biochem. Physiol.* **18:** 745–766.

Werman, R. 1972. CNS cellular level: membranes. *Ann. Rev. Physiol.* **34:** 337–374.

Westermann, E. O., R. P. Maickel and B. B. Brodie. 1962. On the mechanism of pituitary-adrenal stimulation by reserpine. *J. Pharmacol. Exptl. Ther.* **138:** 208–217.

Westman, A. and D. Jacobsohn. 1942. Die Wirküng transorbital an das Tuber cinereum injizierten Novocains auf die Ovulation. *Acta Obstet. Gynecol. Scand.* **22:** 16–23.

White, C. S., R. A. Levitt and S. Boyer. 1972. Drinking elicited by CNS injection of angiotensin in the rat. *Psychon. Sci.* **26:** 283–284.

White, N. M. and A. E. Fisher. 1969. Relationship between amygdala and hypothalamus in the control of eating behavior. *Physiol. Behav.* **4:** 199–205.

White, R. P. 1956. Relationship between behavioral changes and brain cholinesterase activity following graded intercerebral injection of DFP. *Proc. Soc. Exptl. Biol. Med.* **93:** 113–116.

White, R. P. and H. E. Himwich. 1957. Circus movements and excitation of striatal and mesodiencephalic centers in rabbits. *J. Neurophysiol.* **20:** 81–90.

Whittier, J. R., S. E. Graham and N. Kopeloff. 1949. Paresthesia in a rhesus monkey associated with a thalamic lesion, and its alleviation by postcentral cortical excision. *J. Neuropath. Exp. Neurol.* **8:** 93–99.

de Wied, D. 1964. The site of the blocking action of dexamethasone on stress-induced pituitary ACTH release. *J. Endocrinol.* **29:** 29–37.

de Wied, D. 1966. Opposite effects of ACTH and glucocorticosteroids on extinction of conditioned avoidance behavior. *Excp. Med. Int. Cong.* **132:** 945–951.

Wilder, B. J. 1972. Projection phenomena and secondary epileptogenesis—mirror foci, pp. 85–111. *In* D. P. Purpura, J. K. Penry, D. B. Tower, D. M. Woodbury and R. D. Walter (eds.) *Experimental Models of Epilepsy.* Raven Press, New York.

Wilder, B. J., R. L. King and R. P. Schmidt. 1969. Cortical and subcortical secondary epileptogenesis. *Neurology.* **19:** 643–652.

Wilkinson, H. A., V. H. Mark and R. Wilson. 1971. Sleep induced by focal brain suppression using anesthetic gases. *Exptl. Neurol.* **30:** 30–33.

van Wimersma-Greidanus, Tj. B. and D. de Wied. 1969. Effects of intracerebral implantation of corticosteroids on extinction of an avoidance response in rats. *Physiol. Behav.* **4:** 365–370.

van Wimersma-Greidanus, Tj. B. and D. de Wied. 1971. Effects of systemic and intracerebral administration of two opposite acting ACTH-related peptides on extinction of conditioned avoidance behavior. *Neuroendocrinology.* **7:** 291–301.

Winson, J. and J. L. Gerlach. 1971. Stressor-induced release of substances from the rat amygdala detected by the push-pull cannula. *Nature New Biol.* **230:** 251–253.

Winson, J. and N. E. Miller. 1970. Comparison of drinking elicited by eserine or DFP injected into preoptic area of rat brain. *J. Comp. Physiol. Psychol.* **73:** 233–237.

Winterstein, H. 1961. The actions of substances introduced into the cerebrospinal fluid and the problem of intracranial chemoreceptors. *Pharmacol. Rev.* **13:** 71–107.

Wise, C. D. and L. Stein. 1969. Facilitation of brain self-stimulation by central administration of norepinephrine. *Science.* **163:** 299–301.

Wise, R. A. 1972. Rebound eating following carbachol-induced drinking in rats. *Physiol. Behav.* **9:** 659–661.

Wiśniewski, H., W. Karczewski and K. Wiśniewska. 1966. Neurofibrillary degeneration of nerve cells after intracerebral injection of aluminum cream. *Acta Neuropathol.* **6:** 211–219.

Wolf, A. V. 1958. *Thirst.* Charles C Thomas, Springfield. pp. 1–536.

Wolf, G. and N. E. Miller. 1964. Lateral hypothalamic lesions: effects on drinking elicited by carbachol in preoptic area and posterior hypothalamus. *Science.* **143:** 585–587.

Wood, C. D., L. D. Seager and G. Ferrell. 1964. Influence of autonomic blockade on aconitine induced pulmonary edema. *Proc. Soc. Exptl. Biol. Med.* **116:** 809–811.

Woodruff, G. N. 1971. Dopamine receptors: a review. *Comp. Gen. Pharmacol.* **2:** 439–455.

Yahr, P. and D. D. Thiessen. 1972. Steroid regulation of territorial scent marking in the mongolian gerbil (*Meriones unguiculatus*). *Horm. Behav.* **3:** 359–368.

Yaksh, T. L. and R. D. Myers. 1972a. Neurohumoral substances released from hypothalamus of the monkey during hunger and satiety. *Amer. J. Physiol.* **222:** 503–515.

Yaksh, T. L. and R. D. Myers. 1972b. Hypothalamic "coding" in the unanesthetized monkey of noradrenergic sites mediating feeding and thermoregulation. *Physiol. Behav.* **8:** 251–257.

Yamada, T. 1959a. Studies on the mechanism of hypothalamic control of thyrotropin secretion: effect of intrahypothalamic thyroxine injection on thyroid hypertrophy induced by propylthiouracil in the rat. *Endocrinology.* **65:** 216–224.

Yamada, T. 1959b. Studies on the mechanism of hypothalamic control of thyrotropin secretion: comparison of the sensitivity of the hypothalamus and of the pituitary to local changes of thyroid hormone concentration. *Endocrinology.* **65:** 920–925.

Yamada, T. and M. A. Greer. 1959. Studies on the mechanism of hypothalamic control of thyrotropin secretion: effect of thyroxine injection into the hypothalamus or the pituitary on thyroid hormone release. *Endocrinology.* **64:** 559–566.

Yamaguchi, N., G. M. Ling and J. Marczynski. 1964. The effects of chemical stimulation of the preoptic region, nucleus centralis medialis, or brain stem reticular formation with regard to sleep and wakefulness, pp. 9–20. *In* J. Wortis (ed.) *Recent Advances in Biological Psychiatry*. Plenum Press, New York.

Yanagida, H. and H. Yamamura. 1971. Electroencephalographic study of the local injections of central nervous stimulants into the brain. *Adv. Neurol. Sci. (Tokyo)*. **15**: 988–991.

Zanchetti, A. 1967. Subcortical and cortical mechanisms in arousal and emotional behavior, pp. 602–614. *In* G. C. Quarton, T. Melnechuk and F. O. Schmitt (eds.) *The Neurosciences. A Study Program*. The Rockefeller University Press, New York.

Zeisberger, E. and K. Brück. 1971a. Effect of intrahypothalamic noradrenaline-injection on the threshold temperatures for shivering and non-shivering thermogenesis. *J. Physiol. (Paris)*. **63**: 464–467.

Zeisberger, E. and K. Brück. 1971b. Central effects of noradrenaline on the control of body temperature in the guinea-pig. *Pflügers Arch.* **322**: 152–166.

Zeisberger, E. and K. Brück. 1971c. Comparison of the effects of local hypothalamic acetylcholine and RF-heating on non-shivering thermogenesis in the guinea pig. *Int. J. Biometeor.* **15**: 305–308.

Zimmerman, E. and V. Critchlow. 1969. Effects of intracerebral dexamethasone on pituitary-adrenal function in female rats. *Amer. J. Physiol.* **217**: 392–396.

Zumpe, D. and R. P. Michael. 1970. Redirected aggression and gonadal hormones in captive rhesus monkeys (*Macaca mulatta*). *Anim. Behav.* **18**: 11–19.

Author Index

Subject Index*

Ablation, 3, 69, 630
Acetoxycycloheximide, 634
Acetylcholine (ACh), 13, 20, 44, 90, 93, 100,
    104, 140–142, 220, 221, 239, 245, 248,
    250, 251, 254, 255, 258, 261, 262, 286–
    288, 321, 325, 374–376, 383, 385, 387,
    390, 392, 406, 411, 434, 438–445, 447,
    449, 469–471, 474, 477, 482, 488, 492,
    494, 501, 502, 513, 515, 516, 518, 524,
    525, 557, 560, 564, 571, 572, 574, 578,
    579, 584–587, 600, 602, 603, 636, 638,
    652, 653, 656–658, 661–669
  and eserine, 255, 258, 260, 325, 387, 406
  in heat production, 252
  physostigmine, 575, 590
  release of, 254, 657, 658, 667, 668
^{3}H-Acetylcholine, 60
Acetylcholinesterase, 32, 100, 663
Acetylstrophanthidin, 281
Aconitine, 100, 101, 277
Actinomycin D, 213, 633–635
Adenohypophysis, 178, 224
Adenosine 3',5'-monophosphate (Cyclic AMP),
    219, 412, 438, 518
Adenyl cyclase, 662
Adipsia, 335, 407
Adrenal
  activation, 148
  ascorbic acid, 144
  atrophy, 124
  axis, 142, 160
  corticosteroid, 128
  gland, 118, 134

  mechanisms and learning, 624
  response, 121
Adrenalectomy, 123–125, 134
Adrenaline (*See* Epinephrine)
Adrenergic
  action, 89
  hunger system, 400
  mechanism of drinking (*See* Drinking)
  pathway, 141
  receptors, 331, 352
  satiety mechanism, 405
  stimulation, 139, 339
  system, 606
Adrenocorticotrophic hormone (ACTH), 117,
    127, 129, 133, 136, 137, 161, 457, 624,
    625
  excitatory pathway, 142
  feedback
    control, 122
    inhibition, 124
    suppression, 126
  pathway, 142
  suppression, 126
  release, 121, 126, 133, 138, 154, 182, 194,199
  secretion, 123, 124, 139, 142
[D-phe^7]-ACTH-(1-10), 625
Aggression, 553, 571, 576, 587
  defense, 556
Aggressive behavior, 556, 575, 578, 580, 583,
    586
Alloxan, 309
Alpha adrenergic
  blocking agent, 20

*Citations in the Master Summary Table at the end of each chapter are not included in this subject index.

746